Feeding Poultry

The Classic Guide to Poultry Nutrition

NORTON CREEK CLASSICS

Older books about agriculture often have special significance to today's small-scale farmers, who find themselves facing problems similar to those surmounted by our grandparents and great-grandparents. Many books published between 1900 and 1960 have crucial information that is unavailable elsewhere. However, these books have been out of print for decades. They are hard to find and almost entirely forgotten.

The Norton Creek Classics represent a few carefully selected volumes from the treasure trove of our agricultural heritage.

Feeding Poultry

The Classic Guide to Poultry Nutrition

G. F. HEUSER

PROFESSOR OF POULTRY HUSBANDRY, NEW YORK STATE COLLEGE OF AGRICULTURE AND THE SCHOOL OF NUTRITION, AND POULTRY HUSBANDMAN, AGRICULTURAL EXPERIMENT STATION, CORNELL UNIVERSITY, ITHACA, NEW YORK

Second Edition

A Norton Creek Classic

Norton Creek Press
36475 Norton Creek Road
Blodgett, Oregon 97326

http://www.nortoncreekpress.com

Feeding Poultry
The Classic Guide to Poultry Nutrition.
Second Edition.
by G. F. (Gustave Frederick) Heuser

Published by Norton Creek Press, 2003.

Originally published: New York: John Wiley & Sons, 1955.

ISBN 0-9721770-2-7

PREFACE

As stated in the first edition, this book is a product of the direct responsibilities that I have had in connection with instruction and research in poultry nutrition. During this period of nearly forty years most of my time and my efforts have been applied specifically to the field of poultry feeding. I have also been privileged to visit most of the experiment stations in the United States and Canada as well as a number in Europe.

The material here presented covers my experience in Cornell University as well as reports from the Agricultural Experiment Stations and other public institutions. Such technical journals as *Poultry Science*, *Journal of Nutrition*, *Journal of Biological Chemistry*, and *Archiv für Geflügelkunde*, as well as such trade journals as *Feedstuffs*, *Flour and Feed*, and *The U. S. Egg and Poultry Magazine* have been drawn upon for source material.

Many changes in the feeding and management of livestock have taken place over the period of years, and many of these changes have been very extensive. In the present century feeding has become a science. Much of this knowledge, for lack of time or information, is not available to the practical poultryman or even to many persons in institutional work. It is the object of this book to make this information more generally available.

The field of poultry nutrition is a rapidly changing one. The present edition includes the information dealing with the recent advances, such as the use of antibiotics. Much of the material has been rewritten. For convenience and also ease of comparison the recommended rations have been grouped in an appendix.

Both the scientific and practical facts relating to poultry feeding are presented in this book. Information dealing with poultry nutrition is quite extensive. However, much of it is scattered and much is contradictory. Because of the latter fact, it frequently must be evaluated, and this I have attempted to do. Usually a summary has been made of the available data, using as much detail as is necessary for illustrative material. In most cases, the references have been cited so that the reader, if he wishes to do so, can obtain more details than are given in the book.

This book is designed to meet the needs of poultry students, practical poultrymen, feed dealers, and all other persons interested in poultry feeding.

I wish to acknowledge the assistance of all those persons who have been associated with me in teaching and experimental work. I also wish to acknowledge my indebtedness to many friends for various kinds of assistance, support, and inspiration.

G. F. HEUSER

Cornell University
Ithaca, New York

January, 1955

CONTENTS

CHAPTER 1

THE FEEDING PROBLEM

The existence of problems in poultry feeding cannot be denied. At any meeting of poultrymen many questions are raised concerning this important phase of management. The problems are relatively more pressing today than they were a generation ago. Many phases of the feeding problem need solution or clarification.

CHANGED CONDITIONS

There are definite reasons for the existence of feeding problems which can be traced to changed conditions under which the poultryman operates. Many of these problems did not exist a few generations ago. At that time there were comparatively few hens, in fact usually not any larger number than could find their own living on the farm. They were allowed, to a large extent, to take care of themselves. This is shown by the following excerpts taken from books dealing with poultry. In The American Poulterer's Companion,[1] published by C. N. Bement in 1856, we find the following:

> Fowls are, of all birds, the most easy to feed. Every alimentary substance agrees with them, even when buried in manure; nothing is lost to them; they are seen the whole day long incessantly busied in scratching and picking up a living.
>
> The finest, the most imperceptible seed cannot escape their piercing eye. The fly that is most rapid in flight cannot screen itself from the promptitude with which she darts her bill; the worm that comes to breathe at the surface of the earth has no time to shrink from her glance—it is immediately secured by the head and drawn up.
>
> It is customary to throw to the fowls in a poultry-yard, once or twice a day, a quantity of grain, generally corn, and somewhat less than that which they would consume if they had an abundance.
>
> There is no sort of insect, perhaps, which fowls will not eat. They are exceedingly fond of flies, beetles, grasshoppers, crickets, and every sort of grub and maggot. We found it quite advantageous in the summer to open our gates occasionally and give the fowls a run in the garden or surrounding field an hour or so, in the afternoon, when insects and grasshoppers are plenty.

In The Business Hen,[2] published in 1892, H. W. Collingwood gives the following information on feeding as applying to the general farm condition:

There is no kind of food, animal or vegetable, that is not acceptable to the hen. She will pick up the hardest, flinty substances, seize all kinds of insects, regale herself on seeds of every description, and finds a variety in the leaves of the grasses and weeds. All kinds of refuse and waste material from every source, as well as the droppings of cattle, afford her luxuries that would possess but little attraction for larger stock.

Special foods in the summer season are unnecessary, as the hen is capable of selecting and securing a sufficiency of all that is required for supplying her needs; but there are periods when it becomes necessary to assist her, as the production of substances that are to be deposited separately from the body demands certain elements that may be beyond the power of the hen to procure during those seasons when she is really a prisoner and deprived of her liberty.

The hens that thrive on a diet of corn during the summer do not derive their nutriment from the corn alone, but from the variety of forage secured, and as the hen is more prolific during the warmer season she keeps in better condition for laying by the rapid conversion of the food into eggs instead of into fat; but overfeeding will eventually result in fatty degeneracy of the liver.

Among the foods sometimes allowed that may be considered out of the regular course are sunflower seeds, linseed meal (or oil cake), rape seed and millet seed, which, though highly nitrogenous, contain large proportions of oil, and are therefore fattening also; while the oils from them induce the shedding of the feathers, causing premature molting.

The most important of all foods is finely chopped clover hay scalded and fed in troughs. It is rich in mineral matter, nitrogenous, contains a large proportion of carbonaceous matter, and by its bulk reduces or dilutes the concentrated grain food. It is very necessary that a plentiful supply of sharp, gritty material be always kept within reach of the hens, as they can not derive full benefit from any kind of food unless complete mastication results.

However, concentrated poultry production with more attention to feeding was already developing. In the same book Mr. Collingwood gives the accompanying tabulation to show the ration that had given the best results for egg production for 600 hens, this being the method used by C. H. Wyckoff at Groton, New York.

1. Morning, by weight all they can eat of the following mixture: One-half bran, one-fourth corn and one-fourth oat-meals mixed with hot water or milk, with ½ pint of salt, 1 quart of charcoal and 1 bushel of clover hay cut fine. If there be no milk add 16 pounds of chopped meat and 1 bushel of beets cut fine.

2. Noon, whole grain by measure. One part oats, 1 buckwheat, and 1 wheat; give 1 quart to 50 hens in chaff.

3. Night, the same as No. 2, all they will eat.

4. Drink, milk or pure water.

At the turn of the century the hens did not lay large numbers of eggs, and most production usually took place during the spring of the year. The important condition, however, was the fact that the number of hens was not much greater than the natural food supply on the farm. They fed upon such protective feeding stuffs as greens and milk and also consumed considerable whole animal life, for example, bugs and worms. They lived outdoors to a large extent and benefited by direct sunshine.

From this condition the poultry industry in all its phases has developed until at the present time we have fairly definite and often quite complex systems and methods. The number of hens has greatly increased, and they have been so concentrated that they have far exceeded the natural food supply. The birds have been bred for increased production to the extent of obtaining high flock averages as well as individual records. Combined with this we have a greater proportion of the production out of the natural season. Not only table eggs but also hatching eggs are being produced the year round. Early fall production from pullets requires earlier hatching in the spring. Furthermore, many flocks are being kept in more or less close confinement, or even in complete confinement, throughout the entire laying year.

The same situation applies to the young. Larger numbers of chicks are being produced, many of them out of the natural season or at those times of the year when conditions are not favorable. There has been greater development along the lines of mass production of chicks under factory methods. Hundreds of thousands of birds, especially broilers, are raised in batteries under conditions of strict confinement.

Whenever animals are made to produce out of their natural season, it is necessary to introduce artificial methods to a greater or lesser degree. This introduces factors which complicate the problem. A comparison of conditions today, as contrasted with those of a few generations ago, helps to give one an appreciation of some of the factors that are helping to make poultry feeding a more complicated problem.

It must also be borne in mind that the natural foods and those consumed more or less in their entirety were complex when viewed from their feeding value. In substituting for those feeds we run the risk of omitting some of the factors supplied in them. Furthermore, modern methods of manufacture are changing the nature of some feeds. A ration that contains degerminated cereals or cereal by-products might be deficient in vitamins whereas the same mixture with regular products would supply plenty. Meat scraps is a variable product depending upon the nature of the raw material and the process of manufacture. In recent years most of the organs of the animal, such as the liver, are diverted to other channels so that at the present time larger proportions of connective tissue and bone and other less valuable portions are forming the raw material for meat scraps. The method of preparing any feed and the conditions of temperature and oxidation to which it is subjected will affect the feeding value. In the more intensive manufacturing processes, there is a greater likelihood of destruction of some factor. But the important point is that these changes, which are altering the feeding value of products, often cannot be detected by analysis or inspection. Neither does the average feeder know or realize that the nature of many feeds is changing.

There is also the possibility that some of our feeds are undergoing change in composition owing to changes in the supply of the elements in the soil. Depletion of minerals or conversion of them into an insoluble form might render them less available to the plant. It is suspected furthermore that conditions of drought might influence the nutritive value of the feed produced.

EVOLUTION OF MODERN METHODS

At the present time there are in use certain systems of feeding practice. They are the result of development or evolution, based more or less on experience. This development has proceeded along certain lines, which have been influenced by certain facts and conditions. Practically all the knowledge that we have of scientific feeding has been secured within comparatively recent years. As late as the latter part of the last century, poultry was fed by rule almost entirely. The method was one which some one had stumbled upon by accident, but it seemed to get results.

Previously only feeds grown on the farm were used. The ration was thus restricted to the grains produced and to any waste products or by-products of the farm or of the home. Now we have developed a considerable number of specially prepared poultry feeds, which have no restrictions of ingredients, since modern development in transportation has linked all parts of the world and made practically any product available.

There has also been a development in methods of feeding and feeding practices. At first, the hens more or less fed themselves, very little attention being given to any definite or regular system of feeding. Gradually more attention was given to the birds. At first they were hand fed practically entirely on grain. Then systems of hopper feeding developed in which the hens could help themselves.

The hopper itself has undergone considerable changes. In some cases the hoppers were made large enough to hold supplies of mash for a month or more. It is doubtful whether that is the best practice since it encourages neglect of close observation of the birds and also increases the chance of spoilage of the feed. The present-day tendencies are to practice a closer check-up on feeding. This practice has eliminated the very large hoppers and substituted smaller ones of thc open type.

The introduction of ground feeds, fed as mashes, was a distinct advance in poultry feeding. Man found out that he could assist the hen by furnishing part of the grain already ground. So we have systems of feeding ranging from all grain to all mash, with nearly all the possible combinations of proportions of grain and mash between these extremes.

Another variation was the condition in which the mash should be fed, that is, wet or dry. The wet mash was probably fed first. Later the dry mash system of feeding was introduced and used exclusively in many cases. At present the generally recommended system is more likely to be a combination of the two. The dry mash is kept available all the time and may be supplemented with a wet mash when it is necessary to increase mash and food consumption.

When hoppers were introduced in poultry feeding they were used for grain as well as for mash. The hopper system of feeding grain was soon abandoned because it was believed that the hens did not get sufficient exercise. Grain, therefore, was fed in a litter of some kind, the depth of which has also gone through various evolutions. Recently the swing has been back again to hopper feeding of grain, chiefly because of the sanitary advantages that it offers. The ground feed is almost universally fed in hoppers. Hopper feeding of dry mash gives all the hens a more nearly equal chance, allowing them an opportunity to eat at any time and preventing crowding, incidental to feeding a wet mash to larger flocks.

Can a hen balance her own ration? Many theories and opinions have been advanced. As a matter of fact, she comes very near to doing it when she is given a choice of grain and mash. The mash, if properly composed, is rich in protein, vitamins, and minerals while the grain contains more of the energy nutrients. Therefore, the hen eats from both the grain and mash as much as she wants of each and balances her own ration fairly satisfactorily. But the question has not yet been settled as to whether the hen should eat each of the different feeds separately. Feeding each ingredient separately has been tried, but in most cases has not proved satisfactory.

Other practices have been evolved, and no doubt the future holds in store still more. At the present time there is a further development of the all-mash system, which endeavors to obtain some of the advantages of grain feeding. There are cubed feeds or pellets and kernels, which consist of binding an all-mash combination into larger particles. Also, systems of cooking, predigesting, and other methods of processing foods have been tried to a greater or lesser extent and will need to be given further consideration in the future.

CAUSES OF EVOLUTION OR CHANGES IN FEEDING

No doubt there are many reasons for the changes and developments just discussed. Increased population and concentration of population in cities, where eggs and poultry cannot be produced in sufficient amounts, have resulted in an increased demand for the products. This increased demand for poultry products has resulted in an increased number of hens. The increase in the number of hens has made it necessary to introduce other systems of feeding because the number of hens on the farm has got beyond the natural food supply.

The development of the industries supplying human food has had an influence on animal feeding. It is only within the past few generations, for example, that the production of prepared cereals has developed extensively. This preparation of cereals has given rise to a considerable supply of by-products which have merit and are valuable from the feeding standpoint.

The milling industry has long been furnishing wheat by-products which are utilized in animal feeding. But, owing to changes in manufacture, changes have also occurred in the nature of these feeds. The present-day products are milled more closely than previously. Particularly is there a change in the amount of germ that is contained.

We also have the by-products of the packing industries, which enter largely into our poultry feeding, especially as a source of protein feeds. The same may be said of the fish and milk indus-

The maintenance requirement of poultry is very considerable. This requirement takes the major proportion of the feed consumed. If the mature hen is out of production nearly all the feed is used for this purpose. Even if the hen is in heavy production, probably at least 70 to 80 per cent of her food is needed for maintenance. Joshi, Shaffner, and Jull[9] reported that, with hens laying at the rate of 72 per cent, approximately 71 per cent of the food consumed was used for body maintenance, 27 per cent for the production of eggs, and 2 per cent for increase in body weight. Brody, Funk, and Kempster[5] report the gross energetic efficiency (the percentage of the feed energy which appears in the egg) for Leghorns as follows:

	Percentage
100-egg producers	11
150-egg producers	14
200-egg producers	17
250-egg producers	20
360-egg producers	27

For young stock, the proportion of feed needed for maintenance is smallest early in life when the chick is growing rapidly and increases as the chick grows older and the rate of growth is slowed down. Records of experiments with White Leghorn chicks at Cornell University indicate approximately 65 per cent of the food used for maintenance the first month, 75 per cent the second, 80 per cent the third, 85 per cent the fourth, and 90 per cent the fifth month.

After the animal is maintained, an increase in tissue can occur. In young stock this is called growth; in mature birds it might be fattening. Growth in the young animal is chiefly an increase in water, protein, and minerals; in the mature animal it might be fat.

Excess food may also be used for the production of a useful product and for reproduction (the development of a new individual). These two are mentioned together because, in the case of the fowl, production and reproduction are the same process. That is not true of other farm animals. Milk production in the dairy cow is a separate process from reproduction.

Production or reproduction in poultry must not take place before growth is well advanced; otherwise there is danger of stunting. Reproduction necessitates complete production; and, so far as the hen is concerned, she will endeavor to produce a complete egg, which is capable of reproducing herself. The animal in a reproductive state is more intensely nervous. Since abundant production is desired, there is obviously an intense strain on the vitality of the bird. Unless there is an abundant and proper feed supply to keep up body reserves and maintain health and vitality, we shall fail to get not only hatching quality but production as well.

SOME PRINCIPLES OF FEEDING POULTRY

Food furnishes the fuel which is burned in the body. An essential part of this burning process is oxygen. The amount of oxygen needed depends upon the chemical composition of the material that burns in the animal. The rate of metabolism regulates the amount of oxygen absorbed and the carbon dioxide given off.

The phenomena of life are composed of phenomena of motion due to the liberation of energy locked up in the feed. These motions are manifested chiefly as heat, mechanical energy, and electric currents.

The feeding of poultry involves certain special considerations not encountered in feeding other farm animals. First, there are the physiological considerations. All the body processes are conducted in shorter time. Digestion is more rapid. Respiration and circulation are faster. The body temperature is 8 to 10 degrees higher. A greater amount of body surface is exposed per unit of weight. The individuals show greater activity. They are more sensitive to external influences. They mature early. Production is always full and complete, or there is none. The hen does not lay half an egg. The young stock has wonderfully quick growth, the young chick often increasing its weight ten times or more in 5 weeks.

All these facts indicate that in poultry we are dealing with animals that require a high rate of metabolism. It must, therefore, be kept in mind that the requirements are thus more exacting and the balance or equilibrium more easily disturbed.

There are also certain anatomical considerations which must be kept in mind. The hen grinds all her feed in the gizzard. Since the capacity of the digestive tract is limited and since fiber is practically indigestible, there is danger of a lack of sufficient nutriment when the feeds are very coarse. To avoid this danger more concentrated feeds must be fed, which might introduce other difficulties. It is necessary, therefore, to maintain a proper balance between the bulky and the concentrated feeds.

Certain management considerations are also involved when

comparing the feeding of poultry with the feeding of the larger farm animals. A greater number of individuals are represented per man unit, increasing the need for closer scrutiny and observation of condition of the animals. Furthermore, the birds are fed collectively rather than individually, as the larger animals are. In the flock birds of many states of nutrition are likely to be represented, and they require different rations or methods of feeding. Management that gets the best results from one part of the flock will not get the best from another part and might actually be detrimental. However, in order to overcome this difficulty to the greatest degree, there is need for flock segregation in which birds nearly alike in physical condition, age, sexual maturity, and production, and therefore in nutritive requirements, are placed in separate units and fed accordingly.

REFERENCES

1. Jordan, W. H. The feeding of animals. The Macmillan Co. New York 1906.
2. Jennings, R. D. Feed consumption by livestock 1910-1941. Relation between feed, livestock, and food at the national level. U.S.D.A. Circ. 670. 1943
3. Halnan, E. T. Poultry as food converters. Nature 148:335. 1941.
4. Almquist, H. J. Conversion of feed to food. Flour and Feed 44(8):16. 1944.
5. Brody, S., E. M. Funk, and H. L. Kempster. Growth and development with special reference to domestic animals. XLIV. Energetic efficiency of egg production and the influence of live weight thereon. Mo. Res. Bul. 278. 1938.
6. Bird, S., and J. W. Sinclair. A study of the energy required for maintenance, egg production, and changes in body weight in the domestic hen. Sci. Agr. 19:542. 1939.
7. Hess, C. W., and M. A. Jull. A study of the inheritance of feed utilization efficiency in the growing domestic fowl. Poultry Sci. 27:24. 1948.
   McCartney, M. G., and M. A. Jull. Efficiency of feed utilization in New Hampshires to ten weeks. Poultry Sci. 27:17. 1948.
8. Fronda, F. M. Temperature studies in poultry. Thesis, Cornell University. 1922.
9. Joshi, B. C., C. S. Shaffner, and M. A. Jull. Efficiency of feed utilization in relation to body weight and egg production. Poultry Sci. 28:301. 1949.

CHAPTER 3

COMPOSITION OF PLANTS, ANIMALS, AND RATIONS

THE FEED NUTRIENTS AND THEIR FUNCTIONS

All feeds are composed of several distinctly different groups of substances, which are called nutrients. These nutrients have definite functions or uses in the body. A continued deficiency of them will result in general debility, which finally will end in death.

In practical feeding, it is not the separate nutrients which are dealt with, because most natural feeds are mixtures of nutrients. No two feeds are alike in that they contain these nutrients in the same proportions. Each feed is likely to contain a larger proportion of one or more of the nutrients. These differences make it necessary to regulate the amount of the different feeds used so that the total of each nutrient furnished by the ration as a whole will be correct.

Most of our feeding stuffs come from plant material. The plant tissues are derived from the inorganic matter of the soil and air with the aid of energy from the sun. Approximately twenty different chemical elements are generally found in plant and animal tissues. They are combined into the compounds known as nutrients. The recognized nutrients are carbohydrates, fats, minerals, proteins, vitamins, and water.

WATER. Water is a compound composed chemically of 2 parts of hydrogen and 1 of oxygen. The amount which occurs in feeds is quite variable. Green or succulent feeds may contain as much as 80 to 90 per cent of water. In kiln-dried feeds, the amount present may be as low as 5 per cent, whereas the ordinary grains usually contain 10 to 12 per cent of water.

A large proportion of both the body of the fowl and the egg is composed of water. More than half of the body and 2/3 of the egg are water. Since the body of the hen and likewise her product, the egg, contain more water than solid material, water is an important ingredient of any poultry ration. The ordinary poultry ration is composed of feeds containing a relatively small amount of water, which will supply only a part of the requirement for this nutrient. Hence special attention must be given to the water supply. Water is necessary for all the body activities. It is the medium in which the different body processes take place. It also regulates the body temperature.

Very often the water supply is neglected. It is just as essential as feed. In fact, a hen can live for a longer period without feed than she can without water. It is not possible to supply sufficient water to the hen by giving her access to it once or twice a day, as is done with the larger farm animals. Hens must have a continuous supply of water for they drink only a small amount at one time. Especially with dry-mash feeding, it is necessary to have water available whenever feed is available. During freezing weather and where artificial illumination is used, some provision should be made to keep the water from freezing. The hens will also appreciate having the chill removed from the water and will consume larger amounts of it.

MINERALS.[1] The mineral portion of the feed or animal body is also known as the ash or inorganic matter. Only about a dozen, or perhaps fifteen, are thought to be necessary for the animal body. The inorganic matter appears chiefly as phosphates, sulphates, carbonates, chlorides, nitrates, iodides, or silicates of sodium, potassium, calcium, magnesium, iron, copper, manganese, or zinc.

Minerals are important to the animal, but they must be present in the right concentrations. The animal body can tolerate some variation in this respect, but considerable departure from the normal is likely to be detrimental.

Some minerals, such as manganese, cobalt, copper, iodine, and iron, are required only in very small amounts and are called trace minerals.

Location of Minerals. Minerals enter into the composition of all body tissues. Their distribution, however, is not uniform since one finds concentrations of certain minerals in different tissues. For example, the bones are a storehouse for minerals, especially calcium, phosphorus, and magnesium. The shell of the egg is made up largely of calcium. On the other hand, the yolk of the egg has larger proportions of phosphorus and sulfur. Potassium is found abundantly in such tissues as muscles, glands, and nerves. Sodium is found in large amounts in blood and lymph. Phosphorus and sulphur enter into the composition of proteins. Chlorine is a constituent of the hydrochloric acid of the gastric juice. Iron is concentrated in the hemoglobin of the blood. Iodine is found chiefly in the thyroid gland; silicon in the feathers. Cobalt is an integral part of vitamin B_{12}.

Function of Minerals. The various minerals are intimately bound up with animal life. They furnish building materials, as a part of bones they provide rigidity to the body, and they help to control the various life processes. They aid in digestion, assimilation, distribution of food nutrients in the body, and excretion. Some of them act as catalysts. Others function as buffers in the blood and tissues. Some are connected with enzyme activation, oxidation processes, and cell regulation. Minerals might also be involved in the activity of the intestinal flora.

Calcium, phosphorus, and magnesium are essential for bone formation. Their utilization is dependent upon the presence of sufficient vitamin D. Calcium is also essential for clotting of the blood. Magnesium is connected with nerve and muscle activity. Phosphorus also functions in the metabolism of carbohydrates and fats. All the common forms of calcium appear to be well utilized. However, some forms of phosphorus are not available to poultry.[2] This is true especially for the phosphorus in feedstuffs of vegetable origin which is largely in the form of phytin. Inorganic phosphorus is readily available. In the ration for the growing chick a ratio of calcium to phosphorus of 1.5:1 is desirable.

Sodium chloride (salt) is the chief inorganic constituent of the blood plasma. The addition of salt to poultry rations is a common practice. Salt metabolism is related to water balance. The amounts should be restricted since excess salt will cause wet droppings and hence wet litter. Excessive amounts of salt are toxic to chickens. (See Chap. 5, section on minerals.)

Sulfur is an essential mineral and is accounted for almost entirely by the sulfur which occurs in organic combination in the amino acids, methionine, and cystine. Inorganic sulfur has little value in the poultry ration.

Iron and copper are necessary for hemoglobin formation. They function in connection with oxygen transfer.

Iodine is necessary for the normal functioning of the thyroid gland. Most of the iodine of the body occurs in thyroxin, the hormone secreted by the thyroid gland, which regulates body metabolism.

Potassium[3] as well as sodium helps to regulate the osmotic pressure in cellular tissue and body fluids. Symptoms of potassium deficiency in the chick include retarded growth, weakness, loss of use of legs, and the excretion of large amounts of urates. Death was preceded or accompanied by tetanic seizures in which the muscles were unable to relax. Bone calcification was influenced by the amount of potassium in the diet. Electrocardiograms of chickens produced on a potassium deficient ration were abnormal.

Mineral Relationships. Certain mineral metabolism relationships exist, for there must be a proper balance of minerals in the body. To some extent the animal can excrete excesses. The bones act as a storehouse for some of the minerals. Calcium is more effectively assimilated in the presence of vitamin D; magnesium salts cause a loss of calcium. Potassium increases sodium elimination, and calcium increases phosphorus elimination. An excess of phosphorus also increases the need for manganese. On the other hand, copper has a favorable reaction in sparing iron. The best results are secured when an optimum ratio of certain of the minerals is maintained, such as a balance between calcium and phosphorus, and between calcium and sodium and potassium.

Acid-Base Balance. Some of the minerals such as sulfur, phosphorus, and chlorine are acid in reaction, whereas others such as calcium, magnesium, sodium, and potassium are basic. It is thought best to use feeds containing these minerals in such proportions as to provide a proper acid-base balance.

Lack of Minerals. Mineral starvation of chickens, due either to an actual lack of minerals in the ration or to their unavailability, results in weak limbs and improper bone development. A general irritability or excitability and even spasms or convulsions may result from a lack of minerals. Where the minerals have specific functions, a lack of them will produce specific deficiencies, such as anemia when iron is deficient, goiter when iodine is lacking, and perosis when there is not enough manganese present. A deficiency of magnesium[4] might cause convulsions accompanied by gasping. Calcium and phosphorus are required in largest amounts in the ration because of the needs for bone and eggshell formation. These minerals function in connection with vitamin D. When not present in sufficient amounts, weak eggshells will be produced and rickets will develop. (See vitamin D, p. 41.)

Other minerals, needed only in small amounts but important to the animal, are the minor elements, manganese[5] and iodine. With shortages of these minerals, specific nutritional deficiency conditions develop.

Perosis and Manganese Deficiency. Perosis[6] is a nutritional deficiency condition due to a lack of manganese and possibly some other factors, such as choline, biotin, or folic acid. It is sometimes called slipped tendon or enlarged hock disease, owing to the slipping of the tendon and the enlargement of the hock which causes crippling of the bird (Fig. 1). Perosis usually appears when the chicken is 3 to 5 weeks old.

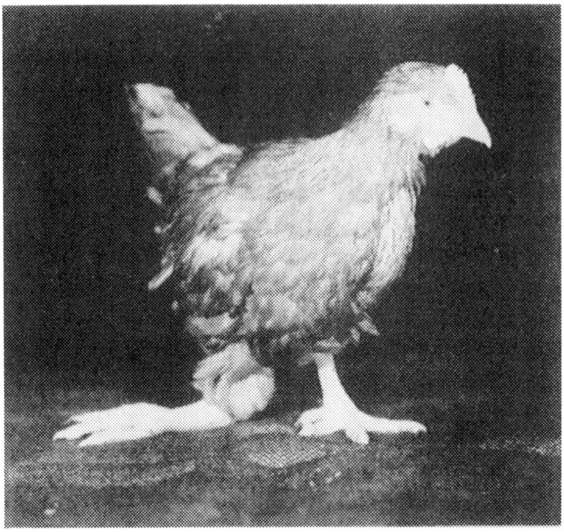

Fig. 1. Perosis. Perosis or slipped tendon resulting from a manganese deficiency. Note the flattened hock and the deformed leg. (Courtesy Cornell University.)

Perosis is a malformation of the bones of chicks. The symptoms usually observed are swelling and flattening of the hock joint, with subsequent slipping of the Achilles' tendon from its condyles. The tibia and tarsometatarsus may exhibit bending near the hock joint and lateral rotation. One or both legs may be affected, but as a rule lameness develops in one leg only. A shortening and a thickening of the long bones of the wings and legs are also observed. The disorder, so far as manganese is concerned, is aggravated by excessive quantities of calcium and phosphorus in the ration.

In laying and breeding birds[7] a manganese deficiency results in lowered egg production, lowered eggshell strength, and lowered hatchability. Numerous embryos that die as a result of manganese deficiency exhibit chondrodystrophy, a condition characterized by a parrot-like beak, wiry down, and shortening of the long bones. This condition is not, however, specific for a manganese deficiency.

An ataxia[8] characterized by a tetanic spasm and due to a manganese deficiency in the maternal diet has also been reported.

Goiter.[9] A deficiency of iodine in the ration affects the functioning of the thyroid gland, causing an enlargement known as goiter. The thyroid gland increases to many times the normal size. Histological examinations of the enlarged thyroid glands show an absence of colloid and a hyperplasia of the living cells of the follicle.

Iodine might be deficient, especially if the amounts of fish meal and other marine products are limited. It has also been observed that soybeans have a goitrogenic effect. The addition of 0.5 per cent of iodized salt to poultry rations is adequate to meet the iodine requirements.

Anemia.[10] A deficiency of iron or copper in poultry rations results in anemia. Certain vitamins or organic factors, such as folic acid, have been reported as also being essential for the prevention of anemia in growing chicks.

Probable Mineral Deficiencies. The ration must contain a suitable inorganic content. However, the practical poultryman is concerned only with the minerals that might be deficient in his ration. If a good ration, made up of natural feeding stuffs, is fed, the minerals that are likely to be found deficient are sodium, chlorine, calcium, and phosphorus.

The sodium and chlorine are furnished by adding common salt. Usually one-half to one per cent is included in the ration. Calcium for eggshell formation is best supplied in the carbonate form. Oyster shells and limestone will furnish this mineral. Where wheat by-products, meat scraps, and milk are used, there will usually be enough phosphorus. When necessary to supply phosphorus, bone meal, dicalcium phosphate, or defluorinated rock phosphate are added to the ration.

Manganese might sometimes be deficient. Only small amounts of the manganese salts will supply the need. A common practice of commercial mixers is to add about one quarter pount of manganese sulphate to each ton of mash.

Possible Mineral Excesses. Where minerals are necessary, they usually need to be added in only comparatively small quantities. Some are detrimental in large amounts. For instance, too much calcium[11] will retard growth and increase mortality in chicks and decrease production and hatchability. In the body certain minerals are balanced by other minerals, and excesses of some might use up the others so as to cause a deficiency. This is true of phosphorus which will combine with manganese.

Excess magnesium in the chick ration has resulted in deformed bones.[12] The use of dolomite limestone containing a high percentage of magnesium[13] has caused egg production to decrease and the shells of the eggs to become progressively thinner. The hens also developed diarrhea and became extremely irritable and easily frightened.

An excess of fluorine[14] has resulted in retarded growth in young chicks and lower egg production and loss of weight in laying hens.

An excess of selenium is also harmful.[15] It has produced retarded growth, ruffled feathers, and irritability in chicks and delayed and reduced egg production and poor hatchability in hens. Many of the embryos which failed to hatch were deformed.

Thus minerals require as much good judgment and as many precautions in their use as other constituents of the ration.

Mineral Mixtures. In general, the use of complex mineral mixtures is not suggested. On the other hand, it is recommended that additions of minerals be specific for definite deficiencies and that such minerals be used singly rather than in combinations. The addition will depend upon the deficiency, and hence each ration is likely to require its own mineral mixture addition.

Grit.[16] Grit may function as a source of minerals when it is furnished in soluble form. It functions as a grinding material only when insoluble. Limestone grit, oyster shells, and rock phosphate furnish minerals but also act as grinding agents. Their life as grinding agents is relatively short. Hens and chicks will benefit by the presence of a grinding material in the gizzard, especially when coarse materials are consumed. Larger and heavier gizzards have been reported for birds receiving insoluble grit. Grit apparently is not necessary when the ration is all mash. When grain is fed, the presence of a grinding material will increase the feed efficiency. The common practice is to supply a grinding material such as grit when grain and other coarse materials are consumed.

CARBOHYDRATES. The carbohhydrates are organic compounds composed of carbon, hydrogen, and oxygen. They are formed in the plant by photosynthesis as follows: $6CO_2 + 6H_2O + \text{energy from the sun} = C_6H_{12}O_6 + 6O_2$. The monosaccharides or simple sugars include glucose, fructose, and galactose. The disaccharides or compound sugars comprise such compounds as sucrose, maltose, and lactose. The polysaccharides include such substances as the hemicelluloses, cellulose, dextrin, starch, and lignin.

From the feeding standpoint, the carbohydrates consist of nitrogen-free extract (N.F.E.) and fiber. The nitrogen-free extract consists mainly of starches, sugars, and a large part of the hemicelluloses. It makes up the so-called soluble portion of the carbohydrates. The fiber, the woody portion or cellulose tissue of the plant, consists of cellulose, hemicellulose, and lignin. In the fowl, fiber is digested, if at all, to only a slight degree. It, therefore, should not be fed in large amounts.

Carbohydrates are used by the body as a source of heat and energy. Any excess may be stored in the body as fat. The yolk of the egg, which is largely fat, may be derived from excesses of carbohydrates in the ration.

FATS. Lipids (fat and fat-like substances) are organic compounds soluble in such organic solvents as ether, chloroform, or benzine, and composed of glycerol and fatty acids (commonly stearic, palmitic, and oleic acids). Like carbohydrates, they contain the three elements carbon, hydrogen, and oxygen. They function the same as carbohydrates in that they serve as a source of heat and energy in the body and of fat in the body and the egg yolk. Fats, however, are so constructed as to liberate more heat upon burning or when digested. They contain approximately two and one fourth times as much energy as carbohydrates. Therefore, less fat is required to serve the same function.

Recent evidence indicates that chickens also have a specific requirement for certain of the unsaturated fatty acids[17] which would then become essential fatty acids.

In the feeding of poultry, carbohydrates, rather than fats, are fed as the principal source of energy. This is true because carbohydrates are usually cheaper and are very easily digested, absorbed, and transformed into fat. Feeds which contain large amounts of fat are likely to become rancid in hot weather, and rancid feed may be injurious to poultry by oxidizing some of the vitamins. Small amounts of fat, however, are desirable since they are carriers of the fat-soluble vitamins and aid in their absorption.

Most of the feeds used in poultry rations do not carry too much fat. Those feeds which are high in fat, such as flaxseed, cottonseed, sunflower seed, and soybeans, are usually extracted for their oil and the remaining meal used for animal feeding.

PROTEINS. Proteins are complex organic compounds made up chiefly of amino acids, present in characteristic proportions for each specific protein. This nutrient always contains carbon, hydrogen, oxygen, and nitrogen, and in addition usually contains sulfur and frequently phosphorus. Proteins are composed of many simpler units called amino acids, of which twenty-three are known. The amino acids are sometimes referred to as the building stones of the proteins. The value of protein depends upon its amino acid composition. The feed proteins are broken down into amino acids by digestion. They are then absorbed and distributed by the blood stream to the body cells which rebuild these amino acids into body proteins.

Essential Amino Acids. Certain of the amino acids are called essential amino acids, because they are indispensable to the animal and cannot be synthesized by the body, and hence must be included in the diet. When the protein contains all the necessary amino acids and will maintain the animal and promote normal growth, it is called a complete protein. Some proteins may be deficient in one or more of the essential amino acids. Such proteins are sometimes called incomplete proteins. A combination of incomplete proteins may supply proteins of good quality in a ration because of their supplementary effects. The deficiency of amino acids in one protein is made up for by the presence of these amino acids in the other protein or proteins.

Amino Acids. The known amino acids which are involved in nutrition are: tryptophan, lysine, methionine, histidine, leucine, isoleucine, phenylalanine, threonine, valine, arginine, glycine, cystine, alanine, norleucine, tyrosine, serine, aspartic acid, glutamic acid, hydroxyglutamic acid, proline, hydroxyproline, iodogorgoic acid, and thyroxine. Of these, the first eleven have been shown to be essential for chickens. Methionine and cystine are sulfur-bearing amino acids. Thyroxine and iodogorgoic acid contain iodine. Cystine can substitute for part of the methionine. Glycine or arginine are precursors of creatine and, with cystine, are essential for feather development and also prevent a certain type of paralysis.[18] Lysine has been reported as being needed for feather pigment formation in turkeys[19] (Fig. 2).

Proteins are widely distributed in plants, which build them up from simple sources in the soil and air. Proteins are the main constituents of animal tissues, which must derive them directly or indirectly from plant tissues. Animal protein feeds are generally of higher quality than vegetable protein feeds because they contain a larger amount of the essential amino acids as well as other necessary nutrients.

Moderate heat treatment improves the quality of soybean protein, whereas prolonged heat treatment decreases the quality.

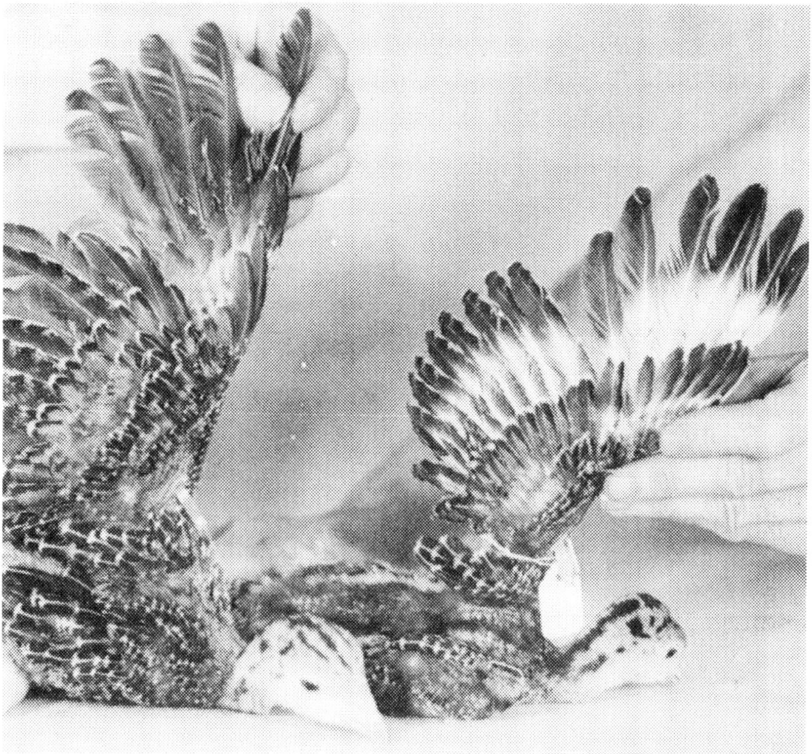

Fig. 2. White-feather syndrome caused by feeding a lysine-deficient diet (right). 7-week old poults. (Courtesy Ontario Agricultural College.)

This is probably due largely to the effect of the heat treatment upon the availability of such amino acids as methionine, lysine, and tryptophan.

Requirements for Proteins. Birds require proteins in their ration for the construction of body tissues. Tissues which are mainly protein are muscles, nerves, cartilage, skin, feathers, and beak. The albumen of the egg is also largely protein. Protein may also enter into the composition of enzymes, hormones, and vitamins.

Proteins also have definite physiological effects. One of these effects is the specific dynamic action of proteins, in which the cell activity is stimulated, and the heat production thereby increased. The animal can take care of a considerable excess of protein, but sometimes overfeeding of proteins may affect the kidneys.

The prime function of protein in the animal body is to supply the amino acids. Any amino acids that are left over, after the requirement has been met, are destroyed in the liver. In this process, a part of each amino acid is turned into fuel, and the remainder is excreted by the kidney. Hence proteins in the ration can also serve as a source of energy. However, because proteins are usually expensive, carbohydrates or fats are more economical to use as a source of energy.

Continued health and physiological efficiency are possible over a wide range of protein intake. However, with proteins, perhaps as with no other nutrient, the body is on continual guard against possible deleterious action of its intermediate digestion products, bacterial end products, and intermediate metabolites.

VITAMINS. Vitamins are those substances which occur in natural feeds in relatively small amounts but are absolutely necessary for growth, reproduction, and the maintenance of health. A prolonged deficiency of many of the vitamins will develop a nutritional deficiency disease.[20] The symptoms of some of these are characteristic so that an experienced observer has little difficulty in recognizing them. Some of these deficiency diseases have been known throughout medical history, such as scurvy, rickets, beriberi, and pellagra.

Formerly the only method of distinguishing the different vitamins was to observe the effects of rations, deficient in one of these nutritive factors, on rats, guinea pigs, pigeons, chickens, and other animals. Until recently, very little has been known regarding the chemical or physical properties of the vitamins. However, in recent years a number of these vitamins have been isolated chemically and synthesized. At the present time, many of the vitamins can be distinguished by chemical and physical properties, as well as by biological and bacteriological assay.

Chemically the vitamins include a variety of compounds. However, they are usually classified as fat-soluble and water-soluble vitamins. Unlike the other classes of nutrients, which are comparatively stable chemical compounds, many of the vitamins are more or less unstable. They are destroyed by exposure to air, heat, light, enzymes, acids, and alkalis. Because of this instability, care must always be taken to insure an ample supply of vitamins in poultry rations. An excess can in certain cases be stored in the animal tissues and in the egg. Many of the pure vitamins have crystals of characteristic color and shape.

A number of different vitamins are recognized. At first, they were named by letter or after the effect upon the animal. Where the chemical name is known, this nomenclature is preferred. Besides the known vitamins, the existence of others is strongly suspected, as several investigators have reported the presence of substances in feedstuffs, which are vitamin-like in nature and possess characteristics that fail to correspond to those of the known vitamins.

Vitamin A.[21] Vitamin A is necessary for maintenance of healthy epithelia in various parts of the body as in the eyes, respiratory tract, and intestinal tract. In vitamin A deficiency, the secretions of the intestinal mucous glands, the tear glands, and the salivary glands fail. Certain tissues, such as the margins of the eyelids, become granular. An opaque appearance, caused by keratinization of the third eyelid, may be observed. Infection may set in and, where it attacks the eyes, a viscous

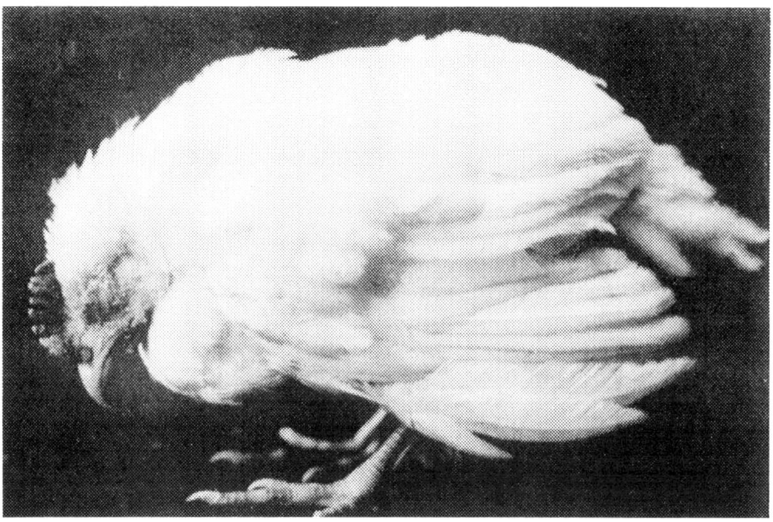

Fig. 3. Vitamin A deficiency. Note the exudate from the eye and the general ruffled appearance. (Courtesy Cornell University.)

fluid is produced which causes the eyelids to stick together (Fig. 3). In some animals, a white film gathers over the center of the eyeball and blindness results. When these symptoms occur, the disease is generally called xerophthalmia. Vitamin A is also necessary for the normal adaptation of the eye to darkness. A low intake of this vitamin results in night blindness.

Pathological lesions, observed on autopsy, are confined largely to the mucous membranes of the mouth, pharynx, esophagus, and respiratory and urinary systems. Creamy white pustules are often found on the roof of the mouth and along the esophagus, sometimes extending into the crop. Urates accumulate in the ureters and in the kidney tubules, so that these organs are enlarged and creamy white in color. This urate accumulation is easily detected on gross examination because of its whitish appearance.

In mature fowl, the symptoms noted for chicks may develop much more slowly, but the eye disorder often becomes more acute. A cheesy exudate from the eyes often is observed, as well as a sticky discharge from the nostrils. The disease is sometimes referred to as nutritional roup because of its similar appearance to roup, a true disease due to other agents. Egg production and hatchability are markedly reduced. It has been reported that blood-spot incidence decreased as the level of vitamin A was increased.

On a severely deficient chick diet, the symptoms of vitamin A deficiency may appear in 2 to 3 weeks. Growth is markedly retarded, the chicks show general weakness, emaciation, and ruffled plumage. Afflicted birds walk in a peculiar weaving or zigzag manner and finally are unable to stand. After this, death soon occurs.

The symptoms of a vitamin A deficiency in turkey poults are, in general, similar to those described for chicks, but are usually much more acute.

Vitamin A, a fat-soluble vitamin, has been chemically identified but not yet given a chemical name. Plants contain precursors, that is, substances that are transformed into the vitamin in the animal body. The pigments carotene and cryptoxanthin are precursors of vitamin A. Carotene is associated with yellow pigments in plants. When vitamin A and carotene are exposed to the air, particularly at warm temperatures, they are gradually destroyed. Hence vitamin A may be lost during storage. The chief sources of vitamin A are fish oils, some animal fats, green grasses, properly dried grasses, yellow corn, and synthetic vitamin A.

Vitamin B Complex. The original vitamin, known as vitamin B, has been found to be composed of a large number of vitamins or vitamin-like factors. This condition has made the terminology confusing. Some of these factors have been isolated and recognized; others are still not so well known.

Vitamin B_1 (Thiamin).[22] Vitamin B_1, known chemically as thiamin, is necessary for maintenance of the appetite and preservation of the health of nervous tissue. Vitamin B_1 deficiency results in loss of appetite, emaciation, general weakness and inability to stand, frequent convulsions, and finally death. It is known technically as polyneuritis or beriberi. In the acute stages of polyneuritis, the head may be drawn over the back (Fig. 4).

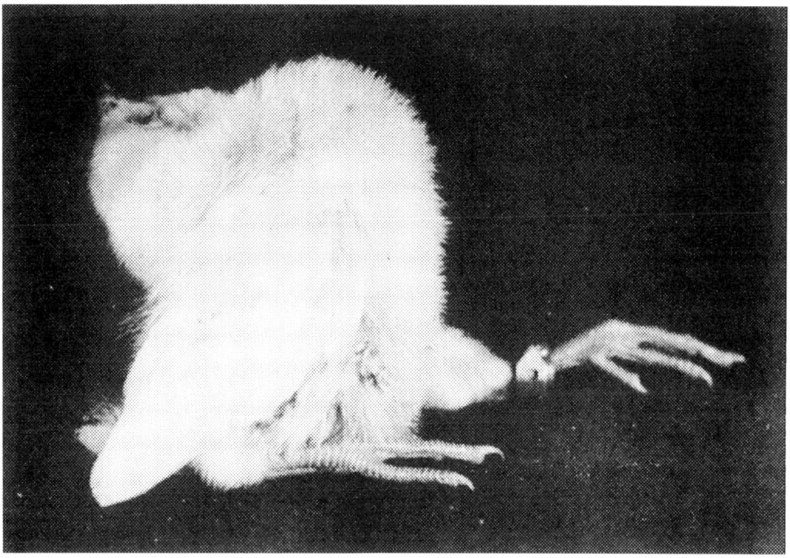

Fig. 4. Vitamin B_1 deficiency (polyneuritis). Note typical head retraction. (Courtesy Cornell University.)

Thiamin is found in the germ and bran of all grains, as well as in yeast, alfalfa, green pasture, and milk products. Hence it is plentifully supplied in every ordinary poultry ration and does not need to be fed in extra quantities by providing special supplements. It is soluble in water and alcohol and is very stable. Exposure to air and moderate dry heat do not destroy it.

Riboflavin (Vitamin B_2 or G). Vitamin B_2 (G), known chemically as riboflavin, is required for the formation of an enzyme present in all living cells. It is necessary for growth, preserves the health of the peripheral nerves, prevents leg paralysis (curled toe paralysis), and is essential for hatchability.

A lack of riboflavin in the diet of young chicks results in diarrhea, retarded growth, and paralysis of the legs, sometimes called nutritional leg paralysis.[23] It involves the legs and feet and occurs in two stages, a preliminary stage which is curable and an acute stage which is incurable. Nutritional paralysis is characterized by chicks suddenly walking on their hocks, with toes curling inward. Otherwise the chicks appear to be in excellent health. The disease ordinarily appears when the chicks are 3 to 4 weeks old. There may be some trembling of the legs (Fig. 5). Chicks receiving rations only partially deficient in this factor often recover spontaneously. The severe cases of the

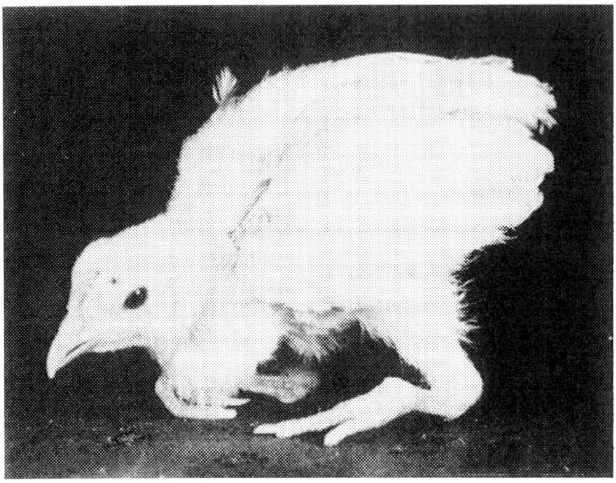

Fig. 5. Riboflavin deficiency in a young chick. Note the position of the hocks, with the toes curled inward. (Courtesy Cornell University.)

paralysis show very marked hypertrophy and softening of the brachial and sciatic nerves, which are usually discernible by inspection. The symptoms are most pronounced and most often observed in the sciatic nerves. These nerves occasionally reach a diameter four to five times normal size.

In breeding birds[24] a deficiency of riboflavin results in poor hatchability. The requirement for hatchability is considerably higher than for egg production and maintenance of health. The embryos that fail to hatch as a result of a riboflavin deficiency are dwarfed, show a high incidence of edema, degeneration of the Wolffian bodies, and a characteristically defective down development, termed clubbed down. On a ration moderately deficient in riboflavin, many embryos die during the second week of incubation. The mortality reaches a peak at about the eleventh day of development.

Riboflavin is a water-soluble vitamin, is fairly stable to heat, but is destroyed by irradiation.

The chief sources of riboflavin for poultry rations are milk products, yeast, liver, alfalfa meal, cereal grass, green pastures, and by-products of the fermenting and distilling industries.

Pantothenic Acid. Pantothenic acid, known also as the anti-dermatitis vitamin or the filtrate factor, preserves the health of the skin and spinal cord. A pantothenic acid deficiency in young chicks[25] results in retarded growth and extremely ragged feather

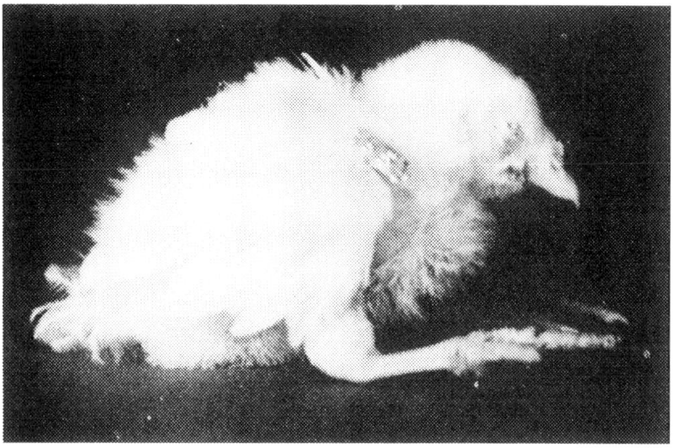

Fig. 6. Pantothenic acid deficiency. Note the lesions at the corners of the mouth, on the eyelids, and feet. (Courtesy Cornell University.)

development (Fig. 6). Within 12 to 14 days, a pellagra-like syndrome develops. The eyelids become granular and stick together as a result of a viscous exudate. Crusty scabs appear at the corners of the mouth and around the vent. Dermatitis of the feet, involving thickening and fissuring of the skin on the bottoms of the feet, causing an awkward gait, is sometimes observed in pantothenic acid deficiency, though the lesions are seldom as severe as those brought about by a biotin deficiency. Liver damage and changes in the spinal cord may be seen on post-mortem examination.

Lesions in adult fowls, similar to those of growing chicks, have usually not been observed although a deficiency of pantothenic acid results in lower hatchability.[26]

Pantothenic acid is supplied chiefly by milk products, yeast, liver, cane molasses, peanut meal, distillers' solubles, alfalfa meal, green pasture, and grains and grain by-products.

Vitamin B_6 (Pyridoxine). Vitamin B_6, known chemically as pyridoxine, is necessary for growth and maintenance of appetite and the prevention of a certain type of convulsions.[27] Chicks fed a pyridoxine-deficient diet show a small initial gain, then cease to grow, or grow very slowly. Some chicks show abnormal excitability and somewhat jerky convulsive movements. Chicks suddenly may run about aimlessly, often flopping their wings and keeping their heads down. Later, convulsions occur. During these convulsions, the chick may rest on its breast, raise its feet off the floor, and flop its wings. Chicks may fall on their sides, roll over on their backs, and rapidly paddle their feet. The head often jerks up and down or retracts, as in polyneuritis, and sometimes moves convulsively in an up-and-down movement with the neck distended or twisted. Complete exhaustion follows one of these convulsions, which are frequently fatal (Fig. 7).

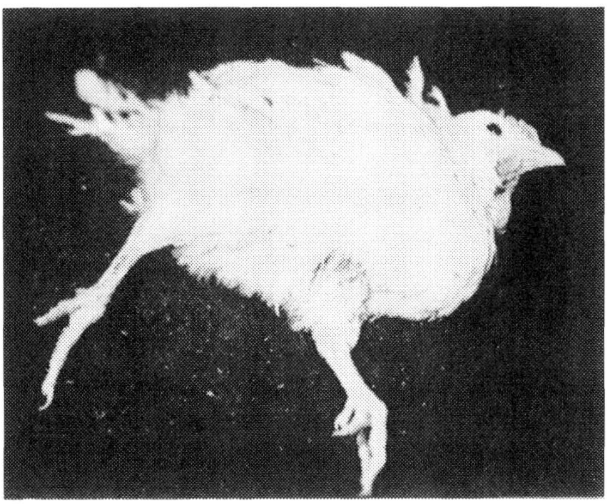

Fig. 7. Pyridoxine deficiency. Note loss of control of the legs and the head retraction. (Courtesy Cornell University.)

Pyridoxine deficiency in mature birds is characterized by loss of appetite, followed by rapid loss of weight, and death. Egg production and hatchability are reduced markedly.[28]

The chief sources of pyridoxine in the ration are grains, wheat by-products, rice by-products, yeast, liver, cane molasses, distillers' solubles, alfalfa meal, and cereal grass.

Vitamin B_{12} (Cobalamin).[29] Vitamin B_{12} is necessary for growth, feather development, and hatchability. Hemoglobin and red cell counts on vitamin-B_{12}-supplemented embryo blood were reported higher than on blood of B_{12}-deficient embryos. Vitamin

B_{12} also appears to be connected with protein metabolism. The response of "animal protein factor" supplements was due chiefly to their content of this vitamin.

Vitamin B_{12} is supplied by special fermentation products, liver, fish meal, fish solubles, meat scrap, and milk products.

Niacin (Nicotinic Acid). Niacin, formerly known as nicotinic acid, is necessary for growth and feather development. It prevents inflammation of the mouth cavity, esophagus, and crop, and scaly dermatosis of the skin and feet.[30]

A deficiency of niacin in the diet of the chick results in "Blacktongue," a condition characterized by inflammation of the tongue and mouth cavity. Beginning when the chick is about 2 weeks old, the entire mouth cavity of the deficient chicks, as well as the upper part of the esophagus, become distinctly inflamed with a deep red color, in contrast to the normal pink of

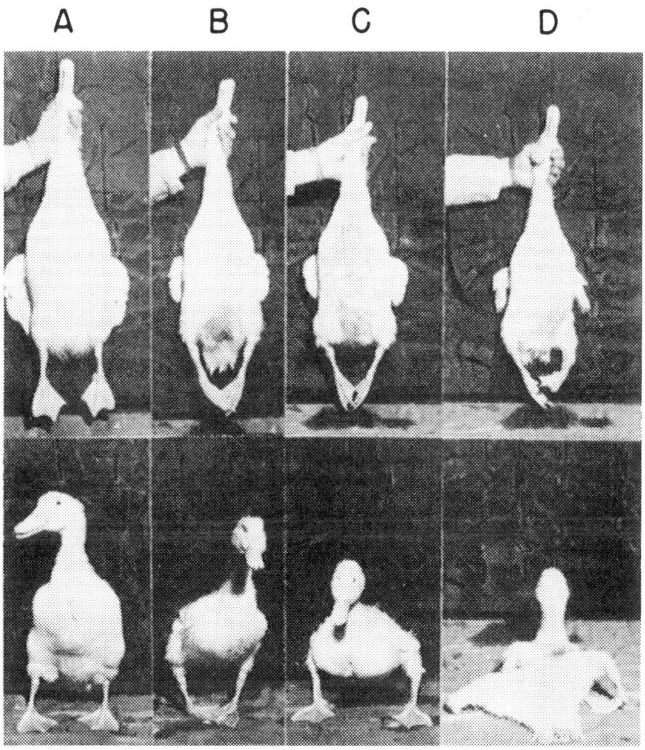

Fig. 8. Bowed legs in ducks due to a niacin deficiency. A = normal, B = bowed, C = very bowed, D = crippled. (Courtesy Cornell University.)

the healthy chick. Growth is retarded and feed consumption is reduced. Poor feather development and occasionally scaly dermatitis of the feet and skin are also observed.

Bowed legs in ducks caused by muscle deterioration has also been attributed to a niacin deficiency[31] (Fig. 8).

Pellagra in human beings and a similar condition in dogs, known as blacktongue, are prevented by niacin.

The chief sources of niacin in the ration are liver, yeast, wheat by-products, rice by-products, peanut meal, distillers' solubles, corn gluten feed, cereal grass, barley, and synthetic niacin.

Biotin. Biotin (formerly sometimes called vitamin H) is necessary for growth and hatchability. It is also involved in the prevention of perosis and a dermatosis similar to pantothenic acid deficiency.

In biotin deficiency in chicks[32] lesions first appear in about 3 weeks, although considerable variation in the time of appearance has been noticed. The bottoms of the feet become rough and calloused and may be severely affected before mandibular lesions are apparent. As the syndrome progresses, the entire bottom of the foot becomes encrusted, and hemorrhagic cracks appear. The toes may become necrotic and slough off, but the top of the foot and the legs usually show only a dry scaliness. The mandibular lesions, which first appear in the corners of the mouth, spread to include the area around the beak, and the eyelids eventually become swollen and stick together (Fig. 9). In contradistinction to these symptoms, the lesions in pantothenic acid deficiency are first evident in the corners of the mouth and eyes, and only in extreme cases do the lesions of the feet become so severe.

Biotin has been reported to be one factor necessary for the prevention of perosis[33] in chicks and in turkeys. Turkey poults exhibit symptoms very similar to those described for chicks when fed a biotin-deficient ration.

Feeding mature fowl[34] a biotin-deficient ration causes reduced hatchability while egg production is not adversely affected, indicating that the requirement for the production of hatching eggs is much higher than necessary for maintenance of good health and egg production. In hens, no dermatitis similar to that of chicks fed biotin-deficient rations has been observed.

The chief sources of biotin in the ration are grains, liver, yeast, cane molasses, alfalfa meal, green pasture, and distillers' solubles.

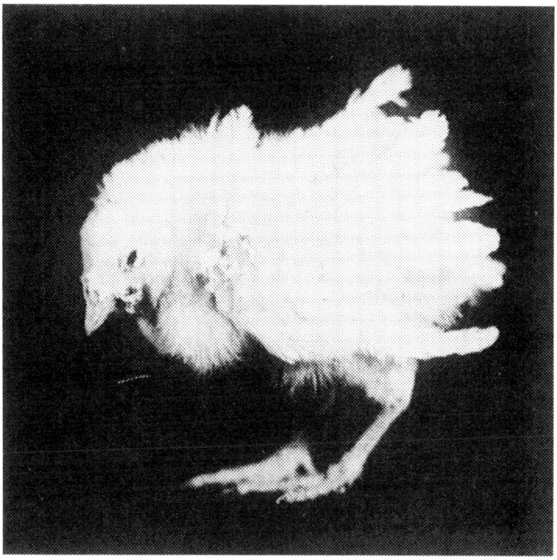

Fig. 9. Biotin deficiency. Note lesions on the feet and at the corner of the mouth. (Courtesy Cornell University.)

Choline.[35] Choline is necessary for growth, bone development, and egg production. A lack of choline in the diet of young chickens and turkeys results in retarded growth and perosis. In ducklings a choline deficiency has also been reported as causing fatty infiltration of the liver. Choline deficiency in mature birds has been reported to result in increased mortality and lowered egg production, with an increased abortion of egg yolks from the ovary.

Choline is supplied by grains, wheat by-products, liver, meat scraps, fish meal, milk products, soybean meal, peanut meal, distillers' solubles, and choline concentrates.

Folic Acid[36] (Pteroylglutamic Acid, Folacin). Folic acid is necessary for growth, maintenance of weight, hemoglobin formation, egg production, and hatchability. It is also involved in good feather formation and the prevention of perosis. In turkeys and geese its absence will cause cervical paralysis (Fig. 10).

The chief sources of folic acid are soybean meal, peanut meal, yeast, distillers' solubles, alfalfa meal, cereal grass, green pasture, and liver.

Other Organic Factors. Inositol,[37] which has been reported necessary for growth, is present in grain, wheat by-products, alfalfa meal, milk products, yeast, and liver.

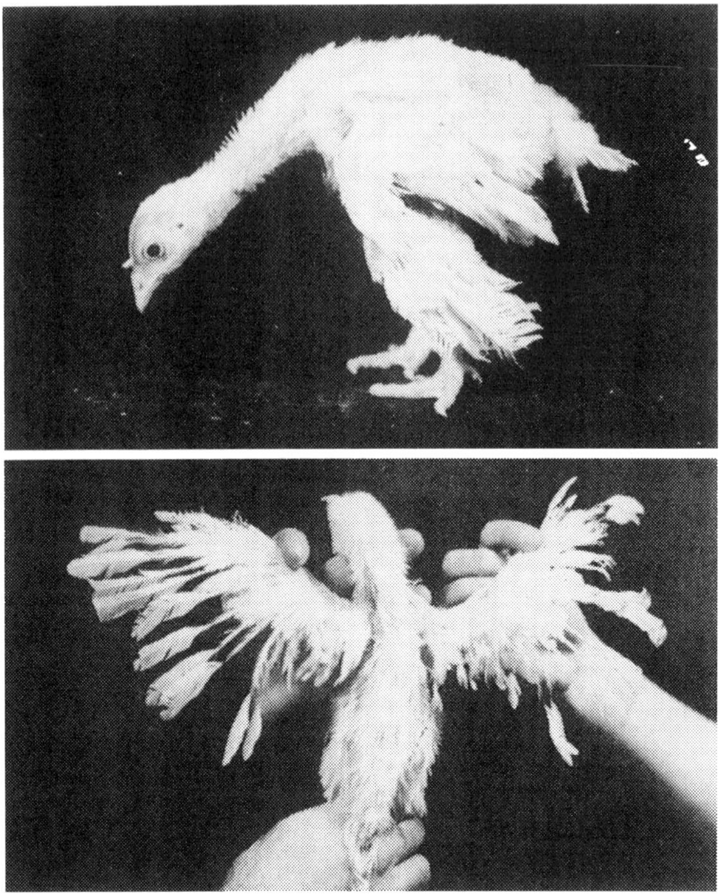

Fig. 10. Folic acid deficiency. Top, cervical paralysis in a turkey. Bottom, poor feathering in a chick. (Courtesy Cornell University.)

Glucuronic acid,[38] which has been reported necessary for growth, is found in oats, wheat by-products, liver, meat scraps, and fish meal.

The antigizzard erosion factor[39] has not been identified chemically. It prevents crater-like lesions and eroded areas on the secreted lining of the gizzard. It is present largely in alfalfa meal, green grass, wheat by-products, oats, and fresh milk. Cholic acid of the bile is an effective preventive of gizzard lesions.

Vitamin C (Ascorbic Acid). Vitamin C is not needed in the poultry diet. Apparently birds are able to make this substance

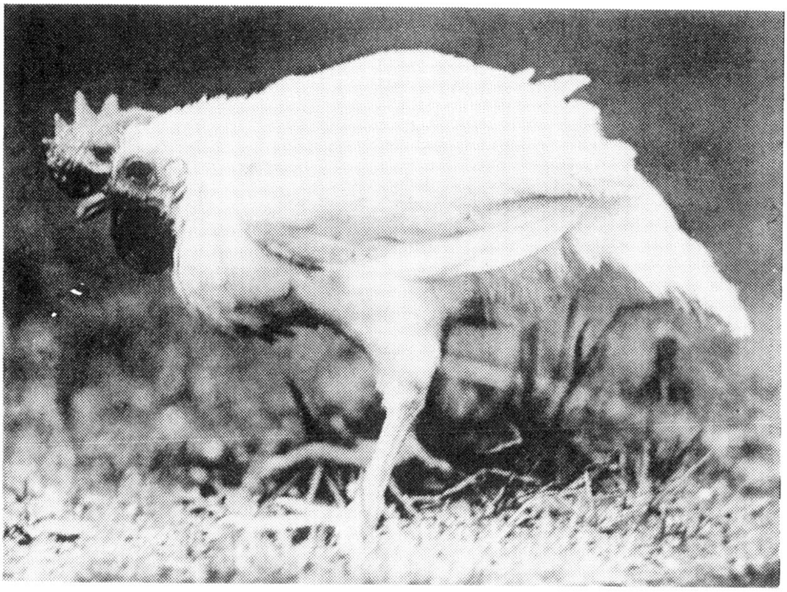

Fig. 11. Vitamin D deficiency (rickets). Note the ungainly manner of balancing the body and initial swelling of the hock joint. (Courtesy Cornell University.)

in their own bodies. In those species which require vitamin C a deficiency of it will produce scurvy.

Vitamin D. Vitamin D is necessary for calcium amd phosphorus utilization. It prevents rickets, the laying of thin-shelled eggs, and failure in egg production and hatchability.

A lack of vitamin D, in the absence of direct sunlight, results in the nutritional deficiency rickets.[40] The chicks are retarded in growth, show a disinclination to walk, or walk with a lame, stiff-legged gait, and have an ungainly manner of balancing the body (Fig. 11). The chicks appear generally unthrifty. In this disorder, an upset occurs in the mechanism involving the absorption and retention of calcium and phosphorus, as a result of which these minerals are not deposited in normal amounts in the bony structure of the body (Fig. 12). Abnormal bone development may be detected most readily in the legs and at the junction of the ribs on the side of the breast. The spinal column may be curved, and the sternum usually shows acute lateral bending or depression. Enlargement of the hock joints and beading of the rib ends become apparent. The beak is soft and rubbery and may be easily bent.

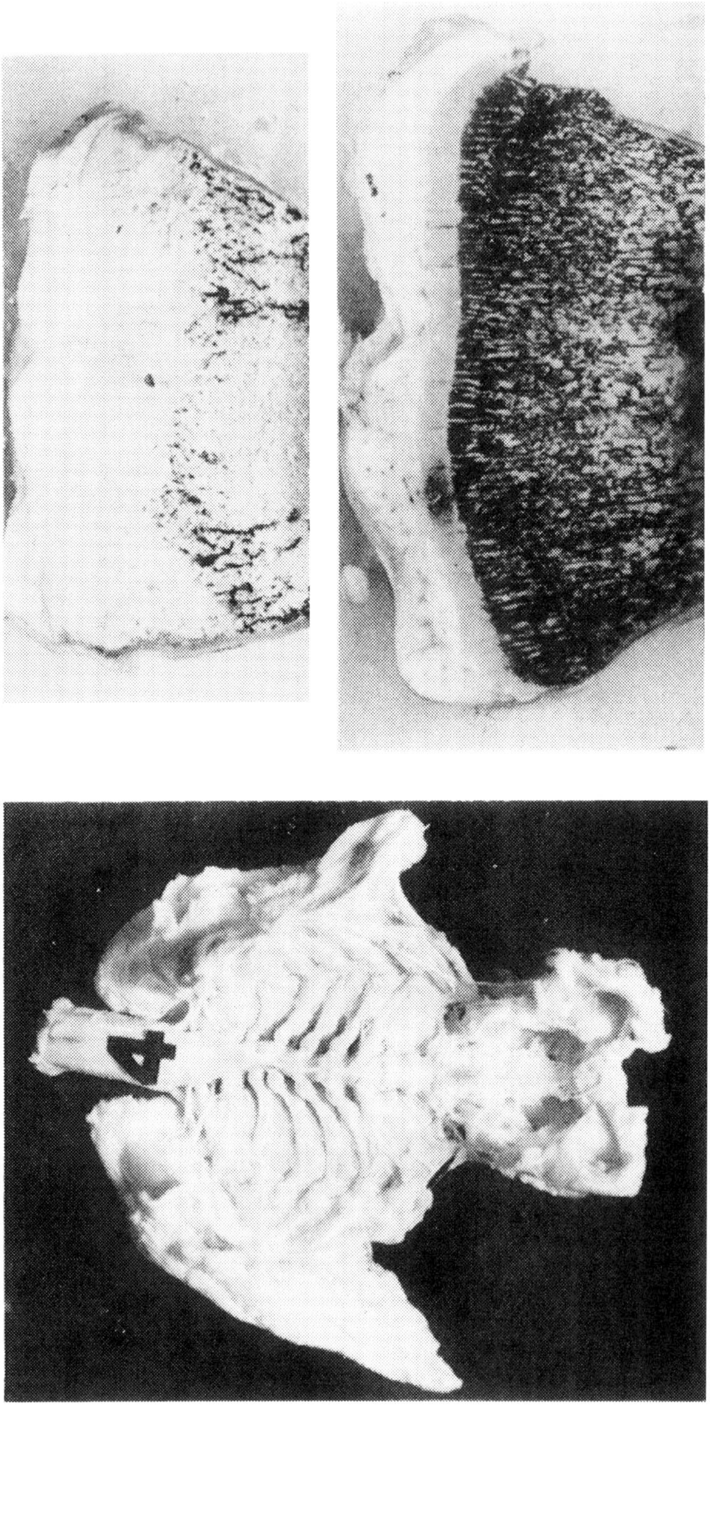

Fig. 12. Vitamin D deficiency. Left, poor skeletal formation. Note beading and bending of the ribs, spinal curvature, and crooked breastbone. Right, poor bone formation. Top, rachitic bone. Note wide band of cartilage and lack of calcification. Bottom, normal bone. (Courtesy Cornell University.)

In mature laying birds, the first symptom of a vitamin D deficiency is the laying of thin-shelled eggs, followed very shortly by decreased egg production. The breast bone becomes soft and rubbery, and the bones of the legs and wings become fragile and easily broken. Birds may lose, temporarily, the use of their legs and squat in a "penguin-like" manner, a symptom which sometimes has been called "egg paralysis." Hatchability is reduced markedly.

The symptoms of a vitamin D deficiency in turkeys are very similar to those described for chickens.

A deficiency of vitamin D has been reported as causing black pigmentation in buff feathers.[41]

Vitamin D is a fat-soluble vitamin, somewhat more stable than vitamin A. However, it is slowly affected by heat and exposure to air. There are a number of different forms of vitamin D. Vitamin D_3 or activated 7-dehydrocholesterol is the form which is most effective for chickens. This is the form found in fish liver oils and irradiated animal sterols. When incorporated in the ration, vitamin D is supplied usually as fish oils or activated animal sterol.

Vitamin D intended for poultry use was formerly expressed as A.O.A.C. (Association of Official Agricultural Chemists) chick units which represented the activity for chicks of 1 unit of vitamin D in U.S.P. Reference Cod Liver Oil. The International unit was used to express vitamin D potency for man and four-footed animals. The A.O.A.C. unit measured vitamin D_3. The U.S.P. unit measured vitamin D_2. These could not be used interchangeably because the effectiveness of these two forms was considerably different for poultry. Now vitamin D unitage has been standardized by an international committee. The International or U.S.P. unit for man and four-footed animals is the same as the International chick unit for poultry. They represent the activity of 0.025 microgram crystalline vitamin D_3 (activated 7-dehydrocholesterol). In order to interpret A.O.A.C. values in terms of the International chick unit, the A.O.A.C. values must be reduced by 25 per cent.

Vitamin D is perhaps the most peculiar of the vitamins since it may be supplied by certain light rays.[42] These rays are usually referred to as the ultraviolet rays or ultraviolet light. They are rays of comparatively short wave length, found in sunlight, and may be produced artificially by mercury vapor or carbon arc lamps. They synthesize the vitamin in the body by activating cholesterol in the skin to the active form of the vitamin.

Vitamin E. Vitamin E, known chemically as alpha-tocopherol, preserves the health of the reproductive organs and of the cerebellum and cerebrum of the brain. It prevents nutritional encephalomalacia (crazy chick disease), failure in hatchability, and loss of fertility in males.[43]

A lack of vitamin E in the ration of growing chicks results in the condition known as nutritional encephalomalacia. Chicks afflicted with this deficiency disease suddenly become prostrated, lying with legs outstretched and spastic, and toes flexed. The head is retracted and often twisted laterally. Before the chicken becomes completely prostrated, its gait and other movements are often incoordinate (Fig. 13). Upon autopsy, lesions are found

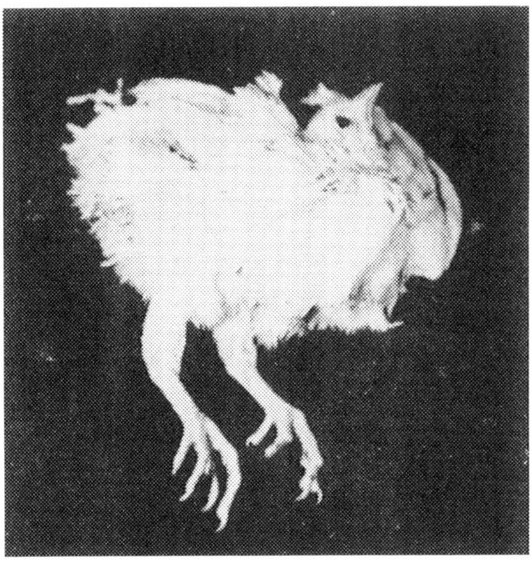

Fig. 13. Vitamin E deficiency in the chick. Note prostrated chick with retracted head. (Courtesy Cornell University.)

in the cerebellum and sometimes in the cerebrum. In many chicks, the chronic reddish or brownish areas on the surface of the cerebellum can be seen by inspection. Under some conditions, vitamin E deficiency results in subcutaneous edema and edema of the heart and pericardium.

In mature fowls, a prolonged vitamin E deficiency results in sterility in the male and reproductive failure in the female. Degenerative changes in the testes of the male may occur, resulting in permanent sterility. In females egg production apparently is not affected by a vitamin E deficiency, but hatchability is reduced markedly. During incubation the rate of growth and differentiation are slow, and many embryos die during the first 2 days of development because of a circulatory failure. A definite critical period in the development of the embryo occurs about the fourth day.

In poults, a deficiency of vitamin E results in the condition known as nutritional myopathy. This condition is characterized by lesions in the muscular wall of the gizzard. These lesions appear as circumscribed gray areas which often are of firmer texture than normal muscle and in some cases suggest scar tissues. It may also be involved in the production of enlarged hocks.

Vitamin E, a fat-soluble vitamin, is very stable. It is found largely in grains, wheat by-products, alfalfa meal, green pasture, cereal grass, and wheat germ oil. It is usually present in these feeds to such an extent that the fowl's needs seem to be completely supplied by ordinary rations.

Vitamin K. Vitamin K, which has been chemically identified but not named and is also known as the antihemorrhagic vitamin, is necessary to preserve the clotting power of blood.[44] It does prevent death from hemorrhage.

A lack of vitamin K greatly delays the clotting time of the blood. Chicks fed a deficiency ration may bleed to death from any injury or bruise which causes rupture of blood vessels. Hemorrhages may occur subcutaneously, intramuscularly, intraperitoneally, or in any part of the chick's body (Fig. 14). The hemorrhages vary in size and appear to be the only symptom of the deficiency.

In mature birds, vitamin K may be synthesized to some extent, as they do not seem to be subject to the acute deficiency. It has been shown, however, that laying birds fed a diet low in vitamin K produce eggs low in vitamin K. When these eggs are incubated, chicks are hatched which have very low reserves of vitamin K, with an accompanying prolonged blood-clotting time. Chicks may bleed to death from an injury such as may result from wing banding.

Vitamin K is a stable, fat-soluble vitamin. It is found chiefly in alfalfa meal, cereal grass, green pasture, meat scrap, and fish products.

Other Vitamins. A number of other vitamins have been reported, but their importance in poultry feeding has not yet been shown. They might include some of the other B vitamins, factor S,[45] the whey factor,[46] the grass juice factor,[47] and perhaps others.

Recent reports from a number of experiment stations indicate

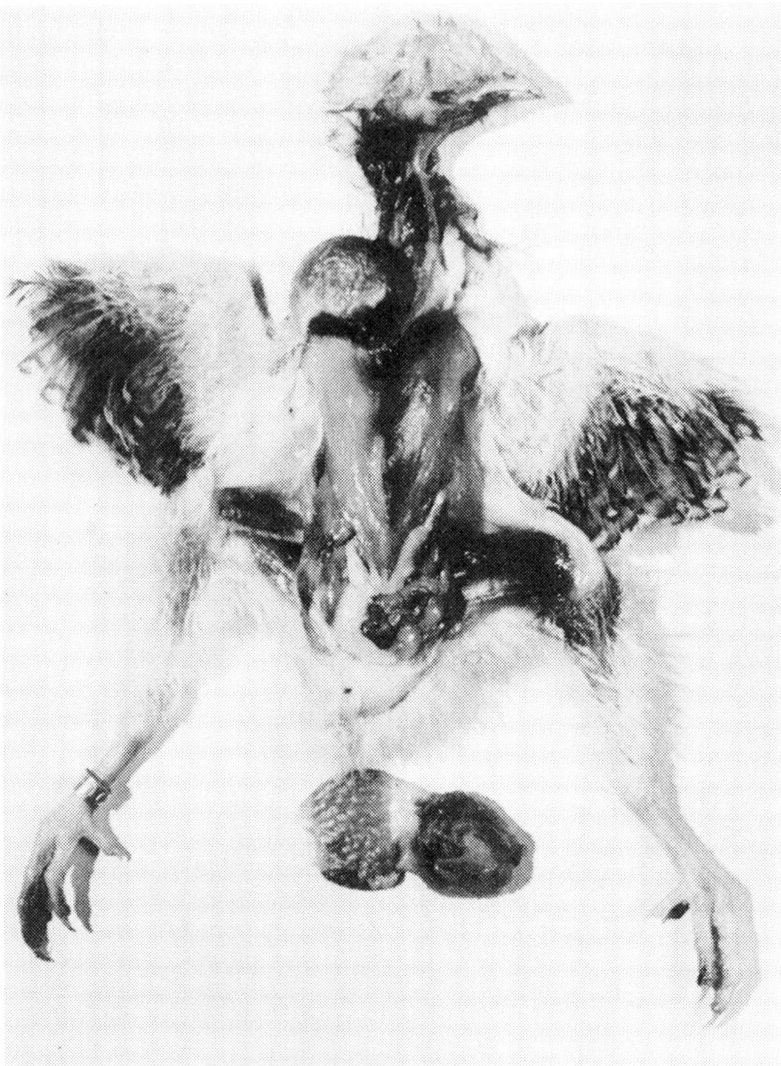

Fig. 14. Vitamin K deficiency. Note general hemorrhages. (Courtesy Cornell University.)

unidentified factors[48] in such ingredients as alfalfa, corn molasses (hydrol), dried distillers' solubles, dried yeast, fish products (including fish meal and fish solubles), liver, meat scrap, and peanut meal.

Requirements for Vitamins. The ration must contain sufficient vitamins. There is a difference in the requirements of different species for the various vitamins. In general, the principles, from a qualitative standpoint, can be applied from one species to another. However, quantitatively, the various species differ, and the actual requirements must be determined by using the species in which one is interested. The quantitative requirements, therefore, for chickens should be determined with chickens as the experimental animal. The quantity of any of the vitamins required varies with the age, sex, and condition of the birds. Chicks and laying hens usually have a larger vitamin requirement than do nonproducers. Generally, too, the requirements for hatchability are greater than the requirements only for egg production. Also turkeys differ from chickens in their needs.

ANTIBIOTICS

One of the most spectacular recent developments in nutrition science is the discovery that antibiotics[49] have growth-stimulating properties when fed to chickens, turkeys, and swine. Few nutritional discoveries have been so quickly and universally applied to feeding practice. The finding came as a result of the use of by-products from antibiotic production as sources of vitamin B_{12}.

It had been repeatedly shown that a ration whose protein is derived from vegetable source will not produce as good growth or hatchability as a ration containing animal proteins. Much interest was therefore shown in the so-called APF (animal protein factor) supplements. This name was derived from the fact that these materials were added to rations from which the animal protein feeds were removed and this probably supplied a factor or factors furnished by animal protein concentrates. They usually supplied vitamin B_{12} and as yet unidentified factors. After the discovery of vitamin B_{12} it was shown that one big difference between these rations is that the vegetable protein diet contains much less of this vitamin. It was also shown that by-products of antibiotic production and other fermentation products were good sources of vitamin B_{12} and could be used for this purpose to supplement rations whose protein was largely or entirely derived from vegetable source.

After synthetic vitamin B_{12} became available it was observed that at times the feeding of antibiotic by-products produced greater growth-promoting activity than could be attributed to their vitamin B_{12} content. It was suspected therefore that some other factor, probably the antibiotic, was producing the extra growth stimulus. This was confirmed by the use of pure antibiotics such as penicillin, aureomycin, terramycin, bacitracin, streptomycin, and others when added to rations containing sufficient vitamin B_{12} and other nutrients.

GROWTH STIMULATION. The increase in growth rate obtainable by antibiotic feeding varies with the type of animal, being greatest for turkeys, somewhat less for chickens and goslings, and least for ducks. The differences are greatest in the early growth period and decrease with age. Increases in early growth rate (during the first month) for chickens has been reported to be about 10-15 per cent. Failure to differentiate clearly between growth response due to vitamin B_{12}, or other essential nutrients, and that due to antibiotics (when the source of the antibiotic was the by-product) has led in some cases to an exaggerated concept of the antibiotic effect.

The feeding of antibiotics has had a growth-stimulating effect with rations containing animal protein feeds as well as those composed entirely or largely of protein from vegetable source. The fact that the relative stimulation is greater on an all-vegetable ration indicates that the antibiotic tends to spare or reduce the requirement for some unidentified nutrient associated with animal proteins. Actually best growth is generally obtained when an antibiotic is added to a ration which contains animal protein and which is complete in all known respects.

If the antibiotic supplement is withdrawn during the period of greatest growth stimulation, a growth retardation usually occurs which largely cancels out the weight advantage obtained up to that time. In no case has the retardation been sufficient to result in slower growth than the corresponding control groups which never received antibiotic supplementation. In broiler production, where weight gains are of major importance, it appears advisable to continue antibiotic supplementation throughout the growth period.

EFFECT ON FEED EFFICIENCY. Research on the effect of antibiotic feeding on the efficiency of feed utilization shows that a small improvement in the efficiency of feed conversion (pounds of feed required to produce a pound of meat) accompanies the growth stimulation; as the growth stimulation disappears, the improvement in feed utilization likewise tends to disappear. It would appear, therefore, that the efficient use of antibiotics covers only the period during which the actual growth stimulation is evident, and that the prolonged use of antibiotics beyond this period does not produce any return to the feeder.

AMOUNT NEEDED. Levels as low as 1 to 2 grams of some pure antibiotics per ton of feed have produced effective growth stimulation, although considerably larger amounts (50 or more grams per ton) have no harmful effects. Lower levels of an antibiotic have produced as effective stimulation as higher levels in experiments with the four major antibiotics generally used (penicillin, aureomycin, terramycin, and bacitracin). In the main no advantage is shown by a combination of antibiotics. The level of use of a specific antibiotic should be in accord with the manufacturer's recommendations.

OTHER EFFECTS. Besides the strictly nutritional effects, as expressed in increased growth, antibiotics have been shown to be effective in preventing such conditions a necrotic enteritis in swine. Hence there may also be some therapeutic value due to the feeding of the antibiotic. This might account for those reports which indicate lower mortality, generally better health or condition, greater uniformity, better feathering, and consequently improved performance and appearance. It might also account for those reports which showed greater benefit from the use of antibiotics under field conditions with the birds managed on the floor or ground as compared with birds kept on wire or in batteries under good conditions of management. Antibiotics are also effective in the control of specific diseases.

HENS. Antibiotics for laying and breeding hens are generally ineffective, having little or no effect upon egg production, hatchability, body weight, feed consumption, egg weight, egg quality, sexual maturity, or mortality.

MECHANISM OF EFFECT. Most investigators believe that the antibiotics exert their nutritional effect through changing the types and numbers of intestinal microorganisms. This might be accomplished by (1) suppression of inhibitory or "toxin-producing" microorganisms, (2) stimulation of microorganisms which manufacture known or unidentified vitamins which can subsequently be used by the host animal, (3) suppression of microorganisms which compete with the host animal for certain essential food nutrients, (4) suppression of "disease level" by eliminating pathogenic organisms from the intestinal tract.

Although each of these hypotheses is plausible, no single explanation seems to serve all cases, and it is not unlikely that several mechanisms may operate in various situations. A part of the growth-stimulating effect may be accounted for by appetite stimulation resulting in greater feed intake. The growth-stimulating effect of antibiotics is most spectacular when observed under conditions which greatly retard the growth of animals fed the usual type of practical rations.

In general, the levels of antibiotics used in practical poultry feeding are too low to have a specific effect on recognized infection, or on the intestinal microorganism population. When higher levels are fed, reported research indicates correlated changes in intestinal microorganisms; these studies, however, have not clearly shown whether the shifts in intestinal flora are responsible for any or all of the growth-stimulating effect of antibiotics.

GROWTH PROMOTERS

Growth stimulation has also been accomplished in other ways. Arsonic acid derivatives[50] have been reported to produce growth stimulation. Detergents[51] or surface acting agents, called "surfactants," have also been reported as being effective in this respect. Results, however, have not been consistent. Why they produce the results has not been explained.

Free methionine added to the ration in relatively small amounts has in some cases produced added growth and increased the efficiency of feed utilization.[52]

INTERRELATIONSHIPS OF DIETARY FACTORS

Nutrition workers have long recognized the existence of interrelationships of dietary factors. More of these are becoming apparent, and they frequently help to explain unexpected results.

One of the earliest relations reported was that of a balance between minerals, especially calcium and phosphorus.

Many of the interrelations involve vitamins. Vitamin E has been reported as sparing vitamins A and D. A sparing action has been noted between vitamin B_{12} and pantothenic acid. The vitamin B_{12} requirement is also influenced by the protein level and the amounts of methionine and choline present in the ration. The vitamin D required is related to the amounts of calcium and phosphorus supplied. Choline, biotin, and folic acid are involved in perosis and manganese metabolism. Thiamin has a relationship with the carbohydrate requirement. Niacin can spare the amino acid tryptophan. Ascorbic acid to a certain extent corrects the harmful effect of excess tyrosine.

The presence of labile methyl groups are necessary for nutrition. A certain amount of shifting can take place for this purpose between choline, methionine, and betaine.

A certain amount of substitution can take place between the amino acids. Cystine can in this way replace part of the methionine.

There is also some interrelationship between the vitamins, enzymes, and hormones. The function of these depend upon a proper balance in the body.

There exists a relationship between the requirement of the chick in early life and the amount of carry-over of nutrients from the egg. Hence, the diet of the dam influences the reaction of the chick. This might be considered a delayed nutritional effect.

The interrelations between nutrients are particularly important in the case of borderline or partial deficiencies.

Some nutritive factors will alter the microflora of the intestinal tract which will have an effect on the synthesis of nutrients which might have a direct effect upon the response of the bird to certain types of rations.

The feeding of animals is sometimes complicated by the presence in the ration of antimetabolites. The avidin of raw egg albumen will tie up the biotin and hence cause biotin deficiency. Heat treatment to inactivate the avidin will result in a normal response without any other change in the ration. The deficiency might also be overcome by the addition of more biotin. Similarly an antithiamin factor in raw fish has been the cause of thiamin deficiency in fur-bearing animals. Antimetabolites have also been reported for some of the other vitamins.

ENERGY

All energy comes from the sun. Energy might be defined as the ability or power to do work. In feeding stuffs, it is present as chemical or stored energy, expressed in this way by Liberty Hyde Bailey: "The blazing log gives back the glow of summer suns of long ago." In the formation of plant tissues, energy from the sun is stored in them. When the feed is consumed by the animal, it is broken down and the energy released. Carbohydrates and proteins are approximately equivalent in their energy values, producing 4 calories per gram. On the other hand, fats produce more energy per unit volume, the value of fats being 9 calories per gram.

A deficiency of energy[53] results in lower growth, poorer feathering, and reduced efficiency of feed utilization in chicks as well as poorer weight maintenance and lower egg production in hens. Increasing the energy content of some rations has resulted in improvement because energy rather than any of the other nutrients was the limiting factor. This largely explains the favorable results of the "high energy" rations.

The young chick compensates for a reduced dietary energy level by increasing feed consumption. Energy levels seem to be the major factor in controlling feed intake. Reduction of the dietary energy level is reflected in changes in the fat content of the carcass. Although large amounts of indigestible fibrous materials can be incorporated in a diet without affecting weight gains of young birds, body composition is greatly changed. Hence weight gains are not a satisfactory criterion in determining energy requirements for growth. Higher energy rations are necessary for higher fat content of the carcass, which influences the degree of pigmentation and appearance of the skin which are major factors in determining market quality.

Available energy values of feedstuffs as reported by Fraps[54] are given in Table 3. In general as the fiber of the feed increases, the energy value is lowered.

Sunshine or light has many effects upon the animal body. The antirachitic value of the ultraviolet rays has already been referred to in connection with vitamin D. The far-ultraviolet rays also are reported to have an antiseptic value. It has also been reported that bactericidal ultraviolet radiation[55] exerted a stimulatory effect upon egg production. The infrared rays have certain heat effects upon the body. The red rays of the visible spectrum are effective in the use of artificial illumination by stimulation of the pituitary gland, which in turn stimulates the reproductive system.

VARIATION IN COMPOSITION OF PLANTS

In dealing with feedstuffs, we must keep in mind the fact that they are mixtures of nutrients. In fact, most feeds contain all or most of the nutrients in varying proportions. No two feeds are alike in their composition. Variations will be found in the water content, ash, crude proteins, fiber, carbohydrates, and fats as well as in the various mineral constituents, vitamins, and amino acids. The problem in compounding a ration is to make a combination of ingredients in such a manner that these various nutrients and constituents are furnished in quantities to meet the requirements for them. It not only is important to furnish a sufficient amount of each of the constituents but, in the case of those which might be harmful or which are very expensive, too great an excess must also be avoided.

RELATIONS BETWEEN PLANT AND ANIMAL TISSUES

CHEMISTRY OF ANIMAL LIFE. The relative proportion of the nutrients as found in animal tissues is shown in Table 1. Water comprises the largest single nutrient of both the fowl and the egg. Protein is also an important nutrient. Fat appears in fairly large quantities in the egg and in certain kinds of fowl. In the animal body, there is an inverse relation between fat and moisture. For example, analysis indicates a larger proportion of fat in the Plymouth Rock capon than in the Leghorn hen. This increase in fat is almost entirely at the expense of the water content. Carbohydrates are present in the body only in small amounts. They occur in the glucose of the blood and the glycogen of the liver and muscles.

The dry matter of the body is made up largely of carbon, oxygen, hydrogen, and nitrogen. Of the mineral elements, phosphorus and calcium are present in largest amounts, and sulfur, potassium, chlorine, sodium, magnesium, and iron in much smaller quantities.

COMPARISON OF PLANT AND ANIMAL TISSUES. There are a number of important differences in the composition of plants and animals. Poultry rations are made up largely of cereals and cereal by-products. A comparison, therefore of corn and the body of the hen will show these differences (Table 1).

One difference between these two is that corn is relatively low in water, whereas the animal body is made up of a large percentage of water. The body of the fowl contains more mineral matter,

TABLE 1. COMPOSITION OF PLANT AND ANIMAL TISSUES

	Corn, %	Leghorn Hen, %	Plymouth Rock Capon, %	Egg, %
Water	11.3	55.8	41.6	73.7
Protein	9.3	21.6	19.4	13.4
Fat	3.8	17.0	33.9	10.5
Carbohydrates	75.3	traces	traces	....
Mineral matter	1.3	3.8	3.7	1.0

proteins, and fat. On the other hand, the corn is composed largely of the carbohydrates.

Similarly, we find differences in the make-up of the amino acids. The animal proteins usually contain larger amounts of such amino acids as lysine, arginine, tryptophan, and histidine than the grains. There are also differences in the mineral constituents, the greatest difference occurring in the calcium content, which is high in the body of the hen and low in the grain.

CYCLE OF LIFE. A study of the composition of the animal body shows the end or aim of feeding. The presence of different elements and compounds in the body indicate that they must be supplied from some source. That source is the feed which the animal eats. Most of this food comes from plant substances.

The transformation and use of the food nutrients or the relation of food nutrients and the animal products derived therefrom are shown in Table 2.

In general, the nutrients found in the body of the fowl or the egg must appear in the ration. A common saying is that we must "feed a part to make a part." In the main, one nutrient cannot be substituted for another. There are, however, a few exceptions to this general statement. For example, carbohydrates can be used in part for fats, and fat can be substituted in part for the carbohydrates. Similarly, proteins can function the same as

TABLE 2. THE TRANSFORMATION AND USE OF THE FOOD NUTRIENTS OR THE RELATION OF FOOD NUTRIENTS AND THE ANIMAL PRODUCTS DERIVED THEREFROM

Kernel of Grain	Chemist's Report	Body of Fowl	Egg
Water	Moisture	Body fluids (water)	Water
Minerals	Ash	Bones (Ca, P) Body tissues (K, S, P) Blood (Fe)	Shell (Ca) Egg contents (P, S, K)
Proteins (gluten)	Crude protein or N × 6.25	Muscles Blood Nerves Feathers	Albumen Yolk proteins
Carbohydrates:		Glycogen	Yolk fat
Starches, sugars	Nitrogen-free extract	Fat (energy)	
Cellulose	Crude fiber		
Lipids	Ether extract	Fat (energy)	Yolk fat
Vitamins		Vital organs Enzymes	Vitamins

carbohydrates and fats in furnishing energy. However, the reverse is not true, because carbohydrates and fats cannot function in place of the proteins.

FEED ANALYSES

The ordinary report of the chemist on feed analyses usually gives water or moisture, crude protein, fat or ether extract, crude fiber, mineral matter or ash, and nitrogen-free extract. All these are determined directly with the exception of the nitrogen-free extract, which is determined by difference. That is, the other nutrients for which direct analyses are made are added together and subtracted from 100. The nitrogen-free extract represents the difference between their sum and 100 per cent.

It is possible also to make other determinations in the laboratory, but they are usually not part of the routine analyses of feeds. Some of the vitamins can be measured chemically or microbiologically in the laboratory in a comparatively short time. Analyses can also be made for most of the mineral elements. It is also possible to make an energy determination of the feed.

In most states, a guaranteed analysis of feeding stuffs is required by law. This analysis must accompany the feed, and usually must include a guarantee of the minimum amount of protein and fat and the maximum amount of fiber. In animal protein feeds, the maximum amount of phosphorus or P_2O_5, which represents the amount of bone present, must also be given. For example, a meat scrap guaranteed to contain 50 per cent protein, 6 per cent fat, 3 per cent fiber, and 8 per cent phosphorus must contain at least 50 per cent protein, at least 6 per cent fat, and not more than 3 per cent fiber, or 8 per cent phosphorus.

COMPOSITION OF FEEDS

When formulating poultry rations, it is necessary to have information on the composition of feeds. In tables 3 and 4 the average composition of feeds commonly used in poultry ratios is given. Table 5 shows the vitamin content of ingredients commonly used in poultry feeding. Table 6 gives the approximate amino acid composition of certain feedstuff proteins.

TABLE 3. AVERAGE COMPOSITION OF ORGANIC NUTRIENTS AND AVAILABLE ENERGY OF FEEDS USED IN POULTRY RATIONS

Feeding Stuff	Protein, %	Fat, %	Fiber, %	N-Free Extract, %	Digestible Protein, %	Total Digestible Nutrients	Energy, cal./lb.
Alfalfa leaf meal, good	21.2	2.8	16.6	39.7	16.1	56.7	314
Alfalfa leaf meal, high in fiber	19.6	2.7	20.7	38.9	14.3	53.2	. . .
Alfalfa, green	4.5	0.9	7.2	10.4	3.4	14.7	. . .
Barley	12.7	1.9	5.4	66.6	10.0	77.7	811
Barley, Pacific Coast	8.7	1.9	5.7	70.9	6.9	78.7	. . .
Bone meal, steamed	7.1	3.3	0.8	3.8	. . .	. . .	202
Buckwheat	10.3	2.3	10.7	62.8	7.4	62.2	700
Buttermilk	3.5	0.6	. . .	4.5	3.3	9.1	. . .
Buttermilk, condensed	10.9	2.2	. . .	12.6	9.8	26.5	241
Buttermilk, dried	32.4	6.4	0.3	43.3	29.2	84.0	707
Corn, dent, Grade 2	8.6	3.9	2.0	69.3	6.6	80.1	1145
Corn feed meal	9.8	4.7	2.9	69.2	7.5	83.1	1145
Corn gluten feed	25.5	2.7	7.6	48.8	21.9	76.0	565
Corn gluten meal	43.1	2.0	4.0	39.8	36.6	80.2	839
Cottonseed meal, 43% protein	42.7	6.4	10.6	27.0	34.2	72.6	694
Dried distillers' solubles	26.7	7.9	2.6	48.4	19.5	77.1	853
Fish meal, all analyses	63.9	6.8	0.6	4.0	56.2	72.8	898
Fish meal, menhaden	62.2	8.5	0.7	4.2	50.4	71.6	. . .
Fish meal, sardine	67.2	5.0	0.6	5.4	55.1	68.9	823
Fish solubles, condensed	29.3	8.4	. . .	2.2	26.1	42.3	. . .
Hominy feed	11.2	6.9	5.2	64.2	8.0	84.5	866
Linseed meal, solvent process	36.9	2.9	8.7	36.3	31.0	72.3	586
Meat scraps, 55% protein	55.6	10.9	1.2	0.5	47.3	67.9	724
Meat and bone scraps, 50% protein	51.0	10.1	2.1	1.6	41.8	64.6	724
Milo grain	11.3	2.9	2.2	71.3	8.8	80.1	1144

TABLE 3 (Concluded)

Feeding Stuff	Protein, %	Fat, %	Fiber, %	N-Free Extract, %	Digestible Protein, %	Total Digestible Nutrients	Energy, cal./lb.
Molasses, cane	2.9	. . .	. . .	62.1	. . .	54.0	714
Oats	12.0	4.6	11.0	58.6	9.4	70.1	817
Oats, Pacific Coast	9.0	5.4	11.0	62.1	7.0	72.2	. . .
Oat kernels, without hulls	16.3	6.1	2.1	63.7	14.7	92.0	1155
Pea seed, field	23.4	1.2	6.1	57.0	20.1	77.9	888
Peanut-oil meal, o.p. 43% protein	43.1	7.6	13.9	23.0	39.2	82.0	731
Rye	12.6	1.7	2.4	70.9	10.0	76.1	817
Skimmilk	3.6	0.1	. . .	5.1	3.4	8.7	. . .
Skimmilk, dried	34.7	1.2	0.2	50.3	31.2	80.7	525
Soybean oil meal, hydraulic or expeller	44.3	5.3	5.7	29.6	37.2	78.4	674
Soybean oil meal, solvent	46.1	1.0	5.9	31.8	42.4	78.5	565
Sunflower seed	16.8	25.9	29.0	18.8	13.9	76.3	950
Tankage, 60% protein	60.6	8.5	2.0	1.8	51.5	68.4	676
Wheat	13.2	1.9	2.6	69.9	11.1	80.0	1024
Wheat, soft Pacific Coast	9.9	2.0	2.7	72.6	8.3	79.9	. . .
Wheat bran	16.9	4.6	9.6	52.9	13.7	67.2	478
Wheat flour middlings	18.3	4.2	3.8	59.8	16.1	78.9	720
Wheat standard middlings	18.1	4.8	6.5	55.8	15.0	77.2	581
Wheat red dog	18.2	3.6	2.6	61.9	16.0	85.6	1020
Whey, dried	12.2	0.8	0.2	70.4	11.0	78.3	490
Yeast, dried brewers'	49.3	1.0	3.7	31.9	42.4	70.5	476

Reproduced with the permission of the Morrison Publishing Company, Ithaca, N. Y., from *Feeds and Feeding*, 21st. Ed., 1948, by F. B. Morrison, Appendix, Table I. Energy values are taken from *Texas Agr. Exp. Sta. Bul.* 678, 1946, by G. S. Fraps.

TABLE 4. MINERAL MATTER CONTENT OF FEEDS USED IN POULTRY RATIONS

Feeding Stuff	Mineral Matter, %	Calcium, %	Phosphorus, %	Manganese, mg. per lb.
Alfalfa leaf meal, good	12.0	1.69	0.25	27.6
Alfalfa leaf meal, high in fiber	10.9	. . .	. . .	. . .
Alfalfa, green	2.3	0.35	0.07	5.6
Barley	2.8	0.06	0.37	8.0
Barley, Pacific Coast	2.6	. . .	. . .	. . .
Bone meal, steamed	81.3	29.30	15.10	5.1
Buckwheat	1.9	0.09	0.31	15.4
Buttermilk	0.8	0.14	0.08	. . .
Buttermilk, condensed	4.0	0.44	0.26	. . .
Buttermilk, dried	10.0	1.36	0.82	. . .
Corn, dent, Grade 2	1.2	0.02	0.27	2.5
Corn feed meal	2.0	0.03	0.34	. . .
Corn gluten feed	6.3	0.48	0.82	11.2
Corn gluten meal	2.5	0.13	0.38	3.4
Cottonseed meal, 43% protein	5.8	0.23	1.12	. . .
Dried distillers' solubles	7.4	0.30	1.41	29.6
Fish meal, all analyses	17.6	4.14	2.67	13.5
Fish meal, menhaden	18.0	5.30	3.38	10.2
Fish meal, sardine	14.9	4.21	2.54	10.3
Fish solubles, condensed	9.6	. . .	. . .	. . .
Hominy feed	2.9	0.22	0.71	6.9
Linseed meal, solvent process	5.6	0.39	0.87	18.4
Meat scraps, 55% protein	26.3	8.33	4.04	8.2
Meat and bone scraps, 50% protein	29.1	9.71	4.81	5.3
Milo grain	1.7	0.03	0.28	5.9

TABLE 4 (Concluded)

Feeding Stuff	Mineral Matter, %	Calcium, %	Phosphorus, %	Manganese, mg. per lb.
Molasses, cane	9.0	0.74	0.08	. . .
Oats	4.0	0.09	0.34	19.9
Oats, Pacific Coast	3.7	. . .	. . .	. . .
Oat kernels, without hulls	2.2	0.08	0.46	16.8
Pea seed, field	3.0	. . .	. . .	. . .
Peanut-oil meal, o.p. 43% protein	5.2	0.16	0.54	. . .
Rye	1.9	0.10	0.33	37.0
Skimmilk	0.7	0.13	0.10	0.1
Skimmilk, dried	7.8	1.30	1.03	0.8
Soybean oil meal, hydraulic or expeller	6.0	0.29	0.66	13.6
Soybean oil meal, solvent	5.8	0.30	0.66	13.8
Sunflower seed	3.1	. . .	0.55	9.8
Tankage, 60% protein	20.2	6.37	3.23	10.0
Wheat	1.9	0.04	0.39	19.9
Wheat, soft Pacific Coast	1.9	. . .	. . .	. . .
Wheat bran	6.1	0.14	1.29	51.5
Wheat flour middlings	3.1	0.09	0.71	. . .
Wheat standard middlings	4.4	0.09	0.93	49.4
Wheat red dog	2.7	0.07	0.51	16.3
Whey, dried	9.9	0.86	0.72	2.0
Yeast, dried brewers'	7.9	0.13	1.56	2.5
Limestone	. . .	38.30	. . .	. . .
Oyster shell	. . .	37.90	. . .	. . .

Reproduced with the permission of The Morrison Publishing Company, Ithaca, N. Y., from <u>Feeds and Feeding</u>, 21st. Ed., 1948, by F. B. Morrison, Appendix, Tables I and IV.

TABLE 5. VITAMIN CONTENT OF INGREDIENTS COMMONLY USED IN POULTRY FEEDING

Feedstuff	Vitamin A Activity, I.U. per lb.	Riboflavin, mg. per lb.	Pantothenic Acid, mg. per lb.	Niacin, mg. per lb.	Thiamin, mg. per lb.	Biotin, mg. per lb.	Choline, mg. per lb.	Folic Acid, mg. per lb.	Pyridoxine, mg. per lb.
Alfalfa leaf meal, dehydrated	113,667	8.7	15.3	18.0	2.5	0.15	?	?	?
Alfalfa leaf meal, sun cured	50,000	7.2	12.6	24.1	2.0	. . .	. . .	. . .	. . .
Alfalfa meal, dehydrated	72,333	6.7	17.4	?	2.0	?	462	3.93	?
Alfalfa meal, sun cured	27,667	5.4	12.0	17.7	1.4	. . .	. . .	. . .	. . .
Barley	317	0.6	3.0	27.2	2.6	0.06	450	0.27	1.62
Brewers' yeast, dried	0	18.6	54.0	228.1	35.0	?	1,635	?	?
Buckwheat	0	0.7	5.7	9.1	2.1	. . .	. . .	. . .	. . .
Buttermilk, dried	0	14.9	15.8	3.7	1.6	?	500	?	?
Corn, yellow	3,667	0.5	2.3	9.0	1.9	0.03	200	0.14	?
Corn, yellow, stored 2 yrs.	1,833	?	?	?	?	. . .	. . .	. . .	. . .
Corn gluten meal	16,667	0.6	5.3	23.4	0	?	135	0.10	?
Cottonseed meal	150	2.2	5.0	14.5	3.3	?	320	1.04	?
Distillers' dried solubles	?	5.2	8.9	54.3	2.7	1.26	1,500	?	?
Fish meal, menhaden	?	2.2	?	25.9	0.2	. . .	. . .	. . .	. . .
Fish meal, sardine	?	2.5	3.2	11.4	0.4	?	1,500	?	?

TABLE 5 (Concluded)

Feedstuff	Vitamin A Activity, I.U. per lb.	Ribo-flavin, mg. per lb.	Panto-thenic Acid, mg. per lb.	Niacin, mg. per lb.	Thiamin, mg. per lb.	Biotin, mg. per lb.	Choline, mg. per lb.	Folic Acid, mg. per lb.	Pyri-doxine, mg. per lb.
Fish solubles, condensed	?	9.8	18.9	166.5	2.0	0.06	1,800	?	5.68
Meat and bone scrap	0	2.1	1.5	21.4	?	?	900	?	?
Meat scrap (55%)	0	2.1	1.8	20.2	0.5	?	1,300	?	?
Oats	83	0.5	6.0	6.3	2.8	0.13	435	0.10	?
Peanut meal	133	1.1	24.1	77.5	3.3	?	840	?	?
Rice bran	0	1.0	10.3	129.1	10.3	. . .	. . .	. . .	. . .
Skimmilk, dried	0	9.5	15.6	6.2	1.6	?	612	0.27	?
Soybean oil meal, solvent	?	1.9	7.3	14.5	0.8	?	1,285	?	?
Wheat	0	0.5	6.3	24.1	2.3	0.04	458	0.20	?
Wheat flour middlings	. . .	0.8	4.5	44.2	6.0	?	450	?	?
Wheat standard middlings	0	0.8	9.3	44.3	5.8	?	547	0.41	?
Wheat bran	133	1.4	10.6	63.5	3.9	?	502	0.10	?
Whey, dried	0	13.0	22.4	5.1	1.8	?	1,635	?	?

Reproduced with the permission of the Morrison Publishing Company, Ithaca, N. Y., from Feeds and Feeding, 21st. Ed., 1948, by F. B. Morrison, Appendix, Tables V and Va.

TABLE 6. AMINO ACID COMPOSITION OF POULTRY FEEDSTUFFS

	Percentage of Feedstuffs						
	Crude Protein	Arginine	Lysine	Methionine	Cystine	Tryptophan	Glycine
Alfalfa meal	20	1.0	1.0	0.36	0.38	0.35	?
Alfalfa meal	18	0.9	0.9	0.32	0.34	0.32	?
Barley	12	0.5	0.3	0.13	0.20	0.13	?
Barley	9	0.4	0.2	0.10	0.15	0.10	?
Blood meal	84	3.0	7.2	1.00	1.50	1.18	trace
Buttermilk, dried	32	1.0	2.2	0.67	?	0.41	0.2
Corn	9	0.4	0.2	0.21	0.15	0.07	0.4*
Corn gluten meal	42	1.3	0.7	0.97	0.68	0.33	2.1*
Cottonseed meal	43	3.5	1.6	0.71	0.97	0.46	2.3
Distillers' solubles, dried	26	0.8	0.8	0.41	0.26	0.12	?
Fishmeal	70	5.0	6.4	2.20	1.18	0.98	4.7
Fishmeal	65	4.6	5.9	2.00	1.10	0.91	4.4
Fishmeal	60	4.0	5.4	1.80	1.00	0.84	4.0
Fish solubles, condensed	35	1.5	1.7	0.60	0.21	0.12	2.3
Linseed meal	35	2.7	1.1	0.84	0.66	0.56	1.8*
Meat scrap	55	3.9	3.4	1.10	0.77	0.44	2.2*
Meat scrap	50	3.0	2.7	0.70	0.60	0.35	2.0*
Milo	11	0.4	0.3	0.16	0.20	0.09	?
Oats	12	0.7	0.4	0.23	0.19	0.14	?
Oats	9	0.5	0.3	0.17	0.14	0.10	?

TABLE 6 (Concluded)

	Percentage of Feedstuffs						
	Crude Protein	Arginine	Lysine	Methionine	Cystine	Tryptophan	Glycine
Peanut meal	44	4.4	1.3	0.49	0.70	0.44	2.5
Peas, dry	24	1.7	1.4	0.19	0.34	0.19	?
Rye	12	0.5	0.4	0.16	?	0.16	?
Skimmilk, dried	35	1.1	2.5	0.81	0.42	0.45	0.2
Soybean meal	45	2.8	2.7	0.62	0.66	0.53	7.6
Sunflowerseed meal	45	3.7	1.9	1.53	0.72	0.59	2.2*
Wheat	13	0.5	0.3	0.21	0.24	0.14	
Wheat	10	0.4	0.3	0.16	0.19	0.11	?
Wheat bran	15	0.9	0.5	0.17	0.19	0.21	?
Wheat middlings	16	0.9	0.4	0.14	0.19	0.14	?
Whey, dried	12	0.4	1.0	0.32	0.41	0.18	0.0
Yeast, dried brewers'	45	2.0	3.1	0.84	0.54	0.55	?

*Minimum value based on feeding tests.

Taken from Table 6 "Recommended Nutrient Allowances for Domestic Animals," Number 1. Recommended Nutrient Allowances for Poultry, A report of the Committee on Animal Nutrition of the National Research Council, Washington, D. C., revised March, 1950.

REFERENCES

1. Branion, H. D. Minerals in poultry nutrition. Sci. Agr. 18:217. 1938.
2. Gillis, M. B., L. C. Norris, and G. F. Heuser. The utilization by the chick of phosphorus from different sources. Jour. Nutr. 35: 195. 1947.
   Gillis, M. B., L. C. Norris, and G. F. Heuser. Studies of the relative value of phytin and inorganic phosphorus in chick nutrition. Poultry Sci. 27:664. 1948.
   Gillis, M. B., L. C. Norris, and G. F. Heuser. The effect of phytin on the phosphorus requirement of the chick. Poultry Sci. 28:283. 1949.
   Gillis, M. B., L. C. Norris, and G. F. Heuser. Biological availability of inorganic phosphates. Poultry Sci. 30:914. 1951.
3. Gillis, M. B. Potassium requirement of the chick. Jour. Nutr. 36: 351. 1948.
   Gillis, M. B. Further studies on the role of potassium in growth and bone formation. Jour. Nutr. 42:45. 1950.
   Sturkie, P. D. Abnormal electrocardiograms of chickens produced by potassium deficiency and effects of certain drugs on the abnormalities. Jour. of Physiol. 162:538. 1950.
4. Almquist, H. J. Magnesium requirement of the chick. Proc. Soc. Exp. Biol. & Med. 49:544. 1942.
   Bird, F. H. Magnesium supplementation in relation to a previously reported cerebellar disorder in chicks. Poultry Sci. 25:396. 1946.
   Bird, F. H. Magnesium deficiency in the chick. I. Clinical and neuropathological findings. Jour. Nutr. 39:13. 1949.
   Van Reen, R., and P. B. Pearson. Magnesium deficiency in the duck. Jour. Nutr. 51:191. 1953.
5. Wilgus, H. S., L. C. Norris, and G. F. Heuser. The role of manganese in poultry nutrition. Rept. Seventh World's Poultry Congress. 171. Cleveland. 1939.
6. Titus, H. W. Perosis, or deforming leg weakness, in the chicken. Poultry Sci. 11:117. 1932.
   Hunter, J. E., H. C. Knandel, and R. A. Dutcher. Factors involved in the experimental production and prevention of hock disease in battery brooded chicks. Proc. Fifth World's Poultry Congress III:184. Rome. 1933.
   Wilgus, H. S., Jr., L. C. Norris, and G. F. Heuser. The role of manganese and certain other trace elements in the prevention of perosis. Jour. Nutr. 14:155. 1937.
7. Lyons, M., and W. M. Insko, Jr. Chondrodystrophy in the chick embryo produced by manganese deficiency in the diet of the hen. Ky. Bul. 371. 1937.
   Gallup, W. D., and L. C. Norris. The effect of a deficiency of manganese in the diet of the hen. Poultry Sci. 17:83. 1939.
   Caskey, C. D., and L. C. Norris. Micromelia in adult fowl caused by manganese deficiency during embryonic development. Proc. Soc. Exp. Biol. and Med. 44:332. 1940.

8. Caskey, C. D., L. C. Norris, and G. F. Heuser. A chronic congenital ataxia in chicks due to manganese deficiency in the maternal diet. Poultry Sci. 23:6. 1944.

9. Kernkamp, H. C. H. Goiter in poultry. Am. Vet. Med. Assn. Jour. 67:223. 1925.

Patton, A. R., H. S. Wilgus, Jr., and G. S. Harshfield. The production of goiter in chickens. Science 89:162. 1939.

Gassner, F. X., and H. S. Wilgus, Jr. Congenital goiter in chicks. Poultry Sci. 19:349. 1940.

Wilgus, H. S. Jr., F. X. Gassner, A. R. Patton, and R. G. Gustavson. The goitrogenicity of soybeans. Jour. Nutr. 22:43. 1941.

Nicholson, L. W., and W. R. Breneman. Goiterogenic diets and their effects on thyroid hyperplasia and vital organs of the chick. Poultry Sci. 24:426. 1945.

Hollander, W. F., and O. Riddle. Goiter in domestic pigeons. Poultry Sci. 25:20. 1946.

10. Elvehjem, C. A., and E. B. Hart. The relation of iron and copper to hemoglobin synthesis in the chick. Jour. Biol. Chem. 84:131. 1929.

Hart, E. B., C. A. Elvehjem, A. R. Kemmerer, and J. G. Halpin. Does the practical chick ration need iron and copper additions to insure normal hemoglobin building? Poultry Sci. 9:92. 1930.

11. Black, D. J. G. A comparison of some methods of supplying calcium to intensively kept chicks. Jour. Agr. Sci. 36:199. 1946.

Gutowska, M. S., and R. T. Parkhurst. Studies in mineral nutrition of laying hens. 2. Excess of calcium in the diet. Poultry Sci. 21: 321. 1942.

Heuser, G. F., and L. C. Norris. Calcite grit and granite grit as supplements to a chick starting ration. Poultry Sci. 25:195. 1946.

Holmes, C. E., C. A. Herrick, and G. L. Ott. Studies in coccidiosis in chickens. Calcium carbonate additions and coccidia. Poultry Sci. 16:335. 1937.

Migicovsky, B. B., and A. R. G. Emslie. Interaction of calcium, phosphorus and vitamin D. I. Influence of calcium and phosphorus on body weight and bone ash of chicks. Arch. Biochem. 13:175. 1947.

Prentice, J. H. The relation of the calcium content of the ration to mortality in the chicken. Jour. Min. Agr. of N. Ire. 6:69. 1938.

Robertson, E. I., M. Brin, and L. C. Norris. The use of dehydrated beet leaves in chick rations. Poultry Sci. 26:582. 1947.

Titus, H. W., T. C. Byerly, N. R. Ellis, and R. B. Nestler. Effect of the calcium and phosphorus content of the diet of chickens on egg production and hatchability. Poultry Sci. 16:118. 1937.

12. Buckner, G. D., J. H. Martin, and Wm. M. Insko Jr. The effect of magnesium carbonate when added to diets of growing chicks. Poultry Sci. 11:58. 1932.

Mussehl, F. E., R. S. Hill, M. J. Blish, and C. W. Ackerson. Utilization of calcium by the growing chick. Jour. Agr. Res. 40:191. 1930.

Schaible, P. J., J. M. Moore, and R. A. Conolly. Factors influencing the incidence of perosis in Barred Rock chicks. Poultry Sci. 12:324. 1933.

13. Alder, B. The use of calcite and other natural deposits of calcium

carbonate in the ration of laying hens. Proc. Third World's Poultry Cong. 231. London, 1927.
Kennard, D. C. A device for testing the breaking strength of shell eggs. U. S. Egg & Poultry Mag. 51:86. 1945.
14. Gerry, R. W., C. W. Carrick, R. E. Roberts, and S. M. Hauge. Phosphate supplements of different fluorine content as sources of phosphorus for chickens. Poultry Sci. 25:401. 1946.
Halpin, J. G., and A. R. Lamb. The effect of ground phosphate rock fed at various levels on the growth of chicks and on egg production. Poultry Sci. 11:5. 1932.
Hauck, Hazel M., H. Steenbock, J. T. Lowe, and J. G. Halpin. Effect of fluorine on growth, calcification, and parathyroids in the chicken. Poultry Sci. 12:242. 1933.
Kick, C. H., R. M. Bethke, B. H. Edgington, O. H. M. Wilder, P. R. Record, W. Wilder, T. J. Hill, and S. W. Chase. Fluorine in animal nutrition. Ohio Agr. Exp. Sta. Bul. 558. 1935.
Kick, C. H., R. M. Bethke, and P. R. Record. Effect of fluorine in the nutrition of the chick. Poultry Sci. 12:382. 1933.
McConnell, E. S., W. M. Insko Jr., and G. D. Buckner. Fused rock phosphate for chicks. Ky. Agr. Exp. Sta. Bul. 455. 1944.
Phillips, P. H., G. Bohstedt, J. M. Fargo, E. B. Hart, and J. G. Halpin. Our changing agriculture. Learn limitations of rock phosphate as a mineral feed. Wisc. Agr. Exp. Sta. Bul. 428:9. 1934.
Phillips, P. H., H. English, and E. B. Hart. The augmentation of the toxicity of fluorosis in the chick by feeding dessicated thyroid. Jour. Nutr. 10:399. 1935.
15. Franke, K. W., A. L. Moxon, W. E. Poley, and W. C. Tully. Monstrosities produced by the injection of selenium salts into hens' eggs. Anat. Record 65:15. 1936.
Franke, K. W., and W. C. Tully. A new toxicant occuring naturally in certain samples of plant foodstuffs. V. Low hatchability due to deformities in chicks. Poultry Sci. 14:273. 1935.
Franke, K. W., and W. C. Tully. A new toxicant occurring naturally in certain samples of plant foodstuffs. VII. Low hatchability due to deformities in chicks produced from eggs obtained from chickens of known history. Poultry Sci. 15:316. 1936.
Kohlmeyer, W., and A. L. Moxon. Selenium toxicity in turkeys. Poultry Sci. 27:670. 1948.
Moxon, A. L. Alkali disease or selenium poisoning. S. Dak. Agr. Exp. Sta. Bul. 311. 1937.
Poley, W. E., and A. L. Moxon. Tolerance levels of seleniferous grains in laying rations. Poultry Sci. 17:72. 1938.
Poley, W. E., A. L. Moxon, and K. W. Franke. Further studies of the effects of selenium poisoning on hatchability. Poultry Sci. 16:219. 1937.
Poley, W. E., W. O. Wilson, A. L. Moxon, and J. B. Taylor. The effect of selenized grains on the rate of growth in chicks. Poultry Sci. 20:171. 1941.
Stenn, F. "Alkali disease"—selenium poisoning. Arch. Path. 22:398. 1936.

Tully, W. C., and K. W. Franke. A new toxicant occurring naturally in certain samples of plant foodstuffs. VI. A study of the effect of affected grains on growing chicks. Poultry Sci. 14:280. 1935.

16. Black. D. J. G. A comparison of some methods of supplying calcium to intensively kept chicks. Jour. Agr. Sci. 36:199. 1946.

Cooney, W. T. Influence of various grits on battery-raised broilers. Oregon Circ. 139. 1941.

Ferber, K. E., and H. Brüggemann. Die Zugabe von Kalksteingrit und Flintgrit zum Futter bei der Yungmast von Hähnchen. Archiv für Geflügelk. 7:363. 1933.

Heuser, G. F., and L. C. Norris. Oyster shells, calcite grit, ground limestone, and granite grit in rations for hens. Poultry Sci. 25: 173. 1946.

Heuser, G. F., and L. C. Norris. Calcite grit and granite grit as supplements to a chick starting ration. Poultry Sci. 25:195. 1946.

Jull, M. A. The value of grit in poultry feeding. Jour. Am. Assn. Inst. & Inv. in Poultry Husb. 2:14. 1915.

Kennard, D. C., and V. D. Chamberlin. New findings in poultry feeding and management. Ohio Agr. Exp. Sta. Farm & Home Res. Bimo. Bul. 248:193. 1947.

Mangold, E. Die Bedeutung von Steinchen und Sand im Hühnermagen. Archiv. für Geflügelk. I:145. 1927.

MacIntyre, T. M., and C. D. T. Cameron. Clam shell, limestone and oyster shell with and without insoluble grit as a source of calcium for the growing chick. Sci. Agric. 31:429. 1951.

MacIntyre, T. M., and M. H. Jenkins, Clam shells, limestone and oyster shells as sources of calcium in the ration of laying hens. Sci. Agric. 32:650. 1952.

Tepper, A. E., R. C. Durgin, and C. A. Bottorff. Fine versus coarse grit as a feed ingredient for poultry. N. Hamp. Agr. Exp. Sta. Circ. 56. 1939.

Wheeler, W. P. Ash and grit for growing chicks. New York (Geneva) Agr. Exp. Sta. Bul. 242. 1903.

17. Carver, D. S., and E. L. Johnson. Unidentified growth factors for the chick in vegetable oils and fatty acid concentrates. Poultry Sci. 32:701. 1953.

Carver, D. S., and E. L. Johnson. Unsaturated fats as sources of unidentified chick growth factors. Poultry Sci. 32:892. 1953.

Reiser, R. Fatty acid changes in egg yolk of hens on a fat-free and a cottonseed oil ration. Jour. Nutr. 40:429. 1950.

Reiser, R. The essential role of fatty acids in rations for growing chicks. Jour. Nutr. 42:319. 1950.

Reiser, R. The metabolism of polyunsaturated fatty acids in growing chicks. Jour. Nutr. 42:325. 1950.

Reiser, R., and J. R. Couch. The essential role of fat in the rations of growing chicks. Poultry Sci. 28:781. 1949.

18. Hegsted, D. M., G. M. Briggs, C. A. Elvehjem, and E. B. Hart. Role of arginine and glycine in chick nutrition. Jour. Biol. Chem. 140: 191. 1941.

Briggs, G. M., Jr., T. D. Luckey, C. A. Elvehjem, and E. B. Hart. The effectiveness of a mixture of arginine, glycine, and cystine in the prevention of the so-called vitamin B_4 deficiency in the chick. Jour. Biol. Chem. 150:11. 1943.

19. Fritz, J. C., J. H. Hooper, J. L. Halpin, and H. P. Moore. Failure of feather pigmentation in Bronze poults due to lysine deficiency. Jour. Nutr. 31:387. 1946.

Funk, E. M., and H. L. Kempster. The use of vegetable protein concentrates for raising turkeys. Mo. Agr. Exp. Sta. Bul. 414. 1940.

German, H. S., B. S. Schweigert, R. M. Sherwood, and L. E. James. Further evidence of the role of lysine in the formation of normal Bronze turkey feathers. Poultry Sci. 28:165. 1949.

Kratzer, F. H., D. E. Williams, and Blanche Marshall. The relation of lysine and protein level in the ration to the development of feather pigment in turkey poults. Poultry Sci. 29:285. 1950.

Slinger, S. J., K. M. Gartley, W. F. Pepper, and D. C. Hill. The influence of animal protein factor supplements and antibiotics on the incidence and severity of white feathers in turkeys. Jour. Nutr. 43:345. 1951.

20. Norris, L. C., and G. F. Heuser. The importance of vitamins in feeding poultry. Cornell Bul. 348. 1936.

Titus, H. W. Nutritional diseases of poultry. "Keeping Livestock Healthy." U.S.D.A. Yearbook 1942:1075.

Recommended nutrient allowances for domestic animals. Number I. Recommended nutrient allowances for poultry. Rept. Com. Animal Nutr., National Research Council, Washington, D. C. 1944. (Revised March 1950.)

Biester, H. E., and L. H. Schwarte. Diseases of Poultry. Chap. 7. The Iowa State College Press, Ames, Iowa. 1952.

21. Beach, J. R. Studies on a nutritional disease of poultry caused by vitamin A deficiency. Calif. Bul. 378: 1924.

Bearse, G. E., C. F. McClary, and H. C. Saxena. Blood-spot incidence and the vitamin A level of the diet. Poultry Sci. 32:888. 1953.

Chapman, M. P. A avitaminosis in chicks. Vet. Med. 33:173. 1938.

Durrell, W. B. Avitaminosis "A" in poultry. Canad. Jour. Comp. Med. & Vet. Sci. 9:163. 1945.

Elvehjem, C. A., and V. F. Neu. Studies on vitamin A avitaminosis in the chick. Jour. Biol. Chem. 97:71. 1932.

Hinshaw, W. R., and W. E. Lloyd. Vitamin A deficiency in turkeys. Hilgardia 8:281. 1934.

Jungherr, E. Nasal histopathology and liver storage in subtotal vitamin A deficiency of chickens. Conn. Bul. 250. 1943.

Seifried, O. Studies on A avitaminosis in chickens. I. Lesions of the respiratory tract and their relation to some infectious diseases. Jour. Exp. Med. 52:519. 1930.

Seifried, O. Studies on A avitaminosis in chickens. II. Lesions of the upper alimentary tract and their relation to some infectious diseases. Jour. Exp. Med. 52:533. 1930.

22. Carrick, C. W. The feeding of corn and its parts to mature cockerels in confinement. Poultry Sci. 4:199. 1925.

Carrick, C. W., and R. H. Carr. The antineuritic properties of corn germs. Poultry Sci. 5:26. 1925.

Shaw, J. H., and P. H. Phillips. Neuropathologic studies of acute and chronic thiamine deficiencies and of inanition. Jour. Nutr. 29:113. 1945.

Swank, R. L. Avian thiamine deficiency. Jour. Exp. Med. 71:683. 1940.

Swank, R. L., and O. A. Bessey. Avian thiamine deficiency. III. Characteristic symptoms and their pathogenesis. Jour. Nutr. 22: 77. 1941.

Vedder, E. B., and E. Clark. A study of polyneuritis gallinarum. Philippine Jour. Sci. 7:423. 1912.

23. Norris, L. C., G. F. Heuser, and H. S. Wilgus, Jr. Study of vitamins in chick rations. Is the chief value of milk for feeding poultry due to the presence of a new vitamin? Ext. Service News 12:78. N. Y. State College of Agriculture. 1929.

Norris, L. C., G. F. Heuser, and H. S. Wilgus, Jr. Is the chief value of milk for feeding poultry due to the presence of a new vitamin? Poultry Sci. 9:133. 1930.

Norris, L. C., G. F. Heuser, H. S. Wilgus, Jr., and A. T. Ringrose. The occurrence in chicks of a paralysis of nutritive origin. Poultry Sci. 10:93. 1931.

Lepkovsky, S., and T. H. Jukes. The response of rats, chicks, and turkey poults to crystalline vitamin G (flavin). Jour. Nutr. 12: 515. 1936.

Phillips, P. H., and R. W. Engel. Neuromalacia associated with low riboflavin diets, a preliminary report. Poultry Sci. 17:463. 1938.

Phillips, P. H., and R. W. Engel. The histopathology of neuromalacia and "curled-toe" paralysis in the chick fed low riboflavin diets. Jour. Nutr. 16:451. 1938.

Bethke, R. M., and P. R. Record. The relation of riboflavin to growth and curled-toe paralysis in chicks. Poultry Sci. 21:147. 1942.

24. Davis, H. J., L. C. Norris, and G. F. Heuser. The role of vitamin G in reproduction in poultry. Poultry Sci. 17:81. 1938.

Lepkovsky, S., L. W. Taylor, T. H. Jukes, and H. J. Almquist. The effect of riboflavin and the filtrate factor on egg production and hatchability. Hilgardia 11:559. 1938.

Schumacher, A. E., and G. F. Heuser. The importance of riboflavin in reproduction in poultry. Poultry Sci. 18:369. 1939.

Engel, W. R., P. H. Phillips, and J. G. Halpin. The effect of a riboflavin deficiency in the hen upon embryonic development. Poultry Sci. 19:135. 1940.

Romanoff, A. L., and J. C. Bauernfeind. Influence of riboflavin deficiency in eggs on embryonic development (Gallus domesticus) Anatomical Rec. 82:11. 1942.

25. Ringrose, A. T., L. C. Norris, and G. F. Heuser. The occurrence of a pellagra-like syndrome in chicks. Poultry Sci. 10:166. 1931.

Phillips, P. H., and R. W. Engel. Some histopathologic observations on chicks deficient in the chick antidermatitis factor or pantothenic acid. Jour. Nutr. 18:227. 1939.

Ram, T. A histopathologic study of chicks deficient in pantothenic acid. Poultry Sci. 28:425. 1949.

26. Bauernfeind, J. C., and L. C. Norris. The antidermatosis vitamin required for reproduction in the domestic fowl. Science 89:416. 1939.

Gillis, M. B., G. F. Heuser, and L. C. Norris. The need for pantothenic acid and an unidentified factor in reproduction in the domestic fowl. Jour. Nutr. 23:153. 1942.

Gillis, M. B., G. F. Heuser, and L. C. Norris. Pantothenic acid in the nutrition of the hen. Jour. Nutr. 35:351. 1948.

27. Carter, C. W., and J. R. O'Brien. Vitamin B complex in relation to the nutrition of the chick and pigeon. Seventh World's Poultry Congress Proceedings, 126. Cleveland, 1939.

Jukes, T. H. Vitamin B_6 deficiency in chicks. Proc. Soc. Exp. Biol. and Med. 42:180. 1939.

Hogan, A. G., L. R. Richardson, H. Patrick, B. L. O'Dell, and H. L. Kempster. Vitamin B_6 and chick nutrition. Poultry Sci. 20:180. 1941.

Lepkovsky, S., and F. H. Kratzer. Pyridoxine deficiency in chicks. Jour. Nutr. 24:515. 1942.

Bird, F. H., F. H. Kratzer, V. S. Asmundson, and S. Lepkovsky. Pyridoxine deficiency in turkeys. Proc. Soc. Exp. Biol. and Med. 52:44. 1943.

Hegsted, D. M., and M. M. Rao. Nutritional studies with the duck. II. Pyridoxine deficiency. Jour. Nutr. 30:367. 1945.

28. Cravens, W. W., E. E. Sebesta, J. G. Halpin, and E. B. Hart. Effect of vitamin B_6 on egg production and hatchability. Poultry Sci. 22: 94. 1943.

Cravens, W. W., E. E. Sebesta, J. G. Halpin, and E. B. Hart. Studies on the pyridoxin requirements of laying and breeding hens. Poultry Sci. 25:80. 1946.

29. Bird, H. R. Vitamin B_{12} in poultry nutrition. Proc. Cornell Nutr. Conf.: 31. 1949.

Briggs, G. M., E. G. Hill, and M. J. Giles. Vitamin B_{12} in all-plant rations for chicks and sparing activity of methionine and choline. Poultry Sci. 29:723. 1950.

Carver, J. S., and J. McGinnis. Effect of vitamin B_{12} and APF supplements on hatchability of chicken eggs. Poultry Sci. 30:752. 1950.

Hsu, J. M., J. R. Stern, and J. McGinnis. The effect of vitamin B_{12} deficiency on erythrocyte count and hemoglobin levels of chick embryo blood. Arch. Biochem. and Biophys. 38:261. 1952.

Lillie, R. J., C. A. Denton, M. W. Olsen, and H. R. Bird. Vitamin B_{12}. Assay methods and role in reproduction of chickens. Abstracts of papers 116th Meeting American Chem. Soc.:37. 1949.

Olcese, O., and J. R. Couch. Effect of injecting vitamin B_{12} into eggs from hens fed a diet low in vitamin B_{12}. Poultry Sci. 29:612. 1950.

Olcese, O., J. R. Couch, J. H. Quisenberry, and P. B. Pearson. Congenital anamolies in the chick due to vitamin B_{12} deficiency. Jour. Nutr. 41:423. 1950.

Ott, W. H., E. L. Rickes, and T. R. Wood. Activity of crystalline vitamin B_{12} for chick growth. Jour. Biol. Chem. 174:1047. 1948.

Peterson, C. F., A. C. Wiese, C. E. Lampman, and R. V. Dahlstrom. Role of crystalline vitamin B_{12} for hatchability. Poultry Sci. 29: 618. 1950.

Yacowitz, H., R. F. Miller, L. C. Norris, and G. F. Heuser. Vitamin B_{12} studies with the hen. Poultry Sci. 31:89. 1952.

30. Briggs, G. M., Jr., R. C. Mills, C. A. Elvehjem, and E. B. Hart. Nicotinic acid in chick nutrition. Proc. Soc. Exp. Biol. and Med. 51:59. 1942.

Briggs, G. M., Jr., T. D. Luckey, L. J. Teply, C. A. Elvehjem, and E. B. Hart. Studies on nicotinic acid deficiency in the chick. Jour. Biol. Chem. 148:517. 1943.

31. Scott, M. L., and G. F. Heuser. Studies in duck nutrition. 4. Bowed legs in ducks caused by niacin deficiency. Poultry Sci. 31:752. 1952.

Heuser, G. F., and M. L. Scott. Studies in duck nutrition. 5. Bowed legs in ducks, a nutritional disorder. Poultry Sci. 32:137. 1953.

32. Hegsted, D. M., J. J. Oleson, R. C. Mills, C. A. Elvehjem, and E. B. Hart. Studies on a dermatitis in chicks distinct from pantothenic acid deficiency. Jour. Nutr. 20:599. 1940.

Eakin, R. E., W. A. McKinley, and R. J. Williams. Egg white injury in chicks and its relation to a deficiency of vitamin H (biotin) Science 92:224, 1940.

Ansbacher, S., and M. Landy. Biotin and scaly dermatosis of the chick. Proc. Soc. Exp. Biol. and Med. 48:3. 1941.

Patrick, H., R. V. Boucher, R. A. Dutcher, and H. C. Knandel. Biotin and prevention of dermatitis in turkey poults. Proc. Soc. Exp. Biol. and Med. 48:456. 1941.

Hegsted, D. M., R. C. Mills, G. M. Briggs, Jr., C. A. Elvehjem, and E. B. Hart. Biotin in chick nutrition. Jour. Nutr. 23:175. 1942.

33. Jukes, T. H., and F. H. Bird. Prevention of perosis by biotin. Proc. Soc. Exp. Biol. & Med. 49:231. 1942.

Richardson, L. R., A. G. Hogan, and O. N. Miller. The relation of biotin to perosis in chicks. Missouri Agr. Coll. Res. Bul. 343.

34. Cravens, W. W., E. E. Sebesta, J. G. Halpin, and E. B. Hart. Effect of biotin on reproduction in the domestic fowl. Proc. Soc. Exp. Biol. and Med. 50:101. 1942.

Couch, J. R., W. W. Cravens, C. A. Elvehjem, and J. G. Halpin. Relation of biotin to congenital deformities in the chick. Anat. Rec. 100:29. 1948.

35. Jukes, T. H. Prevention of perosis by choline. Jour. Biol. Chem. 134:789. 1940.

Jukes, T. H. Effect of choline and other supplements on perosis. Jour. Nutr. 20:445. 1940.

Abbott, O. D., and C. V. DeMasters. Choline in the diet of chickens. Jour. Nutr. 19:47. 1940.

Jukes, T. H. Studies of perosis in turkeys. I. Experiments related to choline. Poultry Sci. 20:251. 1941.

Hegsted, D. M., R. C. Mills, C. A. Elvehjem, and E. B. Hart. Choline in the nutrition of chicks. Jour. Biol. Chem. 138:459. 1941.

Record, P. R., and R. M. Bethke. Further observations on yeast and choline in chick nutrition. Poultry Sci. 21:271. 1942.

Lucas, H. L., L. C. Norris, and G. F. Heuser. Observations on the choline requirements of hens. Poultry Sci. 25:373. 1946.
Bernard, R., and J. M. Demers. Lipotropic activity of choline, betaine, and methionine in ducklings. Canad. Jour. Res. E27:281. 1949.
36. Briggs, G. M., E. G. Hill, and T. H. Canfield. The need for choline, folic acid, and nicotinic acid by goslings fed purified diets. Poultry Sci. 32:678. 1953.
Campbell, C. J., R. A. Brown, and A. D. Emmett. Influence of crystalline vitamin B_c on hematopoiesis in the chick. Jour. Biol. Chem. 152:483. 1944.
Couch, J. R., and H. L. German. Pteroylglutamic acid studies with the mature fowl. Poultry Sci. 29:539. 1950.
Cravens, W. W., and J. G. Halpin. Folic acid needed for good hatchability. Wisc. Bul. 472:56. 1947.
Cravens, W. W., E. E. Sebesta, J. G. Halpin, and E. B. Hart. Effect of lactobacillus casei ϵ eluate fraction on reproduction in the domestic fowl. Proc. Soc. Exp. Biol. & Med. 51:106. 1942.
Daniel, L. J., F. A. Farmer, and L. C. Norris. Folic acid and perosis. Jour. Biol. Chem. 153:349. 1946.
Frost, D. V., F. P. Dann, and F. C. McIntire. Adequacy of the known synthetic vitamins for normal feathering and pigmentation in chicks. Proc. Soc. Exp. Biol. and Med. 61:65. 1946.
Hogan, A. G., and E. M. Parrott. Anemia in chicks caused by a vitamin deficiency. Jour. Biol. Chem. 132:507. 1940.
Lillie, R. J., and G. M. Briggs. Studies on folic acid in the prevention of abnormal feather pigmentation. Poultry Sci. 26:475. 1947.
Lillie, R. J., G. F. Combs, and G. M. Briggs. Folic acid in poultry nutrition. II. Effect of maternal diet and chick diet upon mortality, growth, and feathering of progeny. Poultry Sci. 29:122. 1950.
Luckey, T. D., P. R. Moore, C. A. Elvehjem, and E. B. Hart. The activity of synthetic folic acid in purified rations for the chick. Science 103:682. 1946.
Robertson, E. I., L. J. Daniel, F. A. Farmer, L. C. Norris, and G. F. Heuser. The folic acid requirement of chicks for growth, feathering and hemoglobin formation. Proc. Soc. Exp. Biol. & Med. 62:97. 1946.
Robertson, E. I., L. J. Daniel, F. A. Farmer, L. C. Norris, and G. F. Heuser. Folic acid requirement of growing chicks. Poultry Sci. 25:411. 1946.
Russell, W. C., M. W. Taylor, and J. V. Derby, Jr. The folic acid requirement of turkey poults on a purified diet. Jour. Nutr. 34:621. 1947.
Stokstad, E. L. R., and P. V. D. Manning. Evidence of a new growth factor required by the chick. Jour. Biol. Chem. 125:687. 1938.
Sunde, M. L., W. W. Cravens, C. A. Elvehjem, and J. G. Halpin. The effect of folic acid on embryonic development of the domestic fowl. Poultry Sci. 29:696. 1950.
Taylor, L. W. The effect of folic acid on egg production and hatchability. Poultry Sci. 25:412. 1946.
37. Hegsted, D. M., G. M. Briggs, R. C. Mills, C. A. Elvehjem, and E.

B. Hart. Inositol in chick nutrition. Proc. Soc. Exp. Biol. and Med. 47:376. 1941.

38. Almquist, H. J., E. L. R. Stokstad, E. Mecchi, and P. D. V. Manning. Identification of the rice factor. Jour. Biol. Chem. 134:465. 1940.

39. Almquist, H. J. Influence of bile acids on erosions of the chick gizzard lining. Science 87:538. 1938.

Almquist, H. J., and E. Mecchi. The influence of bile on erosions of the chick gizzard lining. Jour. Biol. Chem. 126:407. 1938.

Almquist, H. J., and E. L. R. Stokstad. A nutritional deficiency causing gizzard erosion in chicks. Nature 137:581. 1936.

Almquist, H. J., and E. L. R. Stokstad. The gizzard factor of the chick. Jour. Nutr. 13:339. 1937.

Bird, H. R., O. L. Kline, C. A. Elvehjem, E. B. Hart, and J. C. Halpin. The distribution and properties of the anti-gizzard-erosion factor required by chicks. Jour. Nutr. 12:571. 1936.

Kline, O. L., H. R. Bird, C. A. Elvehjem, and E. B. Hart. An improved synthetic ration for vitamin B_4 studies. Jour. Nutr. 11: 515. 1936.

Lansing, A. I., D. Miller, and H. W. Titus. The formation of erosions of the gizzard lining in the young chick. Poultry Sci. 18: 475. 1939.

Lansing, A. I., and D. Miller. Dysfunction of the biliary system and hemorrhages in the gizzard of the chicken. Poultry Sci. 19:258. 1940.

Mushett, C. W., and W. H. Ott. Influence of crystalline vitamin B_{12} on gizzard erosions in chicks. Poultry Sci. 28:850. 1949.

40. Hart, E. B., J. G. Halpin, and H. Steenbock. Nutritional requirements of baby chicks. II. Further study of leg weakness in chickens. Jour. Biol. Chem. 52:379. 1922.

Dunn, L. C. Effect of cod-liver oil in various amounts and forms on the growth of young chickens. Jour. Biol. Chem. 61:129. 1924.

McGowan, J. P., and A. R. G. Emslie. Rickets in chickens, with special reference to its nature and pathogenesis. Biochem. Jour. 28:1503. 1934.

41. Decker, A., and J. McGinnis. Black pigmentation in feathers of Buff Orpington chicks caused by vitamin D deficiency. Proc. Soc. Exp. Biol. & Med. 66:224. 1947.

Glazener, E. W., and G. M. Briggs. Further studies in abnormal blackening of feathers of vitamin D deficient chicks. Poultry Sci. 27:462. 1948.

Lillie, R. J., and H. R. Bird. A breed difference in feather pigmentation of vitamin D deficient chicks. Poultry Sci. 28:140. 1949.

42. Hart, E. B., H. Steenbock, S. Lepkovsky, and J. G. Halpin. The nutritional requirements of baby chicks. III. The relation of light to the growth of the chicken. Jour. Biol. Chem. 58:33. 1923.

Hart, E. B., H. Steenbock, S. Lepkovsky, S. W. F. Kletzien, J. G. Halpin, and O. N. Johnson. The nutritional requirement of the chicken. V. The influence of ultraviolet light on the production, hatchability, and fertility of the egg. Jour. Biol. Chem. 65:579. 1925.

Hughes, J. S., L. F. Payne, and W. L. Latshaw. Influence of ultraviolet light on leg weakness in growing chicks and on egg production. Poultry Sci. 4:151. 1924.

Hughes, J. S., C. Nitcher, and H. W. Titus. Relative value of ultraviolet light and irradiated air in preventing rickets in chick. Jour. Biol. Chem. 63:205. 1925.

43. Card, L. E., H. H. Mitchell, and T. S. Hamilton. Chickens need vitamin E to produce normal hatches. Ill. Rept. 1930:101. 1930.

Adamstone, F. B. The effects of vitamin E deficiency on the development of the chick. Jour. Morph. and Phys. 52:47. 1931.

Wolf, A., and A. Pappenheimer. The histopathology of nutritional encephalomalacia of chicks. Jour. Exp. Med. 54:399. 1931.

Pappenheimer, A. M., and M. Goettsch. Nutritional encephalomalacia in chicks. Proc. Fifth World's Poultry Congress III:179. Rome. 1933.

Jungherr, E., and A. M. Pappenheimer. Nutritional myopathy of the gizzard in turkeys. Proc. Soc. Exp. Biol. and Med. 37:520. 1937.

Pappenheimer, A. M., M. Goettsch, and E. Jungherr. Nutritional encephalomalacia in chicks and certain related disorders of domestic birds. Conn. Bul. 229. 1939.

Pappenheimer, A. M. Prevention of nutritional myopathy of ducklings by alpha-tocopherol. Proc. Soc. Exp. Biol. and Med. 45:457. 1940.

Dam, H. Studies on vitamin E deficiency in chicks. Jour. Nutr. 27: 193. 1944.

Dam, H., and H. L. Segal. Dietary gizzard ulcers in chicks. Acta Physiol. Scand. 10:295. 1945.

Adamstone, F. B. Histologic comparison of the brains of vitamin A-deficient and vitamin E-deficient chicks. Arch. Pathol. 43: 301. 1947.

Hepding, L. Vitamin E-Mangel bei Hühnerküken, insbesonder über Therapieversuche mit Vitamin E bei den zerebellaren Störungen. Berliner u. Münchener Tierärztl. Wochensch. No. 8:88. 1947.

44. Dam, H., and F. Schönheyder. A deficiency disease in chicks resembling scurvy. Biochem. Jour. 28:1355. 1934.

Dam, H. The antihemorrhagic vitamin of the chick. Biochem. Jour. 29:1273. 1935.

Almquist, H. J., and E. L. R. Stokstad. Hemmorrhagic disease of dietary origin. Jour. Biol. Chem. 111:105. 1935.

Dam, H. The antihemmorrhagic vitamin of the chick. I. Occurrence and chemical nature. Nature 135:652. 1935.

Cravens, W. W., S. B. Randle, C. A. Elvehjem, and J. G. Halpin. Vitamin K studies. I. Effect of the vitamin K content of the hen's ration on the clotting of the chick blood. Poultry Sci. 20:313. 1941.

Griminger, P., H. Fisher, W. D. Morrison, J. M. Snyder, and H. M. Scott. The influence of different levels of alfalfa meal added to a corn-soybean meal type of ration on blood clotting time. Poultry Sci. 32:902. 1953.

45. Bauernfeind, J. C., A. E. Schumacher, A. Z. Hodson, L. C. Norris, and G. F. Heuser. A new factor required for growth and reproduction in the domestic fowl. Proc. Soc. Exp. Biol. and Med. 39: 108. 1938.

Schumacher, A. E., G. F. Heuser, and L. C. Norris. The complex nature of the alcohol precipitate factor required by the chick. Jour. Biol. Chem. 135:313. 1940.

Hill, F. W., L. C. Norris, and G. F. Heuser. Studies of unidentified vitamins required by the chick. Jour. Nutr. 28:175. 1944.

Scott, M. L., L. C. Norris, and G. F. Heuser. The probable identity of strepogenin with factor S and the importance of this factor in chick nutrition. Jour. Biol. Chem. 167:261. 1947.

46. Hill, F. W. The multiple nature of the deficiency of unidentified nutrients in crude all-vegetable protein chick starter rations. Poultry Sci. 27:536. 1948.

Reed, J. R., Jr., R. L. Atkinson, and J. R. Couch. Dried whey as a source of unidentified factors for the growing chick. Jour. Nutr. 43:501. 1951.

47. Kohler, G. O., and W. R. Graham, Jr. A chick growth factor found in leafy green vegetables. Poultry Sci. 30:484. 1951.

48. Arscott, G. H., and G. F. Combs. Effects on growth of various crude supplements added to corn-soybean meal chick rations adequate in vitamin B_{12}. Poultry Sci. 29:746. 1950.

Atkinson, R. L., J. H. Quisenberry, and J. R. Couch. A factor in liver necessary for hatchability of turkey eggs. Poultry Sci. 32:887. 1953.

Briggs, G. M. A review of recent developments in poultry nutrition; vitamin B_{12}, antibiotics and new growth factors. Trans. Am. Assn. Cereal Chemists 10:31. 1952.

Camp, A. A., and E. L. Stephenson. An unidentified chick growth factor found in corn hydrol. Poultry Sci. 31:910. 1952.

Carlson, C. W., R. F. Miller, H. T. Peeler, L. C. Norris, and G. F. Heuser. The complex nature of the animal protein factor. Poultry Sci. 28:750. 1949.

Combs, G. F. Unidentified factors required for chick growth. Ninth World's Poultry Congress Rept. (2):35. 1951.

Edwards, H. M., R. Dam, L. C. Norris, and G. F. Heuser. Probable identity of unidentified chick growth factors in fish solubles and penicillin mycelium residue. Poultry Sci. 32:551. 1953.

Fisher, H., H. M. Scott, and R. G. Hansen. Further studies on the alfalfa factor and its relation to the liver and whey factors. Jour. Nutr. 52:13. 1954.

Fuller, H. L., C. W. Carrick, and S. M. Hauge. A comparison of B_{12}, fish solubles, and whey in the growth of chicks. Poultry Sci. 31:473. 1952.

Halbrook, E. R., A. F. Beeckler, and E. P. Smith. The value of fish solubles and a vitamin B_{12}-antibiotic supplement in chicken and turkey mash mixtures containing ten per cent meat scraps. Poultry Sci. 32:1058. 1953.

Heuser, G. F., and L. C. Norris. An unknown nutritive factor in feeds of animal origin. Poultry Sci. 30:470. 1951.

Lillie, R. J., J. R. Sizemore, and H. R. Bird. Development of a chick assay for an unknown growth factor. Poultry Sci. 31:923. 1952.

Lillie, R. J., J. R. Sizemore, and H. R. Bird. Unidentified factors

in poultry nutrition. I. Development of chick assay. Poultry Sci. 32:855. 1953.
McGinnis, J., L. R. Berg, J. R. Stern, M. E. Starr, R. A. Wilcox, and J. S. Carver. Additional evidence for an unidentified growth promoting factor for turkeys and chicks. Poultry Sci. 31:100. 1952.
Menge, H., G. F. Combs, P. T. Hsu, and M. S. Shorb. Unidentified growth factors required by chicks and poults. I. Studies with chicks using purified diets. Poultry Sci. 31:237. 1952.
Petersen, C. F., A. C. Wiese, and A. R. Pappenhagen. Chick growth response to an unidentified factor in fish solubles, dried whey, and other supplements. Poultry Sci. 32:921. 1953.
Scott, H. M., H. Fisher, and J. M. Snyder. Alfalfa meal as a source of unidentified growth factors. Poultry Sci. 32:555. 1953.
Savage, J. E., B. L. O'Dell, H. L. Kempster, and A. C. Hogan. The requirement of the chick for an unrecognized growth factor. Poultry Sci. 29:779. 1950.
Sunde, M. L., W. W. Cravens, C. A. Elvehjem, and J. G. Halpin. An unidentified factor required by chicks fed practical rations. Poultry Sci. 29:204. 1950.
Vavich, M. G., A. Wertz, and A. R. Kemmerer. Growth-stimulating factors in alfalfa for chicks. Poultry Sci. 32:433. 1953.
Young, R. J., M. B. Gillis, and L. C. Norris. An unidentified factor in peanut meal required by the chick. Jour. Nutr. 50:291. 1953.
49. Anderson, G. W., J. D. Cunningham, and S. J. Slinger. Effect of protein level and penicillin on growth and intestinal flora of chickens. Jour. Nutr. 47:175. 1952.
Anderson, G. W., S. J. Slinger, and W. F. Pepper. Bacterial cultures in the nutrition of poultry. I. Effect of dietary bacterial cultures on the growth and cecal flora of chicks. Jour. Nutr. 50:35. 1953.
Atkinson, R. L., and J. R. Couch. Vitamin B_{12}, an APF concentrate, aureomycin, streptomycin, Liver "L," and fish meal and fish solubles in the nutrition of the poult. Jour. Nutr. 44:249. 1951.
Atkinson, R. L., and J. R. Couch. Crystalline antibiotics in the nutrition of poults kept on raised screen floors. Poultry Sci. 31: 115. 1952.
Berg, L. R., J. S. Carver, G. E. Bearse, and J. McGinnis. Antibiotics in the nutrition of laying hens. Washington Bul. 534. 1952.
Biely, J., and B. March. The effect of aureomycin and vitamins on the growth rate of chicks. Science 114:330. 1951.
Bird, H. R., R. J. Lillie, L. J. Machlin, and C. A. Denton. Antibiotics in poultry nutrition. Report Ninth World's Poultry Congress. Vol. II:46. Paris, 1951.
Branion, H. D., and D. C. Hill. The comparative effect of antibiotics on the growth of poults. Poultry Sci. 30:793. 1951.
Brown, J. A., A. R. Robblee, and D. R. Clandinin. The use of penicillin in breeding rations. Poultry Sci. 32:576. 1953.
Carlson, C. W., W. Kohlmeyer, D. G. Jones, and A. L. Moxon. Aureomycin and vitamin B_{12} supplements in a turkey breeder diet. Poultry Sci. 30:909. 1951.
Coates, M. E., D. C. Dickinson, G. F. Harrison, S. K. Kon, S. H.

Cummins, and W. F. J. Cuthbertson. Penicillin procaine. Pharmacology (growth). Mode of action of antibiotics in stimulating growth of chicks. Nature 168:332. 1951.

Coates, M. E., C. D. Dickinson, G. F. Harrison, S. K. Kon, and M. E. Mann. Antibiotics and the animal protein factor in chick growth. Report Ninth World's Poultry Congress. Vol. II:101. Paris, 1951.

Davis, R. L., and G. M. Briggs. Studies with antibiotics in chick and poult starting rations. Poultry Sci. 30:767. 1951.

Elam, J. F., L. L. Gee, and J. R. Couch. Effect of feeding penicillin on the life cycle of the chick. Proc. Soc. Exp. Biol. & Med. 77:209. 1951.

Elam, J. F., R. L. Jacobs, and J. R. Couch. The effect of prolonged feeding of antibiotics upon the performance of laying hens. Poultry Sci. 32:792. 1953.

Groschke, A. C., and R. J. Evans. Effect of antibiotics, synthetic vitamins, vitamin B_{12}, and an APF supplement on chick growth. Poultry Sci. 29:616. 1950.

Halick, J. V., and J. R. Couch. Antibiotics in mature fowl nutrition. Proc. Soc. Exp. Biol. & Med. 76:58. 1951.

Heuser, G. F., and.L. C. Norris. Some results of feeding antibiotics to chickens. Poultry Sci. 31:857. 1952.

Heywang, B. W. The effect of antibiotics on the growth of White Leghorn pullets. Poultry Sci. 31:581. 1952.

Machlin, L. J., C. A. Denton, W. L. Kellogg, and H. R. Bird. Effect of dietary antibiotic upon feed efficiency and protein requirement of growing chickens. Poultry Sci. 31:106. 1952.

Matterson, L. D., and E. P. Singsen. A comparison of several antibiotics as growth stimulants in practical chick-starting rations. Conn. Agr. Exp. Sta. Bul. 275. 1951.

McGinnis, J., J. R. Stern, R. A. Wilcox, and J. S. Carver. The effect of different antibiotics on growth of turkey poults. Poultry Sci: 30:492. 1951.

Moore, P. R., H. Evenson, T. D. Luckey, E. McCoy, C. A. Elvehjem and E. B. Hart. Use of sulfasuxidine, streptothricin, and streptomycin in nutritional studies with the chick. Jour. Biol. Chem. 165:437. 1946.

Nordskog, A. W., and E. L. Johnson. Breed differences in response to feeding antibiotics. Poultry Sci. 32:1046. 1953.

Oleson, J. J., B. L. Hutchings, and A. R. Whitehill. The effect of feeding aureomycin on the vitamin B_{12} requirement of the chick. Arch. Biochem. 29:344. 1950.

Patrick, H. Vitamin B_{12} and antibiotics in turkey poult nutrition. Poultry Sci. 30:549. 1951.

Saxena, H. D., L. G. Blaylock, W. J. Stadelman, J. S. Carver, and J. McGinnis. Effect of penicillin on growth, feed efficiency and fattening of turkeys. Poultry Sci. 32:721. 1953.

Sieburth, J. N., J. Gutierrez, J. McGinnis, J. R. Stern, and B. H. Schneider. Effect of antibiotics on intestinal microflora and on growth of turkeys and pigs. Proc. Soc. Exp. Biol. & Med. 76:15. 1951.

Slinger, S. J., K. M. Gartley, W. F. Pepper, and D. C. Hill. The influence of animal protein factor supplements and antibiotics on the incidence and severity of white feathers in turkeys. Jour. Nutr. 43:345. 1951.

Slinger, S. J., A. M. Morphet, E. C. Hunt, and W. F. Pepper. Effect of penicillin on the reproductive performance of turkeys. Poultry Sci. 32:660. 1953.

Slinger, S. J., M. M. Hauser, and W. F. Pepper. The correlation between feed consumption and fecal flora in chicks. Poultry Sci. 32:925. 1953.

Stokstad, E. L. R., and T. H. Jukes. Growth-promoting effect of aureomycin on turkey poults. Poultry Sci. 29:611. 1950.

Stokstad, E. L. R., and T. H. Jukes. Further observations on the "animal protein factor". Proc. Soc. Exp. Biol. & Med. 73:523. 1950.

Stokstad, E. L. R., and T. H. Jukes. Effect of various levels of vitamin B_{12} upon growth response produced by aureomycin in chicks. Proc. Soc. Exp. Biol. & Med. 76:73. 1951.

Stokstad, E. L. R., T. H. Jukes, J. Pierce, A. C. Page, Jr., and A. L. Franklin. The multiple nature of the animal protein factor. Jour. Biol. Chem. 180:647. 1949.

Sunde, M. L., J. G. Halpin, and W. W. Cravens. The effect of vitamin B_{12} supplements and antibiotic feed supplements on egg production and hatchability. Poultry Sci. 31:617. 1952.

Waibel, P. E., M. L. Sunde, and W. W. Cravens. Effect of addition of penicillin to the hen's ration on biotin and folic acid content of eggs. Poultry Sci. 31:261. 1952.

Whitehill, A. R., J. J. Oleson, and B. L. Hutchings. Stimulatory effect of aureomycin on the growth of chicks. Proc. Soc. Exp. Biol. & Med. 74:11. 1950.

50. Bird, H. R., A. C. Groschke, and M. Rubin. Effect of arsonic acid derivatives in stimulating growth of chickens. Jour. Nutr. 37:215. 1949.

Milligan, J. L., J. E. Marr, H. L. Wilcke, R. M. Bethke, and A. W. McKinney. Arsonic acid in commercial broiler rations. Poultry Sci. 32:916. 1953.

Morehouse, N. F. Accelerated growth in chickens and turkeys produced by 3-nitro-4-hydroxyphenylarsonic acid. Poultry Sci. 28:375. 1949.

Wharton, F. D., and J. E. Fritz. Studies on the effect of an arsenical in the diet of the immature and mature chicken. Poultry Sci. 32: 1014. 1953.

51. Ely, C. M. Chick growth stimulation produced by surfactants. Science 114:523. 1951.

Ely, C. M., and S. Schott. Surface acting agents as growth stimulators in chick rations. World's Poultry Sci. Jour. 8:133. 1952.

52. German, H. L., and J. R. Couch. Supplementary values of amino acids in broiler rations. Texas Nutr. Conf. P. 29. Nov., 1950.

Hill, F. W. New information on lysine and methionine requirements of chicks. Proc. Cornell Nutr. Conf. for Feed Manufacturers. P.44. Nov., 1953.

Hill, F. W., and L. C. Norris. Methionine in rations for broilers. Cornell Feed Service 41:6. 1953.

Johnson, J. E. The supplementary value of methionine in poultry feeds. Texas Nutr. Conf. P. 28. Nov. 1950.

Saxena, H. C., and J. McGinnis. Effect of DL-methionine on feed utilization by chicks and turkey poults. Wash. Agr. Exp. Sta. Circ. 197. 1952.

Slinger, S. J., W. F. Pepper, and D. C. Hill. Value of methionine supplementation of chick and poult diets containing a high percentage of wheat. Poultry Sci. 32:573. 1953.

53. Dansky, L. M., and F. W. Hill. The effect of energy level and physical nature of the diet on growth and body composition of chicks. Poultry Sci. 30:910. 1951.

Heuser, G. F., L. C. Norris, H. T. Peeler, and M. L. Scott. Further studies on the apparent effect of digestibility upon growth, weight maintenance, and egg production. Poultry Sci. 24:142. 1945.

Hill, F. W. Energy requirements of chickens. Proc. Cornell Nutr. Conf. for Feed Manufacturers. P. 26. 1952.

Hill, F. W., and L. M. Dansky. The influence of diet on body composition of growing chicks. Proc. Cornell Nutr. Conf. for Feed Manufacturers. P. 27. 1951.

Panda, J. N., and G. F. Combs. Studies on the energy requirement of the chick for rapid growth. Poultry Sci. 29:774. 1950.

Robertson, E. I., R. F. Miller, and G. F. Heuser. The relation of energy to fiber in chick rations. Poultry Sci. 27:736. 1948.

Scott, H. M., L. D. Matterson, and E. P. Singsen. Nutritional factors influencing growth and efficiency of feed utilization. I. The effect of the source of carbohydrate. Poultry Sci. 26:554. 1947.

Scott, M. L., G. F. Heuser, and L. C. Norris. Energy, protein, and unidentified vitamins in poult nutrition. Poultry Sci. 27:773. 1948.

Williams, M. A., and C. R. Grau. Effects of variations in dietary energy on food intake and utilization of lysine-deficient protein. Poultry Sci. 32:928. 1953.

54. Fraps, G. S. Composition and productive energy of poultry feeds and rations. Tex. Agr. Exp. Sta. Bul. 678. 1946.

55. Barott, H. G., L. G. Schoenleber, and L. E. Campbell. The effect of ultraviolet radiation on egg production of hens. Poultry Sci. 30:409. 1951.

CHAPTER 4

MEASURING THE VALUE OF FEEDS

In order to be of use to the animal, the feed which is eaten must be digested, absorbed into the body proper, and then made use of by the body.

DIGESTION

PHYSIOLOGY OF THE DIGESTIVE TRACT OR ALIMENTARY CANAL

The alimentary canal is a long tube passing from the mouth to the vent, with certain enlargements for the storage of food and waste. The digestive tract of the fowl is composed of the following parts (Fig. 15).

MOUTH. The mouth is the first part of the digestive tract. It is the place where the food enters. A distinctive character of the mouth of the bird is the absence of lips and teeth.

ESOPHAGUS OR GULLET AND CROP. Upon leaving the mouth, the feed is forced into the gullet by the tongue. The gullet itself serves only as a passage for the food. However, immediately before entering the body cavity, the esophagus enlarges to form a pouch, called the crop. The crop functions as a storage place for feed. Hard material, like grain, might remain in the crop for 12 hours or more. While in the crop the food becomes softened.

PROVENTRICULUS. The proventriculus is the secretory part of the hen's stomach. It is called the glandular stomach because its thickened walls contain the gastric glands, which secrete the gastric juice. The feed is not kept in the proventriculus for any length of time, but the gastric juice is secreted and mixed with the feed as it passes through it.

GIZZARD. The second part of the hen's stomach is the gizzard. The gizzard is oval, with two openings on its upper side, one connecting with the proventriculus and the other with the small intestine. The gizzard is made up of two thick, red, powerful muscles covered internally with a thick horny epithelium.

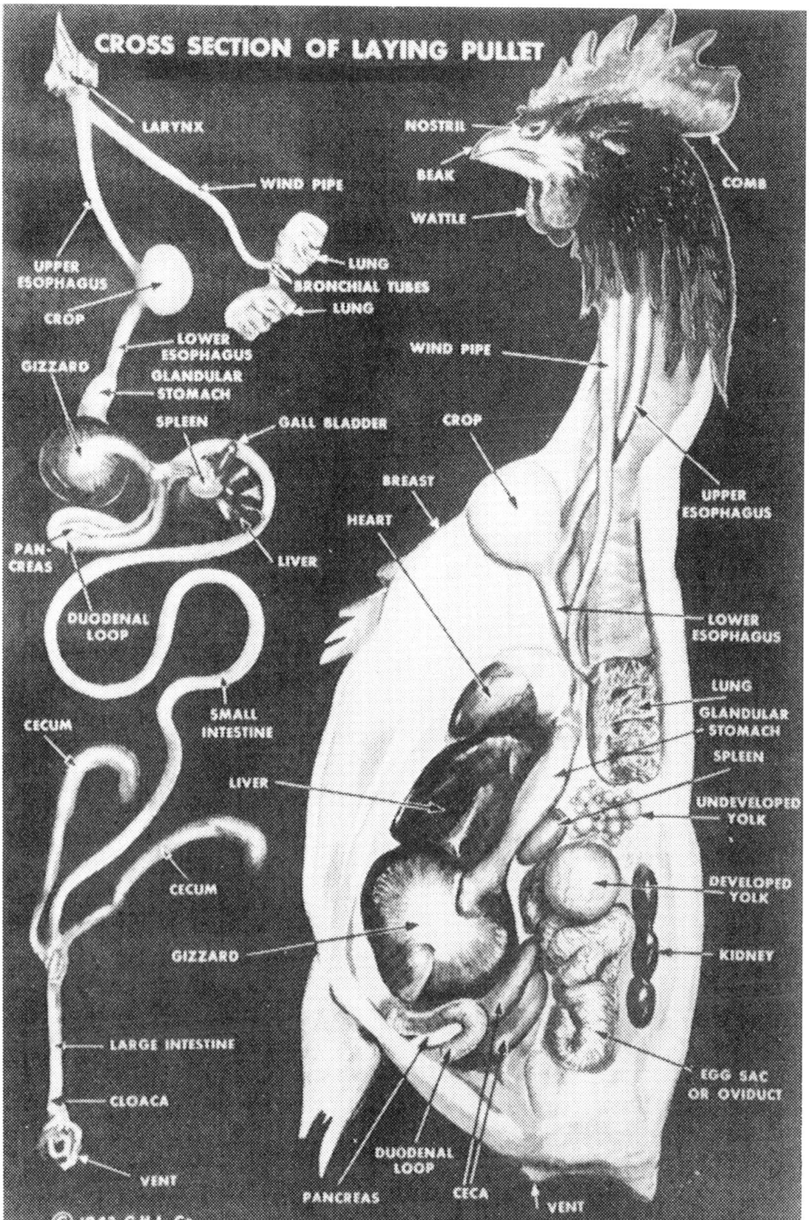

Fig. 15. Cross section of a laying pullet showing the digestive tract.

The function of the gizzard is to grind the food. The grinding action is aided by the presence of grit in the gizzard.

SMALL INTESTINE. From the gizzard, the feed, which has been thoroughly ground and partially digested, passes into the small intestine. The upper portion of the small intestine, which forms a U-shaped loop, is known as the duodenum. Most of the gastric digestion takes place in the duodenum. Further digestion of the feed and absorption of the nutrients take place in the lower intestines.

CECA. At the juncture of the small and large intestines are two blind pouches, called the ceca. They are usually 4 to 6 inches long and are more or less completely filled with fecal matter. It is believed that some bacterial digestion of fiber occurs in the ceca. Some absorption also takes place here.

LARGE INTESTINE OR RECTUM. The large intestine in fowls is relatively short. Its chief function seems to be to absorb moisture from the intestinal content.

CLOACA. The alimentary canal is terminated by the cloaca, a chamber common to the digestive and the genito-urinary systems. The cloaca opens externally at the anus.

ORGANS ASSOCIATED WITH THE ALIMENTARY CANAL. The liver is a bilobed organ, brown in color, which elaborates the bile. The bile functions in the digestion of fat. Bile is stored in the gall bladder and is emptied through the bile ducts into the distal lobe of the duodenum.

The pancreas is a long flesh-colored organ lying in the loop of the duodenum. It secretes the pancreatic juice, which contains ferments that act upon the proteins, carbohydrates, and fats.

THE DIGESTIVE PROCESS

Digestion includes all those physical and chemical processes by means of which the ingested food is broken down and rendered soluble, ready for absorption into the body proper. It includes such physical processes as swallowing, peristalsis, and the grinding action of the gizzard, as well as such chemical processes as the solvent action of water, the action of various ferments or enzymes, and the action of bacteria.

Digestion of feed is usually not complete. The part of the feed that has not been digested is excreted in the feces.

THE DIGESTIVE JUICES

The action of the ferments or enzymes constitute the most important part of digestion. The digestive juices are fluids, excreted from the walls of the digestive tract or associated organs and containing water, enzymes, and other products necessary for rendering the foods soluble.

THE SALIVA. Saliva is not an important digestive juice for the hen because it is secreted in very small quantities. It contains ptyalin, which converts some of the starch to maltose. The saliva also helps to moisten the food.

THE GASTRIC JUICE. The gastric juice is composed of water, hydrochloric acid, and enzymes, such as pepsin and rennin. It is acid in reaction and functions mainly in breaking down proteins.

THE INTESTINAL JUICES. The intestinal juices are composed of water, bile, pancreatic juice, and the intestinal juice. The bile emulsifies and helps digest the fat. The pancreatic juice contains the enzyme trypsin, acting upon proteins, amylopsin, acting upon starch, and steapsin, acting upon fat. The intestinal juice contains erepsin, which breaks down proteins, and invertases, which act upon the sugars.

THE DIGESTION OF FOOD COMPOUNDS

CARBOHYDRATES. The carbohydrates must be converted to single sugars before they can be absorbed by the animal body. The ptyalin of the saliva and the amylopsin of the pancreatic juice act upon starch, changing it to dextrin and then to maltose. The invertases of the intestinal juice act upon the maltose and similar sugars, changing them to the single or glucose-like sugars.

Fiber is digested only to a small extent in poultry. The breakdown of fiber is thought to be accomplished by means of bacterial fermentation, which takes place chiefly in the ceca.

PROTEINS. Proteins must be converted to amino acids before they can be absorbed by the animal body. In this process a number of cleavage products are produced. Primary protein derivatives, which are insoluble, are mostly metaproteins and coagulated proteins. The secondary protein derivatives are soluble and are composed chiefly of proteoses, peptones, and peptides.

The enzymes of the gastric juice act upon the proteins, changing them to metaproteins, proteoses, peptones, and peptides.

The trypsin of the pancreatic juice acts in the same way as the gastric juice, except that peptones and peptides are further partially hydrolyzed to amino acids. The digestion of the protein is completed by the erepsin of the intestinal juice, which converts the proteoses, peptones, and peptides to amino acids.

FATS. The fats must be converted to fatty acids and glycerol in order to be absorbed by the body. The bile, which contains alkaline salt, saponifies, emulsifies, and dissolves the fats and fatty acids. The steapsin of the pancreatic juice can then convert the fat to fatty acids and glycerol.

SUMMARY OF THE DIGESTION OF ORGANIC NUTRIENTS. The digestion of feed as it passes through the digestive tract is summarized in Table 7.

TABLE 7. DIGESTION OF THE ORGANIC NUTRIENTS

Region	Secretion	Enzyme	Substance Affected	Products Formed
Mouth	Saliva	Ptyalin	Starch	Maltose*
Proventriculus	Gastric juice and HCl	Pepsin	Protein	Intermediate* N products
Small intestine	Pancreatic juice	Amylopsin	Starch	Maltose*
		Steapsin	Fat	Fatty acids and glycerol†
		Trypsin	Protein and intermediate N products	Amino acids†
	Intestinal juice	Erepsin	Intermediate N products	Amino acids†
		Invertases	Sugars*	Single sugars†

* Intermediate products.
† Final or absorption products.

COMPARISON OF DIGESTION IN DIFFERENT ANIMALS

DIFFERENCES IN STRUCTURE. The viscera in poultry are less complex than in mammals. This is especially true of the genito-urinary organs. In poultry, the urine is not stored in a bladder, but is poured into the cloaca, where it comes in contact with the feces. The urine is excreted in the form of uric acid, which appears as whitish crystals. In mammals, the urine is excreted as soluble urea.

An outstanding feature of the fowl is the relative shortness of the large intestine. The ratio of the large to the small intestines is about 1 to 30. For the farger farm animals this ratio is about 1 to 3 or 4.

The general structure of the digestive tract of the fowl suggests rapid digestion. The shortness of the tract is a carnivorous characteristic, whereas the nature of the diet and the thorough grinding of feed in the gizzard are herbivorous characteristics.

The stomach of the hen is composed of two parts as compared with a single stomach for the horse and the pig, and a stomach with four divisions for the ruminant.

Fowls secrete very little saliva and the concentration of ptyalin is very low. In ruminants, the amount of saliva secreted is large and the concentration of ptyalin is not great. In swine, saliva secretion is fairly large and the concentration of ptyalin is also appreciable.

DIFFERENCES IN DIGESTION OF NUTRIENTS. The digestibility of the different nutrients varies with the different farm animals.[1] This is illustrated in Table 8.

TABLE 8. ORDER OF EFFICIENCY OF DIGESTION OF THE NUTRIENTS BY VARIOUS ANIMALS

	Protein	Ether Extract	Nitrogen-Free Extract	Crude Fiber
Ruminant	5	4	4	1
Horses	3	5	3	2
Rabbits	4	3	2	4
Swine	1	2	1	3
Hens	2	1	5	5

The nutrient which is digested to the greatest extent by poultry is the nitrogen-free extract. Next in order of digestibility are fat, protein, and fiber.

Fiber is digested to a considerable extent by the other farm animals. In ruminants, this takes place in the rumen, in the horse and swine, in the large intestine. Poultry digests fiber only to a very limited extent, and digestion is thought to occur in the ceca. The amount of fiber digested varies with different feeds. Many show no digestion of fiber at all, and in any feed it rarely goes over 15 per cent. A larger percentage of the fiber of thin-husked varieties of oats is digested than of oats with thick hulls.

The digestion of fats also varies with different feeds. The fat of corn seems to be much more digestible than the fat of oats or barley or wheat.

Organic matter low in fiber is digested to nearly the same extent in all animals.[1] However, with an increase in crude fiber the digestion coefficient of the organic matter decreases rectiliniarly for all animals. The unit decrease, however, is greatest for hens and swine and least for ruminants, so that with a feed containing 35 per cent of fiber, ruminants would digest about 60 per cent of the organic matter, whereas hens would digest 20-25 per cent. With feeds containing very little fiber the different species of animals would all digest approximately 90 per cent of the organic matter. For the best digestibility of organic matter, the feed for hens should not exceed 5 per cent of fiber.

The digestibility of feed does not seem to be affected to any extent by grinding. Cooking increases the digestibility of some of the nutrients, particularly starch. The digestibility of proteins decreases with feeds of low protein content.

TIME REQUIRED FOR FOOD TO PASS THROUGH THE INTESTINAL TRACT. The time required for food to pass through the intestinal tract depends upon the type of feed and the condition of the bird. The North Carolina and California experiment stations[2] report that it took approximately 4 hours for feed to pass through the intestinal tract of laying hens and growing fowl. For nonlaying hens, this time was extended to 8 hours,and, for broody hens, to approximately 12 hours.

The first appearance of any soft foods in the feces has been reported to be 2 to 3 hours after ingestion; for the appearance of grains, this time is extended to 2½ to 3½ hours.

As already indicated, feed is stored in the crop of the bird. The time required for the feed to leave the crop will depend upon the type and condition of the feed. The disappearance of grains from the crops of hens is similar for the various types of grain, except that oats are retained in the crop longer than corn and wheat. Whole corn remains in the crop longer than cracked corn, which in turn is retained longer than corn meal. Boiled oats are not retained in the crop as long as dry oats. Wet mash passes from the crop more rapidly than a dry mixed mash. Experiments at Cornell[3] indicated that approximately the following percentages of a given grain intake were present in the crop:

	Per Cent
After 4 hours	70-80
After 8 hours	55-65
After 12 hours	35-45
After 16 hours	25-35
After 20 hours	10-20
After 24 hours	0-10

Results from Germany[4] indicated that it took 50 to 70 hours entirely to clear the digestive tract of corn, 102 hours for wheat, and 120 hours for barley and oats.

ASSIMILATION

Absorption of the food material takes place largely in the small intestine. Some absorption occurs in the large intestine and in the ceca. In order to be absorbed, the feed must be in a liquid form.

The food nutrients are absorbed through the epithelium of the digestive tract by a process similar to osmosis. The glucose-like sugars, the amino acids, and the mineral matter enter directly into the blood system. The fatty acids and glycerol enter the lymphatic system, which later combines with the blood system.

METABOLISM

Metabolism consists of all those chemical changes which food nutrients undergo from the time they are absorbed into the body proper until they appear as excretory products. Metabolism includes the distribution of the absorbed food, the building of body tissues, the breaking down of body tissues, and the absorption or release of energy. The building of body tissues is a synthetic process called anabolism. The breaking down of body tissues is an oxidative process called catabolism.

DISTRIBUTION OF FOOD NUTRIENTS. The end products of fat digestion, namely, soaps, organic acids, and glycerol, are taken into the epithelial cells, which reconvert them into fat. The fat then passes through the lacteals into the lymphatic vessels, then into the veins and arteries to the capillaries, the lymph spaces, and then to the body cells.

The glucose-like sugars, after passing through the epithelium, are taken up by the capillaries, transported to the veins, and to the liver, where they might be converted into glycogen. The glycogen is reconverted to glucose, which is carried by the veins to the arteries, then to the capillaries, the lymph spaces, and to the cells, where it is utilized or where it might be converted and stored as glycogen.

The amino acids and mineral matter are taken up by the capillaries, transported to the veins, then to the liver, then through the veins and arteries to the capillaries, the lymph spaces, and to the cells, where they are used.

ANABOLISM. The building up processes, involving glucose, consist of its conversion to glycogen or to fats or, with the addition of ammonia, to amino acids. The amino acids are converted to proteins, or, if deaminized, to glucose or fats. The fatty acids and glycerol are converted either to fat or to glucose.

CATABOLISM. The breaking-down process of glycogen involves its conversion to glucose and then to carbon dioxide and water, with the release of energy. Fat is broken down to fatty acids and glycerol, which in turn are converted to glucose and then to carbon dioxide and water, with the release of energy. Proteins are broken down into amino acids, and these into ammonia and glucose. The ammonia is converted into uric acid, which is then excreted. The glucose is broken down to carbon dioxide and water, with the release of energy.

EXCRETION OF BODY WASTES. Carbon dioxide and water, in the form of vapor, are excreted from the lungs. Water, ammonia, and, in come cases, minerals are lost through the urine. The remainder of the body wastes is excreted in the feces. This remainder comprises the minerals and some nitrogenous matter.

SOME CONDITIONS AFFECTING METABOLISM. Growth constitutes a storage chiefly of protein tissue and mineral tissue in the body. In fattening, fatty tissue is stored as energy. A hen in production builds up eggs from the simple products derived from the feed. Sometimes stored tissue is used for this purpose. In that case, the bird loses weight. The bird, if starving, will first use the available glycogen for energy, then the body fat, and finally, if necessary, the protein tissues.

THE NITROGENOUS METABOLISM OF BIRDS COMPARED WITH MAMMALS. In mammals, the urine is excreted and can be collected separately. In birds, the uric acid is excreted with the feces.

Uric acid, a highly insoluble compound, is the end product of nitrogenous metabolism in birds. It is believed that the synthesis of the uric acid takes place in the liver. The uric acid has a relatively small amount of water, which evaporates quickly.

In mammals, the urea is a highly soluble compound. The mammalian urine contains a large amount of water and is rich in such salts as chlorides, sulphates, and phosphates of lime and magnesium. The uric acid of birds contains little or none of the minerals, which in their case are excreted into the intestines.

MEASURES OF USEFULNESS OF FEEDS

There are a number of measures or ways in which the value of feeds can be judged. The greater the number of these measures that can be applied, the more nearly can we arrive at the true value of a feed.

TOTAL CHEMICAL COMPOSITION. This measure of feed is valuable in that it tells the total amount of crude nutrients which the feed contains. The chief limitation, however, is that nothing is known about the digestibility or availability of the feed to the animal.

DIGESTIBILITY OF FEEDING STUFFS. This measure tells the amount of the feed which is digested and thus available to the animal. It is secured by means of the digestion trial. There are some limitations to the digestion trials, particularly for birds. Since the urine and feces in birds are excreted together, it is difficult to separate the undigested nitrogen of the feed from the nitrogen waste of the body. There is also likely to be some inaccuracy in digestion coefficients which must be obtained by indirect digestion trials. These indirect digestion trials are made for feeding stuffs that cannot be fed alone but must be mixed with other ingredients. Therefore, the digestibility is not obtained directly but indirectly by difference.

NITROGEN BALANCE. The object of the nitrogen balance is to get an approximate measure of the quality or efficiency of the protein. Young growing birds are used because of their greater requirement for protein. In this measure the nitrogen of the feed intake and the nitrogen of the feces must be determined, from which information the nitrogen retained or stored can be calculated. The relative efficiency of the various proteins is usually expressed in relation to the value of an arbitrary standard, casein, which is indicated as 100. On this basis, with meat scrap having a relative protein efficiency of 82, it would mean that, when feeding the same quantity of casein and meat scrap, the meat scrap would result in only 82 per cent of the gains produced by the casein.

VITAMIN DETERMINATIONS. Before vitamins were indentified and could be determined chemically, frequently determinations of vitamins, which are related to growth, were made in a way similar to the nitrogen balance trials. In this procedure the gains made by the growing chicks determined the relative vitamin content. The values of the various feeds were then related to some arbitrary standard. For example, in riboflavin determinations of poultry feeds, when dried liver was given a value of 100. dried skimmilk rated 20 and alfalfa meal 10. This meant that dried skimmilk contained 1/5 the amount of riboflavin which the dried liver had, and alfalfa meal contained 1/10 that of dried liver or 1/2 the amount found in dried skimmilk.

CARBON BALANCE. This measure requires the use of a respiration apparatus. In it are measured the nitrogen and carbon intake of the feed and the nitrogen and carbon outgo, as represented in the feces, urine, carbon dioxide, methane, and the like. From the difference, which represents the gains by the animal, the amount of protein and fat stored in the body can be calculated.

ENERGY BALANCE. In getting the energy balance of a feed a respiration calorimeter must be used. The intake of calories in the feed is compared with the outgo of calories as represented in the feces, urine, methane, and other waste products. The difference represents the calories stored by the animal.

MINERAL BALANCE. A comparison can be made of the amount of any of the mineral elements ingested, as compared with the amount of the minerals excreted. If the intake is greater than the outgo, some of the mineral is being stored in the body and the animal is said to be in a positive mineral balance. If the reverse is true, the animal is said to be in a negative mineral balance.

FAT BALANCE. Similarly, a feed or combination of feeds may keep the bird in a positive or negative fat balance. In this case the carbohydrates of the feed must also be taken into consideration.

DETERMINING REQUIREMENTS FOR FOOD

The object of determining the requirements for food is to establish standards by which we can feed our animals for specific purposes. Determining the requirements for food, or for the various nutrients, must be done by means of biological analyses, that is, by actual feeding trials. A number of different methods have been used for doing this.

OBSERVATION AND EXPERIENCE. This might be called a trial and error method. Frequently it is an extremely costly method because there are likely to be many mistakes and failures and often misinterpretation. By observation, it is possible to know whether or not we are getting maintenance of the individual, production, or reproduction which are satisfactory. This method frequently causes waste of food by providing rations in which the food nutrients are present in wrong proportions. It does not get at fundamentals. In the long run results may frequently be fairly satisfactory. A conspicuous example of this is the knowledge which we have secured in the feeding of horses.

COMPARATIVE FEEDING TRIALS. Most of the early feeding experiments were of this nature. For example, in comparing the feeding value of corn, wheat, and oats for hens, we might have fed these grains ad libitum and noted the results in gain or loss and production. Or the value of proteins might have been compared by supplying proteins in different forms, such as meat scrap, fish meal, and dried milk. Many of the comparative feeding trials were not very accurate because there were too many variables and because the nutrients must be fed below the minimum amount necessary in order to get a measure of comparative values.

REFINED FEEDING EXPERIMENTS. These represent more nearly controlled feeding trials. In order to get an accurate measure, either purified diets or diets of known values are used. In qualitative feeding experiments, additions of known nutrients, singly and in various combinations, are then made to the basal ration. In this way the nutrient deficiencies of a feed or ration can be determined. In quantitative experiments, the ration must be complete in every known respect, except the nutrient under test. The nutrient then must be fed in amounts both below and above the requirement in order to measure the exact amount that is essential.

SOME ESSENTIAL PROVISIONS FOR CONDUCTING AND INTERPRETING EXPERIMENTS IN POULTRY NUTRITION

In planning experiments in poultry nutrition, the aim should be to establish fundamental principles. In conducting experiments to do this, some essential provisions must be met. These same provisions can be kept in mind as a guide in passing judgment on the value of experimental work.

PROPER EXPERIMENTAL SETUP. An experiment should eliminate all variables, except the one under study. All other known requirements should be adequately met. The stock used should be obtained from the same breed, strain, and source. Parent stock should be fed and managed uniformly. The birds in an experiment should be distributed evenly in respect to such factors as size, age, sexual maturity, inheritance, previous egg production, condition, and health. Chicks hatched in different incubators should also be distributed evenly.

The basal ration should consist of as few ingredients as possible. Only ingredients of known feeding value should be used. Whenever possible, enough of the basal ration should be prepared in advance to last for the entire experiment, except where there is the possibility of nutrient deterioration. The basal ration, when properly supplemented with the variable factors, should produce normal growth, production, or reproduction. A routine chemical analysis should be made of all basal rations and supplements. Analyses should be made also of any other nutritive factors, whenever these are involved in the experiment. In order to obtain proportionate consumption of every ingredient of the ration, it should be given in the form of a single finely ground mixture, except where the mechanical condition of the feed is the factor under study. It is desirable to give fresh feed in such quantities that the birds will consume nearly all of it before the next feeding. The time of feeding should be as regular as possible.

In conducting an investigation which involves several successive experiments it is essential that all conditions in each experiment be similar. This applies particularly to such environmental conditions as length of day, housing, temperature, and the like. The experimental period must be of sufficient length to make it possible to draw accurate conclusions from the results obtained. Experiments should be conducted as long as there is any possibility of obtaining significant differences.

PROPER RECORDS. It is always wise to weigh the feed weekly to obtain records of feed consumption, and it is necessary where conclusions are to be based upon food intake. The cause of all mortality should be determined. Trapnesting is desirable for all egg production studies.

All birds should be identified in some manner and weighed individually at frequent intervals. Individual or replicate records are necessary in order to apply biometrical methods of analysis to the growth results.

All pertinent physiological, histological, and physical studies and chemical analyses should be applied to the experiment.

INTERPRETATION OF DATA. Unless sexed chicks are used, all growth results with chicks should be weighted for sex influence. Sampling of birds for analyses should be representative in age, size, sex, and experimental conditions.

Biometrical methods of analysis should be applied to all results, whenever possible, to determine if differences obtained are significant. Final conclusions should be based on as many methods of measurement as can be applied, in order to avoid wrong interpretation of results and to make them conclusive.

REFERENCES

1. Axelsson, J. New developments in livestock feeding. Rapport 7. Congrès International des Industries Agricoles, Paris, 1948.
2. Kaupp, B. F., and J. E. Ivey. Digestive coefficients of poultry feeds and rapidity of digestion and fate of grit in the fowl. N. C. Tech. Bul. 22. 1923.

   Hillerman, J. P., F. H. Kratzer, and W. O. Wilson. Food passage through chickens and turkeys and some regulating factors. Poultry Sci. 32:332. 1953.
3. Heuser, G. F. The rate of passage of feed from the crop of the hen. Poultry Sci. 24:20. 1945.
4. Habeck, R. Die Durchgangszeiten verschiedener Futtermittel durch den Verdauungskanal bei Hühnern und Tauben. Wissenschaftliches Archiv für Landwirtshaft. Tierernährung und Tierzucht. 626. 1930.

CHAPTER 5

POULTRY FEEDS—CEREALS, SEEDS, AND OTHER MASH INGREDIENTS

The grain and mash mixtures constitute the bulk of the feed consumed by poultry. The mixtures must possess certain desirable characteristics, which in turn are influenced by the nature of the ingredients used. In order to encourage sufficient food consumption, the feeds must be palatable. It does not hold, however, that because a single feed is not entirely palatable, it must be avoided altogether. It may possess other qualities which render it especially valuable, in which case small amounts could be used, particularly when mixed with ingredients that are extremely palatable. It is the nature of the feed as a whole that is important.

The feed must be of a proper mechanical condition as regards size and hardness of particle, bulk, and consistency when mixed with water. The grains should not be too large or too hard. The ground feeds should not be too bulky or too concentrated. They should not be sticky when mixed with water, nor should they be too crumbly. The mash should be ground evenly and be uniform as to color, in order not to encourage picking over and possible wastage by the birds.

USE OF GROUND FEEDS IN POULTRY RATIONS

Sometimes the question is raised as to why a mash is used. Ground feeds are valuable for various reasons. One of the arguments advanced is that this feed saves the gizzard the work of grinding and in that way makes available a larger amount of the feed for useful purposes; or, stated in another way, saves some of the energy required in grinding. That is probably true when we consider the feeding of an entire whole-grain ration, as compared with an entire mash ration. If part of the feed is given as ground feed, as compared to the whole form, the hens will eat a larger amount of feed. This is important when we keep in mind that our results in growth and production depend upon feed consumption. Another reason is that it enables us to make use of by-products that have excellent feeding value and that are comparatively cheap in cost. It provides a convenient way to feed animal protein by using meat, milk, or fish products as mash ingredients. Sometimes it is stated that the feeding of all mash makes it easy to balance the ration. This statement is true if we consider the effect on the nutritive ratio when we use different proportions of grain and mash.

USE OF GRAINS IN POULTRY RATIONS

In the United States corn is the leading grain fed to poultry. This is true of all parts of the country except in the Western States where wheat is more important. Oats are almost as popular as wheat and are most important in the North Central States. Barley is important only in the Western States. Sorghum grains are important only in about a half dozen states where they are grown.

In making up rations for poultry, it is advisable to use largely the grains that are low in fiber, such as corn and wheat. It has been shown by the South Dakota Station[1] that fiber grains alone, such as barley, oats, buckwheat, and emmer, gave poor production and unsatisfactory results, whereas corn and wheat added to the ration gave decidedly better results. Small variations in the rapidity of growth, production, and hatchability were noted when feeding low- and high-test weight corn, wheat, and barley. The amounts of the fiber grains used will depend somewhat upon the fiber content of the ration. In the scratch grain, palatability must also be considered. Probably not more than 1/3 of the scratch grain should consist of high-fiber grains.

The various grains differ in their value for poultry feeding. If used singly in large amounts, the results will be influenced by the nature of the grain. Experiments at the Iowa Agricultural Experimental Station[2] showed that rations consisting largely of ground oats are more satisfactory for chicks than rations containing large amounts of barley, wheat, or corn. The Indiana Station[3] reported little difference in rate of growth and feed efficiency of chicks which received rations containing about 40 per cent of corn, wheat, or half corn and oats.

Harshaw[4] has shown that the different cereals have varying effects upon the composition of the birds, as represented by the total edible portion and fat content of the edible portions. Corn showed a tendency to deposit more fat than oats, wheat, or barley. He suggests that a mixture of two or more cereals is desirable in feeding poultry for market.

The various grains differ also in their relative value. Experiments with laying hens, reported from Germany,[5] group the four cereals in the following order with regard to their general utility —wheat, oats, rye, barley.

From a review of published data, Crampton[6] indicates that the cereals may be rated in the following order. For growth: oat groats, barley, maize, wheat, rye; for laying and breeding: maize, barley, wheat, oats, rye; for fattening: maize, barley, wheat, oats. When the ration is scientifically balanced, the differences between barley, maize, and wheat are very small and likely to be masked in many cases by differences in the quality of different samples of grains.

Comparing digestible nutrients present in feed grains, Biely[7] gives the following ratings: corn, 100%; wheat, 95.5%; rye, 94.0%; barley, 87.5%; and oats, 84.3%.

It is possible to use a large proportion of a single grain. The Wyoming Station[8] reported that pullets laid equally well and maintained normal health on mash and grain rations containing 65 to 70 per cent of a single cereal grain. The Indiana Station[9] concluded that either wheat or corn was satisfactory with a mash made up of ground wheat, ground oats, meat scrap, and alfalfa leaf meal. The Wisconsin Station[10] obtained severe feather picking when yellow corn was fed as the only grain. Satisfactory growth may be obtained with rations consisting of either corn or wheat.[11]

The results have usually been improved where a variety of grains have been fed. Corn, wheat, and oats, as grains, have been reported better than corn alone by the Ohio[12] and Kentucky[13] stations. The Missouri Station[14] obtained an increase in egg production when the percentage of wheat products was increased up to the point where the ratio between corn and wheat was equal. Experiments at Cornell[15] demonstrated that a laying ration, made up largely of a combination of wheat and corn, gave better results than rations composed largely of either grain alone. Better results were secured at the Oklahoma Station[16] where three grains were fed in the scratch mixture than where it was restricted to one.

COMMONLY USED POULTRY FEEDS *

A large variety of feeds are used in poultry rations. The ones used most commonly are discussed herewith.

* Definitions used here, and inclosed in quotation marks, are those given in the Official Publication of the Association of American Feed Control Officials, Incorporated, 1954.

ALFALFA PRODUCTS. "Alfalfa Meal is the product obtained by grinding alfalfa hay which is reasonably free of other crop plants, weeds, and mold. It must contain not more than 33 per cent of crude fibre."

"Alfalfa Leaf Meal is the ground product consisting chiefly of alfalfa leaves. It must be reasonably free of other crop plants and weeds and shall contain not less than 20 per cent crude protein and not more than 18 per cent of crude fibre."

The word "dehydrated" may precede the definition of alfalfa products, provided the product has been artificially dried.

Where alfalfa products are used in the mash, it is desirable to use the leaf meal or a screened product in order to reduce on the fiber. It will be noticed that the leaf meal, at its best, is high in this respect. Alfalfa meal[17] has been used widely in poultry rations and has shown benefits because it contains valuable nutrients. It is included primarily for its vitamin A and vitamin K values. It may also contribute appreciable amounts of the water-soluble vitamins. It is not palatable and consequently large amounts should not be used. The requirements for the nutrients can be met with amounts not over 5 per cent. There is no particular advantage in feeding larger amounts. On the other hand, the feeding of alfalfa meal has certain limitations. There may be some disadvantages such as the effect on the color of egg yolks and the increase in fiber and bulk which might affect growth and production.

Some experiments have reported a depression[18] in the growth of chicks due to a factor in alfalfa meal. Most of the reports indicate no depressed growth until more than 5 per cent is fed and usually much higher levels are necessary. On the other hand, higher levels frequently have not shown depression. The factor is believed to be a saponin which has hemolytic (i.e., red-blood-cell-dissolving) properties. This action is counteracted by cholesterol and other sterols.

Alfalfa meal is usually limited to 5 per cent in chick rations. With good dehydrated alfalfa the nutritive requirements for vitamins A and K can be met by including much less than 5 per cent in the ration. Mature chickens can tolerate much higher levels, in some cases as much as 10 per cent being fed. Turkeys apparently can efficiently utilize greater amounts than chickens.[19] Unfavorable results, whether caused by any specific harmful fraction, by increasing fiber and decreasing energy, or by the action of some other factors such as palatability, have been reported only with the higher levels of alfalfa, in many instances considerably above the commonly recommended maximum levels.

BARLEY AND ITS PRODUCTS. Barley is used in poultry grain mixtures. It is not quite so palatable as wheat nor does it contain quite the desirable characteristics that wheat does. Except for its higher fiber, it compares very favorably with wheat in its composition.

"Rolled or Crimped Barley is heavy barley that has been rolled to desired thickness after tempering so as not to crumble. It shall contain not less than 90 per cent pure barley and not more than 10 per cent weed seeds or other foreign materials and not more than 6 per cent crude fiber."

"Ground Barley is the entire product obtained by grinding clean sound barley, containing not less than 90 per cent of pure barley and not more than 10 per cent of other grains, weed seeds, and other foreign material and not more than 6 per cent of crude fibre; provided that no portion of this stated 10 per cent of other grains, weed seeds, or foreign material shall be intentionally added."

Barley and ground barley are used quite extensively in regions where barley is grown. Ordinarily, ground oats and ground barley are used more or less interchangeably. Their compositions are comparable, except that barley contains much less fiber than ground oats. Ground barley should be fine ground when included in the mash.

Good results have been reported for barley[20] as a principal ingredient in poultry rations. Because of its low vitamin A value, when barley is used in place of corn, the ration must make special provision for this deficiency, usually by a liberal supply of alfalfa leaf meal or green food.

"Barley Feed is the entire by-product resulting from the manufacture of pearl barley from clean barley." Since the pearl barley is made up of most of the kernel, the feed consists of the outer portions of the grain. It contains too much fiber to be of value as a poultry feed.

"Barley Mixed Feed is the entire offal from the milling of barley flour from clean barley and is composed of barley hulls and barley middlings." It is also too bulky for poultry rations.

"Barley Hulls is the product consisting of the outer coverings of the barley." They are of little value for poultry.

BREWERS' PRODUCTS. "Malt Sprouts is the product obtained by the removal of the sprouts from malted barley together with the malt hulls, other parts of malt, and foreign material unavoidably present. It shall contain not less than 24 per cent of protein. The term 'Malt Sprouts' when applied to a corresponding portion of other malted cereals shall be used in qualified form, as for example: 'Rye Malt Sprouts,' 'Wheat Malt Sprouts,' etc.'' They are a light, bulky feed, only moderately palatable, and would lighten the mash much the same as wheat bran.

''Brewers' Dried Grains is the dried extracted residue of barley malt alone or in mixture with other cereal grain or grain products resulting from the manufacture of wort.'' They are composed largely of barley. They are high in protein and fat but are rather shucky and contain considerable fiber.

DISTILLERS' PRODUCTS. ''Corn Distillers' Dried Grains are obtained in manufacturing distilled liquors and alcohol from corn, or from a grain mixture in which corn predominates, by drying that portion of the whole stillage retained by screens.''

''Rye Distillers' Dried Grains is the product obtain in the manufacture of distilled liquors and alcohol from rye, or from a grain mixture in which rye predominates, by drying that portion of the whole stillage retained by screens.''

''Wheat Distillers' Dried Grains is the product obtained in the manufacture of distilled liquors and alcohol from wheat, or from a grain mixture in which wheat predominates, by drying that portion of the whole stillage retained by screens.''

''Grain Sorghum Distillers' Dried Grains is the product obtained in the manufacture of distilled liquors and alcohol from grain sorghum, or from a grain mixture in which grain sorghum predominates, by drying that portion of the whole stillage retained by screens.''

The distillers' dried grains are fairly high in protein and fat and, like the brewers' dried grains, are chaffy.

''Corn Distillers' Dried Solubles is the product obtained in the manufacture of distilled liquors and alcohol from corn, or from a grain mixture in which corn predominates, by condensing and drying the screened stillage obtained therefrom.''

''Rye Distillers' Dried Solubles is the product obtained in the manufacture of distilled liquors and alcohol from rye, or from a grain mixture in which rye predominates, by condensing and drying the screened stillage obtained therefrom.''

''Wheat Distillers' Dried Solubles is the product obtained in the manufacture of distilled liquors and alcohol from wheat, or from a grain mixture in which wheat predominates, by condensing and drying the screened stillage obtained therefrom.''

"Grain Sorghum Distillers' Dried Solubles is the product obtained in the manufacture of distilled liquors and alcohol from grain sorghum, or from a grain mixture in which grain sorghum predominates, by condensing and drying the screened stillage obtained therefrom."

"Grain Sorghum Distillers' Dried Grains with Solubles is the product obtained in the manufacture of distilled liquors and alcohol from grain sorghum, or from a grain mixture in which grain sorghum predominates, by drying that portion of the whole stillage retained by screens to which condensed screened stillage has been added so that the final product contains not less than 3/4 of the solids content of the whole stillage."

"Corn Distillers' Dried Grains with Solubles is the product obtained in the manufacture of distilled liquors and alcohol from corn, or from a grain mixture in which corn predominates, by drying that portion of the whole stillage retained by screens to which condensed screened stillage has been added so that the final product contains not less than 3/4 of the solids content of the whole stillage."

"Rye Distillers' Dried Grains with Solubles is the product obtained in the manufacture of distilled liquors and alcohol from rye, or from a grain mixture in which rye predominates, by drying that portion of the whole stillage retained by screens to which condensed screened stillage has been added so that the final product contains not less than 3/4 of the solids content of the whole stillage."

"Wheat Distillers' Dried Grains with Solubles is the product obtained in the manufacture of distilled liquors and alcohol from wheat, or from a grain mixture in which wheat predominates, by drying that portion of the whole stillage retained by screens to which condensed screened stillage has been added so that the final product contains not less than 3/4 of the solids content of the whole stillage."

"Molasses Distillers' Condensed Solubles is the product obtained by condensing to a syrupy consistency the residue from the yeast fermentation of molasses after the removal of the alcohol by distillation."

"Molasses Distillers' Dried Solubles is the product obtained by drying the residue from the yeast fermentation of molasses after the removal of the alcohol by distillation."

Distillers' products and especially the dried distillers' solubles have increased in importance in poultry rations. They furnish protein, many of the vitamin B-complex factors, and possibly some unidentified factors. They have been shown to be satisfactory for growth, feed efficiency, and feather development, as well as for egg production and hatchability.[21]

Most of the experiments included 5 to 10 per cent of the distillers' dried solubles, although in some instances higher quantities have been fed. When distillers' dried grains with solubles were fed, a larger amount was used, usually 10 to 20 per cent of the ration.

In the feeding of distillery slop to chicks, the workers at the Kentucky Station[22] found that thin distillery slop proved unsatisfactory as a supplement to an all-mash ration but with thick distillery slop, containing 8.5 to 9 per cent solids, as much as 4/5 of the corn in the mash could be replaced.

Other fermentation products,[23] such as molasses and grain butyl and ethyl fermentation solubles have been satisfactorily fed to poultry. Many of these have been particularly valuable as riboflavin supplements.

BUCKWHEAT AND ITS PRODUCTS. Buckwheat as a grain is of more or less local importance, being fed in those sections where it is grown. Buckwheat has certain undesirable characteristics such as the heavy husk which gives it a larger fiber content and the dark color of the kernel which makes it unattractive to the birds. It is not so palatable as corn or wheat, but is much the same as oats in this respect. Again it is usually used in the winter ration. There is greater difficulty in keeping it over summer, because it is likely to get musty in the bin. It is not a substitute for wheat. Except for the fiber content, its composition resembles corn more than wheat. When used in the grain mixture, it should not make up more than 1/4 of the mixture. Sometimes it is hopper fed in addition to the regular scratch grain. Ground buckwheat may be used in the mash mixture, replacing ground oats.

"Buckwheat Middlings is that portion of the buckwheat grain immediately under the hull after separation of the flour. It shall contain no more hulls than are obtained in the usual process of buckwheat milling, and must not contain more than 10 per cent of crude fibre." A good grade of buckwheat middlings is a valuable fattening feed, producing good quality white flesh. They are high in protein and fat and can be used the same as wheat middlings.

"Buckwheat Feed is a mixture of buckwheat middlings and buckwheat hulls. It must not contain more than 30 per cent of crude fiber."

Rye Buckwheat, which is also called India wheat, Egyptian wheat, Duck wheat, and Bloomless, Mountain, Marino, Tartary, Siberian, and Calentta buckwheat, has a smaller kernel than ordinary buckwheat. It is grown when other more valuable grain crops cannot be grown. It is dull grayish brown in color, with slightly roughened surfaces. It is a grain of low protein content and has a large percentage of hard hull. Its feeding value is probably not much different from buckwheat.

CORN AND ITS PRODUCTS. Corn is the most important crop of American agriculture. It is the most popular grain in the poultry ration in all parts of the country except the West. It is the most widely used single grain in poultry feeding. Of the feed fed to chickens it has been estimated that nearly 1/3 is corn. Wheat is next in importance, comprising about 10 per cent. Its extensive use is the result of a combination of desirable characteristics. Usually, it is as cheap a grain as we can obtain, but it is not only its cheapness that recommends it for poultry feeding. It is attractive in color, extremely palatable, and contains a large amount of digestible nutrients. It can be easily raised and stored; and where it is raised it fits well in crop rotation. It can be fed in a number of ways. To some extent it is fed on the cob, although this is not desirable. Quite a large amount of it is fed as whole corn. In fact, this practice is increasing with the idea of saving the germ and because the quality of the corn can be more readily determined. Gowell[24] indicated that there was nothing to show that it was necessary or advisable to crack corn for hens, and that the danger of heating and souring was less with whole corn. Perhaps larger amounts are fed as cracked corn or as corn meal. A larger amount of it is probably fed as cracked corn than as whole corn, because the corn kernel itself is a little bit larger than is adaptable to poultry in its natural state, and it is also believed that the cracked corn gives a little more exercise to the bird in its consumption. Just how important this factor of exercise is remains to be seen.

Both dent corn and flint corn are used, although the latter is preferable for commercial grain mixtures because it cracks cleaner and thus gives a better appearance. As far as the feeding value is concerned, there is probably little or no difference between the two.

Corn has a wide nutritive ratio, containing a large proportion of the carbohydrates and fat in comparison with the protein. We cannot expect to feed corn alone to poultry and produce growth and eggs, because it is deficient in ash, protein, and vitamins.[25]

Maize is not sufficient alone as a feed for poultry, but where grown it must remain the principal element in poultry feeding. It can be fed heavily, however, when properly balanced.[26]

Some experiments indicate an advantage is using a larger amount of corn, and no gain in feeding a variety ration in place of a simple one composed largely of corn.[27]

Other experiments indicate an advantage in replacing some of the corn with other grains. On a corn-skimmilk ration, the Kentucky Station[13] reports better egg production when part of the corn is replaced by wheat or oats or a combination of the two. Heuser[15] found that a laying ration made up largely of a combination of wheat and corn gave better results than rations composed largely of either grain alone. Ohio[28] reports improvement in the ration when 20 per cent or more of corn was replaced with a like amount of oats. Prentice[29] indicated that maize meal, replacing Sussex ground oats in a laying ration, produced greater gain in body weight and a higher rate of egg production.

The California Station[30] concluded that a ration composed of a high proportion of corn, fed continuously during the first 18 months of life, produced a significantly higher laying-hen mortality than a similar ration in which a large part of the corn had been replaced by barley and alfalfa meal. Differences in mortality were primarily accounted for by an increase in pathological conditions of the reproductive tract, such as ruptured and flabby ova, occluded oviducts, reverse peristalsis, and prolapsus. The corn ration, when fed only during the rearing period or only during the first laying year, did not significantly increase either the laying-hen mortality or reproductive types of pathology, although heavier losses occurred than in the barley-fed lots. More rapid and earlier sexual maturity were produced by the corn ration. Surviving birds produced as many eggs in the corn-fed lots as in the barley-fed lots. Hence the differences in production index were entirely due to the differential mortality.

Jeffrey[31] concluded that the nutrition of the chicken during the growing period had a bearing on adult mortality and suggested that oats, wheat, and barley should be given preferred ratings over yellow corn in compounding rations, especially growing rations. He also called attention to the fact that yellow corn is deficient in the factor, resulting in smooth feathering in chickens, and produces oily and curly or rough feathering, in contrast to smooth and glossy feathering produced by oats, oat hulls, and wheat bran. It is suggested that cannibalism, particularly feather picking, is worse on corn diets because the birds are more inclined to pick at oily, curled feathers than at smooth, glossy ones.

Corn is recognized as one of our best fattening feeds and is used extensively in the fattening industry in this country. It has even been used exclusively as the cereal for this purpose.[32]

Yellow corn is preferable to the white corn because of its higher vitamin content, particularly of the vitamin A. Red corn with a yellow endosperm is equal to yellow corn in vitamin A activity. After the birds become accustomed to red corn, they will eat it readily.

The yellow corn gives yellow color to the flesh of the bird, which is desirable and preferable in poultry markets in this country. In England, where white color is desirable, fattening rations are made up very largely of fine ground oats, which, of course, helps to maintain white color in the carcass. Yellow corn produces a deeper color in the yolk. It also has a tendency to make white-plumaged birds creamy.

GRADES FOR CORN *

No. 1. Cool and sweet, not less than 55 pounds to the bushel, not over 14 per cent moisture; not more than 2 per cent foreign material and not more than 2 per cent of damaged corn; there shall be no heat damage.

No. 2. Cool and sweet, not less than 53 pounds to the bushel, not over 15.5 per cent moisture; not more than 3 per cent foreign material and not more than 4 per cent damaged corn; not more than 0.1 per cent heat damage.

No. 3. Cool and sweet, not less than 51 pounds to the bushel, not over 17.5 per cent moisture; not more than 4 per cent foreign material and 6 per cent damaged corn; not more than 0.3 per cent heat damage.

No. 4. Cool and sweet, not less than 49 pounds per bushel, not over 19.5 per cent moisture; not more than 5 per cent foreign material and 8 per cent damaged corn; not more than 0.5 per cent heat damage.

No. 5. Cool and sweet, not less than 47 pounds per bushel, not over 21.5 per cent moisture; not more than 6 per cent foreign material and 10 per cent damaged corn; not more than 1 per cent heat damage.

No. 6. Cool but may be musty or sour, not less than 44 pounds per bushel not over 23 per cent moisture; not more than 7 per cent foreign material and 15 per cent damaged corn; not more than 3 per cent heat damage.

Sample grade. Sample grade shall be corn which does not come within the requirements of any of the grades 1 to 6, inclusive, or which has any commercially objectionable foreign color, or is heating, hot, infested with live weevils or other insects injurious to stored grain, or is otherwise of distinctly low quality.

* Taken from _U. S. D. A. Handbook of Official Grain Standards_.

Popcorn. The question of the use of popcorn often arises. Where popcorn waste has been tried, it has been found that it does not seem to be very palatable and hence would not be a wise inclusion in the ration.[33]

Sweet Corn. Dried sweet corn can be fed to poultry either as a grain or as the meal. The amounts that can be used will depend upon their consumption by the birds.

"Corn Meal is finely ground, unbolted corn."

"Corn Chop, Ground Corn, or Cracked Corn is the entire product made by grinding, cutting or chopping the grains of sound Indian corn, and may be fine, medium, or coarse. It must not contain more than 4 per cent of foreign material."

"Screened Corn Chop, Screened Ground Corn, or Screened Cracked Corn is the coarse portion of corn chop, ground corn, or cracked corn from which most of the fine particles have been removed. It must not contain more than 4 per cent of foreign material."

Corn meal or ground corn is one of the widely used ingredients of the poultry mash, having the same desirable qualities as listed for the grain. It has the desirable characteristic of not being sticky when mixed with water, and ordinarily will give a good physical condition to the mash mixture. Care must be taken in storing the meal because of heating.

"Corn Feed Meal is the fine siftings obtained in the manufacture of screened corn chop, screened ground corn, or screened cracked corn with or without its aspiration products added."

Since it is not a whole grain ground, there is likely to be considerable variation in this product. It often is a bulkier, chaffier feed because of the larger amounts of bran that it contains. It might also contain more fat because of germs that are lost in cracking. It can be satisfactorily used if it does not contain too much of the fiber.

"Corn Bran is the outer coating of the corn kernel, with little or none of the starchy part or germ." It consists mainly of cellulose and makes up about 6 per cent of the grain. As far as the composition is concerned, it does not differ widely from wheat bran. It does not contain the minerals that wheat bran does, has less protein, and more fiber. Poultry usually is not fed corn bran, although some of it could be fed in the same way as wheat bran, for lightening the ration. Corn bran has been reported as much better than rice bran, but decidedly inferior to corn meal.[34]

"Hominy Feed is a mixture of corn bran, corn germ, and a

part of the starchy portion of either white or yellow corn kernels or mixture thereof as produced in the manufacture of pearl hominy, hominy grits, or table meal, and shall contain not less than 5 per cent of crude fat. If prefixed with the words 'white' or 'yellow,' the product must correspond thereto."

The hominy products are thus made up of all the corn kernel, except part of the interior of the corn or endosperm. They are, therefore, composed of the bran, the germ, and part of the starchy portion of the kernel. Their composition compares favorably with that of corn meal. Hominy has a little more fiber and minerals, since part of the starch has been taken out. There is not much difference so far as the protein is concerned, but as it contains the germ it is higher in fat. The hominy can be used in much the same way as corn meal[35] and can be substituted pound for pound for the corn meal, where it is available at a price not to exceed that of corn meal. It is especially desirable for fattening, since it produces good-quality flesh and fattens quickly. Its use is limited because it is a by-product and is not readily available in large quantities. The yellow hominy products contain vitamin A and are preferable in that respect.

"Corn Germ Meal is ground corn germ cake."

"Corn Germ Cake consists of corn germ with other parts of the corn kernel from which part of the oil has been pressed and is the product obtained in the dry milling process of manufacture of corn meal, corn grits, hominy feed, and other corn products."

"Corn Oil Meal is ground oil cake or flakes. Its name must include one of the terms (hydraulic, expeller, or solvent extracted) to indicate the method of manufacture of the source material."

"Corn Oil Cake and Corn Oil Flakes consist of the corn germ from which most of the oil has been removed by hydraulic, expeller, or solvent extraction and are the products obtained in the wet milling process of manufacture of corn starch, corn syrup, and other corn products. For each product, the designating name must include a term (hydraulic, expeller, or solvent extracted) descriptive of the process of manufacture, and the product must correspond thereto."

These germ products, composed chiefly of the germ which makes up about 10 per cent of the grain by weight, are rich in fat and vitamins and are good feeds. Usually they are more expensive than the other products and are not extensively used. Corn oil meal has the valuable characteristic of being able to absorb large quantities of liquids. When corn oil meal is saturated with liquids, it swells and thickens, enabling it to hold other feeds in a mixture in suspension. For this reason, corn oil meal is a very desirable ingredient in fattening rations.

"Corn Gluten Meal is that part of commercial shelled corn that remains after the extraction of the larger part of the starch and germ, and the separation of the bran by the processes employed in the wet milling manufacture of corn starch or syrup. It may or may not contain one or more of the following: corn solubles, corn oil meal."

"Corn Gluten Feed is that part of commercial shelled corn that remains after the extraction of the larger part of the starch and germ by the processes employed in the wet milling manufacture of corn starch or syrup. It may or may not contain one or more of the following: corn solubles, corn oil meal."

The corn gluten products are high in protein and are thus one of our vegetable protein concentrates (see Chap. 7). When made from yellow corn, they are also rich in vitamin A. Corn gluten meal has been reported to be six times as potent as yellow corn in vitamin A. Gluten meal contains more protein and less fiber than the gluten feed because the bran is not included in the former. In some cases, gluten has had an unfavorable effect upon the kidneys of the birds. It might be possible that in those cases there was not a proper balance of the rest of the ration or too much was fed. The gluten meal seems to be palatable and, where used in moderate amounts, will be satisfactory. The yellow pigments in corn gluten meal promote the desirable yellow coloring in the skin and shanks of the birds.

"Corn Grits or Hominy Grits is the product consisting of fine or medium sized, hard, flinty portions of sound Indian corn containing little or none of the bran or germ."

This is really the hominy used for human food and is ordinarily too expensive to use for poultry feeding, even for the young chicks. There is no advantage gained for poultry over straight cracked corn.

"Flaked Corn is the product obtained by running cracked corn which has been aspirated and properly tempered over smooth flaking rolls and subsequently dried and cooled."

"Ear Corn Chops is corn and cob chopped, without the husk, with no greater proportion of cob than occurs in the ear corn in its natural state." The Ohio[36] Station reported the following results when corn-and-cob meal was used as a substitute for ground shelled corn. During the first 8 to 10 weeks there was

TABLE 9. COMPOSITION OF CORN PRODUCTS*

	Fiber	Protein	Fat	N-Free Extract
Corn meal	2.0	8.6	3.9	69.3
Corn bran	9.2	9.7	7.3	62.0
Hominy feed	5.2	11.2	6.9	64.2
Gluten feed	7.6	25.5	2.7	48.8
Gluten meal	4.0	43.1	2.0	39.8

* _Feeds and Feeding_, Morrison, 1950. (See Table 3.)

little difference in mortality, but in general there was a slightly lower rate of growth. In the growing rations the corn-and-cob meal had a value equal to or greater than ground or whole shelled corn. With layers the corn gave slightly higher production, lower feed consumption, and higher returns. However, a noticeably better plumage condition, with little or no feather picking and cannibalism, was observed with the corn-and-cob meal.

COTTONSEED PRODUCTS. "_Cottonseed Meal_ is a product of the cottonseed only, composed principally of the kernel with such portion of the hull as is necessary in the manufacture of oil; provided that nothing shall be recognized as cottonseed meal that does not conform to the foregoing definition and that does not contain at least 36 per cent of protein. Cottonseed meal shall be graded and classed as follows:

"_Cottonseed Meal, Prime Quality_—must be finely ground, not necessarily bolted, not have a sour or musty odor, reasonably bright in color, yellowish, not brown or reddish, free from excessive lint, and shall contain not less than 36 per cent protein. It must be designated and sold according to its protein content. Cottonseed meal with 36 per cent protein must be termed '36 per cent Protein Cottonseed Meal, Prime Quality,' and higher grades must be similarly designated as '43 per cent Protein Cottonseed Meal, Prime Quality,' etc.

"_Cottonseed Meal, Off Quality_—Cottonseed meal not fulfilling the above requirement as to color, odor, or texture must be graded '36 per cent Protein Cottonseed Meal, Off Quality,' and higher grades similarly designated. It must be designated and sold according to its protein content."

"_Solvent Extracted Cottonseed Flakes_ is the product obtained after solvent extraction of the oil from cottonseed kernels and such portions of the hull as is necessary in the manufacturing process."

"Solvent Extracted Cottonseed Meal is the product resulting from grinding solvent extracted cottonseed flakes. It must be designated and sold according to its protein content."

"Degossypolized Cottonseed Meal shall mean cottonseed meal from which the gossypol has been deactivated, so as to contain not more than 0.04 per cent free gossypol."

Cottonseed meals are vegetable protein concentrates and thus contain a large amount of protein. The chief deficiencies of cottenseed meal are lysine and vitamin B_{12}.[37] The lysine deficiency causes the production of white feathers in bronze turkeys. They also contain considerable fiber. The feeding results have been variable (see Chap. 7).

GRAIN SORGHUMS. Kafir Corn in its composition resembles corn quite closely, except that it contains slightly more fiber. As far as the kernel is concerned, it is of favorable size, has a light husk, has good color, and is relatively soft and palatable. It is used commonly in sections where it is grown. Its use in other sections is not very extensive because it usually costs more than the corn and does not have quite the feeding value. Still kafir corn or red milo can be used to advantage in poultry feeding.[38] In using kafir corn, the lighter, namely the white, or yellow round kernels of the kafir group are desirable because they contain very little of the tannin or bitter property found in darker kernels.

The sorghums are likely to be deficient in vitamin A and hence must be supplemented with green food or some source of this vitamin. When thus supplemented, kafir or hegari may replace yellow corn.[39] It has also been reported that grain sorghum[40] can replace wheat and other grains in poultry rations. The Oklahoma Station[16] reports that feterita and hegari were not so good as yellow corn, and that kafir is more efficient than darso, but that both could be fed. Mitchell[41] reported that the grain sorghum hegari, in starting rations, showed poorer growth and higher mortality and produced white-shanked birds. The palatability of the ration was affected. Fronda, Zialcita, and Basio[42] concluded that broom corn seeds were not so palatable or so efficient for egg production as corn grains. Ackerson and coworkers[43] reported that kalo could be substituted for corn in an otherwise complete ration for growing chicks, but that the instances of cannibalism were confined to the kalo-fed lot. McClymont[44] concluded that grain sorghum should not make up more than 15 to 25 per cent of the ration as higher levels depress growth and increase mortality.

CLASSIFICATION OF GRAIN SORGHUMS

Kafir
- Seeds white—round
  - White kafir
  - Blackhull kafir

Durra
- Seeds white—flattened
  - White durra
  - Blackhull durra
- Seeds yellowish or reddish—slightly flattened
  - Yellow milo
  - Brown durra

Broom Corn
- Seeds reddish brown—round
  - Broom corn
- Seeds white to buff—round
  - Shallu
- Seeds white, brown or red—round
  - Kowliang

Kafir Meal. Its qualities are the same as kafir grain, and would be used in the ration similarly to corn meal.

LINSEED PRODUCTS. "Linseed Oil Meal is the product obtained by finely grinding the cake, chips, or flakes, according to the process employed, in the production of linseed oil. It must be designated and sold according to its protein content, and its name must include one of the terms 'hydraulic,' 'expeller,' or 'solvent extracted' to specify the method of manufacture of the source material."

"Linseed Feed is the product obtained by mixing one or more linseed oil meals with flaxseed screenings oil feed with or without other flaxseed by-products. It must be designated and sold according to its protein content."

Linseed oil meal is quite laxative, probably because of the oil. It is also very sticky when moistened, which renders it unpalatable. Both these characteristics indicate that, where it is used in the mash, the quantity needs to be very much restricted. Where it is included, probably not more than 5 per cent of the mash should be made up of this product. Oil meal is used as a basis for a good many of the so-called tonics. The protein of oil meal is of low biologic value. (See Chap. 7.)

MILLET. Millet is not a valuable feed for poultry. It has a high fiber content. It is often included in small chick grain mixtures for its appearance. It is shiny and very attractive, but because of its hard, heavy husk it often passes through the digestive tract without even being broken down. Besides, it is usually rather expensive. The kernel is too small for the feeding of mature birds.

Proso, also called broom corn millet and hog millet, belongs in the group of millets cultivated for grain production. The seeds are very hard and have a high fiber content. It is very similar to buckwheat in composition and feeding value.

The feeding value of proso millet has compared favorably with that of corn in starting, growing, and laying rations[45, 46] as well as in the ration for growing turkeys.[47]

MINERALS. Common Salt is sodium chloride with impurities not exceeding commercial grade.

"Iodized Salt is common salt (NaCl) containing not less than 0.007 per cent of iodine uniformly distributed."

Salt functions in various ways.[48] This may have some bearing upon the levels recommended. Cereals and cereal by-products are low in sodium. Salt helps to supply sodium and chlorine. Poultry rations to which a small amount of salt was added have given better growth and more efficient utilization of food as well as more satisfactory egg production and better body weight. It has also been reported that salt appeared to improve the utilization of dietary nitrogen.

It has been frequently noted that high salt diets increase the water consumption which has an effect on the consistency of the droppings and results in the litter having to be changed more frequently.

Salt has also been recommended by the Wisconsin Station[49] as a means of preventing cannibalism. The treatment consisted in dissolving a tablespoonful of salt in each gallon of drinking water for one forenoon, and three days later repeating the treatment for another half day.

Too much salt is toxic (see Chap. 11). Much more salt can be fed than is necessary. The Wisconsin Station[50] reported that 5 per cent of salt in the ration is more than is desirable; that 2 per cent is not injurious; that birds getting more than 1 per cent of salt in the ration consumed more than a normal amount of water, with the result that the litter has to be changed more frequently. The Illinois Station[51] indicated that chickens could be raised from 9 to 21 weeks on rations containing as much as 8 per cent of salt, with no apparent detrimental effect on their condition. The Maryland Station[52] found that mortality was not excessive until the level of salt in the ration was greater than 5 per cent by weight and that chicks were able to endure salt levels as high as 30 per cent for short periods of time.

The amount of salt that is required may be influenced by a number of factors. There seem to be some interrelationships[53] between salt and certain minerals such as potassium, calcium, phosphorus, and manganese as well as the nature of the feed ingredients. Because of some of the possible disadvantages it is desirable not to add too much salt to poultry rations.

Phosphorus Carriers. It is frequently necessary to increase the phosphorus content of the ration, particularly when the amounts of meat scrap and fish meal are limited. It is possible to supply phosphorus in a number of forms.

"Steamed Bone Meal is the dried, ground product suitable for animal feeding obtained by cooking bones with steam under pressure."

"Special Steamed Bone Meal is the dried, ground product suitable for animal feeding, obtained by cooking dried bones after the removal of grease and meat fibre with steam under pressure in the process of obtaining gelatin or glue."

"Bone Charcoal or Bone Black is the product obtained by charring bones in closed retorts. It shall contain not less than 14.7 per cent of phosphorus (P)."

"Spent Bone Black is the product resulting from the repeated charring of bone charcoal or bone black after use in clarifying sugar solutions. It shall contain not less than 11.5 per cent of phosphorus (P). The label shall show a guarantee for calcium (Ca) and phosphorus (P)."

"Bone Ash is the ash obtained by burning bones with free access of air, and containing a minimum of 15.3 per cent of phosphorus (P). The label shall show a guarantee for calcium (Ca), and phosphorus (P)."

"Defluorinated Phosphate includes either calcined, fused, or precipitated calcium phosphate. It shall contain not more than one part of fluorine (F) to 100 parts of phosphorus (P). The minimum percentage of calcium (Ca) and phosphorus (P) and the maximum percentage of fluorine (F) shall be stated on the label. The term 'Defluorinated' shall not be used as a part of the name of any product containing more than one part of fluorine (F) to 100 parts of phosphorus (P)."

The inorganic phosphorus carriers vary considerably in their availability.[54] Bone meals, defluorinated phosphates, mono, di-, and tricalcium phosphates, orthophosphates, and Curacao Island phosphate showed generally satisfactory availability. Phosphate rock, phosphate slag, and metaphosphates were generally inferior. "Colloidal" phosphate and pyrophosphates were poor in availability.

Calcium Carriers. Most rations need some addition of calcium. It can be provided in various forms.

"Calcite, Ground Limestone, Chalk Rock, Precipitated Chalk, Oyster Shell Flour, Shell Flour, and Precipitated Calcium Carbonate are acceptable sources of calcium carbonate. They shall in each instance be true to name and shall contain not less than 33 per cent calcium (Ca). They shall be declared as ingredients only by the names listed above.

"Calcium Carbonate is a product containing not less than 38 per cent calcium (Ca)."

"Magnesium Limestone or Dolomitic Limestone is acceptable as a source of magnesium and calcium carbonates. The terms are synonymous and designate a native mineral composed of mixtures of magnesium carbonate ($MgCO_3$) with calcium carbonate ($CaCO_3$). It shall contain not less than 10 per cent magnesium (Mg) and shall be declared as an ingredient only by one of the names listed above."

A number of workers[55] have shown that in rations for chicks the various forms of calcium salts are available for bone formation. For eggshell formation, the carbonate form has proved most effective. Calcium phosphate and rock phosphate[56] have been shown to be definitely inferior as a source of calcium for laying hens.

Most of the forms of calcium carbonate have proved satisfactory as long as they did not contain too large amounts of magnesium, such as is found in dolomitic limestone.[57] Oystershells have been looked upon as the standard for laying hens. Other substances that have been used satisfactorily for this purpose are limestone,[58] marl,[59] mussel shells,[60] coquina shell,[61] cockle shell,[62] coral sand,[63] clam shells,[64] and eggshells.[65]

OATS AND THEIR PRODUCTS. Oats make a desirable grain for poultry feeding, but they should be restricted to plump heavy oats. For poultry feeding, they should weigh 40 pounds or better to the bushel. Light oats are practically valueless. Even with a heavy oat, there is a large amount of husk or fiber, constituting on the average about one-third of its weight. A big difference is found in the amount or proportion or thickness of the husk in different varieties. Dodd and Telford[66] report a variation in the proportion of husks or "hulls" ranging from 20.1 to 45.7 per cent. The fiber content was reported as ranging from 8.5 to 14 per cent. Even in the heavy, favorable oats there is a high fiber content, usually about 10 per cent. The thin-hulled varieties should be chosen. The kernel itself is a desirable feed so that if the husk is taken away, the kernel that is left makes a very good feed. Some feeders say that oats seem to have a stimulating effect upon the nervous system. They are not so palatable as wheat or corn, which are usually eaten first. For that reason, oats are looked upon by some feeders as an indicator of the fowl's appetite.

To the mature birds, the heavy oats and clipped oats are ordinarily fed. However, hulled oats or oat groats of larger size are often fed, although they probably should not be included if they increase the cost materially. The hulled products as pinhead oats, oat groats, or oat flakes are the forms fed to chicks.

Because of the higher fiber content, oats should not compose more than 1/3 of the scratch grain. Ohio[28] reported that the ration was improved when 20 to 40 per cent of corn was replaced with a like amount of oats. There was practically no difference according to the form in which they were fed. Feeding whole oats, mixed with the all-mash mixture, was the easiest and least expensive way of feeding this grain, although a few more eggs were secured when finely ground oats were fed. The difference did not pay for the cost of grinding. With the free choice system of feeding whole oats, troubles such as feather picking, cannibalism, and pick-outs largely disappeared. The time and care required for germinating oats did not seem to be justified by the results obtained.

The results of experiments at the Western Washington Experiment Station[67] show that the cannibalism-preventing properties of oats is due to the fiber fraction of the oat hulls.

When fed as the exclusive grain in the ration, experiments at the Iowa Station[68] showed that oats ranked first for poultry feed in comparison with corn, wheat, and barley. The chicks grew faster and feathered more rapidly, there was less mortality, and cannibalism and feather picking were reduced. It was suggested that up to 40 per cent, or perhaps even more, of the ration of the growing chick, the laying hen, and the turkey could be made of oats, when the quality is good and the price justifies it.

The results of feeding experiments in Germany[69] and Australia[70] indicate that oats can be used in place of wheat, as grain food for laying hens. The digestible foodstuffs in oats can be utilized in the same way as those in wheat. Oat feeding will not be uneconomical when the cost of five parts of oats is the same as four parts of wheat. Care should be taken, however, to use, as far as possible, full-grain, heavy, and fine-husk oats.

The South Dakota Station[71] has also shown that whole or ground oats may be used quite extensively in growing rations for turkeys from 12 to 28 weeks of age. As high as 80 per cent oats were fed.

"Oat Groats are the kernels produced from cleaned and dried oats in the process of manufacturing oat meal."

"Hulled Oats or Undried Oat Groats are the kernels produced from the undried grain in the process of hulling oats."

Pinhead oatmeal consists of oat groats, usually of small oats, so that we have the whole oat kernel. Steel-cut oats consist of larger oat groats that have been cut into several pieces by means of steel knives. Clipped oats are oats which have had the end or tip of the hull broken off. In this process part of the husk or fiber is removed and usually also the light oats are removed. Thus clipping makes the oats a better product for poultry feeding. Frequently oat flakes are used in chick starters.

Some poultrymen have reported trouble from chicks "pasting up behind" with such feeds. In that case the chick has probably picked out the oats. In rats restricted to an oat diet one of the physiological effects reported is pasty feces.

GRADES FOR WHITE OATS*

No. 1. Cool, sweet, not less than 32 pounds to the bushel, not less than 98 per cent sound; with not more than 0.1 per cent heat damage, 2 per cent foreign material, 2 per cent wild oats, or 2 per cent of other color oats.

No. 2. Cool and sweet, may be slightly stained, not less than 29 pounds to the bushel, not less than 95 per cent sound; with not more than 0.3 per cent heat damage, 2 per cent foreign material, 3 per cent wild oats, or 5 per cent of other color oats.

No. 3. Cool and sweet, may be stained, or slightly weathered, not less than 26 pounds to the bushel, not less than 90 per cent sound; with not more than 1 per cent heat damage, 3 per cent foreign material, 5 per cent wild oats, or 10 per cent of other color oats.

No. 4. Cool, may be musty, weathered, or badly stained, not less than 23 pounds to the bushel, not less than 80 per cent sound; with not more than 6 per cent heat damage, 5 per cent foreign material, 10 per cent wild oats, or 10 per cent of other color oats.

"Oat Chop, Ground Oats, Pulverized Oats, Crushed Oats, or Crimped Oats consists of the entire product made by chopping, cutting, grinding, crushing, or crimping whole oats. It shall contain not more than 10 per cent of other grains, weed seeds, and other foreign material."

*Taken from U.S.D.A. Handbook of Official Grain Standards.

Ground oats should be included in restricted amounts since they are a light, bulky food, high in fiber. Ordinarily, they should not constitute more than 20 or 25 per cent of the mash. The Indiana Station[72] reports that oats proved to be an efficient substitute for bran and middlings in rations for chicks when up to 30 per cent ground oats were used in place of 15 per cent each of wheat bran and wheat middlings. They should be ground fine enough so as to prevent picking over by the birds. The hammermill process of grinding is preferable. Crushed oats are not so desirable as ground oats because of their physical make-up. They give a coarseness to the mash which might encourage the hens to pick it over.

"Oat Middlings is the product consisting of the floury portions of the oat groat obtained in the milling of rolled oats."

"Oat Shorts is the product consisting of the covering of the oat grain lying immediately inside the hull, being a fuzzy material carrying with it considerable portions of the fine floury part of the groat obtained in the milling of rolled oats."

PEANUTS are not used as such for poultry, chiefly because they are too expensive. For mature turkeys of 20 pounds or more, the feeding of peanuts has been suggested as possible for about 1 month prior to marketing.

"Peanut Cake is the product obtained after the extraction of part of the oil by pressure or solvents from peanut kernels as produced under reasonable milling conditions. It must be designated and sold according to protein content."

"Peanut Meal is ground peanut cake provided that nothing shall be recognized as such that contains more than 11 per cent crude fiber. It must be designated and sold according to its protein content." It contains considerable protein and can be used satisfactorily where the price warrants its use. (See Chap. 7.)

PEAS. Peas are not used very extensively in poultry feeding chiefly because they are usually too expensive. When price is not a factor, there is no reason why they should not be included in the ration. They contain a large amount of protein. Where peas are grown in combination with other grains, such as oats and barley, the mixture can be used in the scratch grain, although it would be better to grind the mixture and use it as a mash ingredient. Whole peas are used in pigeon feeds since pigeons seem to relish them.

RICE AND ITS PRODUCTS. Rice is not used to any extent in feeding poultry, but it is sometimes included in chick grains. It has no special nutritive value. It is sometimes fed as a regulator for bowel trouble. Diarrhea can frequently be relieved by feeding rice which has been boiled nearly dry in milk.

"Rice Bran is the pericarp or bran layer of the rice, with only such quantity of hull fragments as is unavoidable in the regular milling of rice."

"Rice Polishings is a by-product of rice obtained in the milling operation of brushing the grain to polish the kernel."

"Ground Rough Rice is ground rice from which the hull has not been removed or ground paddy rice."

Brewer's Rice consists of the small and cracked polished grains.

Experiments conducted at the Arkansas, California, Hawaii, and Louisiana agricultural experiment stations[73] show that rice products can be included in both the laying and growing rations of chickens with satisfactory results, provided a good source of vitamin A is furnished as a supplement to the rice feeds. Rice by-products, with a good vitamin A supplement, can be used as a satisfactory substitute for corn, wheat, oats, and the products of these grains in the laying and growing rations of chickens, when the relative price of these feeds justifies such a substitution. Brewer's rice can substitute for corn. Rice bran can be used in place of wheat by-products and rice polishings instead of ground oats.

RYE. Rye is one of the least-used grains in poultry feeding. It has good composition, resembling wheat, but it does not seem to be palatable, owing perhaps to the hardness of the kernels. Rye which was infected with ergot fungus has sometimes caused diarrhea in the poultry to which it was fed. Where it is not infected, there is no reason why some rye should not be used. Rye is frequently sown as a cover crop for poultry yards, for the hens seem to be able to eat the sprouted rye without harm.

Various by-products are also obtained in the milling of rye flour, such as rye feed, rye red dog, rye low-grade feed flour, rye middlings, and rye flour middlings, which are good feeds but are not used in poultry feeding, probably because of the prejudice against rye.

"Rye Feed is a by-product obtained in the usual process of the milling of rye flour from cleaned and scoured rye grain, consisting principally of the mill run of the outer covering of the rye grain and the germ with small quantities of flour and aleurone, and must not contain more than 9.5 per cent of crude fibre."

"Rye Red Dog is a by-product obtained in the usual process

of the milling of rye flour, consisting principally of aleurone with small quantities of rye flour and fine rye bran particles and must not contain more than 3.5 per cent crude fibre."

"Rye Low-Grade Feed Flour consists principally of rye flour and small quantities of aleurone and fine rye bran particles and must not contain more than 1.5 per cent of crude fibre."

"Rye Middlings consists of rye feed and rye red dog combined in the proportions obtained in the usual process of milling rye flour and must not contain more than 8.5 per cent of crude fibre."

"Rye Flour Middlings consists of rye feed, rye red dog, and rye flour combined in the proportions obtained in the milling of rye flour and must not contain more than 5 per cent of crude fibre."

Results of feeding rye in Germany[74] show that hens like food with a high percentage of rye (25 per cent in the mash and 50 per cent in the grain), that it is not harmful to the health of the birds, and produces good laying results. Experiments at Wisconsin[75] indicate that rye is unsatisfactory for young chicks, causing trouble with "sticky" droppings, but that it may be used in the ration for growing pullets and laying hens. For the pullets, not more than 30 per cent and, for mature birds, not more than 45 per cent rye should be fed. Wyoming[76] reports that rations containing 20 per cent of rye or less, when substituted for other cereal grains, were found to be practical for chicks. Higher levels caused a laxative condition.

When rye was fed to hens, there was little difference in egg production among the lots fed barley, rye, and oats. The hens fed rye produced eggs with the flattest yolks and watery albumen. The rye had a laxative effect upon the hens but did not appear to injure their health.

In a 9-month experiment with Leghorn pullets, satisfactory results were obtained when 15 or 30 per cent of rye bran replaced ground cereals in the mash. However, a maximum of 20 per cent is recommended.

The Nebraska[77] Experiment Station found that chicks which were fed ground wheat made better gains than chicks fed ground rye when these grains furnished 25 per cent of the protein of the ration.

SOYBEANS AND THEIR PRODUCTS. Soybeans are not fed to any extent to poultry. They are a vegetable protein concentrate but are not so valuable as the soybean oil meal.

"Ground Soybeans is the product obtained by grinding whole soybeans without cooking or removing any of the oil."

"Expeller Soybean Oil Chips is the product obtained after expressing part of the oil from soybeans by crushing, cooking, and mechanical pressure using an expeller, screw press, or any other mechanical press. It shall be designated and sold according to its protein content."

"Expeller Soybean Oil Meal is the product resulting from grinding expeller soybean oil chips. It shall be designated and sold according to its protein content."

"Hydraulic Soybean Oil Cake is the product obtained after expressing part of the oil from soybeans by crushing, cooking, and hydraulic pressure. It shall be designated and sold according to its protein content."

"Hydraulic Soybean Oil Meal is the product resulting from grinding hydraulic soybean oil cake. It shall be designated and sold according to its protein content."

"Solvent Extracted Soybean Flakes is the product obtained after extracting part of the oil from soybeans by the use of solvents. It shall be designated and sold according to its protein content."

"Solvent Extracted Soybean Oil Meal is the product resulting from grinding solvent extracted soybean flakes. It shall be designated and sold according to its protein content."

"Dehulled Solvent Extracted Soybean Flakes is the product obtained after extracting most of the oil from dehulled soybeans by cracking, heating, flaking, and the use of solvents. After extraction of the oil the product is cooked. It shall contain not more than 3 per cent crude fiber and shall be designated and sold according to its protein content."

"Dehulled Solvent Extracted Soybean Oil Meal is the product resulting from grinding dehulled solvent extracted soybean flakes. It shall contain not more than 3 per cent crude fiber and shall be designated and sold according to its protein content."

Soybean oil meal is the most widely used vegetable protein concentrate in poultry rations (see Chap. 7).

SUNFLOWER SEEDS. Sunflower seeds are not ordinarily used to any extent in poultry feeding because of the very high fiber content and because they are usually too expensive.

Tests made of the value of sunflower seeds, grown in England[78] for poultry feed, found them entirely satisfactory and an excellent substitute for the cereal grains. The seeds were quite digestible, gave more energy than the cereals on an equal-weight basis, and were palatable when fed to the flock under competitive conditions.

When sunflower seeds are fed, they are frequently included in the ration because of the high fat content. Thus their use is usually restricted to the molting season, since it is thought by some that feather growth is aided. They probably help to make the feathers oily or glossy. They are commonly added to commercial mixtures to improve their appearance; usually only 1 to 2 per cent is used.

Sunflowers are frequently grown in the poultry yards to provide shade. They will also help to keep the ground in condition since they are rank feeders. Where they are thus grown in yards, the birds are allowed to harvest the seeds as they become ripe.

VITAMINS. "Cod Liver Oil is the oil obtained from the livers of *Gadus morrhuae* or other species of the family Gadidae, either or both. It must contain not less than 385,900 U.S.P. units of vitamin A per pound (850 units per gram) and not less than 29,510 International chick units of vitamin D per pound (65 units per gram)."

"D-Activated Animal Sterol is a product which is obtained by activation of a sterol fraction of animal origin with ultraviolet light and other means. For label identification it may be followed with the parenthetical phrase ('Source of Vitamin D_3')."

"Vitamin A and D Feeding Oil is either fish or fish liver oil or a blend of two or more of the following: vitamin A and/or D concentrate, synthetic vitamin D, fish liver oil, fish oil, marine animal oil, or edible vegetable oil. The vitamin potency shall be stated in International chick units of vitamin D and U.S.P. units of vitamin A per pound."

"Vitamin D Feeding Oil is either fish or fish liver oil or a blend of two or more of the following: vitamin D concentrate, synthetic vitamin D, fish liver oil, fish oil, marine animal oil, or edible vegetable oil. The vitamin potency shall be stated in International chick units of vitamin D per pound."

"Vitamin A Feeding Oil is either fish or fish liver oil or a blend of two or more of the following: vitamin A concentrate, fish liver oil, fish oil, marine animal oil, or edible vegetable oil. The vitamin potency shall be stated in U.S.P. units of vitamin A per pound."

"Riboflavin Supplement is a feeding material used chiefly for its riboflavin content and shall contain not less than 200 milligrams of riboflavin per pound. The label shall bear a statement of origin."

"Vitamin B_{12} Supplement is a feeding material used for its vitamin B_{12} activity. It shall contain a minimum vitamin B_{12} activity of 1.5 milligrams per pound. The term shall not be applied to products for which there are accepted names and definitions."

"Vitamin E Supplement is a feeding material used for its vitamin E activity. It shall contain a minimum vitamin E activity equal to 10,000 International units of vitamin E per pound. The label shall bear a statement of vitamin E activity in terms of International units of vitamin E per pound."

WHEAT AND ITS PRODUCTS. Wheat is a very good grain for poultry feeding. It is rated by some people as the ideal poultry feed. Because of the demand for wheat for human food, its use has been largely discontinued for other farm animals. Its use for poultry, however, has been continued, probably because it is well adapted to them and because fowls are efficient producers. Wheat has a large number of desirable characteristics. It is the most palatable grain and is adapted to the feeding of fowls because of its favorable size and color and its low fiber content. It compares very favorably with corn in its composition, containing slightly more of the protein and just a little bit more of the fiber. On account of its high protein content it has a slightly narrower nutritive ratio than corn.

Even though wheat has favorable characteristics for poultry feeding, the amounts that are used have been decreasing, probably because of the price. Wheat is more favorably adapted to human consumption than corn and in that respect, where it is used in animal feeding, it is competing with a higher-priced market. For that reason, its use probably will not increase, but is likely to decrease in the future.

Wheat, like corn, can make up a very large proportion of the ration, but it cannot be fed in so large proportions as corn.[79] There is some evidence to indicate that wheat, when fed very heavily, does have detrimental results, probably due to the deficiency of vitamins. In early tests carried on at Ohio[12] there was very little difference in production between corn and wheat rations, but there was a difference in the mortality of the two lots. The corn group lost 8 per cent while in the wheat group the mortality amounted to 52 per cent. In all probability vitamin A was the limiting factor. In feeding wheats of different protein content[80] to chicks it was shown that the differences in growth response were primarily due to differences in the relative proportions of protein contributed and to the differences in the lysine content. McClymont and Hart[81] report that high wheat rations for White Leghorn pullets require a supplement of animal protein, oil meal, riboflavin, and green feed.

Normally, wheat should probably not compose more than 50 to 60 per cent of the laying ration, although larger amounts have been fed satisfactorily. In an experiment conducted at Cornell,[15] a laying ration composed largely of wheat gave better results than a laying ration composed largely of corn. The rations containing wheat resulted in higher grain and total feed consumption, owing to a preference for wheat over corn. The chief factors influencing the results were the nutritive value of wheat and wheat by-products and increased feed intake due to the palatability of the wheat.

In growth trials, normal growth cannot continue long on a heavy wheat diet unless it is properly supplemented. The Indiana Station[82] reported on the substitution of 40 per cent of ground wheat for ground yellow corn in broiler rations. When the ration contained 3 per cent of alfalfa leaf meal, the advantage was in favor of corn. When the ration contained 5 per cent of alfalfa leaf meal, growth was practically the same.

There are many different kinds and varieties of wheat. There is probably not much difference in their feeding values, but practice shows that the soft, plump wheats are more palatable than the harder varieties. Under most conditions, the hen will consume enough feed for her needs, but when food consumption is down this might be a factor to be considered. Goodearl[83] reported that shrunken wheat (40 pounds to the bushel) was not inferior to plump wheat (60 pounds to the bushel) for laying hens when used in equal amounts. However, McArdle[83] reported that as the weight per bushel of wheat fell, egg production decreased.

It is thought by some[84] that wheat may be concerned with the incidence of pullet disease or blue comb. However, all wheats do not seem capable of producing this result. Yet trouble has frequently been reported as the result of feeding new grain. Although the feeding of new wheat is not always fatal and may not prove even noticeably injurious, it seems best not to feed new wheat or other grains, especially those with high moisture content. Birds which are affected show profuse diarrhea, darkened comb, and decided enteritis. The digestive system is usually full of fermented wheat.

Grades of Wheat. There are different classes of wheat, such as hard red spring wheat, durum wheat, hard red winter wheat, soft red winter wheat, and white wheat. Each class has six different grades, the first four of which must be cool and sweet.

The requirements vary with the classes, but the highest grade always has the greatest weight per bushel, the least moisture, and the smallest amount of damaged kernels, heat damage, and foreign material. (For details see U.S.D.A. Handbook of Official Grain Standards.)

Feed Wheat usually has reference to a grade of wheat not accepted for milling purposes. There are several possible reasons for its not being accepted. It may be that the kernels are not large and plump enough; it may be that it contains a large amount of foreign matter, cockle, or other weed seeds; it may be that mold is present or there is too large a percentage of sprouting. Thus feed wheat is a variable product. It may be a favorable feed, or it may be one that is unsatisfactory.

Salvage Wheat ordinarily refers to wheat that has been in an elevator fire. It may be burnt or scorched, and it may be musty because of being soaked with water. If it is not musty, it can be used for poultry feeding; if it is musty, the chances are that it will be unsatisfactory.

Wheat Screenings are ordinarily made up of small, cracked, and shrunken kernels and other foreign material and weed seeds. Wheat screenings are ordinarily made up of refuse of better grades of wheat. Therefore wheat screenings are not considered of much value in poultry feeding, unless they are made up primarily of the smaller and cracked grains.

Elevator Screenings are usually made up primarily of weed seeds and the smaller kernels sifted out. The weed seeds usually are made up of various mustards and cockle. The mustards are usually bitter and, when present in any considerable amount, have a toxic effect by causing irritation of the mucous membrane of the intestines.

Sulfured Wheat is wheat that has been put through a process of bleaching by wetting the wheat, subjecting it to the fumes of sulfur dioxide, and then drying to remove the moisture. Usually the red or durum wheat is thus processed to improve the appearance. Its effect upon the feeding value is not known, but it probably has very little if any effect.

Feeding Wheat. The practice of feeding wheat in the bundle, that is, throwing a sheaf of wheat into the pen and letting the hens thresh it for themselves, can be followed but usually is not reliable because it is hard to tell just how much wheat is being fed. It is difficult to know what amount of grain the birds are getting, and the tendency is to underfeed rather than overfeed. Besides, there is a rapid accumulation of straw which must be removed, frequently before it is necessary to do so for sanitary reasons.

Wheat By-Products. Various by-products of wheat obtained in the manufacture of flour are available for animal feeding. The wheat kernel consists of three rather distinct parts: the outer layers of bran comprise about 16 per cent of the weight of the kernel, the endosperm about 82 per cent, and the germ about 2 per cent. In the milling process much of the bran is removed in layers or flakes, but some is broken into fine particles and becomes mixed with the flour. The by-products removed successively from the outside of the kernel and their approximate percentages are: bran 11 per cent, shorts or middlings 11 per cent, and red dog flour 5 per cent. The remainder, or 72 per cent of the kernel, consisting mostly of starch, is converted into flour. The wheat germ may be included in the by-products or collected separately. The oil may be expressed from the germ and sold as wheat germ oil. The bran layers and germ contain most of the protein, vitamins, fats, and minerals; the endosperm is mostly starch. Since the outer layers contain most of the ash, fiber, and protein, the wheat by-products contain more of these nutrients and less total nutrient than whole wheat.

"Wheat Bran is the coarse outer covering of the wheat kernel as separated from cleaned and scoured wheat in the usual process of commercial milling." Bran is chaffy and bulky and contains considerable fiber. It is also slightly laxative in its nature, owing to its content of crude fiber and pentosans.[85] Its digestibility is low, which, combined with the fiber content, makes it low in total available nutrients. The ash content or mineral content of wheat bran is considered favorable in furnishing phosphorus and manganese.

"Wheat Standard Middlings consist of fine particles of wheat bran, wheat germ, wheat flour, and some of the offal from the 'tail of the mill.' This product must be obtained in the usual process of commercial milling and shall contain not more than 9.5 per cent of crude fibre."

"Wheat Brown Shorts consists of fine particles of wheat bran, wheat germ, and wheat flour and some of the offal from the 'tail of the mill.' This product must be obtained in the usual process of commercial milling and must not contain more than 7.5 per cent of crude fibre."

"Wheat Gray Shorts, Wheat Gray Middlings, or Wheat Flour Middlings consists of the offal from the 'tail of the mill' together with some fine particles of wheat bran, wheat germ, and wheat flour. This product shall be obtained in the usual process of commercial milling and shall contain not more than 6.0 per cent of crude fibre."

"Wheat Red Dog, Wheat White Shorts, or Wheat White Middlings consists of the offal from the 'tail of the mill' together with some fine particles of wheat bran, wheat germ, and wheat flour. This product shall be obtained in the usual process of commercial milling and shall contain not more than 4.0 per cent of crude fibre."

"Wheat Feed Flour consists principally of wheat flour together with fine particles of wheat bran, wheat germ, and the offal from the 'tail of the mill.' This product shall be obtained in the usual process of commercial milling and shall contain not more than 1.5 per cent of crude fibre."

In middlings, we have the standard type and the flour type. These types differ in composition and also in texture because the standard middlings contain a larger proportion of bran particles than the flour middlings.

Wheat middlings and shorts also have a slightly laxative effect. They are sticky when mixed with water and therefore should not constitute large proportions of the feed.

Red dog flour is the product used in poultry feeds. It is low in fiber and has much the same characteristics as flour middlings. It is used to quite an extent in fattening rations.

"Wheat Mixed Feeds consists of the coarse outer covering of the wheat kernel, fine particles of wheat bran, wheat germ, and wheat flour, and the offal from the 'tail of the mill.' This product shall be obtained in the usual process of commercial milling and shall contain not more than 9.5 per cent of crude fibre."

"Wheat Germ Meal consists chiefly of wheat germ together with some bran and middlings or shorts. It shall contain not less than 25 per cent of protein and 9 per cent of fat."

"Wheat Germ Oil Cake is the cake secured in the removal of part of the oil from wheat germ meal and shall contain not less than 29 per cent of protein."

"Wheat Germ Oil Meal is ground wheat germ oil cake."

Part of the wheat germ is sometimes removed so that the by-products contain relatively less of this portion of the grain. It is a valuable part of the grain since several of the vitamins of wheat are located chiefly in this portion. It is desirable that the germ be left in the wheat by-products as otherwise a deficiency of vitamins might result.

Use of Wheat Products. By-Products. The tendency at the

TABLE 10. COMPOSITION OF WHEAT PRODUCTS*

	Fiber, %	Protein, %	Fat, %	N-Free Extract, %
Ground wheat	2.6	13.2	1.9	69.9
Wheat bran	9.6	16.9	4.6	52.9
Wheat standard middlings	6.1	18.1	4.7	56.4
Wheat flour middlings	3.8	18.3	4.2	59.8
Red dog flour	2.6	18.2	3.6	61.9

* Feeds and Feeding, Morrison, 1950 (see Table 3).

present time is to use less of the wheat bran in poultry feeds and more of the middlings and red dog flour. There is considerable variation in the composition of the wheat products, depending upon the source and nature of the grain from which it is made. There is also considerable variation in appearance and texture, depending upon the process of milling and the closeness of milling. For example, a coarse standard winter wheat bran is quite different from a wheat bran obtained from a small local mill.

Wheat by-products have been demonstrated as being important ingredients in poultry rations. The results from tests in Northern Ireland[86] show the value of bran for egg production. Taylor and Lerner[87] concluded that the inclusion of 15 or 25 per cent of wheat bran in the ration resulted in more rapid growth, earlier sexual maturity, and lower egg weight at the beginning of laying. Mussehl, Ackerson, and Blish[88] report a good concentration of a feather-growth factor in wheat bran and state that as much as 40 per cent of bran can be used in chick rations with good results. Embleton[89] concluded that bran was a more economical base for mashes than alfalfa meal, when used to the extent of 20 per cent in the mash.

Bearse[90] reported that replacement, in the rations of laying hens, of as much as 50 per cent of the mash by standard mill run did not seriously interfere with egg-producing ability of the hens or mortality of the chicks. Poley[91] has also reported on the utilization of wheat and wheat by-products in the feeding of young chickens, particularly in respect to furnishing the various components of the vitamin B complex. Carrick and Roberts[92] reported that when 10 per cent each of wheat bran and wheat middlings replaced 20 per cent of ground yellow corn more feed was required per unit of gain, since the rate of growth was reduced and the feed consumption increased.

Hewitt[93] obtained satisfactory egg production in Australian experiments when using various combinations of bran, pollards, ground wheat, oats, barley and maize, and brewer's grains.

Ground Wheat or Wheat Meal is frequently used in place of the wheat by-products. When fed, it should be coarsely ground. Experiments in England[94] indicate that wheat meal can replace up to 80 per cent of the maize meal of an all-mash ration, when the maize constitutes half the mash. The wheat rations produce light-colored yolks and legs. When using wheat meal in place of corn, the vitamin A content of the ration must be checked. Three to 5 per cent of good dehydrated alfalfa meal will prevent this deficiency condition. Twenty per cent of wheat meal has also been satisfactorily substituted for an equal amount of ground oats. South Dakota[95] reported that 30 per cent of ground red durum wheat gave equally satisfactory results, when used to replace 15 per cent each of bran and flour middlings in the mash part of a complete grain and mash ration for laying pullets.

Crushed Wheat has also been used with good results in poultry rations in place of wheat bran and wheat middlings. In experiments reported from Cornell University,[96] growth was greater, egg production was higher, and the body weight of the hen maintained better when crushed wheat replaced wheat bran and middlings. It was concluded that the greater efficiency was probably due to a greater amount of digestible nutrients being made available on the less fibrous rations.

LESS COMMONLY USED POULTRY FEEDS

ALGARROBA FEED consists of the fruit of the algarroba tree processed into a fine meal. It has a high sugar content, satisfactory protein, and high fiber. It is very aromatic and is sometimes used as an appetizer and tonic. Draper[97] suggested that algarroba bean meal could be used in Hawaii to supplement imported feeds for laying hens and for turkeys.

BAKERY REFUSE might consist of any kind of baked goods. Where the product is kiln dried, it can be used as an ingredient of the dry mash. It might also be used as a wet mash, by moistening with milk and feeding as "bread and milk." It might be used in place of part of the wheat products.

BEANS are not usually looked upon as a poultry feed. Cull beans, however, are sometimes fed. It is best to cook them and feed as part of a wet mash. Cull pink beans have been reported as being well utilized up to levels of 10 per cent. Bean meal[98] when included in rations for hens resulted in lower production and smaller eggs.

CHARCOAL. Because charcoal is an absorbent, especially of gases, it was included in poultry rations as an absorbent of gases and an intestinal corrective. Mangold and Damköhler[99] reported some benefit of charcoal in preventing diarrhea. Sipe[100] reported no effect upon egg production, health, or mortality of laying hens.

Experiments, conducted at Cornell,[101] showed that wood charcoal, when used in the feeding of chicks, did not have any effect on growth, mortality, body or shank pigmentation, or condition of feathering. When used in the feeding of laying hens, it did not have any effect on egg production, food consumption, food utilization, mortality, or yolk color. No detrimental results were noted, even when charcoal was incorporated in amounts equal to 8 per cent of the total ration. In most of the trials, the addition of charcoal increased food consumption, usually to the extent of the charcoal included. However, in mild diarrhea, produced by the feeding of dried whey, the condition of the droppings was benefited by charcoal feeding. In severe diarrhea, the consistency of the droppings was not influenced.

On the other hand, Almquist and Zander[102] reported that a chick diet, adequate for normal growth and health, was rendered, in effect, deficient in vitamins A, G, K, and the gizzard factor by the addition of an adsorbing charcoal. These findings point to the possibility of some measure of this effect in practical rations supplemented with charcoal, if the mash does not contain more than adequate levels of these factors, or if the mash consumption is reduced by heavy scratch grain feeding, or if the birds have unlimited access to charcoal. Hence the adsorbing power of charcoals in poultry rations is not necessarily a beneficial property.

Hunt[103] reports that riboflavin added directly to charcoal (Norite A) was 35 per cent available to chicks and that added to bone black it was 85 per cent available. Similar results were obtained in the case of pantothenic acid and niacin. However, if the adsorbents were fed separately from the vitamin, somewhat more was available. In the case of riboflavin, the loss to the chicken was 15 per cent.

COCOA BEAN MEAL has been suggested as a poultry feed. It has been reported that chocolate meal is not eaten readily, is toxic, and at higher levels causes the chicks to lose weight. Temperton and Shaw[104] report that the poisonous effects produced when cocoa wastes are fed are due to the presence of theobromine, the effects of which are cumulative. Fangauf and

Haensel[105] observed unsatisfactory results when 20 per cent of cocoa shell meal was included in the ration of Leghorn hens.

"COCOANUT OIL MEAL or COPRA OIL MEAL is the ground residue obtained after the extraction of part of the oil from the dried meat of the cocoanut. It must be designated and sold according to its protein content." This product contains a considerable amount of protein but is also high in fiber. Its feeding in one trial at the Maryland Station[33] did not give satisfactory results. This was due in part to the fact that it was unpalatable. Temperton and Dudley[106] conclude that, in the event of a shortage of bran, cocoanut cake meal can be used as a substitute, without detriment to the health or productivity of the birds. (See also Chap. 7.)

COWPEAS are not used in poultry rations, although small amounts could be fed in the same way as other leguminous seeds.[107]

ENZYME PRODUCTS have been suggested for the poultry ration, with the idea of furnishing enzymes to aid the digestion and assimilation of the food. Enzymes are found naturally in the digestive tract of the hen.

Improvement of the ration has been reported by the addition to the ration of protozyme,[108] a vegetable enzyme of fungus origin. Observations in regard to enzymes and their action[109] indicate that under normal conditions food utilization is as complete as possible, without the assistance of any enzymes from the outside. It is necessary, therefore, that many more detailed and controlled investigations be carried on with poultry before the use of artificial enzymes can be generally advocated. There is some evidence to indicate that fiber-splitting enzymes might enable the chicken to utilize some nutrients tied up or made unavailable by fiber.

MOLASSES, a by-product of the manufacture of cane sugar or beet sugar, contains a large amount of sugar. It is palatable and liked by farm animals. It is laxative and hence must not be fed in too large quantities.

"Feeding Cane Molasses is a by-product of the manufacture of cane sugar from cane and shall contain 48 per cent or more of total sugars expressed as invert sugar. Its solution in an equal weight of water shall test not less than 39.75 degrees Brix."

"Feeding Beet Molasses is a by-product of the manufacture of beet sugar from sugar beets and shall contain 48 per cent or more of total sugars expressed as invert sugar. Its solution in an equal weight of water shall test not less than 39.75 degrees Brix."

"Feeding Corn Sugar Molasses is a by-product of the manufacture of corn sugar from corn and shall contain 43 per cent or more of reducing sugars expressed as dextrose, and shall contain 60 per cent or more of total carbohydrates (dextrins, and reducing and non-reducing sugars). Its solution in an equal weight of water shall test not less than 39.00 degrees Brix."

"Citrus Molasses is the partially dehydrated juice of citrus fruit. It shall contain not less than 45 per cent of total sugars expressed as invert sugar. Its solution in an equal weight of water shall test not less than 35.5 degrees Brix."

Satisfactory results with molasses have been reported from the Hawaii,[110] Louisiana,[111] Ohio,[112] and Cornell[113] stations. However, Maw[114] gives results from Canada which show that chicks increased food consumption without an increase in weight and that hens showed lower egg production. The Pennsylvania[115] Station also reported that performance was not significantly influenced by including up to 6 per cent of molasses in the rations of growing chickens or hens.

When molasses is used it replaces feeds rich in starch, such as corn. The amounts fed must be restricted as the droppings become very watery, owing in part to increased water consumption. This causes the litter to become damp and soiled. Flies are also attracted and collect in the pens of chickens fed heavily on molasses.

In the feeding of hens 5 to 7 per cent is usually recommended. For the feeding of broilers larger amounts have been used. When mixed with bagasse pith the Hawaii[110] Station has fed levels up to 35 per cent as a source of carbohydrates in layer rations.

Wood sugar molasses[116] prepared by the hydrolization of wood waste has also been satisfactorily substituted for cereal grains in rations for chicks and laying hens.

POTATOES. Small potatoes and potatoes when they are cheap can be used as a poultry feed. It must be remembered, however, that they are composed largely of water. Four to 5 pounds of potatoes are equivalent to 1 pound of grain. On the dry basis, they do not differ greatly from corn or wheat. Rations containing high proportions of cooked potatoes are likely to be deficient in protein, fiber, and the fat-soluble vitamins. The Ohio Experiment Station[117] suggests that potatoes should be cooked since raw potatoes are not satisfactory. The coefficients of digestibility[118] of raw potatoes are lower than those for cooked or ensiled potatoes. After cooking the potatoes should be mashed and mixed with enough of the laying mash to make a crumbly mixture. This can be fed as a moist mash, feeding what the hens will eat in about 15 minutes. One hundred hens will thus consume 6 to 8 pounds of potatoes a day. They seem to like the mash better when it is warm.

Experiments reported from Canada,[119] the Irish Free State,[120] Michigan,[121] Norway,[122] and Wyoming[123] indicate that potatoes make a satisfactory substitute for corn or other feedstuffs rich in carbohydrates.

Results from England[124] show that potatoes were fed in large amounts to all kinds of stock since scarcity of grains and other imported concentrates, owing to war conditions, increased the feeding of home-grown feeds. Large amounts of potatoes (in some cases 50 per cent or more) were included in rations for laying chickens and ducks as well as rations for rearing pullets and ducklings. The feeding of potatoes to breeders and table poultry was not satisfactory.

Potatoes and various potato products have been used extensively in Germany.[125] This interest has been shown because the nutritive yield of potato acreage is greater than that of grain. Freshly steamed potatoes, up to 2½ ounces per day per bird, were given to laying hens. Potato flakes, up to 60 per cent of the food mixture, were fed to hens and chicks with satisfactory results when the ration was properly supplemented. However, high levels of ground, dried, raw potatoes are not recommended for baby chicks. For the fattening of poultry, ducks, geese, and turkeys, potatoes in every form may be made an essential part of the feeding as a supplement to and a substitute for grain fodder. Economic conditions must decide whether potato flakes or cereals are to be used.

The feeding of large amounts of steamed, ensiled potatoes to laying and breeding hens was satisfactory if an adequate amount of protein of high biological value was included in the ration. Similarly, potato-protein flakes, a by-product of starch production, could be used as supplementary protein feed when combined with animal protein feed.

Bolton and Hale[126] reported satisfactory results for egg production when dried potato slices or flakes were fed in amounts as high as 42 per cent of the ration. Results at the Maine[127, 131] Experiment Station indicated that dehydrated potatoes were not satisfactory as a substitute for corn in a chick ration, especially when 50 per cent or more of the corn was replaced. Substitution up to 20 per cent did not affect feed efficiency. The California[128] Experiment Station reported a reduction in growth of both poults and chicks when they were fed sun-dried or oven-dried raw potatoes at a level of 20 per cent. Dried cooked potatoes, however, at that level appeared to be satisfactory. Experiments conducted at Cornell University[129] indicate that 20 per cent of potato meal can be used in place of corn meal or wheat standard middlings in rations for ducklings.

Dried potato solubles,[130] a by-product in starch production, was satisfactorily fed to chicks as a partial substitute for soybean meal. Potato starch pomace,[131] did not prove satisfactory in rations for chicks. The efficiency was very poor due probably to the high level of calcium.

SWEET POTATOES. Sweet potatoes and dehydrated sweet potato meal were used as feed in Louisiana.[132] The hens getting the cooked potatoes ate more than those receiving raw ones. The sweet potatoes were fed to replace green feed, and the egg production was entirely satisfactory. It was also found that sweet potato meal could be used as 20 to 25 per cent of the mash mixture and to replace carbohydrate feeds in chick rations. The Mississippi and Hawaii stations[133] reported poorer growth in chicks when dehydrated sweet potatoes were substituted for corn in the ration. The North Carolina Station[134] reported better gains for poults on a standard turkey starter mash than on the same mash when the principal vitamin A carriers were replaced by sweet potato flour. There was also a reduction in the vitality of those receiving the sweet potato flour in the ration. The South Carolina Station[134] reported dehydrated sweet potatoes as a good source of vitamin A.

SHREDDED WHEAT WASTE can be fed to poultry when it can be obtained cheaply. It can be used in the same way as bakery refuse.

SUGAR may be used as a source of energy, but it is usually too expensive for regular feeding. Because it is primarily carbohydrate, no special advantage has been reported, even by adding it to a ration for finishing broilers.[135] The Hawaii Station[136] indicated that low grade sugar is a potentially good source of carbohydrates for mature chickens.

Sugar Beet Pulp. "Dried Beat Pulp is the dried residue from sugar beets which have been cleaned and freed from crowns, leaves, and sand, and which have been extracted in the process of manufacturing sugar." Ground sugar beets have been successfully adapted as a feed for hens in Germany,[137] but they are not suitable in large quantities for chicks. The feeding of uncooked and steamed sugar beets to laying pullets in England[138] has given satisfactory results. A greater supplement of protein was required for sugar beets than for potatoes. Sugar beet slices are more efficient to use in feeding ruminants and should not be used for poultry except in times of scarcity of carbohydrate-containing food. The apparent digestibility of the dried beet pulp was extremely low.

"VELVET BEAN MEAL is ground velvet beans containing only an unavoidable trace of hulls or pods." It contains a large amount of protein. Special feeding values for poultry have not yet been determined.

YEAST. Dried yeast is the yeast of the botanical classifications Saccharomyces, Torulopsis, or Dandida, which has been separated from the medium in which it was propagated and dried. It shall contain not less than 40 per cent crude protein.

"Irradiated Yeast is yeast which has been subjected to ultraviolet rays in order to increase its antirachitic potency."

"Brewers' Dried Yeast is the dried, nonfermentive, nonextracted yeast resulting as a by-product from the brewing of beer and ale and shall contain not less than 40 per cent of crude protein on the moisture-free basis."

"Dried Torula Yeast is a yeast of the botanical classification Torulopsis which has been separated from the media in which [it was] propagated and dried. It shall contain not less than 40 per cent crude protein on the moisture-free basis."

"Grain Distillers' Dried Yeast is the properly dried yeast resulting from the fermentation of grains and yeast, separated from the mash, either before or after distillation."

"Molasses Distillers' Dried Yeast is the properly dried yeast resulting from the fermentation of molasses and yeast, separated from the medium, either before or after distillation."

Yeast, a rich source of the vitamin B complex, can be used in poultry rations for this purpose. Yeast can also be used to produce a fermented mash.

Adding yeast to a normal chick ration has shown no advantage in some experiments.[139] In some cases[140] the growth rate has been increased owing probably to an increase in some of the nutrients or to increased food consumption.

Some feeding experiments[141] with laying birds showed no apparent advantage in supplementing the regular laying ration witn commercial yeast or diastase from the standpoint of egg production, egg size, body weight, mortality, or cost of feed per dozen eggs. On the other hand, the feeding of yeast-fermented mash and live yeast at the North Carolina Station[142] resulted in higher egg production. The writers indicate that the feeding of yeast-fermented mash stimulated the appetite and led to higher feed consumption and to higher egg production. They also indicated that the enzymes of the live yeast were causative factors for higher production. Temperton and Dudley[143] reported fodder yeast as a satisfactory form for laying pullets.

UNUSUAL POULTRY FEEDS

Besides the more or less commonly used feedstuffs already discussed, a number of unusual products have been used or suggested for poultry rations, either because they were cheap or because the regular ingredients could not be readily obtained.

ACORNS. Temperton[144] concluded that it appeared safe to include ripe, ungerminated acorns up to 20 per cent of feed intake in rations for hens and ducks. When the amount of this type of acorn was increased to 40 per cent of the hens' ration, there was a decrease in egg production and the birds became constipated. No detrimental effect was observed in ducks when acorns made up to 50 per cent of the ration. The production of discolored yolks was attributed to germination of the acorns.

"BABASSU OIL MEAL is the ground residue obtained after the extraction of part of the oil from babassu kernels (*Orbignya speciosa*) by crushing, cooking or mechanical pressure. It must be designated and sold according to its protein content." Babassu meal has been reported by the California Experiment Station as giving satisfactory results when fed at levels up to and including 10 per cent.

BEET SEED.[145] When beet seed was substituted entirely for a grain ration of equal parts of wheat and barley, the hens ceased egg production, lost weight, and were in generally poor condition. However, in three groups of 25 hens each, beet seed successfully replaced 10 and 25 per cent of the grain mixture for 12 weeks, since egg production, egg size, feed consumption, and body weight were not significantly different.

CHEWINGS FESCUE SEED,[146] of such low germination as to be unsuitable for planting, may be used advantageously as a poultry feed. The composition resembles oats, 30 per cent of which was replaced by 30 per cent of the fescue seed.

"DRIED CITRUS PULP, CITRUS MEAL, consists of the dried and ground peel, residue of the inside portions, and occasional cull fruits of the citrus family with or without the extraction of part of the oil of the peel. If calcium oxide or calcium hydroxide is added as an acid in processing, the maximum percentage present, expressed as calcium (Ca), must be stated. If it bears a name descriptive of its kind or origin, it must correspond thereto.

"CITRUS SEED MEAL is a product principally of the seed of oranges and grapefruit singly or mixed, from which the major portion of the oil has been removed, and is composed mostly of kernel with such portion of the hull as is necessary in the manufacture of citrus seed oil. It may contain small amounts of the seed of other varieties of citrus. It must be designated and sold according to its protein content."

The Florida Experiment Station[147] has reported on the use of citrus meal. In general, citrus meal was not a satisfactory component of chick rations. Pullets 8 to 20 weeks old utilized citrus meal fairly well. Up to 15 per cent of citrus meal could be fed to laying pullets with no ill effects. Citrus seed meal proved unsatisfactory for chicks, but when extracted could be fed without apparent ill effects. The California Station reported that orange peel and pulp meal was eaten readily by chicks at levels up to 20 per cent of the ration, but the meal acted like an inert ingredient causing corresponding decreases in gain with increasing amounts of the orange peel and pulp meal.

DRIED COFFEE GROUNDS have been reported by Hammond[148] as being unsuitable for growing chickens. As little as 5 per cent was harmful. The deleterious effect could not be attributed to dilution of the diet.

GARBAGE. The shortage of feeds in England[149] due to the war resulted in the feeding of household garbage to poultry. This product, known as kitchen waste, consisted of unavoidable food waste from households. Vegetable peelings, principally potato, supplied about two-thirds of the fresh material. Reasonably good egg production was obtained when large amounts of the daily dry matter was provided as semi-dried processed food waste. The droppings of the birds eating swill were moister, but looseness was not so pronounced as to cause scouring or to affect the health of the birds. The swill rations were improved by supplementary protein or access to grass runs. The weights of the groups of growing pullets (8 to 21 weeks old) that ate the swill were reasonably satisfactory. Semi-dried town food waste has beed fed with satisfactory results to female ducklings from the age of 2 weeks to the laying stage.

The Hawaii Agricultural Experiment Station[97, 150] reported that raw garbage and processed garbage meal could be used in poultry rations. Satisfactory and economical growth could be obtained by feeding ducks on raw garbage, when properly supplemented with a limited amount of commercial poultry mash or vitamin and mineral concentrates. The feeding of raw garbage necessitates spending considerable time in maintaining satisfactory sanitary conditions about the poultry house. It is essential to clean the feed troughs each day to prevent undesirable odors and attraction of flies.

HEMPSEED MEAL has been reported as efficiently replacing cereal grains up to 20 per cent of the ration.

MANURE. Hammond[151] reported that cow manure had a marked beneficial effect on the growth of chicks if it was added to a diet deficient in riboflavin. It had no deleterious effect on the growth of chicks if it was added to a completely balanced diet. Dried cow manure served as a partial substitute for alfalfa leaf meal. As an ingredient in turkey diets fresh cow manure, dried at 80° and 120° C., was found to be a satisfactory substitute for 10 per cent of alfalfa leaf meal in a diet adequate in vitamin A and nearly adequate in riboflavin. Dried sheep manure[152] has also been reported as a possibility in poultry rations.

"PALM KERNEL OIL MEAL is the ground residue from the extraction of part of the oil by pressure or solvents from the kernel of the fruit of *Elaeis guineensis* or *Elaeis melanococco*." Palm kernel meal, which is not unlike bran in protein and fiber but much less bulky, was reported by Temperton and Dudley[153] as being satisfactory up to levels of 20 per cent as substitutes for concentrated starchy foods.

PERILLA MEAL has been reported by the California Station as being a palatable feed, relatively high in digestible protein and total digestible nutrients.

RUMEN CONTENT. Preliminary experiments reported from Italy[154] on the nutritive value of the contents of the rumen of slaughtered animals, when fed to growing chickens, indicated an increase in growth, when they were added to a diet complete except for a possible deficiency of proteins. Hammond[151] also reported dried rumen contents as a partial substitute for alfalfa leaf meal in rations for chicks.

STRAW EXTRACT. Experiments reported from England[155] show unfavorable results from feeding a caustic soda extract of straw to pullets and ducks. The highest level that could be used without excessive scouring was 6 per cent, but this amount significantly lowered egg production.

SWEET LUPIN SEEDS. The seeds have a high content of crude protein, crude fat, and nitrogen-free extract. Experiments reported from Germany[156] indicate high digestibility of the seeds. In rearing poultry it was found that two-thirds of the animal protein usually used could be replaced by sweet lupins.

TAPIOCA MEAL has a high starch content. Experiments reported from England[157] show that, as a wartime substitute for the more usual kind of poultry food, tapioca meal at a level of 20 per cent proved suitable for the rearing of cockerels and pullets and even at higher levels of 40 and 50 per cent produced no discernible harmful effects but was less satisfactory.

"DRIED TOMATO POMACE is a mixture of tomato skins, pulp, and crushed seeds resulting from the process of extracting the juice from tomatoes." On the basis of its vitamin A, B_1, and B_2 content, Esselen and Fellers[158] suggest that dried tomato pomace should be considered as a desirable feed. It is palatable when fed at 10 to 15 per cent levels.

WOOD SUGAR. Feeding experiments with wood sugar, reported from Germany,[159] indicate that as much as 30 per cent can be included in poultry mashes.

OTHER FEEDS. Many feeds have been used locally in regions where they are produced. For example, the Hawaii Station[160] reports that avocados, bananas, sweet potatoes, and taro waste were found to make economical supplemental feeds. Poi could be used but produced more expensive gains when fed to broilers. In the Philippines[161] palay, tahup, and cassava refuse meal have also been fed to poultry. Other feeds[162] used in poultry rations are adlay cereal, manioc meal, dried penicillin mycelium, algae, and raisins.

Many feeds have been suggested as ingredients of poultry rations which have not proven satisfactory. Besides cocoa bean meal, dried coffee grounds, and straw extract which have been previously mentioned, other feeds[163] which have been shown unsatisfactory are green banana meal, ground carob pod and bean, horse chestnuts and elderberries, dried sewage sludge, and hairy vetch seed.

There are many products that are used occasionally, and undoubtedly other by-products that could be used will appear. Unless there is a shortage of feeds, or unless such products can be obtained at a very low price, have been tried out, and can be obtained in sufficient amounts, it is probably best not to use them. There are normally available a choice of satisfactory feeds that are known and can be obtained in sufficient quantities and at a reasonable price. It is, therefore, usually best to make up a poultry ration of those feeds, the feeding values of which have been demonstrated, unless one is willing to take a chance on the unknown.

REFERENCES

1. Stevenson, G. L. Experiments with poultry at the South Dakota Station. S. Dak. Rept. 1925:33
   Stevenson, G. L. Experiments with poultry at the South Dakota Station. S. Dak. Rept. 1926:32
   Poley, W. E., and W. O. Wilson. Feeding values of low- and high-test weight grains for chickens. S. Dak. Bul. 353:1941.
2. Wilcke, H. L. The relative value of farm grains in poultry nutrition. Jour. Am. Vet. Med. Assn. 90:188. 1937.
   Wilcke, H. L., and J. C. Hammond. Feathering, growth, feed consumption, and rachitogenesis in chicks as influenced by the kind of grain in the diet. Jour. Agr. Res. 61:369. 1938.
   Sanford, P. E., and H. L. Wilcke. Effect of cereal grains and their by-products on plumage development and body growth of the chick. Poultry Sci. 23:298. 1944.
3. Roberts, R. E., and C. W. Carrick. Research solves farm problems. Indiana Rept. 1941:93.
4. Harshaw, H. M. The effect of different cereals on the composition of the edible portions of cockerels. Poultry Sci. 18:486. 1939.
5. Jaeger, J. Die Verwendbarkeit von Weizen, Hafer, Gerste, und Roggen als Körnerfutter an Legehennen. Rept. Sixth World's Poultry Congress. 282. Germany. 1936.
6. Crampton, E. W. The comparative feeding values for poultry of barley, oats, wheat, rye, and corn. A review and analysis of published data. Dominion of Canada. Nat. Res. Council Rept. 29:50. 1936.
7. Biely, J. Cereal grains and wheat by-products in poultry rations. Amer. Miller & Processor 76:66. 1948.
8. North, M. O. Poultry feeding, housing, and lighting experiments at the Wyoming Experiment Station. Wyo. Bul. 203. 1934.
9. Carrick, C. W. Wheat and corn as grain for layers. Indiana Rept. 1938:81.
10. Halpin, J. G. Besides salt, what's needed to prevent cannibalism? Wis. Bul. 455:15. 1942.
11. Biely, J., B. E. March, G. L. Inkin, and G. T. Eedy. Wheat versus corn in the Connecticut broiler ration. Poultry Sci. 30:593. 1951.
    Biely, J., M. Narod, and R. McMillan. Grains in the poultry ration. Feedstuffs 18 (35) :20. 1946.

12. Buss, W. J. Feeding experiments with laying hens. Ohio Bul. 322. 1918.
13. Martin, J. H. Sources of animal protein for laying hens. Ky. Bul. 260. 1925.
14. Kempster, H. L. Wheat as a supplement to yellow corn in rations for egg production. Mo. Bul. 300:92. 1931.
15. Heuser, G. F. Corn and wheat as the main part of the laying rations. Poultry Sci. 22:123. 1943.
16. Penquite, R. M. Grain sorghums are good poultry feeds. Okla. Rept. 1927-1930:87.
17. The effect of different mash levels of alfalfa leaf meal in enhancing hatchability. R. I. Rept. 1938:38.
Hart, C. P., and H. O. Stuart. The effect of different intake levels of alfalfa meal in enhancing hatchability. R. I. Misc. Pub. 20. 1944.
Draper, C. I. A comparison of sun-cured and dehydrated alfalfa meal in the diet of the chick. Poultry Sci. 27:659. 1948.
McGinnis, J. Alfalfa feed for poultry. Flour & Feed. Sept., 1948, 49 (4): 20.
Jensen, L. S. Hens gain on alfalfa. Flour & Feed. Dec., 1949, 50:24.
18. Ayala, E., and E. L. Johnson. Vitamin B_{12} and growth inhibiting properties of the dried juice of alfalfa. Poultry Sci. 30:893. 1951.
Cooney, W. T., J. S. Butts, and L. E. Bacon. Alfalfa meal in chick rations. Poultry Sci. 27:828. 1948.
German, H. L., and J. R. Couch. The effect of feeding varying levels of dehydrated alfalfa leaf meal on the growth of chicks and poults. Poultry Sci. 29:841. 1950.
Heywang, B. W. High levels of alfalfa meals in diets for chickens. Poultry Sci. 29:804. 1950.
Kodras, R., W. T. Cooney, and J. S. Butts. Effect of alfalfa meal, alfalfa leaves, alfalfa stems, and fresh alfalfa on chick growth. Poultry Sci. 30:786. 1951.
Kodras, R., W. T. Cooney, and J. S. Butts. Chick growth depressing factor in sun-cured and dehydrated alfalfa meals. Poultry Sci. 30: 280. 1951.
Lepkovsky, S., W. Shaeleff, D. Peterson, and R. Perry. Alfalfa inhibitor in chick rations. Poultry Sci. 29:208. 1950.
Peterson, D. W. Alfalfa in chick rations: possible control of growth depressing effect of alfalfa indicated by addition of cholesterol to diet of chicks. Calif. Agr. 4:13. 1950.
Peterson, D. W. Some properties of a factor in alfalfa meal causing depression of growth in chicks. Jour. Biol. Chem. 183:647. 1950.
Peterson, D. W. Effect of sterols on the growth of chicks fed high alfalfa diets or a diet containing Quillaja saponin. Jour. Nutr. 42: 597. 1950.
19. Alder, B. Alfalfa meal as a part of a turkey growing ration. Poultry Sci. 27:651. 1948.
20. Elford, F. C. Corn vs. barley. Rept. Dominion Poultry Husbandryman. Ottawa, Canada. 1928:59
Herner, M. C., A. D. Robinson, and C. H. Whidden. Barley vs. corn

research, 1931-32. Proc. Fifth World's Poultry Congress. 647. Rome. 1933.
Moore, J. M. Barley is satisfactory in poultry ration. Mich. Quart. Bul. 12(4):146. 1930.
Moore, J. M. Barley substituted for corn in poultry ration. Mich. Quart. Bul. 13(2):59. 1930.
Morgan, C. L. Poultry feeding experiments. S. C. Bul. 273. 1931.
Hart, E. B., J. G. Halpin, and O. N. Johnson. Milk substitutes and barley in the Wisconsin chick ration. Wis. Bul. 396:51. 1927.
Kohn, F. J. Feeding poultry. Wyo. Rept. 1930:14.
Lomax, E. B. Study of the comparison of barley and wheat as constituents of the scratch grain. Harper Adams Utility Poultry Jour. 14:67. 1928-1929.
Kitto, H. A. Barley for poultry feeding. A comparison with wheat. New Zealand Jour. Agr. 49:156. 1934.
Hinds, H. B. Poultry studies. Ariz. Bul. 158:169. 1937.
Hinds, H. B. Poultry feeding and confinement rearing experiments. Ariz. Bul. 184. 1942.
Tallent, V. K. The production of table ducklings. Harper Adams Utility Poultry Jour. 17:357. 1931-32.
21. Allman, R. T., and H. D. Branion. A preliminary investigation of the value of corn distillers' dried grains in chick rations. Sci. Agr. 18:700. 1938.
Couch, J. R., J. R. Reed, Jr., R. L. Atkinson, and B. E. Welch. Distillers' grain solubles and dried whey with an APF concentrate in broiler feeds. Proc. 6th Dist. Feed Conf: 47. 1951.
Couch, J. R., J. R. Reed, Jr., B. L. Reid, and J. W. Dieckert. Distillers' solubles and other sources of unidentified factors for promoting the growth of chicks and poults. Proc. 7th Dist. Feed Conf: 43. 1952.
D'Ercole, A. D., W. B. Esselen, Jr., and C. R. Fellers. The nutritive value of distillers' by-products. Poultry Sci. 18:89. 1939.
Dickens, F. L., R. T. Parkhurst, and C. R. Fellers. Corn distillers' dried grains with solubles in poultry rations. II. Laying rations. Poultry Sci. 20:536. 1941.
Ely, C. M. Distillers' solubles in broiler rations. Proc. 3rd Dist. Feed Conf.: 76. 1948.
Marvel, J. A., C. W. Carrick, R. E. Roberts, and S. M. Hauge. Distillers' dried solubles in chick rations containing corn and vegetable protein supplements. Poultry Sci. 24:252. 1945.
Matterson, L. D. Distillers' grain solubles in high energy, low fiber broiler rations. Proc. 4th Dist. Feed Conf.:54. 1949.
Matterson, L. D. Distillers' solubles for rapidly growing broilers. Proc. 5th Dist. Feed Conf.:26. 1950.
Morgan, C. L. The effect of various levels of distillers' grain solubles in a broiler mash upon growth, feathering, and litter condition. Proc. 6th Dist. Conf.: 67. 1951.
Nelson, W. L., Frances E. Voltz, R. T. Parkhurst, and L. R. Parkinson. Corn distillers' by-products in poultry rations. I. Chick rations. Poultry Sci. 23:278. 1944.
Novak, A. F., S. M. Hauge, and C. W. Carrick. An unidentified

growth factor in distillers' dried solubles essential for the chick. Poultry Sci. 26:604. 1947.
Parkhurst, R. T., C. R. Fellers, and J. W. Kuzmeski. Corn distillers' by-products in poultry rations. II. Laying and breeding rations. Poultry Sci. 24:8. 1945.
Parkhurst, R. T., and J. W. Kuzmeski. Supplementing distillers' dried by-products in breeding rations. Poultry Sci. 23:554. 1944.
Parkhurst, R. T., and J. W. Kuzmeski. Supplements for distillers' by-products in poultry breeding diets. Poultry Sci. 25:162. 1946.
Rasmussen, R. A. Observations on feeding high levels of distillers' dried solubles to growing chicks. Proc. 3rd Dist. Feed Conf.:79. 1948.
Ruf, E. W., and J. A. Marvel. Turkey feeds containing distillers' grain solubles. Proc. 5th Dist. Feed Conf.:41. 1950.
Schlamb, K. F., and A. R. Winter. An evaluation of dried distillers' feedstuffs fed to chickens throughout their life cycle. I. During the starting and growing period. Poultry Sci. 27:492. 1948.
Schlamb, K. F., and A. R. Winter. An evaluation of dried distillers' feedstuffs fed to chickens throughout their life cycle. II. During the early reproduction period. Poultry Sci. 27:498. 1948.
Scott, H. M., and W. A. Glista. Growth and feed efficiency studies with broilers with special reference to the use of distillers' grain solubles. Proc. 4th Dist. Feed Conf.: 60. 1949.
Shea, K. G., C. R. Fellers, and R. T. Parkhurst. Corn distillers' dried grains with solubles in poultry rations. I. Chick rations. Poultry Sci. 20:527. 1941.
Sloan, H. J. The use of distillers' by-products in poultry rations. Poultry Sci. 20:83. 1941.
Synold, R. E., C. W. Carrick, R. E. Roberts, and S. M. Hauge. Distillers' dried solubles as a vitamin supplement for chick rations. Poultry Sci. 21:478. 1942.
Synold, R. E., C. W. Carrick, R. E. Roberts, and S. M. Hauge. Distillers' dried solubles as a vitamin supplement in chick rations. Poultry Sci. 22:323. 1943.
22. Buckner, G. D., W. M. Insko, Jr., J. H. Martin, and A. Harms. The influence of distillery slop on the production of chicken fat. Poultry Sci. 17:369. 1938.
Insko, W. M., Jr., G. D. Buckner, J. H. Martin, and A. Harms. Distillery slop in chick rations. Ky. Circ. 46. 1937.
23. Bird, H. R., and J. P. Mattingly. Fermentation solubles in diets for growing chickens. Poultry Sci. 24:34. 1945.
Groschke, A. C., and H. R. Bird. Value of a fermentation by-product in poultry feeds. Md. Bul. A-6:145. 1941.
Record, P. R., R. M. Bethke, D. C. Kennard, and V. D. Chamberlin. The value of B-Y riboflavin supplement for replacing dried skimmilk in an all-mash laying ration. Poultry Sci. 21:476. 1942.
24. Gowell, G. M. Poultry experiments. Maine Bul. 144. 1907.
25. McCollum, E. V., N. Simmonds, and W. Pitz. Is lysine the limiting amino acid in the proteins of wheat, maize or oats? Jour. Biol. Chem. 28:483. 1917.
Mussehl, F. E., J. W. Calvin, D. L. Halbersleben, and R. M. Sand-

stedt. Nutrient requirements of growing chicks: Nutritive deficiencies of corn. Jour. Agr. Res. 22:139. 1921.
Mussehl, F. E., R. Hill, and J. A. Rosenbaum. Corn as a nutrient for growing chicks. Poultry Sci. 5:281. 1926.
Nichita, G., N. Tuschak, and G. Iftimescu. Der Nährwert des Maises bei verschiedenen Hühnerrassen. Rept. Sixth World's Poultry Congress. 302. Germany. 1936.
26. Hart, E. B., H. Steenbock, J. G. Halpin, and O. N. Johnson. New chick feeding facts. Wis. Bul. 371, 1924, 4th Rev. 1929.
Wheeler, W. P. Feeding experiments with laying hens. N. Y. (Geneva) Bul. 29, N. S. 1891.
27. Buss, W. J. Experiments with laying hens. Ohio Bul. 291. 1916.
Buss, W. J. Feeding experiments with laying hens. Ohio Bul. 322. 1918.
Roberts, R. E., and C. W. Carrick. Research solves farm problems. Indiana Rept. 1941:93.
28. Kennard, D. C. Oats for laying hens. Ohio Bul. 431:124. 1927-1928.
Kennard, D. C. Oats for layers. Ohio Bimo. Bul. 146:152. 1930.
Kennard, D. C. Rations for layers. Ohio Bimo. Bul. 155:42. 1932.
Kennard, D. C., and R. M. Bethke. Oats for layers. Ohio Bul. 446: 145. 1930.
Kennard, D. C., and V. D. Chamberlin. Oats for chickens. Ohio Bimo. Bul. 181:95. 1936.
Kennard, D. C., and V. D. Chamberlin. Whole oats for layers. Ohio Farm & Home Res. 32:215. 1947.
29. Prentice, J. H. The use of substitutes for Sussex ground oats in the ration of the laying hen. Jour. Ministry Agr. N. Ireland 5:149. 1937.
30. Taylor, L. W., I. M. Lerner, and K. B. DeOme. An effect of ration on mortality of laying hens. Poultry Sci. 23:181. 1944.
31. Jeffrey, F. P. Poultry mortality as affected by diet. Feedstuffs 16(52):30. 1944.
32. Pennington, M. E., H. A. McAleer, A. D. Greenlee, A. W. Broomell, L. E. Harker, and H. L. Shrader. Wheatless ration for the rapid increase of flesh on young chickens. U.S.D.A., Bur. Animal Indus. Bul. 657. 1918.
33. Waite, R. H. Poultry experiments, observations, notes, and plans. Md. Bul. 244. 1921.
34. Tolentino, C. S. The feeding value of corn bran in rations for growing chicks. Philippine Agr. 24:413. 1935.
35. Davidson, J. A., C. M. McCrary, and C. G. Card. Comparison of hominy feed and ground yellow corn in a broiler ration. Mich. State Quart. Bul. 27:313. 1945.
36. Kennard, D. C., and V. D. Chamberlin. Corn-and-cob meal for growth of pullets and egg production. Ohio Bimo. Bul. 231:268. 1944.
Kennard, D. C., and V. D. Chamberlin. Corn-and-cob meal versus ground shelled corn in rations for chickens. Ohio Bimo. Bul. 241:104. 1946.
37. Grau, C. R. Protein concentrates as amino acid sources for the

chick: Corn gluten meal, cottonseed meal, and peanut meal. Jour. Nutr. 32:303. 1946.

Machlin, L. J., C. A. Denton, and H. R. Bird. Supplementation with vitamin B_{12} and amino acids of chick diets containing soybean or cottonseed meal. Poultry Sci. 31:110. 1952.

Richardson, L. R., and L. G. Blaylock. Supplements to soybean and cottonseed meal diets for poults and growing turkeys. Poultry Sci. 29:651. 1950.

Richardson, L. R., and L. G. Blaylock. Vitamin B_{12} and amino acids as supplements to soybean oil meal and cottonseed meal for growing chicks. Jour. Nutr. 40:169. 1950.

38. Berry, L. N. The value of milo for laying hens. New Mexico Press Bul. 1063. 1952.

Hinds, H. B. Poultry studies. Ariz. Bul. 158:169. 1937.

Hinds, H. B. Poultry feeding and confinement rearing experiments. Ariz. Bul. 184. 1942.

Payne, L. F. The comparative nutritive value of sorghum grain, corn, and wheat as poultry feeds. Kans. Bul. 268. 1934.

Serfontein, P. J. Kaffir corn in poultry rations. Farming in South Africa. 12:136. 1937.

39. Heywang, B. W., and R. B. Morgan. The comparative value of yellow corn, yellow milo, and hegari in a diet for growing chicks. Poultry Sci. 11:307. 1932.

Hammond, J. C. Comparison of corn, milo, and hegari in the diet of laying hens. Poultry Sci. 21:410. 1942.

Penquite, R. M. Grain sorghums are good poultry feeds. Okla. Rept. 1927-1930: 87.

Smith, M. C. The feeding value of the grain sorghums, hegari, and yellow milo, compared with yellow corn. Ariz. Timely Hints for Farmers. No. 161.

40. Black, D. J. G., and J. Getty. Sorghum for poultry feeding. Fertilizer, Feeding Stuffs and Farm Supplies Jour. (Eng.) 36:97. 1950.

McClymont, G. L., D. C. Duncan, and S. Wilkins. Grain sorghum can replace wheat in laying rations. Agric. Gaz. New South Wales. 61:656. 1950.

41. Mitchell, R. E. Variations in starting rations. Ga. Bul. 39:20. 1939.

42. Fronda, F. M., L. P. Zialcita, and E. Basio. Broom corn seeds as a grain feed for layers. Philippine Agr. 30:430. 1941.

43. Ackerson, C. W., M. J. Blish, and F. E. Mussehl. The utilization of food elements by growing chicks. VII. A comparison of corn and kalo in a ration for growing chicks. Neb. Res. Bul. 109. 1939.

44. McClymont, G. L. Grain sorghum—unsatisfactory in chicken rations. The Poultry Farmer (Australia) 20(6):13. 1952.

McClymont, G. L. Studies on nutrition of poultry. III. Toxicity of grain sorghum for chickens. Australian Vet. Jour. 28:229. 1952.

45. Wilson, W. O., and W. E. Poley. Proso millet and oats in poultry rations. S. Dak. Bul. 337. 1940.

46. Goodearl, G. P. Comparison of proso millet and yellow corn for feeding laying hens. N. Dak. Bul. 329. 1943.

47. Goodearl, G. P., and F. E. Moore. Turkey feeding. I. Proso Millet

—a substitute for yellow corn in the ration for growing turkeys. N. Dak. Agr. Exp. Sta. Bul. 303. 1941.

48. Barlow, J. S., S. J. Slinger, and R. P. Zimmer. The reaction of growing chicks to diets varying in NaCl content. Poultry Sci. 27: 542. 1948.

Bearse, G. E., and L. R. Berg. Salt and "pasted vent" condition in baby chicks. Wash. Agr. Exp. Sta. Bul. 482:86. 1946.

Burns, C. H., W. W. Cravens, and P. H. Phillips. The requirement of breeding hens for sodium chloride. Poultry Sci. 31:302. 1952.

Heuser, G. F. Salt additions to chick rations. Poultry Sci. 31:85. 1952.

Mitchell, H. H., and G. C. Carman. Does the addition of sodium chloride increase the value of a corn ration for growing animals. Jour. Biol. Chem. 68:165. 1926.

Parthasarathy, D. Influence of salt on the nitrogen retention of laying hens. Poultry Sci. 29:480. 1950.

Prentice, J. H. The role of salt in poultry nutrition. Jour. Ministry Agr. of N. Ireland 4:72. 1933.

Robertson, S. Salt as the sole mineral. Successful new chick mashes from Northern Ireland. Feathered World. Aug. 21, 1931.

Sjollema, B. Studies on the sodium requirement of chickens and on the consequences of a diet almost free of sodium. Tierernährung 7:184. 1935.

49. Halpin, J. G. Besides salt, what's needed to prevent cannibalism? Wis. Bul. 455:15. 1942.

50. Halpin, J. G., C. E. Holmes, and E. B. Hart. Salt requirements of poultry. Poultry Sci. 15:99. 1936.

51. Mitchell, H. H., L. E. Card, and G. G. Carman. The toxicity of salt for chickens. Ill. Bul. 279. 1926.

52. Quigley, G. D., and R. H. Waite. Salt tolerance of baby chicks. Md. Bul. 340. 1932.

53. Burns, C. H., W. W. Cravens, P. H. Phillips, and J. G. Halpin. Sodium requirements and interrelationships with potassium for chickens. Poultry Sci. 30:752. 1950.

Slinger, S. J., W. F. Pepper, and I. Motzok. Factors affecting the salt requirements of chickens. Poultry Sci. 30:780. 1950.

54. Bird, H. R., J. P. Mattingly, H. W. Titus, J. C. Hammond, W. L. Kellogg, T. B. Clark, C. E. Weakley, Jr., and A. H. VanLandingham. Nutritive evaluation of defluorinated phosphates and other phosphorus supplements. II. Defluorinated phosphates as phosphorus supplements for chicks. Jour. Assoc. Off. Agr. Chem. 28: 118. 1945.

Carver, J. S., and R. J. Evans. Phosphorus supplements in the chick starting mash. U. S. Egg & Poultry Mag. Dec., 1943.

Gerry, R. W., C. W. Carrick, R. E. Roberts, and S. M. Hauge. Phosphate supplements of different fluorine content as sources of phosphorus for chickens. Poultry Sci. 26:323. 1946.

Gillis, M. B., L. C. Norris, and G. F. Heuser. The utilization by the chick of phosphorus from different sources. Jour. Nutr. 35: 195. 1947.

Gillis, M. B., L. C. Norris, and G. F. Heuser. Biological availability of inorganic phosphates. Poultry Sci. 30:914. 1951.

Grau, C. R., and P. A. Zweigart. Phosphatic clay as a phosphorus source for chicks. Poultry Sci. 32:500. 1953.

Johnson, E. L., R. E. Phillips, and G. A. Donovan. Utilization of soft phosphate with colloidal clay. Poultry Sci. 32:907. 1953.

Matterson, L. D., E. P. Singsen, and H. M. Scott. Rock phosphates as phosphorus supplements for the growing chick. Poultry Sci. 24:188. 1945.

55. Bethke, R. M., D. C. Kennard, and C. H. Kick. The availability of calcium in calcium salts and minerals for bone formation in the growing chick. Poultry Sci. 9:45. 1929.

Deobald, H. J., C. A. Elvehjem, E. B. Hart, and J. G. Halpin. Availability of calcium salts for bone formation and rickets prevention in chicks. Poultry Sci. 15:42. 1936.

Hunter, J. E., R. A. Dutcher, and H. C. Knandel. Relative utilization from calcium carbonate and calcium gluconate by chickens. Soc. Exp. Biol. and Med. 31:70. 1933.

56. Buckner, G. D., J. H. Martin, and A. M. Peter. Calcium metabolism in the laying hen. Ky. Bul. 250. 1923.

Phillips, P. H., G. Bohstedt, J. M. Fargo, E. B. Hart, and J. G. Halpin. Learn limitations of rock phosphate as a mineral feed. Wis. Bul. 428:9. 1934.

57. Alder, B. The use of calcite and other natural deposits of calcium carbonate in the ration of laying hens. Proc. Third World's Poultry Congress 231. Canada. 1927.

58. Clark, T. B., H. M. Hyre, C. E. Weakley, Jr., and A. H. VanLandingham. West Virginia limestone—A calcium supplement. West Va. Bul. 345. 1951.

Dupras, C. A., W. Robinson, and C. S. Platt. Oystershell and grit supplements for all-mash poultry feeds. N. Jersey Agr. Exp. Sta. Bul. 762. 1952.

Martin, J. H., and W. M. Insko. Feeding trials with laying hens. II. A comparison of a dull-gray limestone and a shiny white limestone as sources of shell-forming material. Ky. Bul. 294. 1929.

Tully, W. C., and K. W. Franke. Comparative metabolism of several calcareous materials used in poultry feeding. S. Dak. Bul. 287. 1934.

Waite, R. H. Poultry observations, notes, and plans. Md. Bul. 244: 18. 1921.

59. Buckner, G. D., W. M. Insko, Jr., and J. H. Martin. Marl for laying hens. Poultry Sci. 14:125. 1935.

60. Edin, H., and A. Anderson. Kalkstengrus, ostronskal och messelskal som Kompletterings-foder till Kalkfattiga foderstater vid hög äggproduktion. Rept. 476. Central Inst. Agr. Res. Stockholm. 60. 1937. (Reference in Nut. Abst. 7:785. 1938.)

Fangauf, R., and O. Brüninghaus. Haben Austernschalen bei der Legehennenfütterung einen besonderen Vorzug gegenüber gewöhnlichen Muschelschalen? Archiv für Geflügelk. 9:180. 1935.

61. Scholes, J. C. Feeding of coquina shell to laying hens. Poultry Sci. 24:53. 1945.

62. Voelcker, J. A. Oystershell and cockle shell for poultry. Jour. Ministry Agr. (London) 37:1002. 1931.
63. Brophy, J., and E. J. Sheehy. Irish coral sand as a source of lime for laying hens. Irish Free State Dept. Agr. Jour. 38:387. 1941.
Tanaka, J., A. L. Palafox, and M. M. Rosengerg. A comparison of three sources of calcium for laying chickens. Hawaii Agr. Exp. Sta. Progress Notes, 68. 1951.
64. Blair, W. S. Oystershell vs. clam shell. Canada Exp. Farms (Kentville, N. S.) Rept. 1923:67.
Miller, M. W., and G. E. Bearse. Mineral supplements for laying hens. Wash. Bul. 320. 1935.
Tully, W. C., and K. W. Franke. Comparative metabolism of several calcareous materials used in poultry feeding. S. Dak. Bul. 287. 1934.
65. Gutteridge, H. S., and J. M. Pratt. Eggshells as a source of calcium for laying birds. Poultry Sci. 24:87. 1945.
66. Dodd, F. R., and A. P. Telford. "Sussex Ground" oats. Harper Adams Utility Poultry Jour. 23:77. 1937-1938.
67. Bearse, G. E., V. L. Miller, and C. F. McClary. The cannibalism preventing properties of the fiber fraction of oat hulls. Poultry Sci. 19:210. 1940.
Miller, M. W., and G. E. Bearse. The cannibalism preventing properties of oats. Poultry Sci. 16:314. 1937.
Miller, M. W., and G. E. Bearse. The cannibalism preventing properties of oat hulls. Poultry Sci. 17:466. 1938.
68. Wilcke, H. L. Oats rank first for poultry feed. Iowa Farm Sci. Reporter. January, 1940.
69. Fangauf, R., and R. Deditius; J. Jaeger and E. Rühle; L. Weinmiller and K. Voigt; K. Richter and H. Brüggemann; H. Bünger, J Schulz, Augustin, and Fissmer. Fütterungsversuche über die Verwendung von Hafer als Körnerfutter bei Legehennen. Archiv für Geflügelk. 9:137. 1935.
70. Hall, M. D., and A. G. Clark. Werribee 1947-48 poultry feeding tests. The Poultry Farmer (Australia). Oct. 9, 1948: 9.
McArdle, A. A. Five years of poultry feeding and housing trials. The Poultry Farmer (Australia) 17 (32):10. 1950.
71. Carlson, C. W., W. Kohlmeyer, D. G. Jones, and A. L. Moxon. Levels of oats in turkey growing rations. Poultry Sci. 30:909. 1951.
72. Carrick, C. W., and R. E. Roberts. Studies on feed efficiency. II. The relative efficiency of corn and oats in chick rations. Poultry Sci. 27:213. 1948.
Roberts, R. E., and C. W. Carrick. Ground oats as a substitute for wheat bran and wheat middlings in rations for chicks. Poultry Sci. 13:135. 1934.
73. Upp, C. W. Rice and rice by-products as feeds for laying hens. La. Bul. 243. 1933.
Palafox, A. L., and M. M. Rosenberg. A comparison of corn, brown rice, and wheat in chick rations. World's Poultry Sci. Jour. 8:6. 1952.

Smith, R. M. Value of rice by-products for laying hens. Ark. Bul. 231:41. 1928.

Smith, R. M. Poultry experiments at the Arkansas Station. Ark. Bul. 246:43. 1929.

Smith, R. M. The value of rice by-products in feeding poultry. Proc. Poultry Science Assn., Ala. Bul. Vol. XXV, No. 1:29. January, 1930.

Smith, R. M. Value of rice by-products for laying hens. Ark. Bul. 257:47. 1930.

Smith, R. M. The value of rice products in the growing ration. Ark. Bul. 268:42. 1931.

Smith, R. M. The value of rice by-products for laying hens. Ark. Rept. 1932:38.

Smith, R. M. Rice by-products in the poultry ration for egg production and growth. Ark. Bul. 304. 1934.

Smith, R. M. Rice products for poultry. Ark. Bul. 464:12. 1946.

Smith, R. M. The use of rice and rice by-products in the laying ration. Ark. Bul. 478. 1948.

Lloyd, W. E. Rice feeds for poultry. Calif. Rept. 1918-1919:81.

Stout, S. R. Value of rice by-products for laying hens. Ark. Bul. 203:26. 1926.

Stout, S. R. Value of rice by-products for laying hens. Ark. Bul. 215:32. 1926.

Stout, S. R. Value of rice by-products for laying hens. Ark. Bul. 221:40. 1927.

74. Zöllner, I. Roggen in Legehennenfütter. Deutsche landwirtschaftl. Geflügelzeitung, p. 852. 1932.

Bünger, H., R. Fangauf, A. Haensel, K. Richter, and H. Brüggemann. Fütterungsversuche mit Roggen als Körnerfütter für Legehennen. Archiv für Geflügelk. 10:33. 1936.

75. Halpin, J. G., and C. E. Holmes. Rye proves unsatisfactory in chick feeding trials. Wis. Bul. 421:129. 1932.

Halpin, J. G., and C. E. Holmes. Rye does not retard egg production of pullets. Wis. Bul. 428:49. 1934.

Halpin, J. G., and C. E. Holmes. Rye satisfactory for growing pullets and laying hens but not for baby chicks. Wis. Bul. 430:148. 1935.

Halpin, J. G., C. E. Holmes, and E. B. Hart. Rye as a feed for poultry. Poultry Sci. 15:3. 1936.

76. North, M. O. The effect of various grains upon egg production. Wyo. Rept. 1932-1933:7

North, M. O. Poultry feeding, housing, and lighting experiments at the Wyoming Experiment Station. Wyo. Bul. 203. 1934.

77. Ackerson, C. W., W. E. Ham, and F. E. Mussehl. The utilization of food elements by growing chicks. XI. A comparison of ground wheat and ground rye in rations for growing chicks. Neb. Sta. Res. Bul. 146. 1946.

78. Halnan, E. T. Digestibility trials with poultry. IX. Digestibility and metabolizable energy of sunflowerseeds. Jour. Agr. Sci. (Eng.) 33:113. 1943.

79. Smith, C. D., and C. S. Brooks. Some experiments with poultry. Mich. Bul. 158. 1898.
80. Biely, J., and B. March. Wheat of different protein content in the chick ration. Poultry Sci. 28:756. 1949.
March, B., J. Biely, and J. Tonzetich. Supplementation of wheat with amino acids in the diet of the chick. Jour. Nutr. 42:565 1950.
81. McClymont, G. L., and L. Hart. Studies on nutrition of poultry. 1. Investigations on the inadequacy of high wheat content rations for hatchability in White Leghorn pullets. Australian Vet. Jour. 23:247. 1947.
82. Roberts, R. E., and C. W. Carrick. Wheat as a substitute for corn in broiler rations. Indiana Rept. 1938:81.
83. Goodearl, G. P. Shrunken wheat for laying hens. N. Dak. Bul. 297. 1941.
McArdle, A. A. Five years of poultry feeding and housing trials. The Poultry Farmer (Australia) 17 (32):10. 1950.
84. Quigley, G. D. The effect of wheat upon the incidence of pullet disease or blue comb. Poultry Sci. 23:386. 1944.
O'Neill, J. B., and W. J. Rae. Is the type of wheat fed a factor in "New Wheat Disease"? Poultry Sci. 23:548. 1944.
Quigley, G. D. Further studies with wheat and pullet disease. Poultry Sci. 27:647. 1948.
85. Falcon-Lesses, M. The cause of the laxative action of bran. Jour. Nutr. 2:295. 1930.
86. The value of bran for egg production. Jour. Ministry Agr., N. Ireland. 4:42. 1936.
87. Taylor, L. W., and I. M. Lerner. Effect of varying levels of wheat bran on age at sexual maturity. Poultry Sci. 18:323. 1939.
88. Mussehl, F. E., C. W. Ackerson, and M. J. Blish. The influence of whole wheat, bran, and shorts on body weight and feather growth in chicks. Neb. Res. Bul. 119. 1940.
89. Embleton, H. Poultry feeding experiments. Ariz. Bul. 177. 1941.
90. Bearse, G. E. Mill run in the breeders' mash. Northwestern Miller 205:31. 1941.
91. Poley, W. E. The utilization of wheat and wheat by-products in the feeding of young chickens. III. Ground wheat, bran, and middlings as sources of the antineuritic vitamin B. Poultry Sci. 17:338. 1938.
Poley, W. E. The utilization of wheat and wheat by-products in feeding young chickens. IV. Ground wheat as a source of vitamin G growth factor. Unknown factors which affect plumage, color, and structure. Poultry Sci. 17:390. 1938.
Poley, W. E. The utilization of wheat and wheat by-products in feeding young chickens. V. Protein supplements for ground wheat. Poultry Sci. 17:399. 1938.
92. Carrick, C. W., and R. E. Roberts. Studies on feed efficiency. I. The relative efficiency of corn and wheat products in chick rations. Poultry Sci. 26:111. 1946.
93. Hewitt, A. C. T. Poultry feeding experiments. The Poultry Farmer: 10:17. New South Wales. 1942.

94. Rhys, I. W. Wheat meal in all-mash rations for poultry. Harper Adams Utility Poultry Jour. 17:352. 1931-1932.
Rhys, I. W. Wheat meal in all-mash rations for poultry. Harper Adams Utility Poultry Jour. 17. Supplement. 1932.
Stewart, W. A. Notes on feeding wheat versus oats in a laying mash. Jour. Ministry Agr. Great Britain. 41:83. 1934-1935.
95. Tully, W. C. Wheat and wheat by-products for laying hens. S. Dak. Bul. 284. 1934.
Poley, W. E. The utilization of wheat and wheat by-products in feeding young chickens. I. The effect of the fineness of grinding wheat. II. Alfalfa leaf meal as a vitamin A supplement for ground wheat. Poultry Sci. 17:331. 1938.
96. Heuser, G. F., L. C. Norris, H. T. Peeler, and M. L. Scott. Further studies on the apparent effect of digestibility upon growth, weight maintenance, and egg production. Poultry Sci. 23:552. 1944. Poultry Sci. 24:142. 1945.
97. Draper, C. I. Algaroba beans, pigeon peas, and processed garbage in the laying mash. Hawaii Progress Notes 44. 1944.
Draper, C. I. Algaroba bean meal in turkey rations. Hawaii Circ. 23. 1945.
98. Parkhurst, R. T. The value of certain vegetable protein feeds supplementing sour skimmilk in a ration for laying hens. Idaho Circ. 43:8. 1927.
99. Mangold, E., and H. Damköhler. Versuche über die Wirkung der Holzkohle bei der Kükenaufzucht sowie auf die Verdauungsfunktionen und Futterausnutzung des Geflügels. Archiv für Geflügelk. 10:289. 1936.
100. Sipe, G. R. Value of charcoal for laying hens. Miss. Rept. 1929: 28.
Sipe, G. R. Charcoal in the ration for laying hens. Miss. Rept. 1938:48.
101. Hodgson, G. C. Wood charcoal as a supplement to poultry rations. Master's Thesis. Cornell University. 1938.
102. Almquist, H. J., and D. Zander. Adsorbing charcoals in chick diets. Proc. Soc. Exp. Biol. and Med. 45:303. 1940.
103. Hunt, C. H. Use of wrong carrier may result in serious vitamin losses. Ohio Farm and Home Research, July–Aug., 1952.
104. Temperton, H., and I. G. Shaw. The toxic principle in cocoa wastes. Harper Adams Utility Poultry Jour. 28:15. 1943.
105. Fangauf, R., and A. Haensel. Bericht über einen Fütterungsversuch mit Kakaoschalenmehl bei Legehühnern. Archiv für Geflügelk. 12:54. 1938.
106. Temperton, H., and F. J. Dudley. Coconut cake meal as a food for laying hens. Harper Adams Utility Poultry Jour. 26:213. 1941.
107. Serfontein, P. J. Cowpeas as a poultry feed. Farming in South Africa, Oct., 1944.
108. Decker, M., and F. H. Clickner. Feeding value of "protozyme" for poultry. N. J. Hints 15 (1). 1926.
Clickner, F. H., and E. H. Follwell. Application of "protozyme" (Aspergillus oryzae) to poultry feeding. Poultry Sci. 5:241. 1926.

109. Holst, W. F. "Artificial" enzymes and poultry feeding. Poultry Sci. 5:261. 1926.
Hastings, W. H. Enzyme supplements to poultry feeds. Poultry Sci. 25:584. 1946.
110. Bice, C. M. Cane molasses in poultry rations. Hawaii Bul. 67. 1933.
Rosenberg, M. M. A study of B-grade and refinery B-molasses in layer rations. Poultry Sci. 32:605. 1953.
111. Black strap molasses in poultry rations. La. Bul. 262:30. 1935.
Snell, M. G., C. W. Upp, and R. H. Lush. Blackstrap molasses as a livestock feed. La. Circ. 19. 1937.
Upp, C. W. Cane molasses in poultry rations. La. Bul. 289. 1937.
112. Winter, A. R. Cane molasses for poultry. Poultry Sci. 8:369. 1929.
113. Norris, L. C., and G. F. Heuser. The nutritive properties of poultry feedstuffs. Cornell Rept. 1935:130.
114. Maw, A. J. G. Feeding cane molasses to growing chicks and laying hens. Sci. Agr. 13:743. 1933.
115. Ott, W. H., R. V. Boucher, and H. C. Knandel. Feeding cane molasses as a constituent of poultry rations. I. Molasses for growing chickens. Poultry Sci. 21:340. 1942.
Ott, W. H., R. V. Boucher, and H. C. Knandel. Feeding cane molasses as a constituent of poultry rations. II. Molasses for adult chickens. Poultry Sci. 21:536. 1942.
116. Cooney, W. T., and J. E. Parker. Wood sugar molasses as a feedstuff for laying hens. Poultry Sci. 31:343. 1952.
Cooney, W. T., and J. E. Parker. Wood sugar molasses in the ration of floor managed layers. Poultry Sci. 32:1039. 1953.
McGinnis, J., H. I. MacGregor, and J. S. Carver. Wood sugar molasses as a feedstuff for chicks. Poultry Sci. 27:459. 1948.
117. Kennard, D. C. Add cooked potatoes to chickens' ration. Ohio Bimo. Bul. 14(1):25. 1929.
Kennard, D. C. Potatoes for chickens. Ohio Bimo. Bul. 182:111. 1936.
Kennard, D. C. Potatoes for chickens. Ohio Bimo. Bul. 31 (243): 176. 1946.
118. Höje, J. Verdauungsversuche über Kartoffelfütterung an Hühnern. Der Geflügelhof 43:678, 1947.
119. Elford, F. C. Potatoes vs. corn meal in fattening. Rept. Dominion Poultry Husband. Ottawa, Canada. 1927:22.
Experimental Station, Frederickton, New Brunswick, Canada. Report of the Superintendent. 1929:50.
120. Sheehy, E. J., and E. M. Burke. Feeding potatoes and oats to growing chickens. Irish Free State Dept. Agr. Jour. 38:361. 1941.
121. Klooster, M. J., and C. G. Card. Potatoes as a feed for chickens. Mich. Sta. Quart. Bul. 19:104. 1936.
122. Finne, I. Foring av verpehons. Norsk Landbruk 2:592. 1936.
Finne, I., and T. B. Hesthamar. Forsok med Norskavlet for til verpehoner. Second Rept. from the State Training School for Teachers to Smallholders. 1939:42.

Finne, I. Potatoes and skimmilk as feed for laying hens. Rept. Seventh World's Poultry Congress. 153. Cleveland. 1939.

Finne, I. Forsok med store mengder poteter til verpehoner. Meld. Stat. Smabr. laeversk 28:59. 1944

123. Kohn, F. J. Feeding poultry. Wyo. Rept. 1930:14.

124. Halnan, E. T. The digestibility and metabolizable energy of raw and cooked potatoes, potato flakes, dried potato slices, and dried potato shreds. Jour. Agr. Sci. (Eng.) 33:139. 1944.

Halnan, E. T., and C. E. Fermor. Surplus potatoes in poultry feeding. Agriculture. 49:175. 1942.

McMillan, A. M., and F. J. Dudley. Steamed potatoes in table poultry rations. Harper Adams Utility Poultry Jour. 25:251. 1939-1940.

Temperton, H., and F. J. Dudley. Steamed potatoes for laying pullets. Harper Adams Utility Poultry Jour. 25:177. 1939-1940.

Temperton, H., and F. J. Dudley. The feeding of high levels of potatoes as the main food for laying pullets. Harper Adams Utility Poultry Jour. 27:175. 1942.

Temperton, H., and F. J. Dudley. The feeding of raw and cooked potatoes and sugarbeet to laying pullets. Jour. Agr. Sci. (Eng.) 33:204. 1943.

Temperton, H., and F. J. Dudley. The feeding of steamed potatoes to breeding stock. Harper Adams Utility Poultry Jour. 28:34. 1943.

Temperton, H., and F. J. Dudley. Rearing pullets from 8 weeks of age on potatoes, alfalfa meal, and meat meal. Harper Adams Utility Poultry Jour. 28:9. 1943.

Temperton, H., and F. J. Dudley. The use of dried grass and potatoes in rations for growing pullets. Harper Adams Utility Poultry Jour. 29:31. 1944.

Temperton, H., and F. J. Dudley. "Free choice" feeding as a method of supplementing swill and potato rations for laying pullets. Harper Adams Utility Poultry Jour. 30:5. 1945.

Wright, M. M., and F. J. Dudley. An experiment on the feeding of steamed potatoes and swedes to laying ducks. Harper Adams Utility Poultry Jour. 25:225. 1939-1940.

Wright, M. M., and F. J. Dudley. Feeding of laying ducks on high levels of steamed potatoes. Harper Adams Utility Poultry Jour. 27:195. 1942.

Wright, M. M., and F. J. Dudley. Rearing ducklings on town food waste and steamed potatoes. Harper Adams Utility Poultry Jour. 29:35. 1944.

Wright, M. M., and F. J. Dudley. Semi-dried town food waste and steamed potatoes for laying ducks reared on these foods. Harper Adams Utility Poultry Jour. 30:19. 1945.

125. Alberti, F., and M. Mehnert. Vergleichenden Fütterungsversuch mit Kartoffelflocken und Maisschrot.. Archiv für Geflügelk. 7:10. 1933.

Bienko, G., and A. Liersch. Zur Frage der Kartoffelfütterung an Legehennen. Archiv für Geflügelk. 7:261. 1933.

Fangauf, R. Kartoffelschnitzelschrot im Kukenfutter. Archiv für Geflügelk. 17:27. 1953.
Fangauf, R., and O. Brüninghaus. Hohe Gaben von Kartoffeln und Zuckerrübenschrot im Mischfutter der Legehennen. Archiv für Geflügelk. 9:269. 1935.
Carstens, P., and J. Prüfer. Ein Beitrag zur Frage der Verfütterung von Magermilch, Kartoffeln, und Kartoffelflocken an Legehennen. Züchtungskunde 10:453. 1935.
Dahmköhler, H. Beobachtungen bei einer Kükenaufzucht mit gekochten Kartoffeln, Haferschrot, und Magermilch. Deutsche Landwirtschaftliche Geflügelzeitung. 28. October, 1937.
Fangauf, R., and R. Deditius. Kartoffelflocken als Ersatz für Maisschrot bei Legehühnern. Archiv für Geflügelk. 6:372. 1932.
Liebscher, W. Fütterungsversuch mit eingesäuerten Kartoffeln bei Lege und Zuchthühnern. Biedermanns Zentralbl (B) Tiernernährung. 10:385. 1938.
Mangold, E. Verdaulichkeit und biologische Wertigkeit von Kartoffeleiweiss beim Schwein und Geflügel. Der Forschungsdienst 5(1). 1937.
Mangold, E. Versuche über Ausnutzung und Futterwert Wirtschaftseigener Futtermittel. Rept. Seventh World's Poultry Congress. 159. Cleveland. 1939.
Mangold, E., and H. Damköhler. Versuche über Kükenaufzucht bis zur Legereife mit den neuen, mit mechanischer Vorentwässerung hergestellten Kartoffelflocken. Archiv für Geflügelk. 10:55. 1936.
Mangold, E., A. Hock, and H. Damköhler. Versuche über die Verdaulichkeit neuer Kartoffeleiweiss Produkte bei Hühnern und über ihre Eignung als Eiweissfutter zur Küken Aufzucht. Archiv für Geflügelk. 11:382. 1937.
Stahl, W. Kartoffelfütterung beim Geflügel. Rept. Sixth World's Poultry Congress. 341. Germany. 1936.
Wehner, A. Kartoffeln im Legehennenfutter. Archiv für Geflügelk. 7:289. 1933.
Weinmiller, L., and K. Voigt. Kartoffelflocken für wachsende Jungtiere. Archiv für Geflügelk. 9:372. 1935.

126. Bolton, W., and R. W. Hale. Dried potato products for egg production: Statistical analysis of a laying experiment. Jour. Agr. Sci. (Eng.) 35:158. 1945.
127. Smyth, J. R., R. W. Gerry, and C. E. Howes. Dehydrated potatoes as a substitute for corn in a chick ration. Maine Bul. 473:66. 1949.
128. Kratzer, F. H., Blanche Marshall, and D. E. Williams. Potatoes for poultry. Value of dried potatoes as feed for chicks and poults investigated. Calif. Agric. 3:10. 1949.
129. Heuser, G. F., M. L. Scott, R. K. Eskew, and P. W. Edwards. Studies in duck nutrition, III. The feeding of potatoes to ducks. Poultry Sci. 30:672. 1951.
130. Musseh1, F. E., R. Borchers, and C. W. Ackerson. Potato byproducts for chicks. Neb. 60th Ann. Report: 69. 1946.

131. Gerry, R. W., J. R. Smyth, and C. E. Howes. Potato products for poultry. 1. The value of a potato starch waste product in rations for growing chicks. Poultry Sci. 30:913. 1951.
Gerry, R. W., J. R. Smyth, C. E. Howes, M. E. Highlands, J. J. Licciardello, J. S. Getchell, and B. E. Plummer, Jr. Potato products as poultry feed. Maine Bul. 491:67. 1951.
132. Sweet potatoes for chickens. La. Bul. 262:32. 1935.
Tillman, A. D., and H. J. Davis. Studies on the use of dehydrated sweet potato meal in chick rations. La. Bul. 358. 1943.
133. Polk, H. D. Dehydrated sweet potatoes for chicks. Miss. Rept. 1943:28.
Rosenberg, M. M., and J. Seu. Sweet potato root meal versus yellow corn meal in the chick's diet. World's Poultry Sci. Jour. 8:93. 1952.
134. Dearstyne, R. S., W. J. Peterson, and W. B. Nesbit. Sweet potato flour in turkey starting mash. Res. and Farming (N. C.) 3, Prog. Rept. 1:6. 1944.
Lease, E. J., and J. H. Mitchell. Biochemical and nutritional studies of dehydrated sweet potato. S. Car. Bul. 329. 1940.
135. Hartwell, B. L., and W. F. Kirkpatrick. Protein concentrates for winter chickens. R. I. Bul. 145. 1911.
136. Rosenberg, M. M. Low grade sugar, a potential carbohydrate feedstuff for laying chickens. Poultry Sci. 31:933. 1952. Poultry Sci. 32:69. 1953.
137. Mangold, E., and H. Rüdiger. Die Verwendung der Steffen'schen Zuckerrübenschnitzel zur Fütterung der Hühner. Archiv für Geflügelk. 6:193. 1932.
Müller, H. Aufzucht mit Wirtschaftseigenen Futtermitteln, Versuch über die Verfütterung von Zuckerschnitzelschrot an Küken. Rept. Seventh World's Poultry Congress. 157. Cleveland. 1939.
138. Temperton, H., and F. J. Dudley. The feeding of raw and cooked potatoes and sugar beet to laying pullets. Jour. Agr. Sci. (Eng.) 33:204. 1943.
Halnan, E. T. Digestibility trials with poultry. VIII. The digestibility of dried molasses sugar-beet pulp. Jour. Agr. Sci. (Eng.) 27:137. 1937.
139. Kempster, H. L., and E. M. Funk. Influence of yeast on growth of White Leghorn chicks. Mo. Bul. 310:49. 1932.
Halpin, J. G., and C. E. Holmes. Yeast fails to improve a good poultry ration. Wis. Bul. 421:127. 1932.
140. Mussehl, F. E., and C. W. Ackerson. The growth promoting value of yeast added to certain chick rations. Poultry Sci. 10:369. 1931.
Grau, C. R., and M. Kamei. Yeast culture investigations. Live yeast culture tested for production efficiency as feedstuff for chicks. Calif. Agric. 3:13. 1949.
141. Cassel, L. W. Feeding experiments with Leghorns. Wash. Bul. 210. 1927.
Carver, J. S. The supplementary value of yeast in the laying ration. Wash. Bul. 354. 1937.
Barton, O. A. Experiments with poultry at the North Dakota Station. N. Dak. Bul. 233:108. 1930.

142. Dearstyne, R. S., and C. O. Bollinger. Some effects of feeding yeast fermented mash to laying pullets. N. C. Bul. 55. 1938.
143. Temperton, H., and F. J. Dudley. Fodder yeast for laying pullets. Harper Adams Poultry Jour. 26:172. 1941.
144. Temperton, H. Feeding of acorns to laying pullets and ducks. Empire Jour. Exp. Agr. 11:175. 1943.
145. Kratzer, F. H., and A. M. Vance. Beet seed tested for poultry feed and litter material in experiments at station. Col. Farm. Bul. 6(5):7. 1944.
146. Whitson, D., N. R. Ellis, and C. A. Cabell. Chewings fescue seed as a feedstuff. Poultry Sci. 23:544. 1944.
147. Driggers, J. C. Citrus seed meal for chicks. Proc. Assn. Southern Agr. Workers, 1950:143.
Driggers, J. C., G. K. Davis, and N. R. Mehrhof. Citrus seed meal for growing chicks. Poultry Sci. 28:762. 1949.
Driggers, J. C., G. K. Davis, and N. R. Mehrhof. Feeding value of citrus meal and citrus seed meal for poultry. Fla. Exp. Sta. Rept. 1947:63.
Mehrhof, N. R., and L. L. Rusoff. Utilization of citrus by-products for poultry. Fla. Rept. 1937:61. Fla. Rept. 1938:69.
Mehrhof, N. R., and L. L. Rusoff. Utilization of citrus meal for poultry. Rept. Seventh World's Poultry Congress. 209. Cleveland. 1939.
148. Hammond, J. C. Dried coffee grounds unsuitable for use in the diet of growing chickens. Poultry Sci. 23:454. 1944.
149. Hunt, K., E. T. Halnan, M. S. Pease, T. Ashton, and D. Page. Feeding trials with household garbage. Harper Adams Utility Poultry Jour. 28:37. 1943.
Temperton, H., and F. J. Dudley. The feeding of town kitchen waste to laying pullets. Harper Adams Utility Poultry Jour. 27:244. 1942.
Temperton, H., and F. J. Dudley. The feeding of high levels of semi-dried town kitchen waste to laying stock. Harper Adams Utility Poultry Jour. 28:49. 1943.
Temperton, H., and F. J. Dudley. Feeding processed kitchen waste to laying pullets. Harper Adams Utility Poultry Jour. 28:59. 1943.
Temperton, H., and F. J. Dudley. Feeding processed food waste (swill) to growing chickens. Harper Adams Utility Poultry Jour. 29:1. 1944.
Temperton, H., and F. J. Dudley. Supplementary protein in swill rations for laying pullets. Harper Adams Utility Poultry Jour. 30:1. 1945.
Temperton, H., and F. J. Dudley. The use of fortified dried food waste for laying pullets reared on diets containing this food. Harper Adams Utility Poultry Jour. 30:50. 1945.
Wright, M. M., and F. J. Dudley. Rearing ducklings on town food waste and steamed potatoes. Harper Adams Utility Poultry Jour. 29:35. 1944.
Wright, M. M., and F. J. Dudley. Semi-dried town food waste and steamed potatoes for laying ducks reared on these feeds. Harper Adams Utility Poultry Jour. 30:19. 1945.

150. Pierson, K. W. Preliminary experiments on feeding processed garbage meal to poultry. *Hawaii Progress Notes* 40. 1943.
Draper, C. I. Utilization of raw garbage by growing ducks. *Hawaii Progress Notes* 42. 1944.
Draper, C. I. Processed garbage meal in the chick ration. *Poultry Sci.* 24:442. 1945.
151. Hammond, J. C. Cow manure as a source of certain vitamins for growing chickens. *Poultry Sci.* 21:554. 1942.
Hammond, J. C. Cow manure as an ingredient of turkey diets. *Poultry Sci.* 23:358. 1944.
Hammond, J. C. Dried cow manure and dried rumen contents as a partial substitute for alfalfa leaf meal. *Poultry Sci.* 23:471. 1944.
152. Cravens, W. W., W. McGibbon, and J. G. Halpin. "Vegetarian" poultry rations a possibility. Wisc. Bul. 469:49. 1946.
153. Temperton, H., and F. J. Dudley. Palm kernel and earthnut meals in the rations for laying pullets. *Harper Adams Utility Poultry Jour.* 25(11). 1940.
Temperton, H., and F. J. Dudley. Nutrition in wartime. *Empire Jour. Exp. Agr.* 9:248. 1941.
154. Usuelli, F., and D. P. Fiorni. Preliminary experiments on the nutritive value of the contents of the rumen on the growth of chickens. *Rept. Seventh World's Poultry Congress.* 203. Cleveland. 1939.
155. Temperton, H., and F. J. Dudley. Feeding straw extract to laying pullets. *Harper Adams Utility Poultry Jour.* 28:18. 1943.
156. Columbus, A. Die Ausnutzung und biologische Wertigkeit der Süsslupinen Körner. *Forschungsdienst.* 1:536. 1936.
157. McMillan, A. M., and F. J. Dudley. Potato meal, tapioca meal, and town waste in chicken rations. *Harper Adams Utility Poultry Jour.* 24:191. 1941.
158. Esselen, W. B., Jr., and C. R. Fellers. The nutritive value of dried tomato pumace. *Poultry Sci.* 18:45. 1939.
159. Fangauf, R., and A. Haensel. Bericht über einen Fütterungsversuch mit Holzzucker bei Hühnern. *Archiv für Geflügelk.* 11:249. 1938.
Weinmiller, L., and K. Mantel. Fütterungsversuch mit Verwendung von Futterzucher. *Archiv für Geflügelk.* 12:47. 1938.
160. Bice, C. M. Poultry feed supplements. *Hawaii Circ.* 4. April 1932.
Bice, C. M., and B. A. Tower. Crossbreeding poultry for meat production, including a feeding test of taro waste and poi. *Hawaii Bul.* 81. 1939.
161. Chan, G. S., and J. D. Guiyab. Comparative studies of the value of corn and palay as feed for chickens. *Philippine Agr.* 23:49. 1934.
Fernandez, C. J. The relative value of tahup sa mais and rice bran in rations for egg production. *Philippine Agr.* 23:529. 1934.
Tabayoyong, T. T. The value of cassava refuse meal in the ration for growing chicks. *Philippine Agr.* 24:509. 1935.
162. Raimo, H. F., and G. L. daRocha. Contribuicao para o estudo dos

substitutos dos farelos de trigo na alimentacao das aves. I. Cereal adlay. Boletim de Industria Animal (Brazil) 11:85. 1950.
Falanghe, O. Substituicao dos farelos de trigo por farelos de arroz e mandioca na alimentacao de poedeiras. Biologica (Sao Paulo) 15:35. 1949.
Schaaffhausen, R. V. Adlay or Job's tears—A cereal of potentially greater economic importance. Economic Botany 6:216. 1952.
Newell, G. W., W. H. Peterson, and C. A. Elvehjem. The value of dried penicillin mycelium as a supplement in practical chick rations. Poultry Sci. 26:284. 1946.
Combs, G. F. Algae (Chlorella) as a source of nutrients for the chick. Science 116:453. 1952.
Kratzer, F. H., and D. E. Williams. Raisins for turkeys. Calif. Agric. 5:13. 1951.
163. Platt, C. S. Green banana meal in the poultry ration. Poultry Sci. 29:614. 1950.
Kratzer, F. H., and D. W. Williams. The value of ground carob in rations for chicks. Poultry Sci. 30:148. 1951.
Temperton, H. Feeding horse chestnuts and elderberries to poultry. Nature 152:345. 1943.
Cravens, W. W., W. McGibbon, and J. G. Halpin. ''Vegetarian poultry rations a possibility. Wisc. Bul. 469:49. 1946.
Thayer, R. H., and V. G. Heller. Vicia Villosa (vetch): Chemical composition and use in poultry rations. Proc. Okla. Acad. Sci. 26:40. 1946.

CHAPTER 6

POULTRY FEEDS—ANIMAL PROTEIN SUPPLEMENTS

Poultry rations are composed largely of cereals and cereal by-products. It is necessary to include some protein concentrates in order to satisfy the protein requirements. A wide variety of ingredients will serve this purpose.

MEAT PRODUCTS

"MEAT is the clean, wholesome flesh derived from slaughtered mammals and is limited to that part of the striate muscle which is skeletal or that which is found in the tongue, in the diaphragm, in the heart, or in the esophagus and does not include that found in the lips, in the snout, or in the ears; with or without the accompanying and overlying fat and the portions of skin, sinew, nerve, and blood vessels which normally accompany the flesh. If it bears a name descriptive of its kind it must correspond thereto.

"The term 'meat' when applied to the corresponding portions of animals other than cattle, swine, sheep, and goats shall be used in qualified form, as, for example, 'horse meat,' 'reindeer meat,' 'whale meat,' etc."

Meat has been used largely in the diet because it possesses many desirable characteristics. It is very palatable, is easily digested, and also has a high nutritive value. It is rich in protein and in such minerals as phosphorus and iron.

Meat scraps and tankage[1] are prepared from the inedible portion of slaughtered animals and from entire carcasses of diseased and dead animals. The material is rendered to extract the fat, and the residues are used for feed or fertilizer. The raw materials may be obtained from (1) slaughter houses, in which case it consists usually of cavity contents, trimmings, and cracklings, (2) dead animal rendering plants, (3) city fat smelters, and (4) hotel and restaurant waste rendering plants.

"MEAT MEAL OR MEAT SCRAP is the finely ground, dry-rendered residue from animal tissues exclusive of hair, hoof, horn, blood, manure, and stomach contents, except in such traces as might occur unavoidably in good factory practice. When these products contain more than 4.4 per cent of phosphorus (P), they shall be designated either 'Meat and Bone Meal' or 'Meat and Bone Scrap.' If the product bears a name descriptive of its kind, composition, or origin it must correspond thereto. It must be designated and sold according to its protein content."

Meat scraps consist only of dry-rendered tissues and contain no blood or "stick." In the dry-rendering process the materials are heated in steam-jacketed tanks. No water is added directly to the materials. The fat is removed, and the remaining cake or cracklings is ground to make the meat scraps. Meat scraps are high in protein, usually having about 45 to 60 per cent. Occasionally a product contains less than 45 per cent, especially when the bone content is unusually high. On the other hand, some meat scraps contain as much as 75 or 80 per cent protein. Ordinarily, the fat content is relatively low, and it should be practically free of fiber.

The nutritive value of these products[2] varies considerably, depending upon the kind of material from which they are made and the conditions of manufacture. For example, the organs of the body have higher feeding value than the other tissues. Meat products are also likely to contain varying amounts of connective tissue, made up largely of collagen or gelatin which is deficient in such amino acids as tyrosine, cystine, and tryptophan. Meat scraps or meat meal from various manufacturers may not give the same rate of growth, even when fed at the same protein level.

The biological value[3] of the nitrogen of pork tenderloin has been reported to be 79, whereas that of pork cracklings, consisting largely of connective tissue, was found to be 25. The biological value of the proteins of meat meals containing no bone was found to be much higher than that of those containing a large proportion of bone.[4]

Wilgus, Norris, and Heuser in tests at Cornell[5] showed that meat scraps were variable in protein efficiency, owing probably to differences in raw materials. There seemed to be a distinct difference in favor of the 55 per cent product as compared with the 50 to 45 per cent products. The rendering process apparently causes little variation in the protein efficiency. There is also considerable variation in the riboflavin content of different samples of meat scraps, depending upon ingredients used and conditions of manufacture.

A high free fatty acid content of meat scraps[6] is not necessarily a true factor for the evaluation of the product, but generally is not desirable. Meat scraps high in free fatty acids have been shown[7] markedly to increase the death rate, to decrease the rate of growth and feed consumption, and to retard calcification. The evidence presented indicates that the inferior results are probably not so much attributable to the free fatty acids, per se, but to an inactivation of vitamin A and, to a lesser degree, of other fat-soluble vitamins, presumably owing to oxidation. The formation of free fatty acids is accelerated by increased temperature, especially when it is accompanied by an increase in the moisture content. It would appear that the acidity of the fat is increased through the presence of fat-splitting enzymes, most active around temperatures of 80° to 90° F. Although a low free acidity of the fat gives no assurance that a meat scrap is desirable in every respect, a high acidity at once indicates an inferior product. To that extent the free fatty acids of meat scraps can be used as a criterion for the quality of the product.

Meat scraps as compared with fish meal are likely to be lower in available lysine, methionine, cystine, and tryptophan.[8]

"DIGESTER TANKAGE, MEAT MEAL TANKAGE, OR FEEDING TANKAGE is the finely ground, dried residue from animal tissues exclusive of hair, hoof, horn, manure, and stomach contents, except in such traces as might occur unavoidably in good factory practise, especially prepared for feeding purposes by tanking under live steam or by dry-rendering or a mixture of the products. When these products contain more than 4.4 per cent of phosphorus (P), they must be designated 'Digester Tankage with Bone,' 'Meat and Bone Meal Digester Tankage,' 'Meat and Bone Meal Tankage,' or 'Feeding Tankage with Bone.' If the product bears a name descriptive of its kind, composition, or origin, it must correspond thereto."

Tankage is similar to meat scraps in that it is also made from the residue of animal tissues. However, it is usually prepared under the wet process known as tanking. The raw material is cooked under live steam; the grease is removed; and the product is dried at a very high temperature and ground to a granular meal. The liquid is evaporated down and is known as "stick." The residue contains about 45 per cent protein and usually has added to it "stick" and blood to raise the protein to about 60 per cent. Tankages are usually the product of the wet process, although they may be that of the dry process to which blood and stick have been added. Tankages ordinarily are very dark colored.

They are also likely to contain more of the fiber because of inclusion of the contents of the digestive tract. As far as protein is concerned, they usually run around 60 per cent, which is somewhat higher than meat scraps.

The tankages are not so palatable as the meat scraps and have generally not given such good results for growth,[9] although very favorable results have been reported for mature birds. The results obtained depend largely upon quality and palatability. The deficiency has been reported as being probably tryptophan.

The question still remains whether meat meal should contain the "stick." Tests at the Institute for Animal Physiology at the Agricultural High School at Berlin[10] indicated that the presence of "stick" or "extract" in animal meal has an irritating effect on the digestive organs of animals. The United States Department of Agriculture[11] reported that liquid stick and a mixture of blood meal and stick in the diet seemed to cause an increased embryonic mortality throughout the incubation period.

There is undoubtedly greater variation in tankages than in meat scraps, ranging all the way from those that are prepared specially for feeding purposes to those that are not fit for feeding purposes and are intended only for fertilizer.

"MEAT BY-PRODUCTS consist of any nonrendered, clean, wholesome part of the carcass of slaughtered mammals other than meat, such as lungs, spleens, kidneys, brains, stomach and intestines free from their contents; it does not include skin, horns, teeth, hoofs, and bones. If it bears a name descriptive of its kind it must correspond thereto.

"The term 'meat by-products' when applied to the corresponding portions of animals other than cattle, swine, sheep, and goats shall be used in qualified form, as, for example, 'horse meat by-products,' 'reindeer meat by-products,' 'crab meat by-products,' etc."

Experiments reported from England[12] showed that hide-fleshings, a by-product of tanneries, contained 66.25 per cent protein and was digested by poultry in the same way as meat-meal protein. Dried muskrat meal[13] was shown to be satisfactory in chick rations.

FRESH MEAT. There is the possibility of fresh meat as a source of animal protein, using meat trimmings or often the carcasses of cows or horses. This is a source that is not very extensive but can be used. In using such meat, ordinarily the best practice is to cook the carcass, grind it, and then feed in with a wet mash.

Jack rabbits have been suggested as a source of fresh meat in New Mexico.[14] The meat was fed by hanging the cleaned carcasses in the yards, where the birds could pick the meat from the bones. Egg production was satisfactory when the laying flock was fed only grain and raw rabbit meat.

LIVER MEALS

"ANIMAL LIVER MEAL is the product obtained by drying and grinding liver from slaughtered mammals. This product must contain at least 27 milligrams of riboflavin per pound."

"ANIMAL LIVER AND GLANDULAR MEAL is the product obtained by drying and grinding liver and other glandular tissue from slaughtered mammals. At least 50 per cent of the dry weight of the product must be derived from liver, and the product must contain at least 18 milligrams of riboflavin per pound."

"EXTRACTED ANIMAL LIVER MEAL is the product obtained by drying and grinding the residue of animal liver tissue from which a large portion of the vitamins and/or minerals have been removed."

MILK PRODUCTS

Milk is valuable for poultry because of its vitamins, lactose, minerals, and proteins.

Skimmilk or buttermilk in any form provides riboflavin and associated factors which are very important, especially for growing chicks.

About one-half the dry matter of skimmilk or buttermilk is composed of lactose or milk sugar. Milk begins to "sour" when certain acid-producing bacteria start a fermentation of the lactose and change a small part of it to lactic acid. Lactose favors the development of acid-producing bacteria in the intestines, and through the multiplication of these "friendly germs" the objectionable putrifactive bacteria are suppressed, thus providing good intestinal hygiene. In tests reported from Ohio[15] the *p*H of the contents of the duodenum and ileum was shown to be increased, while the *p*H of the cecal contents was markedly decreased by the use of milk. The cecal contents present a characteristic firm, brownish, pultaceous mass when birds are fed upon milk-free rations. This invariably changes to a yellow, creamy, frothy mass when birds are fed upon rations containing milk products. Lactose also seems to function in some way in the assimilation of minerals, especially of calcium and phosphorus. It has been suggested,[16] however, that the use of products rich in lactose be restricted, since in the hen glycogen is either not produced from lactose or is produced only in minimal amounts, more than $1/2$ of the lactose being excreted unchanged.

Part of the beneficial action of milk may be due to the improvement of the mineral intake, especially sodium, chlorine, and calcium, in which grains are deficient.

Milk proteins, composed chiefly of casein, lactalbumin, and lactoglobulin, are of excellent quality and easily digested. They function efficiently in supplying the body needs.

Milk in any form adds palatability to a ration and therefore tends to increase the feed consumption, which in turn is likely to increase growth and egg production.

MILK FOR CHICKS. Milk as a part of the chick ration has resulted in many benefits. The early experiments on the feeding of chicks have dealt almost entirely with a comparison of milk and meat scrap as sources of animal protein. A study of 36 early trials reported from various experiment stations[17] showed all in favor of milk. The maximum benefit from milk is obtained during the first 2 months of the chick's life.[18]

The Connecticut Station[19] reported that milk feeding stimulated growth and caused a reduction in deaths from general causes, that the chicks were larger, stronger, and more vigorous, and that there was a reduction in the death rate from bacillary white diarrhea. The Indiana Station[20] reported that milk feeding made the chicks less susceptible to disease and hence lowered mortality, particularly where the chicks were raised in confinement.

A special value of milk, previously important, was its effect upon coccidiosis.[21] This disease is caused by a protozoan parasite which develops and multiplies in the cells of the walls of the intestines, thereby injuring the cells. The beneficial results seemed to be due to the lactose. Coccidiosis is now more economically and effectively controlled by the use of medicants such as sulfaquinoxaline.

The benefits of milk feeding to chicks were due particularly to its vitamin value. Probably the riboflavin is the most important vitamin. The North Carolina Station[22] indicated heavier mortality in a meat-fed lot, as compared to a milk-fed group, in which the losses were due to vitamin A deficiency.

In general, milk fed to chicks has proved to be beneficial when compared with rations containing no milk.[23] However, satisfactory substitutes for dried skimmilk in chick rations have been made by supplying the nutrients furnished in milk. Hammond and Titus[24] used different mixtures of alfalfa leaf meal, dried whey, B-Y feed, fish meal, meat scrap, and peanut meal as substitutes for dried skimmilk. Nikolaiczuk and Maw[25] found that a combination of dried brewers' yeast and fish meal satisfactorily replaced dried skimmilk.

MILK FOR HENS. Milk, including the liquid, condensed, and dried forms, has proved to be a very effective protein feed as far as egg production is concerned. Comparing milk with the meat products, we find that most of the experiments favor the birds receiving milk.

Several stations[26] have reported favorable results on a mashless ration, in which only grain was fed, with an abundant supply of either the liquid milk or semi-solid buttermilk.

The Washington Station[27] reported improved hatchability when powdered whey, condensed buttermilk, and condensed buttermilk containing cereal grasses were fed as supplements to a breeding hen ration. Balance studies[28] to determine the biological values of the proteins in feeds showed that the value of a basal mash plus milk was significantly higher than that of earthnut mash and soy mash.

Milk is also reported as producing larger eggs than meat (see Chap. 9).

LIQUID MILK may be used where it is available on the farm or can be readily obtained near by. It is usually given as a drink. When feeding pullets or laying hens, buttermilk or skimmilk may be used in place of meat scraps, 12 to 14 quarts being allowed for 100 hens each day. It is more economical, however, to keep some protein concentrate in the mash.

In considering the amount of milk to feed, the Kentucky Station reports that 1 gallon of milk had the same value as 1 pound of meat scrap. The Indiana Station[29] reports that Leghorn pullets consumed 93 pounds of skimmilk per year.

Extensive trials conducted in Germany[30] and experiments reported from Norway[31] have shown the value of feeding skimmilk to laying hens.

No different results have been obtained when feeding chickens on sweet milk, naturally soured milk, artificially soured milk, or milk to which lactic acid was added. Sour milk is probably preferable since it is difficult to keep milk sweet when it is exposed to high temperature, and because the acid taste seems to make it more appetizing. The Idaho Station[32] reports sweet skimmilk as having a tendency to cause digestive disorders.

It is more difficult to maintain sanitary conditions when liquid milk is fed. During the summer months, flies are likely to be present around the milk vessels in large numbers. Flies are one of the intermediate hosts of tapeworms. The Kansas Station[33] reported that 91.1 per cent of the hens fed liquid milk were infested with tapeworms as compared with 51.3 per cent of those receiving no liquid milk. The infested birds also showed a higher degree of infestation. The reverse was true for round and ceca worms.

"EVAPORATED BUTTERMILK, CONCENTRATED BUTTERMILK, or CONDENSED BUTTERMILK is the product resulting from the removal of a considerable portion of water from clean, sound buttermilk derived from natural cream to which no foreign substances have been added excepting such as are permitted and necessary in the manufacture of butter. It shall contain not less than .055 per cent of butterfat for each per cent of solids, and not more than .14 per cent of ash for each per cent of solids."

"CONDENSED SKIMMED MILK is the product resulting from the removal of a considerable portion of water from clean, sound skimmed milk. It shall contain not less than 27 per cent of total solids."

"EVAPORATED CULTURED SKIMMED MILK, CONCENTRATED CULTURED SKIMMED MILK, or CONDENSED CULTURED SKIMMED MILK is the product resulting from the removal of a considerable portion of water from clean, sound skimmed milk which has been cultured by a suitable culture of lactic bacteria. It shall contain not less than 27 per cent of total solids."

Condensed buttermilk or skimmilk has been used to advantage as a supplement to the regular mash and grain at the rate of 2 pounds a day for 100 hens. It is often fed in paste form, as it comes from the container. In the summer time, or whenever a wet mash is fed, the milk in condensed form may be diluted with a little water and used to moisten the mash.

"DRIED BUTTERMILK is the product resulting from the removal of water from clean, sound buttermilk derived from natural cream to which no foreign substances have been added, excepting such as are necessary and permitted in the manufacture of butter. It shall contain not more than 8 per cent of moisture, not more than 13 per cent of mineral matter (ash), and not less than 5 per cent of butterfat, as determined by the Roese-Gottlieb method."

"DRIED SKIMMED MILK is the product resulting from the removal of water from clean, sound skimmed milk. It shall contain not more than 8 per cent of moisture."

The Pennsylvania Experiment Station[34] reported that the most efficient gains in body weight, on the basis of dried skimmilk intake, were made by the chicks receiving the 1.25 and the 2.5 per cent levels. From the standpoint of egg production, egg weight, and hatchability, the most efficient performance by laying pullets occurred at the 2.5 and 5 per cent levels. Results at the 2.5 and 3.75 per cent levels were essentially as satisfactory as the higher levels.

"DRIED CULTURED SKIMMED MILK is the product resulting from the removal of water from clean, sound skimmed milk which has been cultured by a suitable culture of lactic bacteria. It shall contain not more than 8 per cent of moisture."

WHEY in liquid form is not much used in poultry rations. It contains little protein. The dry matter of whey is mostly milk sugar. It can be used, when available in the natural state, for moistening mashes or it can be given to the birds as a drink. Results at the Idaho Station[35] show a production of 106 eggs for whey, as against 89 for no animal protein and 146 for the pen receiving skimmilk. It is probable that the vitamin content could be more fully utilized if some compensation were made for the protein.

"DRIED WHOLE WHEY is dried, clean, sound cheese and/or casein whey. It shall contain not less than 65 per cent of lactose." Because of its high milk sugar content, dried whey or milk sugar feed was of special value in rations for the control of coccidiosis. It is an important source of riboflavin and other water-soluble vitamins. It has also been suggested that it contains an unidentified growth factor. Because of its laxative nature the amounts fed must be restricted, 10 per cent being the maximum amount recommended.[36]

"CONDENSED WHOLE WHEY is the product resulting from the removal of a considerable portion of water from clean, sound cheese or casein whey, either or both. It shall contain not less than 62 per cent of total whey solids. When this product contains less than 62 per cent of total whey solids, it shall be designated 'condensed whey, . . . per cent solids.'"

"CONDENSED WHEY SOLUBLES is the product resulting from the removal of albumen and the partial removal of milk sugar from clean, sound whey, to which no foreign substances have been added except such as are necessary in the manufacture of milk sugar."

"DRIED WHEY SOLUBLES is the product resulting from the removal of albumen and the partial removal of milk sugar from clean, sound whey, to which no foreign substances have been added except such as are necessary in the manufacture of milk sugar."

"DRIED MILK ALBUMIN is the dried coagulated protein fraction separated from whey. It shall contain not less than 75 per cent protein (N × 6.25) on a moisture-free basis." Milk albumin results as a by-product in the manufacture of milk sugar. It contains most of the casein and albumin of the milk. It usually contains about 45 per cent protein and 25 to 30 per cent ash, although some products have a much higher percentage of protein. It has been used with favorable results as a source of protein in poultry rations.[37]

"CASEIN (FEEDING) is the product resulting from acid or rennet precipitation of skimmed milk. It must contain at least 80 per cent of crude protein." Its cost limits its use to experimental rations. With a lower relative cost it could be used in poultry rations as a source of protein.[38]

COTTAGE CHEESE is not used to any extent in poultry feeding. It is a valuable feed, however, and can be used. The Arizona Experiment Station[39] reported on a method for preserving skimmilk curd on the farm by adding formalin. Curds, conserved in this way, can be fed to hens and chickens without any danger.

CHEESE MEAL[40] has been reported as giving good results in poultry rations.

Milk can be used in different forms about equally satisfactorily.[41] The forms to use will depend upon convenience of obtaining them, the feeding system, and the cost. The price one can afford to pay for the different forms of milk depends to a large extent on the total solids each contains and the percentage of protein.

Form	Per Cent Solids	Per Cent Protein
Liquid milk	7 to 9	3.6
Condensed milk	28 to 30	12.0
Dried milk	90 to 95	35.0

Any of the various forms of milk can be fed to young stock.[42] Results reported from Nebraska favored dried buttermilk as compared with dried skimmilk. The liquid milk was reported to give better results than the dried product in trials conducted in Scotland and Wisconsin. Card reports no significant difference between liquid, condensed, and dried milk. In feeding chicks at

Cornell, it was found that there was little difference in growth due to the form of milk that was used. The Connecticut Station reports sweet and sour milk of about equal value, with probably a slight preference for the sour milk.

In the comparison of the different forms of milk for hens, there was generally no difference in the results. However, the Washington Station[43] reported liquid skimmilk superior to milk powder and other forms of protein.

MARINE PRODUCTS

In this category the fish meals are the most important. Fish meal was formerly utilized only as fertilizer, but, with improved methods of handling, better products are available.

"FISH MEAL is clean, dried, ground tissues of undecomposed whole fish or fish cuttings, either or both, with or without the extraction of part of the oil. If it contains more than 3 per cent of salt (NaCl) the amount of salt must constitute a part of the brand name, provided that in no case shall the salt content of this product exceed 7 per cent."

"FISH RESIDUE MEAL is the clean, dried, undecomposed residue from the manufacture of glue from non-oily fish. If it contains more than 3 per cent of salt (NaCl) the amount of salt must constitute a part of the brand name, provided that in no case shall the salt content of this product exceed 7 per cent."

The product obtained from fish or fish waste which is suitable for animal consumption is usually called fish meal.[44] The products which are fit only for fertilizer are called fish scrap or fish guano.

CLASSES OF FISH MEAL. Two general classes of fish meal are produced in the United States:

1. White Fish Meal, which is low in fat and hence called lean fish meal, made principally from the cod, halibut, hake or ling, whiting, haddock, plaice, sword, and tuna, utilizing only the non-edible portions of edible fish, such as heads, backs, and fins, or whole unusable or unsalable fish.

2. Dark Fish Meal, which is made from fish rich in oil, such as the herring, menhaden, sardine, pilchard, and mackerel (in which case the whole fish is generally used), and from the wastes from the shrimp- and salmon-canning industry. Oily fish are usually treated to recover a greater or lesser portion of the oil and the residue dried and ground.

COMPOSITION OF FISH MEALS. Fish meal is a feed that

contains a large amount of protein and also a large proportion of ash or bone-forming material. It contains a relatively large amount of iodine. A good fish meal will show approximately the following composition:

	Per Cent
Protein	55-60
Phosphate of lime	18-25
Other minerals	3-5
Oil	2-5
Moisture	10-14

There is considerable variation in composition, mechanical condition, and other physical characteristics, depending upon source of the raw material and the process of manufacture. Meals are produced both by the vacuum and by direct heat processes.

Vacuum-dried cod and vacuum-dried haddock meal have been reported rich in vitamin A, whereas flame-dried and steam-dried menhaden meals supply little if any of this vitamin.[45] Growth experiments showed the protein in the vacuum-dried cod and the vacuum-dried haddock meal to be superior in quality to that of the flame-dried menhaden, while the steam-dried menhaden meal appeared to occupy an intermediate place. There were also indications that the vacuum-dried product was superior in one or more of the substances in the vitamin B complex. The proteins of vacuum-dried meal and steam-dried meal have been reported superior in both digestibility and biological value to those of flame-dried menhaden meal.

Maine[46] white fish, herring, and sardine meal were found to contain vitamin D. The rapid fire-dried sardine meal contained this vitamin at a protective level when fresh. The sample containing the highest percentage of fat was the most potent in vitamin D. The fish proteins, fed as 10 to 12 per cent of the ration by weight, supplied protection against vitamin D and riboflavin deficiencies for the period of 3 to 11 weeks of age.

The relative protein efficiencies of various fish meals (with casein rated as 100) determined at Cornell[5] are: vacuum-dried and steam-dried white fish meals, 104; domestic sardine meal, 98; flame-dried white fish meal, 94; steam-dried menhaden fish meal and Asiatic sardine meal, 91; flame-dried menhaden fish meal, 80. The relative riboflavin content of these meals (with dried skimmilk rated as 19) are: vacuum-dried white fish meal, 10; domestic sardine meal, 9; steam-dried and flame-dried white and menhaden fish meals and Asiatic sardine meal, 5. The Texas Station[47] also reported that vacuum-dried fish meal gave the best results of any of the protein feeds studied, when used as a supplement to any two other protein feeds.

Also in a study to determine the effect of the manufacturing process upon nutritive values, it was shown at Cornell[48] that dry-rendered haddock meals possessed a greater protein value and 50 per cent more riboflavin than those wet-rendered by similar processes of drying. A flame-dried meal was of inferior value. The use of vacuum drying with steam drying materially preserved the riboflavin content but did not improve the relative protein efficiency over that obtained without the use of vacuum. Overheating[49] fish meal during drying depresses the availability of the amino acids.

In comparing salmon fish meals, a Columbia River salmon fish meal, with a high fat content, and secured late in the fall, was distinctly inferior in quality to the other meals.[50]

HERRING MEAL is not so desirable as some others for poultry feeding. It is darker in color, contains more oil, and varies considerably in quality and composition. The two variables are salt and oil, large amounts of either being undesirable.

USE OF FISH MEALS. Fish meals may not be so palatable as some other animal protein concentrates. There is risk of taint to the flesh and product when large quantities are used, especially those with a high oil content. However, they have given good results when used in chick rations.[51]

"CRAB MEAL is the undecomposed ground dried waste of the crab and contains the shell, viscera, and part or all of the flesh. It shall contain not less than 25 per cent of protein. If it contains more than 3 per cent of salt (NaCl) the amount of salt must constitute a part of the brand name, provided that in no case shall the salt content of this product exceed 7 per cent."

Average samples of crab meal run about 28 per cent protein. The calcium carbonate content is high, running over 40 per cent. In feeding trials, it has been shown to compare favorably with meat meal and fish meal.[52] Hairy crabs[53] have been reported as not being satisfactory as an albuminous food, owing probably to the high ash content (about 40 per cent).

"SHRIMP MEAL is the undecomposed ground dried waste of the shrimp and contains the head, hull, or the whole shrimp, either or in mixture. If it contains more than 3 per cent of salt (NaCl) the amount of salt must constitute a part of the brand name, provided that in no case shall the salt content of this product exceed 7 per cent."

Shrimps are a valuable food compared with meat meal.[53] The feeding value of sun-dried shrimp meal for poultry is considerably less than steam-dried (or other unsalted) shrimp meal.[54] The protein content of shrimp meal runs close to 50 per cent, which makes it a valuable concentrate.[55] Shrimps are also rich in iodine. Chicks fed shrimp "bran," to the extent of 10 per cent of a ration, did not grow quite so well as chicks fed fish meals or meat meal.[56]

LOBSTER MEAL is less valuable tham shrimp meal but may be a useful food for poultry.[53]

STARFISH MEAL, prepared from the starfish (*Asterias forbesi*), contains about 28 per cent protein and 60 per cent ash. When the calcium and phosphorus are adjusted, it compares favorably[57] with fish meal and meat scraps in feed efficiency and in the production of shank pigment. The high mineral content limits the quantity that can be used in a chick ration to about 5 per cent. Compared with fish meal, starfish meal contains as much riboflavin but probably less of the nutritional factors that prevent poor feathering and dermatosis of the feet.

DOGFISH MEAL, prepared by dry-rendering methods, was reported by the Washington Station[58] as having little value as a protein feed. On the other hand, wet process meal, prepared with good care and speed, had gross protein values comparable with pilchard fish meal and soybean meal.

WHALE MEAL is prepared from the clean, dried undecomposed flesh of the whale, after part of the oil has been extracted. If it contains more than 3 per cent of salt (NaCl) the amount of salt must constitute a part of the brand name, provided that in no case shall the salt content of this product exceed 7 per cent.

Whale meal of good quality (free from bone and of very low fat content) has been reported to possess good feeding value for poultry.[59]

SHARK MEAL has been reported[60] to increase the egg yield greatly when 10 per cent of this product is added to a cereal ration. It has also given good results as a supplement in chick rations.

COD LIVER MEAL is the ground residue of cod livers after the oil has been extracted. It contains about 50 per cent protein and is ordinarily not used on account of its protein, but it is a possible source of this nutrient. It also contains a large amount of fat, which gives it its antirachitic value. The protein from cod liver meal has been reported to be lower in value than the protein of buttermilk, fish meal, and meat scrap.[61]

"FISH LIVER AND GLANDULAR MEAL is the product obtained by drying the complete coelomic contents of the fish. At least 50 per cent of the dry weight of the product must be derived from fish liver and the product must contain at least 18 milligrams of riboflavin per pound."

"CONDENSED FISH SOLUBLES is the product obtained by condensing the water resulting from the hydraulic extraction of oil from fish."

Favorable results[62] have been reported in the use of condensed fish solubles and other fish water products in chick and poult rations, especially those composed largely of corn and soybean oil meal. The supplementary value of these products was due largely to water-soluble factors, rather than the protein content. Condensed fish solubles contain an unidentified factor not present in vegetable proteins.

CONDENSED WHALE SOLUBLES[63] have also been shown to be of value as a supplement in poultry rations.

"HOMOGENIZED CONDENSED FISH is a partially dehydrated, homogeneous product made from fish and/or fish cuttings, from which a part of the oil may have been removed. It shall contain not less than 50 per cent of total solids."

SHELLFISH MEAL is a product made from blue mussels. It has been reported to give favorable results in poultry rations in Denmark. The protein content is only 11 to 12 per cent.

SEAWEED MEAL containing about 7 per cent protein has been reported as an excellent food for hens in Norway. However, it has considerable fiber and probably cannot be fed in large amounts.

KELP MEAL. Most of the kelp or seaweed meal is manufactured from the giant brown kelp of the Pacific Coast. The kelp is harvested by an especially adapted type of mowing machine. This wet kelp is then dried and ground into meal, which, in appearance, resembles alfalfa meal. Its principal value is as a mineral supplement. When fed to layers at a level of 10 per cent it produced damp droppings.[64] Chicks tolerated up to 10 per cent.

BLOOD PRODUCTS

There is probably nothing that the hen likes better than fresh blood. This great liking for fresh blood often results in severe losses due to various forms of cannibalism.

FRESH BLOOD has been fed to ducks, pullets, and hens.[65] The fresh blood used by the Western Washington Experiment Station was a regular slaughter house product, sold commercially under the term "blood sausage" blood. It was an edible blood produced under government inspection, was practically free of bacteria, and had all the fibrin removed so that it would not coagulate.

"BLOOD MEAL is ground, dried blood."

"BLOOD FLOUR is dried blood, prepared by special processes and reduced to a fine powder."

The dried blood is very high in protein (approximately 70 per cent) but as the only source of protein does not give good results.[66] This failure is probably due to unpalatability, decrease in digestibility attributable to the manufacturing process, and low biological value of its protein. Grau and Almquist[67] reported that the serum and fibrin fractions of beef blood are of much better quality than the blood cell fractions. However, the blood cell fraction will support chick growth when supplemented with isoleucine. Mixtures of blood cells and corn gluten meal gave satisfactory growth results. In the practical tests (20 per cent protein ration) where this mixture furnished 60 per cent of the total protein the gains made were nearly as good as those made when sardine meal furnished the protein.

BONE PRODUCTS

GREEN CUT BONE consists of fresh bones, with more or less adhering meat, put through a special grinder. This is a very palatable feed, comparing very favorably with fresh meat and blood, for hens are cannibalistic enough to like raw meat and fresh blood. Green cut bone makes a good source of animal protein, containing about 30 per cent protein, but there are certain disadvantages which restrict its use. Ordinarily, it is not available regularly and constantly and in sufficient quantities. Then, too, the bones must be free from any contamination or diarrhea and other bowel trouble will result. In warm weather it might be a difficult problem to keep the meat adhering to the bone from becoming tainted. One must also consider the expense of grinding.

Where it was fed in the fresh form and in amounts so that the birds obtained sufficient protein, varying results in production have been obtained. In the main, however, the feeding of fresh cut bone has compared favorably with meat scraps.[68] However, some form of dry animal food is likely to prove safer and more satisfactory and cheaper, or, when available, green cut bone can be used as part of the animal protein.

"Cooked Bone Meal is the dried, ground product, obtained by cooking undecomposed bone in water at atmospheric pressure just enough to remove excess fat and meat. It shall contain not more than 25 per cent protein and not less than 10 per cent phosphorus (P). The label shall include a guarantee for protein, calcium (Ca), and phosphorus (P)."

Bone meal or granulated bone is ordinarily not used as a source of animal protein but is considered as a mineral product furnishing calcium phosphate. The raw bone contains considerable protein, but it is of low biologic value and has not given satisfactory egg production.[69] (For other bone products which are phosphorus carriers see Chap. 7.)

EGG PRODUCTS

EGGS are a possible source of animal protein although they are too costly for this purpose. However, incubator infertiles have long been recognized as a valuable feed for chicks, and are thus used.[70] The infertile eggs can also be boiled hard, run through a food chopper without removing the shells, and mixed with enough mash to keep from being sticky.

ALL-EGG MEAL[71] is a product used with favorable results as a source of protein. It may be made from the by-products of hatcheries consisting of the infertile, dead-germ, and dead-in-the shell eggs. The eggs are boiled, passed through a sausage mill or food chopper, mixed with mash and fed, or dried and re-ground into a meal. The final product contains about 35 per cent protein, 30 per cent fat, and 30 per cent minerals.

MISCELLANEOUS ANIMAL PRODUCTS

INSECTS. On range, the birds have opportunity to eat the natural animal foods, which are insects and worms. Poultry is fond of worms, larvae, grubs, and beetles. They could be used as food, but, naturally, where large numbers of birds are involved, it is not practical to furnish them. It is not advisable that poultry eat too much of this class of food.

LIVE SNAILS, which contain about 20 per cent protein, have been reported as giving favorable results when fed to ducks.[72]

SILKWORM CHRYSALIS FLOUR, a by-product of the silk industry, has been reported from Italy[73] as being an excellent substitute for meat and fish meals. It contains about 54 per cent protein. Unextracted silkworm pupae meal, when used as the sole protein concentrate in Germany,[74] did not prove satisfactory. Since the pupae contain a large amount of fat, the silkworm pupae meal should be fed after the fat has been removed.

ANT EGGS consist really of the pupae and not the eggs. They have been used by game-keepers, especially in Europe.[75] They can be used either fresh or as a semi-dried preserves for poultry or winged game.

LOCUST MEAL,[76] which contains about 45 per cent protein, has been reported as a possible source of protein for chicks, since it has proved to be as palatable as fish meal. However, it is not so efficient as fish meal. The consumption of grasshoppers by turkeys has been reported as causing mortality.[77] This was thought to be due to an enteritis caused by the legs of the insects.

HYDROLIZED TANNERY WASTE, a product obtained by hydrolizing waste resulting from the scraping of hides in tanneries and containing 44.7 per cent crude protein, was reported by the California Station[78] as producing 10 per cent fewer eggs than meat scrap.

HYDROLYZED FEATHERS as a feed for chickens were used at the Kansas Station.[79] It seemed to delay molting in hens for a short time. The conclusions drawn were that hydrolyzation was too expensive and added nothing of importance to present-day rations. The Iowa Station[80] reported that the addition of sodium sulphide-treated feathers to a basal cereal diet resulted in a rate of growth significantly greater than that produced by the basal diet. Feathers contain a large amount of cystine and supplement corn oil meal.

"POULTRY BY-PRODUCT MEAL consists of the nonrendered, clean, wholesome parts of the carcass of slaughtered poultry, such as head, feet, undeveloped eggs, gizzard and intestines exclusive of feathers, and gizzard and intestinal content." Chicken scrap thus produced has been reported as comparing favorably[81] with two other sources of supplementary protein when fed to chicks for 8 weeks.

HOOF MEAL was fed to hens by the Missouri Station[82] but did not prove an adequate source of protein. Production was only 75 eggs as compared with 128 for sour milk.

The Wisconsin Station[83] concluded that chicks are able to utilize powdered swine hoofs when finely ground and mixed with other protein feeds. It "teams" well with soybean oil meal. It appears to be a satisfactory substitute for meat scraps and fish meal in practical chick rations. The Ontario Agricultural College[84] reported that hoof and horn meal was a fairly adequate substitute for 5 per cent of meat meal, when the ration contained

5 per cent of fish meal and 3 per cent of dried buttermilk, but was not satisfactory in the absence of fish meal. It did not exhibit any supplemental effect when fed in combination with corn gluten feed, sunflower seed oil meal, soybean oil meal, or linseed oil meal. All the vegetable proteins were markedly superior to the hoof and horn meal.

PROTOZOA OF THE RUMEN. Experiments, reported from Italy,[85] indicate nutritive values for the dried ciliate infusoria from the rumen of a sheep and from dried bacteria from the same source. The favorable influence is attributed to the protein contributed by the supplements.

UREA. Experiments reported from Germany[86] indicated that amide flakes could not replace or save albumin in rations for hens. High percentages of amide were eaten with relish and did not cause any disturbance of health. The Wisconsin Station[87] reports that simple nitrogen compounds, such as urea, can be used in calf rations as a substitute for protein, but not in rations for chicks, guinea pigs, and rats. The Hawaii Station[88] found definite protein starvation, characterized by retarded growth, when urea was fed as the supplement to a low-protein ration to chicks. Apparently it can be fed only to ruminants, since certain bacteria in the rumen probably use the nitrogen for growth, converting it into protein in their bodies. Then the bacteria pass along the alimentary canal until they are digested. Similarly, the Nebraska and Oklahoma stations[89] showed that amide nitrogen was not utilized by growing chicks.

NECESSITY FOR AND USE OF ANIMAL PROTEIN

The common use of animal protein concentrates in poultry feeding shows the high regard in which they are held, and experimental evidence points to a superiority of animal over vegetable protein concentrates in poultry rations. The difference is probably due to several factors: (1) the quality of protein as represented by the amounts and kinds of amino acids present; (2) the essential mineral elements; (3) the comparative vitamin content. In a National Research Council Report[90] it is concluded that the "available evidence rather clearly demonstrates that the effectiveness of animal protein concentrates, in promoting maximal production in swine and particularly in poultry, is not due primarily to their protein constituents, but rather to their higher contents of certain vitamins, of calcium, of phosphorus, and possibly of some of the micro-nutrients."

Many early reports showed better egg production with rations containting animal protein. However, when the mineral deficiencies of the vegetable protein were made up the results were very satisfactory.

Poor hatchability[91] has been reported for rations not including feeds from animal source. This has usually been due to a deficiency of vitamins, chiefly riboflavin, vitamin B_{12}, and unidentified factors.

Cannibalism, which was reported as the result of a deficiency of animal protein in the diet, was reported cured by the addition of 5 per cent of meal meal to the diet.[92]

The value of animal protein food in chick feeding has long been recognized. As early as 1898, W. P. Wheeler of the New York Experiment Station[93] reported that a ration in which $2/5$ of the protein was supplied by animal food was much more profitably fed than one containing only protein from a vegetable source.

When rations with plant and animal proteins were compared for feeding on range in Bulgaria,[94] little difference in the rate of growth was observed over a period of 100 days. The Nebraska Station,[95] comparing protein concentrates from animal and vegetable sources for growing chicks, reported that the percentage rate of gain, the gain per gram of nitrogen, and nitrogen retention were greater at 60 days of age in the lot fed the animal protein concentrate.

In more recent comparisons the differences between growth of chicks on plant versus animal protein rations are not so great. This is due to more complete information which permits the supplementation of vegetable protein feeds to make up known deficiencies such as calcium, phosphorus, methionine, lysine, riboflavin, vitamin B_{12}, and others. The chief importance or necessity of animal feeds[96] under these conditions lies in unidentified vitamins or factors which they might supply.

AMOUNTS OF ANIMAL PROTEIN

The question arises as to the amounts of animal protein feeds that should be included in poultry rations.

MATURE BIRDS. Some protein concentrates are needed in the ration to give good egg production.[97] In 70 early experiments, comparing rations containing a protein concentrate in the form of animal protein feeds with others not containing the protein concentrate, all favored the feeding of animal proteins. The average increase in egg production was 116 per cent.

Northern Ireland[98] reports a laying mash of cereals, supplemented with 1/2 per cent of common salt, as capable of supporting egg production at a level of more than 200 eggs per bird per annum, with no return from the addition of supplements of soybean meal to the ration.

In the earlier experiments in which animal protein was the only supplementary protein it was necessary to feed sufficient amounts to meet the various requirements such as protein and possibly minerals and vitamins. For that reason egg production was closely related to the consumption of meat scrap or other form of animal protein.[99] Approximately 10 per cent of animal protein in the ration gave the best results with birds in confinement. With birds on free range this amount could be safely and economically reduced. This accounts in part for the almost universal practice in England[100] of reduced amounts of meat or fish in the mash.

A shortage of animal proteins during World War II made it desirable to know to what extent the animal protein could be decreased and the soybean oil meal increased without materially affecting production, hatchability, and feed efficiency. A number of experiments[101] have been reported in which small amounts of animal protein, in combination with soybean oil meal as the protein supplement, have given as good egg production as larger quantities. Usually the hatchability was also satisfactory. In some experiments[102] the egg production has been satisfactory on a high soybean oil meal ration, but hatchability was reduced. In one experiment conducted at Cornell[103] no difference in either egg production or hatchability was obtained between rations supplying all the supplementary protein from soybean oil meal and part from soybean oil meal and part from meat scrap.

GROWING BIRDS. Where no extra protein, as animal protein,[104] is included in the ration, the chicks make very slow growth, lack uniformity, and are not thrifty. For example, in experiments at Cornell, the chicks receiving no animal protein feed had at a certain period the average weight of 0.49 pound, those receiving meat scrap supplement weighed 0.66 pound, and those receiving milk weighed 0.78 pound.

During early life, chicks require more protein than later. Therefore, the protein as supplied by an animal protein concentrate is usually higher in the starting rations.[105] For the later periods, less protein and animal protein feeds are required.[106]

A shortage of animal protein during World War II also made it desirable to known to what extent the animal protein could be decreased in chick rations without affecting growth, mortality, and feed efficiency.[106] A number of reports show very good growth of chicks on rations containing no animal protein supplements. The animal protein itself is not essential for good growth in chickens. It may be easier, however, to provide all the nutritive essentials when some animal protein is included.

Comparing rations containing some animal protein concentrates with those containing all soybean oil meal as the supplementary source of protein, it was found that the results in practically all instances were in favor of the rations containing some animal protein. Summarizing the reports as published by a number of experiment stations, Almquist found that the relative growth on the soybean meal rations represented 55 to 99 per cent of the growth obtained on the good rations. To equal the best growth, the addition of some animal protein concentrates to the soybean oil meal rations seems to be necessary.

COMPARISON OF ANIMAL PROTEIN FEEDS

Differences exist in the results that are obtained when the various kinds of animal protein are fed as the sole source of supplementary protein.

MATURE BIRDS. Representative results of different animal proteins in poultry feeding, as expressed in egg production per hen per year, are shown in Tables 11 and 12.

The evidence tends to indicate that combinations of two or more animal proteins are equally effective and often preferable

TABLE 11. REPRESENTATIVE RESULTS OF DIFFERENT ANIMAL PROTEINS IN POULTRY FEEDING. EGG PRODUCTION PER HEN

Meat Scrap	Liquid Milk	Dried Milk	Tankage	Fish Meal	No Protein	Reference
145	175	...	134	...	113	Idaho Circ. 27, 1922
...	146	...	115	...	89	Idaho Bul. 134, 1924
135	135	...	...	128	33	Ind. Bul. 182, 1915
136	140	...	...	...	61	Ind. Bul. 218, 1918
179	...	...	184	...	60	Ind. Bul. 227, 1919
...	165	189	...	...	57	Ind. Bul. 258, 1921
156	153	165	...	...	..	Ky. Bul. 260, 1925
107	131	...	...	...	55	Mo. Circ. 79, 1916
134	127	...	...	...	60	Mo. Circ. 82, 1917
120	129	...	...	...	57	Mo. Bul. 155, 1918
117	125	112	120	...	61	Mo. Bul. 225, 1924
139	...	140	125	...	..	Mo. Bul. 272, 1929
134	...	171	...	...	..	Pa. Bul. 206, 1926

TABLE 12. COMPARATIVE RESULTS OF DIFFERENT ANIMAL PROTEIN FEEDS IN EGG PRODUCTION

Animal Protein Feed	Exp. 1	Exp. 2	Exp. 3
20% dried buttermilk in mash	166	...	...
20% meat scraps in mash	151	147	150
20% milk albumin in mash	163	...	...
20% dried skimmilk in mash	151	...	...
20% meat meal in mash	...	141	...
20% fish meal in mash	...	137	132
20% meat scrap mash plus liquid milk	165	177	...
20% meat scrap mash plus semi-solid buttermilk	...	161	...
11% meat scrap mash plus liquid milk	...	161	...
Mash plus liquid milk	147	...	...
Mash plus semi-solid buttermilk	164	...	...
Liquid milk (no mash)	...	161	...

All pens received grain.

Comparative Results of Different Animal Protein Feeds in Egg Production, M.S. Thesis, by A. L. Romanoff, Cornell University, 1926.

to using any of them singly.[108] In a comparison of dried milk, meat and bone meal, and combinations of both as protein supplements for egg production, Henderson ranked the groups as follows: "milk," 152 eggs; "combinations," 139 eggs; "meat and bone meal," 121 eggs.

Mortality and the condition of the birds, as well as egg quality, must also be considered. In general, there is not much difference between the various sources of animal protein, except that milk tends to give better average weights of hens, and liquid milk slightly larger eggs.

The cost of the feeds must also be taken into account, since the real measures of the value of the various feeds are the cost per dozen eggs and especially the returns per hen above feed cost. However, it does not cost much more per hen per year to feed the higher-priced feeds, and, if production is enough higher to be significant, the increased number of eggs will probably more than offset the higher feed cost. In most cases combinations of meat and milk products gave higher returns above feed cost than either one used separately.

GROWING BIRDS. Combinations[109] of two or more forms of animal protein feeds, in many cases, have given better growth than one alone. The supplementary value of milk has been especially evident, owing probably, in many cases, to the vitamin B complex. The extent of any benefits of combinations will depend upon completeness of the ration in other respects. It may be desirable that at least two sources of animal protein feeds be included in the ration for young stock.

Where the chicks are reared on good range, it will not be necessary to use so much animal protein feeds. This is particularly true where small numbers are reared, as under general farm conditions.[110]

MEASURING THE VALUE OF PROTEIN CONCENTRATES

The value of any particular product is influenced (1) by the nature of the raw materials and (2) by the conditions of manufacture. Both the quality of the proteins of common protein supplements used in poultry rations and the riboflavin content were reported as being influenced by the process of manufacturing them.[111] Process of manufacture, however, affected the riboflavin content to a greater extent than the protein quality. To maintain maximum riboflavin potency a relatively low temperature and a relatively short time are required in cooking and drying the raw materials. Flame drying, because of the extremely high temperature, was found deleterious to proteins, but the other processes of manufacture did not materially affect protein quality. Dry process meals were found to have a higher protein and a lower ash and ether extract content than wet process meals.

No loss in supplementary protein nutritive value was observed in certain fish meals after 10 months of storage in paper, cotton, and burlap bags.[112]

The relative values of the different protein concentrates must, in the main, be determined by feeding trials.

The Cornell workers,[113] by determining the relative efficiency for growth, suggested relative protein efficiency as an expression of the utilization of the proteins of a protein supplement. The relative protein efficiency was obtained by determining the percentage of protein stored by normal chicks during the seventh week of age, dividing the percentage storage by that of a standard casein diet, and multiplying by 100. The value of the protein is thus expressed in relation to the value of casein, which is represented by 100. On this basis the samples studied showed the following values: casein, 100; dried skimmilk, 100; white fish mean, 104; sardine meal (domestic), 98; Menhaden fish meal (steam-dried), 91; soybean oil meal (expeller), 89; meat scrap (55 per cent protein), 82; meat scrap (50 per cent protein), 73; corn gluten meal, 61; ground soybeans, 58.

The Washington Station[114] has also reported a method for determining the gross value of protein concentrates. This method consists of depleting the protein reserve of the chicks for a period of 2 weeks by feeding a suitable chick ration, complete in all the known nutrients except protein. The level of protein in the depletion ration is 8 per cent and is derived from plant sources. The experimental rations consist of the depletion ration to which is added a sufficient amount of the supplement to bring the protein content to 11 per cent. The experimental period is 2 weeks, and the results are compared with commercial casein, which is given a gross protein value of 100. The gross values for some of the samples studied were: Alaska herring fish meal, 101; dried buttermilk, 91; dried skimmilk, 78; Manchurian soybean meal (hydraulic), 57; domestic soybean meal (expeller), 46; meat meal (Brazilian), 43; meat and bone meal (Brazilian), 32; dried Alaska peas, 27; dehydrated alfalfa, 25.

The Nebraska Station[115] reported the following relative biological values for the different protein concentrates:

Dried buttermilk Fish meal Casein	AA
Meat and bone meal Soybean meal	A
Blood meal Cotton seed meal	B
Linseed oil meal Corn gluten meal	C
Gelatin	D

The California Station[116] has reported on the use of analyses of concentrates considering intact protein, protein decomposition products, indigestible protein, and hot-water-soluble protein. These analytical characteristics were found to exhibit a good correlation with nutritive value for chicks when assigned the relative values of 100, 40, 0, and 40 respectively. Such analytical methods offer a possibility for the rapid laboratory determination of protein quality in commercial concentrates. The cystine, tryptophan, and hydrogen sulphide content of the protein concentrates could not be used as a basis for predicting their nutritive values.

From the results of Canadian reports[117] it would appear that a satisfactory evaluation of the biological value of animal protein concentrates might be obtained from the microbiological assays for amino acid content based on acid hydrolysis of the total protein corrected for the indigestible and nonprotein fractions.

REFERENCES

1. Kraybill, H. R. What are tankage, meat scraps, and meat meal? Poultry Sci. 8:11. 1928.
   Wilder, O. H. M. The use of packinghouse by-products for animal feeds. Food Technology 5:118. 1951.
2. Bronkhorst, J. J. The growth-promoting qualities of various protein concentrates for Leghorn chickens. Onderstepoort Jour. Vet. Sci. 10:481. 1938.
   Gerhardt, W. F. Diermeel en Vleeschmeel in Rautsoenen voor jonge Kiuken. Ned. Indische Bladen voor Diergeneeskunde 45:406. 1933.
   Mussehl, F. E., C. W. Ackerson, and R. L. Borchers. Growth promoting value of meat scraps. Neb. 63rd Ann. Rept. 121. 1950.
   Prange, R. W., C. W. Carrick, and S. M. Hauge. Growth values of proteins from commercial animal products. I. Commercial meat and bone scrap. Poultry Sci. 7:95. 1928.
3. Mitchell, H. H., J. R. Beadles, and J. H. Kruger. The relation of the connective tissue content of meat to its protein value in nutrition. Jour. Biol. Chem. 73:767. 1927.
4. Pope, E. A. Nutritive values of meat meals. New Zealand Dept. Sci. Indus. Res. Bul. 12. 1929.
5. Wilgus, H. S., Jr., L. C. Norris, and G. F. Heuser. The relative protein efficiency and the relative vitamin G content of common protein supplements used in poultry rations. Jour. Agr. Res. 51:383. 1935.
6. Gray, R. E., and H. E. Robinson. Free fatty acids and rancidity in relation to animal by-product protein concentrates. Poultry Sci. 20:36. 1941.
7. Schroeder, C. H., G. K. Redding, and L. J. Huber. Some causes and effects of a high free fatty acid content of the meatscraps in poultry rations. Poultry Sci. 15:104. 1936.
   Schroeder, C. H., G. K. Redding, and L. J. Huber. Conditions influencing the formation of free fatty acids in meatscraps. Report Sixth World's Poultry Congress. 43. Germany. 1936.
8. March, B., J. Biely, and R. J. Young. Supplementation of meat scrap with amino acids. Poultry Sci. 19:444. 1950.
   Kraybill, H. R. Meat scraps and tankage. Flour and Feed 48:16. 1947.
   Patrick, H. Supplements for a "meat-scraps" type chick ration. Poultry Sci. 32:570. 1953.
9. Halpin, J. G., and C. E. Holmes. Tankage compares favorably with meat scraps in chick ration. Wisc. Bul. 428:49. 1934.
   Prange, R. W., S. M. Hauge, and C. W. Carrick. The study of the protein in a commercial meat product. Poultry Sci. 6:302. 1927.

Prange, R. W., S. M. Hauge, and C. W. Carrick. Growth values of proteins from commercial animal products. II. Commercial digester tankage. Poultry Sci. 7:186. 1928.

Prange, R. W., C. W. Carrick, and S. M. Hauge. Growth values of proteins from commercial animal products. III. A commercial meat meal. Poultry Sci. 7:233. 1928.

10. Turck, K. G. Schlachtblut und Abfallsstoffverwertung. Allgemeiner Industrie Verlag. N. 43. Berlin. 1928.

11. Titus, H. W., T. C. Byerly, N. R. Ellis, and R. B. Nestler. Effect of packinghouse by-products, in the diet of chickens, on the production and hatchability of eggs. Jour. Agr. Res. 53:453. 1936.

12. Bondi, A., and H. Meyer. The digestibility of dura, carobs, and hide-fleshings. Jour. Agr. Sci. (Eng.) 34:118. 1944.

13. Goff, O. E. Dried muskrat meal in chick rations. Louisiana Ann. Rept. 1943-44:121.

14. Berry, L. N. Profitable feeding and management practices for poultry. N. Mex. Bul. 286:15. 1942.

15. Ashcraft, D. W. Effect of milk products on pH of intestinal contents of domestic fowl. Poultry Sci. 12:292. 1933.

16. Lenkeit, W., and M. Becker. Beitrag zur Verwertung des Milchzuckers beim Geflügel. Tierernährung und Futtermittelkunde 2:15. 1939.

17. Elford, F. C. Poultry investigations at the Dominion Experimental Farms. Canada Exp. Farms, Poultry Div. Rept. 1925:67.

Rettger, L. F., W. F. Kirkpatrick, and L. E. Card. Milk feeding and its influence on growth and mortality. A comparative study of the value of sweet and sour milk. Conn. (Storrs) Bul. 80. 1915.

Roemer, R. Poultry feeding in Germany. Proc. Third World's Poultry Congress. 239:Canada. 1927.

Fangauf, R., and A. Haensel. Die Milchtränke in der Aufzucht der Kücken. Archiv für Geflügelk. 9:33. 1935.

Anderson, W. B. Skimmilk as food for young growing chickens. Ind. Bul. 71:60. 1898.

Anderson, W. B. Skimmilk as a food for young growing chickens. Ind. Bul. 76:21. 1898.

Do minerals supplement meat scrap rations? Ind. Rept. 1927:47.

Rations for chicks. Iowa Sta. Rept. 1928:25.

Smith, A. D. Drink for brooder chicks. Rept. Northwest Exp. Sta. Crookston, Minn. 1924:73.

Clayton, E. P., and J. P. Clayton. Experiments with poultry, 1920 and 1921. Miss. Bul. 204. 1921.

Kempster, H. L. Experiment in chick feeding. "What the agricultural experiment station is doing for Missouri," Mo. Bul. 179: 43. 1921.

Kempster, H. L. Experiment in chick feeding. "One Year's Work," Mo. Bul. 189:47. 1921.

Kempster, H. L., and E. W. Henderson. The value of sour milk and beef scrap in rations for growing chicks and the cost of growing chicks. Mo. Bul. 197:77. 1922.

Henderson, E. W. Dried skimmilk superior to meat. "Experiment Station Research," Mo. Bul. 285:97. 1930.

Schnetzler, E. E. Dried milk vs. meat scraps. "Progress in Agricultural Research," Mo. Bul. 300:93. 1931.

Kempster, H. L. Meat scrap and milk in chick rations. Mo. Bul. 310:48. 1932.

Lewis, H. R., and W. C. Thompson. Sour skimmed milk for chicks. N. J. Rept. 1916:150.

Lewis, H. R. Protective feeds for poultry. N. J. Hints 7. 1919.

Thompson, W. C. The relative value of meat scrap, powdered buttermilk, powdered skimmilk, and semi-solid buttermilk as developing feeds for White Leghorn pullets. N. J. Rept. 1922:159.

Massengale, O. N. The value of milk and meat proteins in chick rations. Poultry Sci. 8:151. 1929.

Wheeler, W. P. Skimmilk for growing chicks. N. Y. (Geneva) Bul. N.S. 39:11. 1892.

Rice, J. E., and Clara Nixon. Seven methods of feeding young chickens. Cornell Bul. 282. 1910.

Nixon, Clara. Animal food for chick rearing. Cornell Countryman 9:84. 1911.

Rice, J. E., and Clara Nixon. Methods of chick feeding. Cornell Bul. 327. 1913.

Kaupp, B. F. Poultry investigational work. N. C. Rept. 1917:55.

Kaupp, B. F. Feeding and nutritional work. N. C. Rept. 1919:48.

Kaupp, B. F. The rate of growth of Single Comb Rhode Island Reds. Poultry Sci. 1:39. 1921.

Kaupp, B. F. Operation of a four unit farm poultry plant. N. C. Bul. 251. 1927.

Kaupp, B. F. Influence of meat meal vs. milk in chick development. N. C. Rept. 1928:82.

Dearstyne, R. S., H. D. Smith, and H. P. Brigman. Summer broiler production. N. C. Bul. 303. 1936.

Orr, J. B., G. S. Robertson, A. Kinross, G. Lewis, and H. Newbiggin. The nutritive requirement of poultry. Scottish Jour. Agr. 9:392. 1926.

Titus, H. W., and M. A. Jull. The growth of Rhode Island Reds and the effect of feeding skimmilk on the constants of their growth curves. Jour. Agr. Res. 36:515. 1928.

Halpin, J. G., O. N. Johnson, and E. B. Hart. Milk substitutes and barley in the Wisconsin chick ration. Wis. Bul. 396:51. 1927.

18. MacDonald, A. J. The protein requirements of poultry. Harper Adams Utility Poultry Jour. 22:487. 1937.

Ott, W. H., H. C. Knandel, and R. V. Boucher. Dry skimmilk in rations for growing, laying, and breeding fowls. Pa. Bul. 381. 1939.

19. Rettger, L. F., W. F. Kirkpatrick, and L. E. Card. Chickens: Milk feeding and its influence on growth and mortality. A comparative study of the value of sweet and sour milk. Conn. Bul. 80. 1915.

20. Value of animal protein in laying ration determined. Ind. Rept. 1924:32.

21. Beach, J. R. The effect of feeding cultures of Bacillus acidophilus, lactose, dry skimmilk, or whole milk on the hydrogen ion concen-

tration of the contents of the ceca of chickens. Hilgardia 1:145. 1925.

Beach, J. R., and D. E. Davis. The influence of feeding lactose or dry skimmilk on artificial infection of chicks with Eimeria avium. Hilgardia 1:167. 1925.

Beach, J. R., and D. E. Davis. Coccidiosis of chickens. Calif. Circ. 300. 1925.

Powdered buttermilk in the treatment of coccidiosis. Mich. Rept. 1927–1928:25.

22. Kaupp, B. F. Operation of a four-unit farm poultry plant. N. C. Bul. 251. 1927.

23. Fangauf, R., A. Haensel, and M. Harken. Gesteht ein Zusammenhang zwischen Jugendentwicklung und Legeleistung? Archiv für Geflügelk. 10:401. 1936.

Righi, M. L'utilizzazione dei derivati del latte nell' alimentazione del pollame. Rivista di Avicultura 6:309. 1936.

Paci, C. L'Utilizzazione del latte scremato in parziale o totale sostituzione della farina di carne nell' allevamento dei pulcini. Rivista Zootecnia 14:387. 1938.

24. Hammond, J. C., and H. W. Titus. Substitutes for dried skimmilk in the diet of growing chickens. Poultry Sci. 22:411. 1943.

25. Nikolaiczuk, N., and W. A. Maw. Substitutes for dried buttermilk and yellow corn in chick rations. Sci. Agr. 23:496. 1943.

26. Cassel, L. W. Feeding experiments with Leghorns. Wash. Bul. 210. 1927.

Martin, J. H. Sources of animal protein for laying hens. Ky. Bul. 260. 1925.

Walker, A. L. The relative feeding value and cost of milk in egg production. N. Mex. Bul. 150. 1925.

27. Bearse, G. E. A comparison of molasses, whey, condensed buttermilk, and condensed buttermilk containing cereal grasses as supplements to a breeding hen ration. Poultry Sci. 17:433. 1938.

28. Macdonald, A. J., and S. Bose. Studies on the digestibility coefficients and biological values of the proteins in poultry feeds. Poultry Sci. 23:135. 1944.

29. Philips, A. G. The value of meat scrap, fish scrap, and skimmilk in rations for laying pullets. Ind. Bul. 182. 1915.

30. Lang, H. Die Magermilchfrage bei der Hennenfütterung. Archiv für Geflügelk. 8:65. 1934.

Bünger, H., R. Fangauf, and R. Deditius; Jaeger, J., L. Weinmiller and K. Voight; Bünger, H., Dr. Werner, Dr. Schultz, and Dr. Keseling. Fütterungsversuche über den Ersatz des Eiweissfutters im Futter der Legehennen durch Magermilch. Archiv für Geflügelk. 8:1. 1934.

Lang, H. Magermilch und Molkenbestandteile (speziell die Milchsäure) in der Legehennenfütterung. Deutsche Landwirtschaftliche Geflügelzeitung. Aug. 30, 1934.

Fangauf, R., O. Brüninghaus, and A. Haensel. Durch Wieviel Magermilch Kann die normale Fischmehlgabe bei Legehennen ersetzt werden? Archiv für Geflügelk. 9:201. 1935.

Fangauf, R., and A. Haensel. Wieviel milch trinken Legehennen, wenn gleichzeitig Wasser zur Verfügung steht? Archiv für Geflügelk. 10:71. 1936.

Fangauf, R. Die Verfütterung von frischen Milchabfällen. Rept. Sixth World's Poultry Congress. 256. Germany. 1936.

Weinmiller, L., and K. Voigt. Untersuchungen an Hühnern über den Futterwert von Milcheiweiss. Archiv für Geflügelk. 10:78. 1936.

Fangauf, R., and A. Haensel. Molke und Quarg in der Fütterung der Legehühner. Archiv für Geflügelk. 10:129. 1936.

Carstens, P., and J. Prüfer Fütterungsversuch mit Magermilch und Buttermilchquarg an Legehennen. Archiv für Geflügelk. 10: 385. 1936.

Weinmiller, L., and K. Mantel. Molkenkleie als Ersatz für die Milchtränke in der Geflügelfütterung. Forshungsdienst 5:210. 1938.

31. Finne, I. Potatoes and skimmilk as feed for laying hens. Rept. Seventh World's Poultry Congress. 153. Cleveland. 1939.

32. Poultry husbandry. Idaho Bul. 160:27. 1928.

33. Payne, L. F., A. E. Schumacher, and L. D. Bushnell. Milk as a beverage increased tapeworm infestation in poultry. Poultry Sci. 24:93. 1945.

34. Ott, W. H., H. C. Knandel, and R. V. Boucher. Dry skimmilk in rations for growing, laying, and breeding fowl. Pa. Bul. 381. 1939.

35. Parkhurst, R. T. The value of certain protein feeds for production and quality in eggs. Idaho Bul. 134. 1924.

36. Slinger, S. J., F. N. Marcellus, and E. V. Evans. Dried whey as a substitute for dried buttermilk in chick rations. Sci. Agric. 26: 381. 1946.

37. Ott, W. H., and R. V. Boucher. Lactalbumen as a protein supplement for growing chickens. Poultry Sci. 23:497. 1944.

38. Fangauf, R., and E. Kallmann. Kassein im Legehennenfutter. Archiv für Geflügelk. 7:170. 1933.

Zöllner, I. Die Verwendung von Kassein und Lebertran im Legehennenfutter. Archiv für Geflügelk. 7:358. 1933.

39. Davis, R. N. The preservation of skimmilk curd for poultry feeding. Jour. Dairy Sci. 16:495. 1933.

40. Halpin, J. G., and C. E. Holmes. Cheese meal gives good results in poultry rations. Wis. Bul. 435:34. 1936.

Taylor, M. W. P.A.G.B. feeding experiments. Modern Poultry Keeping LV:270. 1946.

41. Card, L. E. A comparison of different forms of milk in a ration for growing chickens. Poultry Sci. 5:199. 1926.

Kaupp, B. F. Experiments with poultry at the North Carolina Station. N. C. Rept. 1925:26.

Roberts, R. E., and C. W. Carrick. Meat scraps and dried milk in rations for starting chicks. Ind. Bul. 421. 1937.

42. Card, L. E. A comparison of different forms of milk in a ration for growing chickens. Poultry Sci. 5:199. 1926.

Halpin, J. G., O. N. Johnson, and E. B. Hart. Milk substitutes and barley in the Wisconsin chick ration. Wis. Bul. 396:51. 1927.

Mussehl, F. E., and C. W. Ackerson. The growth promoting values of dried buttermilk, dried skimmilk and dried whey for chicks. Poultry Sci. 11:69. 1932.

Moir, M., H. Newbiggin, A. Kinross, and G. S. Robertson. The nutritive requirements of poultry. VII. Growth in chickens. Scottish Jour. Agr. 12:291. 1929.

Rettger, L. F., W. F. Kirkpatrick, and L. E. Card. Chickens: milk feeding and its influence on growth and mortality. A comparative study of the value of sweet and sour milk. Conn. Bul. 80. 1915.

Roberts, R. E. Liquid and condensed milk for chicks. Poultry Sci. 11:226. 1932.

43. Cassel, L. W. The value of various proteins and combinations of them for laying pullets. Wash. Bul. 229:42. 1928.

Cassel, L. W. The value of various proteins and combinations of them for laying pullets. Wash. Bul. 237:42. 1929.

44. LeClerc, J. A. Growing commercial importance of fish meal. Memo. S. 287. Bureau of Foreign and Domestic Commerce, Washington, D. C. 1928.

45. Maynard, L. A., and C. M. McCay. Fish-meal studies. N. Y. (Cornell) Rept. (II) 1931:31.

Schneider, B. H. Nitrogen balance studies with various fish meals. Jour. Agr. Res. 44:723. 1932.

46. Dove, W. F. A study of the causes of nutritional deficiency diseases in the livestock and inhabitants of Maine with possible corrective methods secured from the utilization of Maine fishery products and the production of superior foods. Maine Bul. 375. 1934.

47. Sherwood, R. M., and J. R. Couch. Values of various protein feeds for growing chicks. Tex. Bul. 588. 1940.

48. Wilgus, H. S., Jr., L. C. Norris, and G. F. Heuser. Haddock meal. Effect of manufacturing processes upon nutritive values. Ind. Eng. Chem. 27:419. 1935.

49. Clandinin, D. R. The effects of methods of processing on the nutritive value of herring meals. Poultry Sci. 28:128. 1949.

50. Carver, J. S., and V. Heiman. The utilization of fish by-products for poultry. Wash. Bul. 325:55. 1935.

51. Allardyce, W. J., W. Henderson, and V. S. Asmundson. Fish meal supplements for chicks. III. Comparative growth on rations with pilchard meals. Poultry Sci. 12:163. 1933.

Arsenjew, A. F., and N. J. Chlebnikow. Untersuchungen der biologischen Wertigkeit des Fischmehls in Abhängigkeit vom Rohstoffe. Biedermanns Zentralbl. B. Tierernährung. 8:580. 1936.

Johnson, O., and D. Brazie. Comparative value of some commercial protein supplements in the rations of growing chicks. Jour. Agr. Res. 48:183. 1934.

Sherwood, R. M., and J. R. Couch. Comparative values of various protein feeds for growing chicks. Texas Bul. 569. 1939.

52. Manning, J. R. Crab scrap versus meat meal in poultry feeding. Memo. S. 302. Department of Commerce, Bureau of Fisheries, Washington, D. C. 1929.

Byerly, T. C., H. W. Titus, and N. R. Ellis. Production and hatchability of eggs as affected by different kinds and quantities of

proteins in the diet of laying hens. Jour. Agr. Res. 46:1. 1933.
Mangold, E., and A. Hock. Wollhandkrabbenschrot als Eisweissfutter für das Geflügel. I. Die Verdaulichkeit des Wollhandkrabbenschrotes bei Hühnern. II. Mangold, E., and H. Damköhler. Die Eignung des Wollhandkrabbenschrotes als Eiweissfutter für die Kükenaufzucht. Archiv für Geflügelk. 12:97. 1938.
Parkhurst, R. T., M. S. Gutowska, and C. R. Fellers. The use of crab meal in poultry rations. Mass. Bul. 388:97. 1942.
Parkhurst, R. T., J. A. Lubitz, M. S. Gutowska, and C. R. Fellers. The nutritive properties and use of crab meal. Poultry Sci. 21: 475. 1942.
Parkhurst, R. T., C. R. Fellers, F. P. Griffiths, and J. W. Kuzmeski. The nutritive properties and use of fishery by-products in poultry rations. Poultry Sci. 23:554. 1944.
Parkhurst, R. T., M. S. Gutowska, J. A. Lubitz, and C. R. Fellers. Crab meal in poultry rations. II. Chick and broiler ration. Poultry Sci. 23:58. 1944.
Parkhurst, R. T., M. S. Gutowska, and C. R. Fellers. Crab meal in poultry rations. III. Laying and breeding rations. Poultry Sci. 23:118. 1944.

53. Fangauf, R., O. Brüninghaus, and A. Haensel. Garnelen, Langusten, und Wollhandkrabbenmehl als Eiweissfutter bei Legehennen. Archiv für Geflügelk. 9:359. 1935.

54. Upp, C. W. New information about livestock and poultry. La. Bul. 262:31. 1935.

55. Barnett, C. E., and H. D. Polk. Cottonseed meal, shrimp meal, soybean meal, meat scrap for growing chicks. Miss. Farm Research. June, 1942.
Fronda, F. M. The effects of dried shrimps and fish meal as supplements in rations for egg production. Philippine Agr. 18:3. 1930.
Fronda, F. M., A. C. Badelles, and J. S. Padilla. Protein supplements in poultry rations. I. Comparative studies of the effects of shrimp meal, meat scraps, tankage, and fish meal as supplements in rations for growing chicks. Philippine Agr. 22:582. 1934.
Francisco, A. A., G. S. Chan, and F. M. Fronda. Protein supplements in poultry rations. II. Comparative effects of shrimp meal, meat scraps, tankage, and fish meal as supplements in rations for laying hens. Philippine Agr. 22:685. 1934.
Fronda, F. M., and A. E. Kabigting. Protein supplements in poultry rations. III. The optimum amount of shrimp meal to use as supplement in rations for growing chicks. Philippine Agr. 23:652. 1935.
Fronda, F. M., and A. E. Kabigting. Protein supplements in poultry rations. Amount of shrimp meal as supplementary ration for growing chicks. Philippine Poultry Jour. 5(2). 1935.
Polk, H. D., and C. E. Barnett. Broiler production with high protein feeds. Miss. Bul. 374. 1943.

56. Titus, H. W., E. McNally, and F. C. Hilberg. A comparison of shrimp "bran" and two kinds of fish meal when fed at a level of ten per cent in diets for growing chicks. Poultry Sci. 9:219. 1930.

57. Bird, H. R. Dehydrated pea vines and starfish meal in poultry feeds. Poultry Sci. 23:76. 1944.

Morse, R. E., F. P. Griffiths, and R. T. Parkhurst. The value of starfish meal in the poultry starting ration. Poultry Sci. 23:408. 1944.

Parkhurst, R. R., C. R. Fellers, F. P. Griffiths, and J. W. Kuzmeski. The nutritive properties and use of fishery by-products in poultry rations. Poultry Sci. 23:554. 1944.

Studies on the marine resources of southern New England. III. The possibility of the utilization of the starfish (Asterias forbesi desor). Bul. Bingham Oceanographic Collection (Yale University). Vol. IX. Art. 3. 1946.

Bird, H. R. Dehydrated pea vines and starfish meal in poultry feeds. 7.

Heuser, G. F., and J. McGinnis. Starfish meal in chick rations. 10.

Morse, R. E., F. P. Griffiths, and R. T. Parkhurst. Preliminary report on eight weeks of comparative feeding of protein equivalent diets containing fish meal, crab meal and starfish meal to Rhode Island Red chicks. 13.

Ringrose, R. C. Starfish meal feeding experiments with chicks. 17.

Stuart, H. O., and C. P. Hart. Starfish meal as a protein substitute in chick rations. 20.

Whitson, D., and H. W. Titus. The use of starfish meal in chick diets. 24.

Stuart, H. O., and C. P. Hart. Starfish meal as a protein substitute in chick rations. R. I. Misc. Pub. 21:5. 1944.

58. Rhian, M., J. S. Carver, R. W. Harrison, and W. S. Hamm. The value of dogfish meal as a protein supplement. Wash. Bul. 416: 24. 1942.

59. Fangauf, R., and R. Detitius. Die Verfütterung von Walmehl an Legehennen. Archiv für Geflügelk. 8:383. 1934.

Halnan, E. T. The value of whale-meat meal as a constituent of chick diets with a note on the influence of added protein on the efficiency of utilization of the gross energy of a ration. Jour. Agr. Sci. (Eng.) 32:179. 1942.

60. Poultry progress at the Kizimbani Experimental Station. 1932-1935. East African Agr. Jour. Zanzibar 2:90. 1936.

Marshall, S. P., and G. K. Davis. Shark meal as a protein supplement in chick rations. Poultry Sci. 25:381.

61. McFarlane, W. D., W. R. Graham, Jr., and G. E. Hall. Studies in protein nutrition of the chick. I. The influence of different protein concentrates on the growth of baby chicks when fed as the source of protein in various simplified diets. Jour. Nutr. 4:331. 1931.

62. Berry, E. P., C. W. Carrick, R. E. Roberts, and S. M. Hauge. Condensed fish press water and fish liver meal in chick rations. Poultry Sci. 24:270. 1945.

Cravens, W. W., W. H. McGibbon, and J. G. Halpin. The value of certain supplements in practical chick rations containing adequate riboflavin. Poultry Sci. 24:305. 1945.

Pratt, Jean M., and J. Biely. A note on the value of stickwater meal as a riboflavin supplement in poultry rations. Poultry Sci. 24:377. 1945.
Lassen, S., and E. K. Bacon. The use of condensed fish solubles in poultry nutrition. Poultry Sci. 25:486. 1946.
Grau, C. R. Fish solubles for poultry feeding. Flour & Feed 47:46. 1946.
Robblee, A. R., C. A. Nichol, W. W. Cravens, C. A. Elvehjem, and J. G. Halpin. Studies on an unidentified growth factor in fish solubles. Poultry Sci. 26:553. 1947.
Mishler, D. H., C. W. Carrick, and S. M. Hauge. Condensed fish solubles as a supplement for corn and soybean oil meal chick rations. Poultry Sci. 27:263. 1948.
German, H. L., B. S. Schweigert, P. B. Pearson, and R. M. Sherwood. A preliminary study on the value of condensed fish solubles for turkey poults. Poultry Sci. 27:113. 1948.
Hoie, J. Forsok med limvatn til kyllinger. Tidsskrift for det Norske landbruk: 1. 1949.
King, R. H., and S. M. Hauge. Concentration of the unidentified growth factor in condensed fish solubles. Arch. Biochem. 24:350. 1949.
Carrick, C. W., D. H. Mishler, and S. M. Hauge. Fish solubles as supplements in chick rations. Ind. 63rd Ann. Rept: 115. 1950.
Stephenson, E. L., and B. B. Clower. The influence of an unidentified factor found in fish solubles on hatchability. Poultry Sci. 31: 936. 1952.
63. Lassen, S., E. K. Bacon, and H. J. Dunn. An evaluation of condensed whale solubles as a supplement in poultry nutrition. Poultry Sci. 30:422. 1951.
64. McIntyre, T. M., and M. H. Jenkins. Kelp meal in the ration of growing chickens and laying hens. Sci. Agr. 32:559. 1952.
65. Shoup, Mrs. George R. Feeding market egg layers for winter production. Western Wash. Bimo. Bul. XII(3). 1924.
Richter, K., and H. Brüggeman. Fresh slaughter blood for the fattening of swine, ducks, and pullets. Züchtungskunde 11:113. 1936.
66. Winter, A. R. The nutritive value of blood meal protein for growth. Ohio Bul. 436. 1929.
Serfontein, P. J. Blood meal in poultry rations. S. Africa Dept. of Agric. Bul. 280. 1947.
67. Grau, C. R., and H. J. Almquist. Blood proteins for poultry feeding. Flour and Feed 44(2):26. 1943.
Grau, C. R., and H. J. Almquist. Beef blood proteins in chick diets. Poultry Sci. 23:486. 1944.
68. Mass. Rept., Public Document 33:40. 1896.
Mass. Rept., Public Document 33:48. 1897.
Mass. Rept., Public Document 33:41. 1898.
Mass. Rept., Public Document 33:90. 1899.
Brooks, W. P. Poultry keeping for egg production. Mass. Bul. 122: 47. 1908.
Schoppe, W. F. Animal protein for laying hens. Mont. Bul. 161. 1923.

Graham, W. R., and A. C. McCulloch. Animal foods for fowls. Ontario Dept. Agr. Bul. 217. 1913.
Stewart, J. H., and H. Atwood. Poultry Experiments. W. Va. Bul. 71:390. 1900.
Stewart, J. H., and H. Atwood. Poultry Experiments. W. Va. Bul. 83:443. 1902.
69. Clickner, F. H. Animal investigations at the New Jersey Station. N. J. Rept. 1926:380.
70. Halpin, J. G., and E. B. Hart. Feeding eggs to baby chicks gets results. Wis. Bul. 352:7. 1923.
North, M. O., and J. G. Halpin. Poultry research guides farm practice. Wis. Bul. 420:85. 1931.
Halpin, J. G., C. E. Holmes, and M. H. Meshew. Infertile eggs make good chick feed. Wis. Bul. 443:89. 1939.
Halpin, J. G., M. H. Meshew, and C. E. Holmes. Chicks make good use of infertile eggs. Wis. Bul. 449:87. 1940.
Halpin, J. G., and C. E. Holmes. Here's a cheaper way to feed infertile eggs. Wis. Bul. 451:32. 1941.
71. Utilization of by-products from hatcheries. Ohio Bul. 362:45. 1922.
Kennard, D. C., and V. D. Chamberlin. Feed, don't waste, by-product incubator eggs. Ohio Bimo. Bul. 228:186. 1944.
Hammond, J. C., J. C. Fritz, R. B. Nestler, and H. W. Titus. Effect of length of incubation period on gross nutritive value of contents of fertile eggs. Poultry Sci. 23:217. 1944.
Kempster, H. L. The use of dried incubator offal in chick rations. Poultry Sci. 24:396. 1945.
72. Goseco, A. A study of the effects of animal and plant protein feeds on the egg production of ducks. Philippine Agr. 9:197. 1921.
73. Taibell, A. Increase in weight of chicks in relation to the carbohydrates in their ration supplemented by flour of the chrysalis of the silkworm. Proc. Third World's Poultry Congress. 226. Canada. 1927.
Vecchi, A. The utilization of the waste products of the fishing and silk industries in the feeding of poultry. Proc. Third World's Poultry Congress. 247. Canada. 1927.
74. Mangold, E., and H. Damköhler. Versuche über die Eignung der Puppen des Seidenspinners als Eiweissfutter bei Legehühnern. Archiv für Geflügelk. 10:359. 1936.
Mangold, E., H. Stutz, and A. Columbus. Der Nährstoffgehalt der Puppen des Seidenspinners und ihre Verdaulichkeit beim Geflügel. Biedermanns Zentralblatt. B. Tierernährung 8:267. 1936.
Fangauf, R., and A. Haensel. Seidenraupenpuppenschrot als Eiweissfutter für Legehühner. Archiv für Geflügelk. 12:172. 1938.
Lauprecht, E. Vergleich Tierischer Eiweissfuttermittel in der Legehennenfütterung. Rept. Seventh World's Poultry Congress. 148. Cleveland. 1939.
75. Friede, M. Pest that may prove to be a blessing. Poultry Sci. 2: 181. 1923.
76. Nutritive value of locusts. Farming in South Africa 9:232. 1934.
Fronda, F. M. Notes on locust meal as a poultry food. Philippine Agr. 24:425. 1935.

77. Heller, V. G., and L. Morris. Grasshoppers in turkey feeding. Okla. Exp. Sta. Rept. 1934-36:77. 1936.
Wickware, A. B. Grasshoppers; A potential danger to turkeys. Canad. Jour. Comp. Med. & Vet. Sci. 9:80. 1945.
78. Dougherty, J. E., and S. S. Gossman. Hydrolized tannery waste as a feed for poultry and rabbits. Calif. Rept. 1922:140.
79. A study of the use of hydrolyzed feathers as a feed for chickens. Kans. Rept. 1926-1928:102.
80. Draper, C. I. The nutritive value of corn oil meal and feather protein. Iowa Res. Bul. 326. 1944.
81. Stewart, G. F., and F. E. Mussehl. The recovery of by-products from poultry evisceration wastes. Poultry Sci. 20:450. 1941.
82. Kempster, H. L., and E. W. Henderson. Value of sour milk, beef scrap, cottonseed meal, gluten meal and oil meal in rations for egg production. Mo. Bul. 197:76. 1922.
83. Wagner, J. R., and C. A. Elvehjem. Nutritive value of Keratins. I. Powdered swine hoofs. Proc. Soc. Exp. Biol. Med. 51:394. 1942.
Newell, G., and C. A. Elvehjem. Ground hoof makes valuable protein feed. Wis. Bul. 461:11. 1943.
Wagner, J. R., and C. A. Elvehjem. Powdered swine hoofs in poultry rations. Poultry Sci. 22:275. 1943.
Newell, G. W., and C. A. Elvehjem. Nutritive value of keratin. III. Effect of source, particle size, and method of grinding. Jour. Nutr. 33:673. 1947.
84. Slinger, S. J., E. V. Evans, W. I. Kellam, and F. N. Marcellus. The use of a hoof and horn meal to replace animal and vegetable protein in rations for growing chicks. Poultry Sci. 23:431. 1944.
85. Usuelle, F., and P. Fiorini. Esperienze sul valore alimentare della fauna protozoaria del rumine nella crescenza. Boll. Soc. ital. Biol. sper. 13:11. 1938.
86. Carstens, P., and J. Prüfer. Fütterungsversuch mit Amidflocken an Legehennen. Züchtungskunde 13:109. 1938.
87. Hart, E. B., G. Bohstedt, and M. I. Wegner. Urea gives good results as a protein substitute in calf rations. Wis. Bul. 446:31. 1939.
88. Bice, C. M., and L. A. Dean. Utilization of urea nitrogen by growing chicks. Poultry Sci. 21:15. 1942.
89. Ackerson, C. W., W. E. Ham, and F. E. Mussehl. The utilization of food elements by growing chicks. IX. The nitrogen of urea. Neb. Res. Bul. 120. 1940.
Heller, V. G., and R. Penquite. Utilization of casein and amide nitrogen by chickens. Proc. Okla. Acad. Sci. 21:85. 1942.
90. Mitchell, H. H. Is animal protein an essential constituent of swine and poultry rations? Nat. Res. Council Rept. 9. 1944.
91. Parkhurst, R. T.. and J. W. Kuzmeski. Supplementing distillers' dried by-products in breeding rations. Poultry Sci. 23:554. 1944.
Bethke, R. M., D. C. Kennard, and V. D. Chamberlin. Animal protein supplements essential for hatchability. Ohio Agr. Sta. Bul. 665:13. 1946.
Parkhurst, R. T., and J. W. Kuzmeski. Supplements for distillers' by-products in poultry breeding diets. Poultry Sci. 25:162. 1946.

Schlamb, K. F., and A. R. Winter. An evaluation of dried distillers' feedstuffs fed to chickens throughout their life cycle. II. During the early reproduction period. Poultry Sci. 27:498. 1948.

92. Hart, L. Cannibalism in fowls associated with a deficiency of animal protein in the diet. Agr. Gaz. (New South Wales) 45:647. 1934.

93. Wheeler, W. P. The economy of using animal food in poultry feeding. N. Y. (Geneva) Bul. 149. 1898.

Wheeler, W. P. The adaptability of concentrated by-products for poultry feeding. N. Y. (Geneva) Bul. 271. 1905.

94. Tabakoff, I. I. The comparative influence of animal and plant proteins upon the growth of chicks reared on free range. Rept. Sixth World's Poultry Congress. 346. 1936.

95. Ackerson, C. W., M. J. Blish, and F. M. Mussehl. The utilization of food elements by growing chicks. I. A comparison of protein concentrates from animal and vegetable sources. Neb. Res. Bul. 90. 1937.

96. Carrick, C. W. Fish solubles in poultry nutrition. Flour & Feed 50(3):14. 1949.

Emerson, R., J. Houston, R. H. Thayer, and R. MacVicar. Studies on all-vegetable protein rations. Poultry Sci. 28:431. 1949.

Essary, E. O., R. Emerson, R. MacVicar, and R. H. Thayer. Growth factor studies with all vegetable protein chick rations. Poultry Sci. 27:661. 1948.

Heuser, G. F., and L. C. Norris. An unknown nutritive factor in feeds of animal origin. Poultry Sci. 30:470. 1951.

Heuser, G. F., L. C. Norris, and J. McGinnis. Vegetable protein concentrates fed alone and in combination with soybean oil meal and fish meal as the chief supplementary protein in chick starting rations. Poultry Sci. 25:130. 1946.

Insko, W. M. Practical methods of feeding distillers' grain solubles to growing pullets. Proc. 4th Dist. Conf. March, 1949:51.

Schlamb, K. F., and A. R. Winter. An evaluation of dried distillers' feedstuffs fed to chickens throughout their life cycle. I. During the starting and growing period. Poultry Sci. 27:492. 1948.

97. Embleton, H. Poultry feeding experiments. Ariz. Bul. 177. 1941.

Stout, S. R. Comparison of vegetable and animal sources of protein for laying hens. Ark. Bul. 203:26. 1926.

Rugg, W. C., and W. O. Pederick. Poultry feeding experiments. Jour. Dept. Agr. (Victoria) 23:490. 1925.

Pederick, W. O., and A. G. Clark. Poultry feeding experiment: Dried milk vs. meat meal. Jour. Dept. Agr. (Victoria) 26:99. 1928.

Dougherty, J. E. Poultry investigations. Calif. Rept. 1915:37.

Hicks, W. H. Feeding laying pullets. Report of the Superintendent (Agassiz [B.C.] Canada) 1928:35.

Elford, F. C. Skimmilk vs. beef scraps. Rept. Dominion (Canada) Poultry Husbandman 1919.

Elford, F. C. Poultry investigations at the Dominion Experimental Farm. Canada Dominion Exp. Farms Rept. 1923:10.

Elford, F. C. Meat meal vs. fish meal for egg production. Rept. Dominion (Canada) Poultry Husbandman 1928:51.
Straight, E. M. Experiments with poultry at the Sidney Experimental Station. Canada (B.C.) Rept. 1923:38.
Graham, W. R., and A. C. McCulloch. Farm poultry. Ont. Bul. 217. 1913.
Ballantyne, S. Poultry experiments at the Kapuskasing Experimental Station. Canada Exp. Farms (Kapuskasing, Ontario) Rept. 1922: 83.
Ballantyne, S. Experiments with poultry at the Kapuskasing Experiment Station. Canada Exp. Farms (Kapuskasing, Ontario) Rept. 1923:55.
Blair, W. S. Feeding experiments with poultry at the Kentville Experimental Station. Canada Exp. Farms (Kentville, N.S.) Rept. 1923:67.
Baird, W. W. Poultry experiments at the Nappan Experimental Farm. Canada Exp. Farms (Nappan, N.S.) Rept. 1923:47.
Clark, J. A. Poultry feeding experiments at the Charlottetown Experimental Station. Canada Exp. Farms (Charlottetown, P.E.I.) Rept. 1922:57.
Tinline, M. J. Poultry experiments at the Scott Experimental Station. Canada Exp. Farms (Scott, Sask.) Rept. 1922:82.
Tinline, M. J. Experiments with poultry at the Scott Experimental Station. Canada Exp. Farms (Scott, Sask.) Rept. 1923:53.
Munro, W. A. Experimental work with poultry at the Rosthern Experimental Station. Canada Exp. Farms (Rosthern, Sask.) Rept. 1924:46.
Jull, M. A. Concentrates for growing chicks and for laying stock. Jour. Am. Assoc. for Instructors and Investigators in Poultry Husb. 2:66. 1916.
Kirkpatrick, W. F., and L. E. Card. Fourth Annual International Egg Laying Contest. Conn. (Storrs) Bul. 87:197. 1916.
Fangauf, R., and A. Haensel. Die Wirkung von Eiweissgaben auf die Legetätigkeit in Beispielen bäuerlicher Hühnerfütterung. Archiv für Geflügelk. 11:39. 1937.
Parkhurst. R. T. Relative value of certain protein feeds for egg production. Idaho Circ. 27. 1922.
Work and progress of the Agricultural Experimental Station for the year ended Dec. 31, 1923. Idaho Bul. 133:13. 1924.
Parkhurst, R. T. The value of certain protein feeds for production and quality of eggs. Idaho Bul. 134. 1924.
Parkhurst, R. T. Summarized report of 1925-1926 poultry feeding experimental work. Idaho Circ. 43. 1927.
Philips, A. G. The value of meat scrap, fish scrap, and skimmilk in rations for laying pullets. Ind. Bul. 182. 1915.
Philips, A. G. To find the feeding value of skimmilk and meat scraps for White Plymouth Rocks, also for White Leghorns. Ind. Rept. 1918:54.
Philips, A. G. The value of skimmilk and meat scraps for White Plymouth Rocks. Ind. Bul. 218. 1918.

Philips, A. G. Feeding experiments with Leghorns. Ind. Bul. 227. 1919.
Meat scraps in a laying ration for Plymouth Rocks profitable. Feeding value of dried buttermilk as compared with liquid buttermilk in the ration of White Leghorns. Ind. Rept. 1920:30.
Philips, A. G. Feeding experiments with laying pullets. Ind. Bul. 258. 1921.
Feeding for egg production. Iowa Rept. 1922:30.
Comparison of dried buttermilk, fresh buttermilk, tankage, and meat scraps for laying hens. Iowa Rept. 1923:34.
Milk feeds as a source of protein for laying hens. Iowa Rept. 1925: 32.
Martin, J. H. Sources of protein for hens. Ky. Rept. 1919:40.
Martin, J. H. Experimental work with poultry. Ky. Rept. 1920:35.
Martin, J. H. Cottonseed meal, buttermilk, and tankage as sources of protein of the laying hen. Jour. Am. Assoc. of Instructors and Investigators in Poultry Husb. 7:39. 1921.
Martin, J. H. The feeding of skimmilk and semi-solid buttermilk to poultry. Ky. Rept. 1922:41.
Martin, J. H. The feeding of milk in various forms to laying hens. Ky. Rept. 1923:46.
Martin, J. H. Sources of animal protein for laying hens. Ky. Bul. 260:101. 1925.
Clayton, E. P., and J. P. Clayton. Experiments with poultry 1920-1921. Miss. Bul. 204. 1921.
Clayton, E. P. Report of the poultry department. Miss. Rept. 1924:14.
Clayton, E. P. A study in various proteins alone and in combination as egg producers. Miss. Rept. 1927:35.
Kempster, H. L. Sour milk for chicken feeding. Mo. Circ. 79. 1916.
Kempster, H. L., and G. W. Hervey. Meat scrap and sour milk for egg production. Mo. Bul. 155. 1918.
Kempster, H. L. Value of sour milk, beef scrap, cottonseed meal, gluten meal, and oil meal in rations for egg production. Mo. Bul. 172:34. 1920.
Kempster, H. L., and E. W. Henderson. Value of sour milk, beef scrap, cottonseed meal, gluten meal, and oil meal in rations for egg production. Mo. Bul. 197:75. 1922.
Kempster, H. L., and E. W. Henderson. Value of sour milk, beef scrap, cottonseed meal, gluten meal, and oil meal in rations for egg production. Mo. Bul. 210:59. 1924.
Kempster, H. L. The influence of animal and vegetable proteins on egg production. Mo. Bul. 225:16. 1924.
Kempster, H. L. Value of sour milk, beef scrap, cottonseed meal, gluten meal, and oil meal in rations for egg production. Mo. Bul. 236:66. 1926.
Kempster, H. L. Value of sour milk, beef scrap, cottonseed meal, gluten meal, and oil meal in rations for egg production. Mo. Bul. 256:84. 1927.

Kempster, H. L. Value of cottonseed meal, ground soybeans, soybean meal, tankage, meat scrap, and dried buttermilk in rations for egg production. Mo. Bul. 272:77. 1929.
Kempster, H. L. The influence of various protein concentrates on egg production. Mo. Bul. 288. 1930.
Schoppe, W. F. Report of the poultry department. Mont. Rept. 1916:179.
Schoppe, W. F. Animal protein for laying hens. Mont. Bul. 161. 1923.
Lewis, H. R. Skimmilk for laying hens. Jour. Am. Assoc. Instructors and Investigators in Poultry Husb. 2:72. 1916.
Thompson, W. C. Protein of animal origin for poultry feeding. N. J. Rept. 1924:134.
Walker, A. L. The relative feeding value and cost of milk in egg production. N. Mex. Bul. 150:32. 1925.
Wheeler, W. P. Animal food for poultry. N. Y. (Geneva) Bul. 171. 1899.
Heuser, G. F. Effect of certain rations on the efficiency of breeders. Jour. Am. Assoc. for Instructors and Investigators in Poultry Husb. 7:15. 1920.
Brown, F. C. Poultry feeding—meat vs. no meat. New Zealand Jour. Agr. 21:136. 1920.
Kaupp, B. F., and R. S. Dearstyne. Fish meal vs. meat meal in egg production. N. C. Rept. 1926:70.
Kaupp, B. F. Fish meal vs. meat meal in egg production. N. C. Rept. 1927:92.
Kaupp, B. F. Operation of a four unit farm poultry plant. N. C. Bul. 251. 1927.
Kaupp, B. F. Farm flock management. N. C. Rept. 1929:112.
Buss, W. J. Feeding experiments with laying hens. Ohio Bul. 322: 199. 1918.
Kennard, D. C., and P. S. White. Poultry investigations. Ohio Bimo. Bul. IX(7 and 8). 1924.
Kennard, D. C. Meat meal vs. meat scraps for egg production. Ohio Bimo. Bul. 11(6). 1926.
Meat meal vs. meat scrap for egg production. Ohio Bul. 392:62. 1926.
Robertson, G. S., and R. G. Baskett. The feeding of poultry. Jour. Ministry Agr. North Ireland 2:22. 1929.
Kistler, P. T., T. B. Charles, and H. C. Knandel. The effect of various sources of animal protein on the egg production and condition of Single Comb White Leghorn pullets. Pa. Bul. 206:23. 1926.
Fronda, F. M. A study of the effects of animal and plant proteins in rations for laying hens. Philippine Agr. 7:235. 1919.
Fronda, F. M. The effects of dried shrimps and fish meal as supplements in rations for egg production. Philippine Agr. 18:3. 1929.
Morgan, C. L. Fish meal vs. meat scrap for laying hens. S. C. Rept. 1930:90.

Stevenson, G. L. Comparison of high protein feeds. S. Dak. Rept. 1927:29.
Stevenson, G. L. High protein feeds. S. Dak. Rept. 1928:27.
Harvey, R. N. Egg-producing values of some Texas feeding stuffs. Tex. Bul. 220. 1917.
Sherwood, R. M. Comparative influences of various protein feeds on laying hens. Tex. Bul. 317. 1924.
Harvey, R. N. Poultry feeds and feeding results. Tex. Bul. 206. 1927.
Lee, A. R. Experiments in feeding laying hens. Jour. Am. Assoc. for Instructors and Investigators in Poultry Husb. 7:74. 1921.
Byerly, T. C., H. W. Titus, and N. R. Ellis. Production and hatchability of eggs as affected by different kinds and quantities of proteins in the diet of laying hens. Jour. Agr. Res. 46:1. 1933.
Stewart, J. H., and H. Atwood. Poultry experiments—the value of skimmilk for egg production. W. Va. Bul. 102. 1906.
Macdonald, A. J. Meat offals for poultry. Indian Farming 5:509. 1944.
98. Prentice, J. H. The amount of protein-rich supplements required in practical laying rations. Jour. of the Ministry of Agr. N. Ireland 4:116. 1933.
99. Dougherty, J. E. Rept. Calif. Agr. Sta. 1916:58.
Thompson, W. C. Poultry husbandry research program. N. J. Rept. 1929:280.
Knandel, H. C., and T. B. Charles. Effect of different levels of animal protein, supplied by dried skimmilk, on egg production, hatchability of eggs, and condition of Single Comb White Leghorn and Barred Plymouth Rock pullets. Pa. Bul. 230:38. 1928.
Knandel, H. C. Effect of different levels of animal protein, supplied by dried skimmilk, on egg production, hatchability of eggs, and condition of Single Comb White Leghorn and Barred Plymouth Rock pullets. Pa. Bul. 243:28. 1929.
Philips, A. G. Feeding experiments with laying pullets. Ind. Bul. 258. 1924.
Martin, J. H. Sources of animal protein for laying hens. Ky. Bul. 260. 1925.
Kempster, H. L. The influence of animal and vegetable proteins on egg production. Mo. Bul. 225. 1924.
Buss, W. J. Experiments with laying hens. Ohio Bul. 291. 1916.
Buss, W. J. Feeding experiments with laying hens. Ohio Bul. 322. 1918.
100. Parkhurst, R. T. Brief summary of the two years' experiments with certain animal and vegetable protein feeds with and without mineral supplement. Harper Adams Utility Poultry Jour. 15:177. 1930.
Feeding demonstrations. From the Sixth Annual Report of the Herts County Laying Trials—Hertfordshire Institute of Agriculture. The Utility Record. July 1932.
Newman, Tom. Protein levels. Eggs. Oct. 21, 1936.
101. Almquist, H. J. Summary of reports on minimum levels of ani-

mal protein required in supplementation of expeller soybean meal and cereal proteins in poultry mashes. Flour and Feed 44(2):12. 1943.

Hoffman, E., and A. E. Tomhave. Low animal protein laying mash. Feedstuffs 15(15):20. 1943.

Wightman, E. T., T. D. Runnels, and A. H. Van Landingham. Soybean oil meal in laying rations. Poultry Sci. 23:392. 1944.

102. Wilgus, H. S., and D. V. Zander. Minimum levels of animal protein for reproduction. Poultry Sci. 23:344. 1944.

103. Heuser, G. F., and L. C. Norris. Soybean oil meal in hen rations. Poultry Sci. 23:371. 1944.

104. Wheeler, W. P. Animal food for poultry. N. Y. (Geneva) Bul. 171. 1899.

Fronda, F. M., A. C. Badelles, and J. S. Padilla. Protein supplements in poultry rations: I. Comparative studies of the effects of shrimp meal, meat scraps, tankage, and fish meal as supplements in rations for growing chickens. Philippine Agr. 22:582. 1934.

105. Mussehl, F. E., and D. E. Gish. Protein requirements of growing chicks. Poultry Sci. 5:20. 1925.

Animal protein studies with chicks. Ind. Rept. 1927:48.

Roberts, R. E. Liquid and condensed milk for chicks. Poultry Sci. 11:226. 1932.

Roberts, R. E., and C. W. Carrick. Proportions of meat scraps and dried milk in rations for starting chicks. Poultry Sci. 12:223. 1933.

Kempster, H. L., and E. M. Funk. Dried skimmilk in rations for baby chicks. Mo. Bul. 310:49. 1932.

Carver, J. S., and L. W. Cassel. Protein requirements for growing chicks. Wash. Bul. 237:43. 1929.

St. John, J. L., J. S. Carver, J. P. Helphrey, W. Miller, and L. W. Cassel. The effect on growth of various protein levels of dry skimmilk in a chick mash. Poultry Sci. 9:320. 1930.

106. Bronkhorst, J. J. The influence of the protein level of the diet on the growth, egg production, egg weight, and mortality of Single Comb White Leghorn pullets. Onderstepoort Jour. Vet. Sci. and Animal Indus. 10:469. 1938.

Roberts, R. E. Protein requirements of growing pullets. Poultry Sci. 9:19. 1929.

Roberts, R. E., and C. W. Carrick. Reducing protein concentrates in rations of chicks at different ages. Poultry Sci. 14:156. 1935.

107. Pratt, J. M. A biological study of the protein and riboflavin content of British Columbia fish meals. M. S. Thesis, University of British Columbia. 1942.

Carter, C. W. Feeding pullets on less animal protein. Texas Progress Rept. 856.

Carver, J. S., and M. Rhian. Soybean oil meal in the chick starting ration. U. S. Egg and Poultry Mag. 49:131. 1943.

Bearse, G. E., D. Boucher, L. R. Berg, and V. L. Miller. Soybean oil meal in the chick starting ration. U. S. Egg and Poultry Mag. 49:131. 1943.

Carver, J. S., and R. J. Evans. Animal and vegetable protein combinations in chick starting rations. U. S. Egg and Poultry Mag. 49:468. 1943.

Draper, C. I., and R. J. Evans. Soybean oil meal in the broiler ration. Wash. V Circ. 19. 1944.

Brant, A. W., and J. S. Carver. Growing pullets under protein conservation plan. Flour and Feed 44(8):20. 1944.

Marvel, J. A., C. W. Carrick, R. E. Roberts, and S. M. Hauge. A comparison of soybean oils and soybean oil meals in chick rations containing distillers' dried solubles. Poultry Sci. 24:46. 1945.

Scott, H. H., T. B. Avery, and L. D. Matterson, Conservation of animal protein in chick rations. Flour and Feed 43(12):32. 1943.

Sloan, H. J., and L. E. Card. Soybean oil meal a good protein feed for chicks. Ill. Rept. 1937:120.

Bird, H. R., and A. C. Groschke. Feeds for chick mashes. Flour and Feed 43(5):7. 1942.

Bird, H. R. Dehydrated pea vines and starfish meal in poultry feeds. Poultry Sci. 23:76. 1944.

Irwin, M. R., and H. L. Kempster. The value of soybean oil meal in broiler rations. Mo. Bul. 441. 1942.

Heuser, G. F., and L. C. Norris. Effect of the war upon protein needs of poultry. Farm Research (New York State Agricultural Experiment Station) 9:1. 1943.

Norris, L. C., and G. F. Heuser. Studies on the amount of animal protein required in poultry rations. Flour and Feed 43(8):38. 1943.

Heuser, G. F., and L. C. Norris. Soybean oil meal in chick rations. Cornell Bul. 810. 1944.

Winter, A. R. Protein feedstuffs for poultry rations. Flour and Feed 43(10):10. 1943.

Almquist, H. J. Summary of reports on minimum levels of animal protein required in supplementation of expeller soybean meal and cereal proteins in poultry mashes. Flour and Feed 44(2):12. 1943.

Almquist, H. J. Oil-cake meal for poultry feeding. Flour and Feed 43(8):14. 1943.

Wilgus, H. S., Jr., and D. V. Zander. The quantity of animal protein required to supplement soybean oil meal for growth. Poultry Sci. 24:41. 1945.

108. Cassel, L. W. The value of various proteins and combinations of them for laying pullets. Wash. Bul. 229:42, 1928; Wash. Bul. 237:42, 1929.

Graham, W. R., J. B. Smith, and W. D. McFarlane. Results of a three years study of certain poultry rations as they affect the hatching power of hen eggs as well as the number of eggs laid. Ont. Bul. 362. 1931.

Parkhurst, R. T., and E. B. Lomax. Comparative value of various protein feeds for laying hens. Harper Adams Agr. Col. Bul. 4. 1930.

Parkhurst, R. T., and I. W. Rhys. Mixed protein rations for laying hens and breeders. Harper Adams Agr. Col. Bul. 7. 1932.
Leschke, B. The value of various proteins. Zentralblatt für Kleintierzucht, p. 26. 1931.
Weigner, G., and A. Tscherniak. Fütterungsversuche mit Magermilchpulver bei Legenhühnern. Biedermanns Zentralbl B. Tierernährung 7:344. 1935.
Weigner, G., and A. Tscherniak. Wie wirken Magermilchpulver und Dorschmehl als Eiweissbeifutter bei Legehennen? Tierwelt, Zofingen-Schweiz. 45:773. 1935.
Hewitt, A. C. T. Poultry feeding experiments. The Poultry Farmer (New South Wales) 10(9):17. 1942.
Bearse, G. E. Protein supplements for laying hens. Wash. Bul. 347. 1937.
Henderson, E. W. A comparison of dry milk, meat, and bone meal and combinations of both as protein supplements for egg production and a critique of methods. Poultry Sci. 18:106. 1939.

109. Shrimp meal as a protein supplement for chickens. La. Bul. 262: 31. 1935.
Record, P. R., R. M. Bethke, O. H. M. Wilder, and D. C. Kennard. The comparative nutritive value of different fish meals for chicks. Poultry Sci. 13:259. 1934.
Carver, J. S., J. L. St. John, M. W. Miller, and G. E. Bearse. The comparative efficiency of various proteins for growing chicks. Wash. Bul. 321. 1935.
Asmundson, V. S., and J. Biely. Fish meal supplements for chicks. I. Comparative rate of growth to eight weeks on rations supplemented with pilchard, salmon, halibut, dried skimmilk, or with salmon meal and dried skimmilk. Sci. Agr. 12:236. 1932.
Biely, J., and V. S. Asmundson. Fish meal supplements for chicks. II. Comparative rate of growth to eight weeks on rations supplemented with various proportions of fish meal and dried skimmilk. Sci. Agr. 13:435. 1933.

110. Tabakoff, I. I. The comparative influence of animal and plant proteins upon the growth of chicks reared on free range. Rept. Sixth World's Poultry Congress (I) :346. Berlin-Leipzig. 1936.

111. Wilgus, H. S., Jr., R. C. Ringrose, and L. C. Norris. Studies of the essential nutritive properties of common protein supplements used in poultry rations. Proc. Fifth World's Poultry Congress. 541. Rome. 1933.
Record, P. R., R. M. Bethke, and O. H. M. Wilder. Effect of method of manufacture on the nutritive value of fish meals as determined by growth studies with chicks. Jour. Agr. Res. 49: 715. 1934.
Oshima, K., and S. Itaya. The relation of the qualities and the manufacturing method of fish meal and scrap. Jour. Agr. Chem. Soc. Japan 14:512. 1938.
Chlebnikow, N. J., and A. F. Arsenjef. Die technologischen Bearbeitungsbedingungen und die biologische Wertigkeit des Fischmehls. Beidermanns Zentralblatt. B. Tierernährung 8:565. 1936.
Haddock fish meal proteins. Pigs and Pig Products 5:11. 1936

Clandinin, D. R. The effects of methods of processing on the nutritive value of herring meals. Poultry Sci. 28:128. 1949.

112. Evans, R. J., J. S. Carver, and W. S. Hamm. The influence of storage on the supplementary protein nutritive value of certain fish meals. Poultry Sci. 23:491. 1944.

113. Wilgus, H. S., Jr., R. C. Ringrose, and L. C. Norris. Studies of the essential nutritive properties of common protein supplements used in poultry rations. Proc. Fifth World's Congress. 541. Rome. 1933.

Wilgus, H. S., Jr., L. C. Norris, and R. C. Ringrose. Studies of the essential nutritive properties of some common protein supplements used in poultry rations. I. The relative efficiency of the proteins. Poultry Sci. 12:331. 1933.

Wilgus, H. S., Jr., L. C. Norris, and G. F. Heuser. The relative protein efficiency and the relative vitamin G content of common protein supplements used in poultry rations. Jour. Agr. Res. 51:383. 1935.

114. Heiman, V., and J. S. Carver. A method for determining the gross value of protein concentrates. Poultry Sci. 16:359. 1937.

Robertson, E. I., and J. S. Carver. Protein values of concentrates. Wash. Bul. 368. 1938.

Cook, J. W., J. L. St. John, and V. Heiman. A comparison of method for the determination of protein efficiency of protein supplements. Poultry Sci. 17:445. 1938.

Robertson, E. I., J. S. Carver, and J. W. Cook. Gross protein values of some concentrates. Poultry Sci. 17:443. 1938.

Heiman, V., J. S. Carver, and J. W. Cook. A method for determining the gross value of protein concentrates. Poultry Sci. 18:464. 1939.

Robertson, E. I., J. S. Carver, B. B. Bohren, and J. W. Cook. Gross values of combinations of some protein concentrates. Poultry Sci. 18:410. 1939.

Draper, C. I., and M. Rhian. Gross values of combinations of soybean oil with pilchard meal or meat meal. U. S. Egg and Poultry Mag. 48:466. 1942.

115. Mussehl, F. E., and C. W. Ackerson. Utilization of proteins by the growing chick. Neb. Res. Bul. 55, 1931.

116. Almquist, H. J., E. L. R. Stokstad, and E. R. Halbrook. Supplementary values of animal protein concentrates in chick rations. Jour. Nutr. 10:193. 1935.

Almquist, H. J. Chemical estimation of quality in animal protein concentrates. Jour. Nutr. 21:347. 1941.

117. Clandinin, D. R. The effects of methods of processing on the nutritive value of herring meals. Poultry Sci. 28:128. 1949.

March, B. E., D. Stupich, and J. Biely. The evaluation of the nutritional value of fish meals and meat meals. Poultry Sci. 28: 718. 1949.

CHAPTER 7

POULTRY FEEDS

VEGETABLE PROTEIN SUPPLEMENTS

In general, cereal grains alone have not given satisfactory results in growth or egg production, owing largely to deficiencies in protein and minerals. However, with birds on range in Northern Ireland,[1] a production of approximately 200 eggs from White Wyandotte pullets has been reported for a ration of cereals, supplemented only with minerals. The further addition of a protein-rich feed resulted in an additional increase of 13.5 per cent in egg production.

Protein has always been considered an important constituent of the ration. As shown in Chapter 6, animal protein products have consistently given satisfactory results. It is only natural, therefore, to inquire about the value of vegetable protein feeds, particularly where they are home grown or cheaper. Since early feeding trials have generally demonstrated the superiority of protein-rich feeds from animal origin, as compared with those from a vegetable source, it is of value to know to what extent vegetable proteins can be used and to find out in what respects they are deficient.

The results of some of the early experiments[2-6] with vegetable proteins were not favorable, but these could probably be attributed to deficiencies of minerals or amino acids. On the other hand, other experiments[7,8] indicated satisfactory results, particularly for laying hens.

A number of protein-rich vegetable feeds have been used in feeding trials with poultry. However, cottonseed meal and soybean products have been fed most extensively, probably because of the supply of the cottonseed meal, and of the favorable results obtained with the soybean.

COTTONSEED MEAL

COTTONSEED MEAL FOR MATURE BIRDS. A large number of experiments have been conducted using cottonseed meal in rations for mature hens.[9]

Results in Egg Production. A review of the early experiments involving the use of cottonseed meal shows that most of the trials do not give favorable egg production as compared with the trials in feeding some animal proteins, such as meat or milk. It is probable that many of these productions are low because of mineral deficiencies.[10] Table 13 gives some of the results.

TABLE 13. AVERAGE EGG PRODUCTION PER HEN FROM COTTONSEED MEAL TRIALS

Meat	Cottonseed	Cottonseed Plus Minerals	Reference
135	60	83	Mo. Circ. 82
117	48	81	Mo. Bul. 225
107	67	117	Mo. Bul. 236
143	45	136	Mo. Bul. 256
122	49	106	Ohio Monthly Bul. 7-8, 1924
	117	134	
174	97	154	Okla. Rept., 1925-1926
	106	131	

Even though cottonseed meal cannot be used alone as the protein-rich supplement to the mash, it may be possible to use it in combination with animal protein feeds. Several stations report tests where a combination of meat scraps or tankage and cottonseed meal gave better results than either one alone.

Poorer hatchability has been reported for the hens fed cottonseed meal. This has been attributed to the harmful effects of the components of cottonseed pigment glands, including gossypol, and a deficiency of lysine.[11]

Greater mortality and smaller egg size have been reported in some of the trials in the pens receiving cottonseed meal.

Effect of Cottonseed upon Egg Quality. The most serious objection to the use of cottonseed meal in the poultry ration has been its effect upon the quality of the egg,[12] although in many trials this effect is not mentioned. An early report by Roberts and Rice[13] indicated that the eggs laid by nitrogen-fed hens (cottonseed meal ration) were small and had a disagreeable flavor and smell, watery albumen, an especially small, dark-colored yolk, with a tender vitelline membrane, which turned black after being kept several weeks in brine.

Cottonseed meal spots occur on the yolk and can be seen when candled. The market value is thus affected because of the unattractive appearance. Yolks may vary considerably in appearance, ranging from a few tiny brown spots to a condition where the brownish area may cover a large part of the yolk.

In some reports it has been stated that the eggs that were seriously affected with the cottonseed meal spots had a strong flavor which made them objectionable for most uses.

Cottonseed meal affects the keeping quality of eggs in storage,[14] which holds true also for eggs that do not show the cottonseed meal spots. Heavy losses have been reported with eggs held in storage because of dark yolks that resulted from the heavy feeding of cottonseed meal.

Sherwood reported that the substance in cottonseed meal that causes eggs to deteriorate in storage was probably something closely associated with the cottonseed oil. Experiments conducted at the Louisiana Station indicated that gossypol is the factor responsible for olive-colored yolks. The characteristic olive color is due to a chemical combination of gossypol with ferric iron, released from the egg proteins of the yolk. In the fresh yolk insufficient ferric ions are present. During storage, sufficient iron is liberated to form the olive color. The addition of soluble ferric salts to the ration containing cottonseed meal prevents the absorption of gossypol by the hen and the formation of olive yolks in the stored eggs.

The degree of yolk darkening during storage increased as the free gossypol content of the diets increased. Bound gossypol did not cause discoloration of the eggs. Eggs from hens fed gland-free cottonseed flour do not develop egg-yolk discoloration. The storage quality of eggs produced from hens fed screw-pressed cottonseed meal or isopropanol extracted meal was satisfactory whereas olive-colored yolks and pink albumen were observed when a hydraulic meal was fed.

GENERAL SUMMARY. As far as egg production is concerned, the results are variable. The use of cottonseed meal seems to be warranted as a substitute for meat and tankage. Cottonseed meal is useful for the production of eggs when the eggs are to be used fresh but not when they are to be stored because of the effect upon the quality of the eggs. If cottonseed meal is used in the ration for laying hens, adjustment should be made for its mineral deficiency. It is also advisable to use it only to furnish part of the protein-rich feed and not to substitute it entirely for meat scraps or similar feeds.

COTTONSEED MEAL FOR YOUNG CHICKENS. As early as 1899 the New York (Geneva) Experiment Station[15] reported that when the deficiency of mineral matter was made good by the addition of bone ash, the vegetable food ration for chicks equaled or somewhat surpassed in efficiency a corresponding ration containing three-eighths of the protein from animal food.

Workers at the Rhode Island Station[16] reported that the animal protein ration produced faster growth when compared with cottonseed meal, gluten feed, gluten meal, and oil meal. However, the addition of ash constituents greatly improved the vegetable protein feeds.

Some experiments indicated slower growth with a cottonseed meal ration.[17] Other experiments show good results,[18] especially when properly supplemented with animal protein. A combination of protein supplements seems to be more important than the percentage of cottonseed meal used.

The method of processing affects the nutritive value of cottonseed meal.[19] The physiologically deleterious components of cottonseed are segregated in the pigment glands. Hence gland-free meals and some processed meals have supported excellent growth. Solvent meal has been reported slightly superior and hydraulic meal inferior to expeller meal.

SOYBEAN PRODUCTS

Soybeans are being raised in greater abundance, partly because of their value in crop rotations. It is one of the most valuable of the leguminous seeds. The two important commercial products derived from soybeans are soybean oil and soybean oil meal. Soybean oil meal, the product remaining after removal of the oil, should not be confused with soybean meal, which refers to ground whole soybeans.

SOYBEAN OIL MEAL. There are several processes employed in making soybean oil meal: (1) solvent or new process, in which the oil is removed by use of some chemical that will dissolve oil; (2) hydraulic or old process, in which the oil is removed by hydraulic pressure; (3) expeller method, in which the oil is expelled by a friction process which generates heat.

Soybean oil meals, processed from frost-damaged immature beans,[20] have been fed to chicks with results that have compared favorably with results from those fed normal meal.

The soybean contains a high percentage of physiologically good protein, a considerable amount of energy-yielding material, and a fairly liberal supply of the fat-soluble and water-soluble vitamins. The soybean protein has been reported to be quite as valuable as the casein of milk.[21]

The soybean is deficient in minerals, however, and sodium chloride and calcium compounds need to be added. Soybean oil meal is much lower in calcium and phosphorus content than the animal proteins. Hence it was soon discovered that the mineral content of the protein supplements was as important as the protein content.[22]

A ration deriving its protein chiefly from soybean meal has also been shown to be deficient in the sulfur-bearing amino acids, especially methionine.[23]

A ration composed largely of corn and soybean oil meal is likely to be deficient in vitamins,[24] particularly riboflavin, pantothenic acid, niacin, choline, vitamin B_{12}, and unknown factors present in animal products. The vitamin deficiencies have been reported as being corrected by the microbiological action produced in built-up litter.[25]

The variable results obtained with soybean oil meal indicated differences in nutritive value in various samples of the meal depending largely upon the conditions of manufacture.[17,26] Raw soybeans and also soybean oil meals processed at low temperatures contain proteins of low nutritive value, whereas soybean oil meals prepared at higher temperatures contain proteins of higher nutritive value.[27] The color and flavor of the meals are not infallible criteria of their nutritive value, but a raw, beany flavor is indicative of an insufficient amount of heat and a resulting inferior protein efficiency.

The raw soybeans contain a trypsin inhibitor[28] which is inactivated by heating. Heating also renders the soybean nutrients more available or digestible.[29] On the other hand there is the possibility of impairment of feeding value by overheating.[30] The methionine and lysine seem to be particularly affected. Overheating may cause the production of brown-colored substances that appeared to be related to more liquid and sticky droppings produced by the birds.[31]

Experiments conducted at the Colorado Station[32] showed that raw soybeans had a goitrogenic effect when fed to chicks. This effect was partially inactivated by heat. Iodine counteracted the effect on the thyroid. Egg production and hatchability were low, and it is suggested that the poor reproduction was related to the goitrogenicity of soybean meal.

Increasing the level of soybean meal in the diet of broilers has been reported to increase water consumption.[33]

Laboratory estimations of the biological value[34,95] of soybean meal have been reported. Underheated soybean oil meals contain a substance or substances which significantly delay coagulation time of the blood of chicks.

SOYBEAN OIL MEAL FOR HENS. Egg production has been satisfactory when soybean oil meal was used either as a partial source or the sole source of supplemental protein.[35,36] Satisfactory body weight has also been obtained.

The results of some of the early experiments comparing soybean oil meal with meat scrap and fish meal were not favorable for the soybean oil meal because minerals were a limiting factor. When minerals were properly supplemented,[36] the egg production with soybean oil meal was increased and made comparable with that secured with rations containing animal protein. Some of the representative results are shown in Table 14.

TABLE 14. INFLUENCE OF SOYBEAN OIL MEAL ON EGG PRODUCTION

Soybean Oil Meal Plus Minerals	Animal Protein	Source
125	139	Ind. Rept. 1923
151	140	Ind. Bul. 293
125	139	Ind. Bul. 293
144	133	Ind. Bul. 293
138	132	Ind. Bul. 293
173	186	Ind. Bul. 293
135	153	Ind. Bul. 293
139	143	Mo. Bul. 256
132	139	Mo. Bul. 272
133	142	Mo. Bul. 285
223	210	Scottish Jour. Agr. 11
194	232	Scottish Jour. Agr. 11
164	166	Harper Adams Bul. 4

The feeding of soybean oil meal to breeders has shown variable results in hatchability.[37] Soybean oil meal as the only supplemental protein has usually not been satisfactory. However, when hatchability results were unfavorable they could usually be attributed to some deficiency such as riboflavin, vitamin B_{12}, or other essential nutritive factors.

SOYBEAN OIL MEAL FOR FEEDING THE YOUNG STOCK. Soybean Oil Meal. The results from the feeding of soybean oil meal to growing chickens and poults have been very satisfactory. The chick can utilize soybean oil meal protein to advantage. Some trials[38] indicate just as good results with soybean oil meal as with animal protein, provided that the minerals are adjusted and that the protein is the only varying factor. On the other hand, a number of experiments[39] report superior results for animal proteins, such as meat scraps and dried buttermilk. In general, a combination of soybean oil meal and animal proteins or their equivalent has given good growth.[40] This is particularly true for the starting ration.

In rations containing large amounts of soybean oil meal, Hammond[41] concluded that as much as 15 per cent of cottonseed meal, corn gluten meal, peanut meal, or ground hempseed may be used to replace an equal weight of soybean oil meal for growing chickens.

The Western Washington Station[42] reported that rations in which soybean oil meal supplied all the supplemental protein caused "pasting up" in chicks to a much greater extent than did rations in which herring fish meal or casein furnished the supplemental protein. The amount of "pasting up" which occurred varied with different samples of the meal. Less of it was caused by the solvent process meal. The droppings of chicks fed soybean oil meal rations were of a stickier consistency than were those fed fish meal or casein rations. The retardation in growth caused by this condition was only slight at 4 weeks of age.

GROUND SOYBEANS. Ground Soybeans have been used in laying rations. They are not as efficient as the soybean oil meal, however, and in most trials did not give as good results as the soybean oil meal or animal protein.[43] The Delaware Station found that ground soybeans were relished and readily eaten and that they maintained excellent physical condition. It was found furthermore than when the laying ration contained over 7 per cent of ground soybeans, the egg production per hen decreased and mortality increased. On the other hand, the Indiana Station found ground whole soybeans as satisfactory as soybean oil meal. In this work, the hens were allowed free range over a grassy plot at all times.

Ground Soybeans are not so effective in the feeding of young chickens[44] as soybean oil meal, but they can be used if they are relatively cheap. The quantities used, however, must be limited. The Delaware Agricultural Experiment Station concluded that if the ground soybeans, supplemented with bone meal, do not replace more than one-third of the meat scrap, the results will not be seriously affected. Experiments conducted at Cornell[45] and Nebraska[46] showed the relative protein efficiency of ground raw soybeans to be approximately 65 to 70 per cent of that of soybean oil meal, when expressed on the basis of growth response.

Ground whole cooked soybeans effectively replaced 5 per cent of soybean meal and 5 per cent of cottonseed meal when fed at a 20 per cent level in a broiler mash during a 9-week growing period at the Oklahoma Station.[47]

PEANUT PRODUCTS

PEANUT MEAL[48] as a source of protein has generally given satisfactory results, especially when the deficiencies were overcome. The deficiencies of peanut meal are minerals,[49] methionine, and lysine.[50]

Experiments at the Alabama Station[51] showed that the feeding of peanuts, without shells, to either hens or chicks gave poor results, thought to be due to the inability of the chicks to utilize large amounts of fat.

CORN PRODUCTS

GLUTEN FEED[52] has not given good results in egg production, especially in the earlier work, although some improvement has been shown when minerals were added. This is probably due to the fact that gluten feed is deficient in protein quality and in riboflavin. Other results[53] indicate that corn gluten feed is suitable as a partial protein supplement in rations for growing chicks as well as mature birds.

GLUTEN MEAL. Corn gluten meal[54] may be used in rations for laying hens and chicks when properly supplemented to compensate for its deficiencies. It might be lacking in arginine, lysine, and tryptophan[55] and in some of the members of the vitamin B complex. Used in large amounts it is not as satisfactory as soybean oil meal.[56] When corn gluten meal was used in rations for growing chicks and poults the degree of pigmentation of the shanks and skin was markedly increased.[57]

CORN OIL MEAL. Several experiments were conducted at the Iowa Station[58] to determine the nutritive value of corn oil meal and feather protein. The chicks fed a basal diet, supplemented with large quantities of corn oil meal (over 30 per cent), grew at a very slow rate, utilized their feed inefficiently, and suffered a high mortality. The inclusion of up to 30 per cent of corn oil meal did not affect palatability of the feed. The addition of cystine or lysine increased the growth.

LINSEED OIL MEAL

Early experiments with linseed oil meal have not shown good results.[59] The addition of minerals improves linseed meal but does not make it so efficient as animal protein.[60]

Linseed meal is deficient in lysine.[61] It also contains a factor or factors detrimental to the growth and health of chickens. It has been suggested that the presence of mucilage in linseed oil meal is one of the factors.[62] The toxic principal in linseed oil meal has been destroyed by water treatment or overcome by additional pyridoxine.[63] Flaxseed treated with ammonia and stored before processing was found superior to untreated flaxseed meal.[64]

Supplementing the linseed meal with a small amount of fish meal has improved its feeding value.[65]

OTHER VEGETABLE PROTEINS

Other vegetable protein feeds have been used in poultry feeding. The Idaho Station[66] lists pea meal, alfalfa meal, and bean meal in the order mentioned. Bean meal gave smaller eggs than the others.

BROCCOLI MEAL[67] as the only protein supplement did not produce good growth but when combined with soybean oil meal maintained fair growth and livability.

CASTOR BEAN. Castor bean oil meal[68] was toxic when fed to chicks either untreated or after steaming. However, repeated extraction resulted in a meal which gave normal growth.

COCONUT OIL MEAL. "Cocoanut oil meal or copra oil meal is the ground residue obtained after the extraction of part of the oil from the dried meat of the cocoanut. It must be designated and sold according to its protein content." Coconut oil meal, plus minerals, was used by the Pennsylvania Station[69] as a vegetable protein to replace a large part of the animal protein. In the Philippines,[70] copra meal did not prove satisfactory for growing chicks or ducklings. With an increase in the amount of copra meal, mortality increased while food consumption and weight increase diminished. A report from England[71] indicated that coconut meal up to 20 and 25 per cent of the mash was satisfactory for laying hens.

HORSE-BEAN (*Vicia Faba L.*) MEAL[72] as the principal protein source is very deficient in the sulfur-containing amino acids and deficient to a lesser degree in a number of others. However, when properly supplemented improvement in growth and feathering were obtained.

IPIL-IPIL SEED MEAL[73] is not a satisfactory protein supplement for chick rations, but it can be improved by water treatment.

LESPEDEZA SEED. The Missouri Station[74] reported that whole lespedeza seed proved a satisfactory substitute for soybean oil meal in chick rations, when fed at levels not to exceed

15 per cent. More than this amount produced sticky droppings. The whole lespedeza seed proved superior to ground lespedeza seed as a supplement to meat scrap.

MUNGO. The mungo bean has been used in the Philippines[75] in rations for growing chicks. Fair results were obtained by replacing 20 to 40 per cent of the shrimp meal by mungo. Mungo as the sole protein supplement caused high mortality and small size in chicks.

The Oklahoma Station[76] reports satisfactory growth, egg production, and hatchability when mungo beans were properly supplemented. They were also satisfactory as a source of protein for turkey poults.

MUSTARD. Mustard seed oil meal in chick rations has given variable results.[77] O'Neil indicated significantly lower weights with as small quantities as 2.8 per cent. Kondra and Hodgson reported normal growth on mashes containing up to 9 per cent of the meal.

PALM NUT. Corozo palm nut oil meal[78] can be fed to chicks as a partial supply of protein. It was found to supplement sesame oil meal and cottonseed meal.

PEAS. Peas have been used in feeding hens at the Idaho Station.[79] The egg production was better than where no protein concentrate was fed, but not so good as the production in the animal protein lots. Ground peas needed to be supplemented with animal protein to meet the requirements of laying hens. Methionine was shown to be the principal growth-limiting deficiency of pea protein. Pea meal as the main protein source for chicks[80] is unsatisfactory. However, when supplemented with fish meal or casein to supply methionine growth was improved.

RAPESEED OIL MEAL. Rapeseed oil meal[81] is the byproduct in the production of oil from rapeseed. Feeding experiments with hens in Germany indicated that, on the mash containing 15 per cent of rapeseed cake, food consumption was reduced. A maximum of 10 per cent of this ingredient is recommended. Rapeseed oil meal can be fed in limited amounts in chick rations. When larger amounts are included in the ration mortality and a reduction in the rate of growth during the early period of the bird's life resulted. It has been shown that the rapeseed oil meal contains a goitrogenic agent. This meal may be used for growing birds after hot water extraction or when supplemented with iodine. It has been suggested that rapeseed oil meal may be more suitable for fattening and finishing.

SAFFLOWER OIL FEED. Safflower oil feed is the ground

residue obtained after the extraction of the oil from whole safflower seed. Safflower oil meal[82] when properly supplemented gave good growth. It is deficient in lysine and methionine.

SESAME OIL MEAL. "Sesame oil meal is the ground residue obtained after the extraction of part of the oil by pressure from sesame seed as produced under reasonable milling conditions. It must be designated and sold according to its protein content." Poor growth has been reported on sesame protein alone,[83] owing primarily to a deficiency of lysine and vitamin B_{12}, In connection with other proteins (soybean meal and fish meal), relatively richer in lysine, sesame seed is capable of supporting optimal chick growth rates.

Sesame Cake Meal has also given satisfactory results when fed to laying pullets.[84]

SORGHUM GLUTEN MEAL[85] is not satisfactory as a major protein supplement since it is deficient in the amino acids arginine, lysine, methionine, and tryptophan. When properly supplemented it has produced the same results in chick rations as corn gluten meal and could be used in place of it.

SUNFLOWER SEED. Sunflower seed oil meal[86] is the byproduct in the production of oil from sunflower seeds. The chief deficiency appears to be lysine. It has proven satisfactory in chick and turkey starter rations especially when used in combination with other proteins. Sunflower oil cake and meal have also been satisfactorily fed to mature birds.

SWEET LUPINES. Ground sweet lupine seeds, which contain about 45 per cent protein, have been fed to chickens in Germany.[87] It was shown that one-third or more of the usual fish and meat meal could be replaced by ground seeds of yellow sweet lupines.

Sweet blue lupine[88] did not prove satisfactory in replacing part of the soybean oil meal in a chick ration.

TUNG OIL MEAL. Tung oil meal is the residue remaining after the oil has been expressed from ground dehulled tung fruit. It has been reported as being unpalatable and containing some irritating material which has a harmful effect on the mucous membrane of the intestines. The Florida Station[89] reported that feeding tung oil meal to chicks was unsatisfactory.

WHEAT GLUTEN.[90] Wheat gluten meal and wheat gluten feed are deficient chiefly in lysine, but when properly supplemented they can furnish part of the protein in chick rations.

YEAST. Experiments in Poland[91] showed that the protein of yeast had a nutritive value almost equal to that of milk protein and greater than that of all other vegetable proteins. The egg yield was increased 6 to 10 per cent, and the weight of chickens and ducklings 2 to 12 per cent, according to the proportion of yeast-treated feeding stuffs in the ration.

Results from Germany[92] indicate that a 5 per cent yeast-supplemented ration had 17 per cent higher egg production that a similar pen receiving the same amount of skimmilk but no yeast.

Distillery yeast[93] in amounts of 10 to 15 per cent has been reported satisfactory for layers and growing chicks.

The feeding results with torula yeast have been variable,[94] depending to some extent upon the conditions under which it is produced and the wastes utilized in its production. The results indicate that it is a satisfactory source of protein and riboflavin.

NUTRITIVE VALUE OF VEGETABLE PROTEINS

Evans and St. John[95] reported that the chemical protein quality index, as used for animal proteins, appeared to give good indication of the relative protein nutritive value for soybean oil meals, cottonseed meals, and Alaska peas, with the exception of the overcooked soybean oil meals. A coefficient of correlation between gain per unit of supplementary protein and the chemical protein quality index of +0.946 was obtained. A high coefficient of correlation of +0.928 between the gain per unit of supplementary protein and the percentage of glutelin (insoluble in water, saline solutions, or alcohol, but soluble in very dilute acids and alkalies) was obtained for the heat-treated concentrates. A determination of the percentage of glutelin may offer a chemical means of estimating differences in the protein nutritive values of soybean oil meals and, in combination with the percentage of residual protein, the extent of heat denaturation of the soybean proteins.

Laboratory estimations[34] of the value of soybean meal have been reported. Fluorescence and urease activity gave a satisfactory evaluation of the nutritive value for chicks of solvent soybean oil meals but not of expeller meals.

A chemical index (total gossypol content plus N soluble in 0.02 sodium hydroxide) for cottonseed meal[96] gave good correlation with chick growth rate.

GENERAL SUMMARY FOR VEGETABLE PROTEINS

Animal protein feeds have been somewhat more effective than vegetable protein feeds for both young and mature stock. The lack of good results from vegetable proteins has probably been due to a deficiency, chiefly in minerals, certain amino acids, and vitamins. Partial substitutions have given very satisfactory results. With an increasing knowledge of requirements for these factors and a more exact knowledge of the nature of the more common poultry feeds, it should be possible to find combinations of feeds which include larger proportions of vegetable feeds. In general, the vegetable proteins need to be supplemented with minerals, particularly calcium and phosphorus, and vitamins, of which they contain considerably less than the animal proteins.

REFERENCES

1. Prentice, J. H., R. G. Baskett, and G. S. Robertson. The nutrition of the chick and its effect on growth, maturity, egg production, and mortality. Rept. Fourth World's Poultry Congress. 242. London. 1930.
   Robertson, G. S., and R. G. Baskett. The nutritive requirement of poultry. The influence of certain nutritional factors on the size of the egg and the condition of the birds. Scottish Jour. Agr. 11: 176. 1928.
   Robertson, G. S., and R. G. Baskett. The feeding of poultry. Jour. Ministry Agr. N. Ireland 2:1. 1929.
2. Lewis, H. R. The ash and protein factor in poultry feeding. N. J. Bul. 265. 1913.
   Thompson, W. C. Protein of animal origin for poultry feeding. N. J. Rept. 1924:134.
3. Experiments with poultry at the Idaho Station. Idaho Sta. Bul. 160: 27. 1928.
4. Guisti, G. Sulla importanza Delle Proteine Animali Nella Alimentazione Dei Pulcini. Clinica Veterinaria 432. 1930.
5. Hatano, T. Effect of feeding vegetable protein on copulation and fertilization in the fowl. Proc. Fifth World's Poultry Congress (II) :547. Rome. 1933.
   Hatano, T. Effect of feeding vegetable proteins on copulation and fertilization in the fowl. Bul. Agr. Chem. Soc. Japan 11:125. 1935.
6. Byerly, T. C., H. W. Titus, and N. R. Ellis. Production and hatchability of eggs as affected by different kinds and quantities of proteins in the diet of laying hens. Jour. Agr. Res. 46:1. 1933.
7. Fangauf, R., and E. Kallmann. Ölkuchengemisch als teilweiser Ersatz für Fischmehl. Archiv für Geflügelk. 6:353. 1932.
   Weinmiller, L. Pflanzliches Eiweiss im Hühnerfutter. Archiv für Geflügelk. 6:203. 1932.
8. Bird, H. R. Laying mash containing no animal protein. Flour and Feed 44(5) :16. 1943.
   Wilson, W. O. Corn, wheat, and barley for chickens. S. Dak. Bul. 376. 1944.

9. Anderson, C. F. Cottonseed in the poultry ration. The Poultry Farmer (Australia) 17:10. 1949.
Cottonseed meal for laying hens. Miss. Rept. 1931:48.
Kempster, H. L. Influence of animal and vegetable proteins on egg production. Mo. Bul. 225. 1924.
Kempster, H. L. The value of cottonseed meal, soybean meal, dried skimmilk, and dried buttermilk in rations for egg production. Mo. Bul. 300:91. 1931.
Thompson, R. B. Poultry feeding experiment. N. Mex. Bul. 117. 1918.
Morgan, C. L. Poultry feeding experiments. S. Car. Bul. 273. 1931.
Sherwood, R. M. Comparison of the value of protein from vegetable sources with protein from animal sources when fed to laying hens. Tex. Rept. 1927:75.
Ivey, J. E. Experiments with poultry at the Alabama Station. Vegetable protein studies. Ala. Rept. 1927:14.
Embleton, H. R. Poultry feeding experiments. Comparing cottonseed meal, meat scraps, and dried buttermilk as protein supplements for egg production. Ariz. Bul. 143:84. 1933.
Experiments with poultry at the Arkansas Station. Ark. Bul. 203: 26. 1926.
Philips, A. G. Feeding experiments with Leghorns. Ind. Bul. 227: 3. 1919.
Sources and amounts of protein for hens. Ky. Rept. (1) :40. 1919.
Experimental work with poultry. Ky. Rept. (1) :35. 1920.
Martin, J. H. Cottonseed meal, buttermilk, and tankage as sources of protein of the laying hens. Jour. Am. Assoc. Instructors and Investigators Poultry Husb. 7:39. 1921.
Waite, R. H. Poultry experiment observations, notes, and plans. Cottonseed meal feeding experiment with poultry. Md. Bul. 244: 14. 1921.
Morrison, J. K. Cottonseed meal as a feed for laying hens. Miss. Bul. 162. 1913.
Clayton, E. P. Cottonseed meal: A good feed for laying hens. Miss. Bul. 175. 1916.
Clayton, E. P., and J. Clayton. Experiments with poultry. Miss. Bul. 204. 1921.
Clayton, E. P. Poultry feeding experiments at the Mississippi Station. Miss. Rept. 1924:14.
Clayton, E. P. Poultry investigations at the Mississippi Station. Comparing certain proteins as egg producers. Miss. Rept. 1926: 23.
Clayton, E. P. Poultry studies at the Mississippi Station. A study in various proteins alone and in combination as egg producers. Miss. Rept. 1927:35.
Kempster, H. L., and G. W. Hervey. Meat scrap and sour milk for egg production. Mo. Bul. 155. 1918.
Kempster, H. L. Value of sour milk, beef scrap, cottonseed meal, gluten meal, and oil meal in rations for egg production. Mo. Bul. 172:36. 1920.

Kempster, H. L., and E. W. Henderson. Value of sour milk, beef scrap, cottonseed meal, gluten meal, and oil meal in rations for egg production. Mo. Bul. 197:76. 1922.
Kempster, H. L., and E. W. Henderson. Value of sour milk, beef scrap, cottonseed meal, gluten meal, and oil meal in rations for egg production. Mo. Bul. 210:59. 1924.
Kempster, H. L. Value of sour milk, beef scrap, cottonseed meal, gluten meal, and oil meal in rations for egg production. Mo. Bul. 236:66. 1926.
Kempster, H. L. Value of sour milk, beef scrap, cottonseed meal, gluten meal, and oil meal in rations for egg production. Mo. Bul. 256:84. 1927.
Kempster, H. L. Value of cottonseed meal, ground soybeans, soybean meal, tankage, meat scrap, and dried buttermilk in rations for egg production. Mo. Bul. 272:78. 1929.
Kempster, H. L. Value of dried buttermilk, meat scrap, cottonseed meal, soybean meal, and ground soybeans in rations for egg production. Mo. Bul. 285:95. 1930.
Kempster, H. L. Influence of various protein concentrates on egg production. Mo. Bul. 288. 1930.
Lewis, H. R., and W. C. Thompson. Animal vs. vegetable protein. N. J. Rept. 1915:100.
Cottonseed meal feeding. N. Mex. Rept. 1919:21.
Cottonseed meal feeding experiments. N. Mex. Rept. 1925:50.
Cottonseed meal feeding experiments. N. Mex. Rept. 1926:51.
Cottonseed meal feeding experiments. N. Mex. Rept. 1927:63.
Cottonseed meal feeding experiments. N. Mex. Rept. 1928:54.
Cottonseed meal feeding experiment. N. Mex. Rept. 1929:72.
Berry, L. N. Relative value of cottonseed meal and tankage for egg production. N. Mex. Bul. 183. 1930.
Kennard, D. C., and P. S. White. Cottonseed meal vs. meat scraps. Ohio Monthly Bul. IX(7 and 8) :107. 1924.
Ahrens, B. A. A study of the effect of cottonseed meal vs. beef scrap upon the egg production, fertility, and vitality of poultry. Okla. Bul. 112:3. 1917.
Embleton, E. Sources of protein feeds for poultry. Okla. Rept. 1919:50.
Thompson, R. B. Cottonseed meal. Okla. Rept. 1925-1926:52.
Cottonseed meal vs. meat scrap. S. C. Rept. 1929:82.
Comparison of high protein feeds. S. Dak. Rept. 1927:29.
High protein feeds. S. Dak. Rept. 1928:27.
Harvey, R. N. Poultry feeds and feeding results. Tex. Bul. 206:3. 1917.
Harvey, R. N. Egg-producing values of some Texas feeding stuffs. Tex. Bul. 220. 1917.
Comparison of cottonseed meal with animal protein feeds for laying hens. Tex. Rept. 1921:12.
Sherwood, R. M. Comparative influences of various protein feeds on laying hens. Tex. Bul. 317:5. 1924.
10. Thompson, R. B. Cottonseed meal for poultry. Okla. Rept. 1926-1930:103.

11. Heywang, B. W., and H. R. Bird. Supplements for cottonseed meal in diets for chickens. Poultry Sci. 29:486. 1950.

Heywang, B. W., H. R. Bird, and A. M. Altschul. The effect of pure gossypol on hatchability and egg weight. Poultry Sci. 30:763. 1951.

Heywang, B. W., H. R. Bird, and R. P. Kupperman. The loss or inactivation of pure gossypol in a mixed diet. Poultry Sci. 31:35. 1952.

Heywang, B. W., C. A. Denton, and H. R. Bird. The effect of the dietary level of cottonseed meal on hatchability. Poultry Sci. 28:610. 1949.

12. Lamon, H. M., and A. R. Lee. Feed cost of egg production. Results of three years' experiments at the Government Poultry Farms. U.S.D.A. Bul. 561. 1917.

Thompson, R. B. Poultry feeding experiment. N. Mex. Bul. 117. 1918.

Berry, L. N. Relative value of cottonseed meal and tankage for egg production. N. Mex. Bul. 183. 1930.

13. Roberts, I. P., and J. E. Rice. The effect on fowls of nitrogenous and carbonaceous rations. N. Y. (Cornell) Agr. Exp. Sta. Bul. 25:162. 1890.

14. Sherwood, R. M. The effect of various rations on the storage quality of eggs. Tex. Bul. 376. 1928.

Walker, A. L., L. N. Berry, and E. E. Anderson. New Mexico egg storage studies. N. Mex. Bul. 177. 1929.

Effect of cottonseed meal on storage eggs. Miss. Rept. 1930:32.

Sherwood, R. M. The effect of various rations on the storage quality of eggs. Poultry Sci. 8:99. 1929.

Sherwood, R. M. Sources of protein for laying hens. Texas Rept. 1929:88.

Sherwood, R. M. The effect of feeds on the quality of eggs. Texas 43rd Ann. Rept. 1930:82.

Sherwood, R. M. The effect of cottonseed meal and other feeds on the storage quality of eggs. Tex. Bul. 429. 1931.

Smith, R. M. The influence of some factors on the storage quality of eggs. Ark. Bul. 341. 1937.

Fieger, E. A., C. W. Upp, and A. D. Swenson. Biochemical study of olive yolk eggs from hens fed cottonseed meal. Proc. La. Acad. Sci. 7:85. 1942.

Swenson, A. D., E. A. Fieger, and C. W. Upp. The nature of egg yolk discoloration produced by cottonseed meal. Poultry Sci. 21: 374. 1942.

Schaible, P. J., S. L. Bandemer, and J. A. Davidson. Composition of fresh and storage eggs from hens fed cottonseed and noncottonseed rations. I. General observations. Poultry Sci. 25: 440. 1946.

Bandemer, S. L., P. J. Schaible, and J. A. Davidson. Composition of fresh and storage eggs from hens fed cottonseed and noncottonseed rations. II. Ammonia nitrogen content. Poultry Sci. 25:446. 1946.

Schaible, P. J., and S. L. Bandemer. Composition of fresh and storage eggs from hens fed cottonseed and noncottonseed rations. III. Iron content. Poultry Sci. 25:451. 1946.

Bandemer, S. L., and P. J. Schaible. Composition of fresh and storage eggs from hens fed cottonseed and noncottonseed rations. IV. Spectographic examination of the egg whites. Poultry Sci. 25: 453. 1946.

Schaible, P. J., and S. L. Bandemer. Composition of fresh and storage eggs from hens fed cottonseed and noncottonseed rations. V. Cause of discoloration. Poultry Sci. 25:456. 1946.

Brant, A. W., and J. S. Carver. From one day of age through the first laying year on rations containing soybean oil meal as a protein supplement. Poultry Sci. 26:598. 1947.

Heywang, B. W. A comparison of cottonseed and soybean meals in diets for laying chickens. Poultry Sci. 26:442. 1947.

Kuiken, K. A., C. M. Lyman, and F. Hale. The effect of feeding isopropanol extracted cottonseed meal on the storage quality of eggs. Poultry Sci. 27:742. 1948.

Heywang, B. W., C. A. Denton, and H. R. Bird. The effect of the dietary level of cottonseed meal on hatchability. Poultry Sci. 28: 610. 1949.

Stephenson, E. L., and R. M. Smith. The storage quality of eggs produced by hens fed screw-pressed cottonseed meal. Poultry Sci. 31:98. 1952.

15. Wheeler, W. P. Animal food for poultry. N. Y. (Geneva) Bul. 171: 461. 1899.

16. Bolte, J. W. Feeding experiments with chickens, cockerels, and turkeys. R. I. Bul. 126. 1908.

Hartwell, B. L., and W. F. Kirkpatrick. Protein concentrates for winter chickens. R. I. Bul. 145:3. 1911.

Wheeler, H. J. Cottonseed meal compared with beef scraps as a source of protein for chicks. R. I. Rept. (11) :202. 1912.

Hartwell, B. L., and R. A. Lichtenthaeler. The availability of the nitrogen of cottonseed meal and of beef scrap for chicks. R. I. Bul. 156. 1914.

17. Draper, C. I., and R. J. Evans. Gross values of combinations of cottonseed meal, soybean oil meal, and herring meal. Poultry Sci. 23:189. 1944.

Draper, C. I., and R. J. Evans. Plant protein concentrates in the chick ration. Poultry Sci. 23:507. 1944.

18. Annual report of the Mississippi Experiment Station. Miss. Rept. 1929:29.

Polk, H. O., and C. E. Barnett. Broiler production with high protein feeds. Miss. Bul. 374. 1943.

Barnett, C. E., and H. D. Polk. Cottonseed meal, shrimp meal, soybean meal, meat scraps for growing chicks. Miss. Farm Res. 1942.

Philips, A. G., R. H. Carr, and D. C. Kennard. Meat scraps vs. soybean proteins as a supplement to corn for growing chicks. Jour. Agr. Res. 18:391. 1920.

The utilization of food elements by growing chicks. V. A comparison of cottonseed meal and linseed oil meal as portions of the protein concentrate. Neb. Res. Bul. 100. 1938.

Poultry experiments at the Ohio Station. Linseed oil meal vs. meat scraps for layers. Ohio Bul. 417:71. 1928.

Bethke, R. M., G. Bohstedt, H. L. Sassaman, D. C. Kennard, and B. H. Edington. The comparative nutritive value of the proteins of linseed meal and cottonseed meal for different animals. Jour. Agr. Res. 36:855. 1928.

Berry, L. N. A comparison of the nutritive values of cottonseed meal, alfalfa leaf meal, and meat and bone scraps in a ration for growing chicks. N. Mex. Bul. 221. 1934.

Kempster, H. L. Protein concentrates in chick rations. Mo. Bul. 310:47. 1932.

Goff, O. E., and R. Penquite. Cottonseed meal and peanut meal have a place in baby chick feeds in the South. Okla. Rept. 1930-1932:112.

Ringrose, R. C., and C. L. Morgan. The use of cottonseed meal in the chick starting ration. Poultry Sci. 17:109. 1938.

Fraps, G. S., and D. H. Reid. Use of proteins from different sources in feeding baby chicks. Poultry Sci. 8:383. 1929.

Heuser, G. F., L. C. Norris, and J. McGinnis. Vegetable protein concentrates fed alone and in combination with soybean oil meal and fish meal as the chief supplementary protein in chick starting rations. Poultry Sci. 25:130. 1946.

German, H. L., and R. M. Sherwood. A comparison of soybean oil meal and cottonseed meal with various protein supplements in chick starter rations. Poultry Sci. 27:663. 1948.

Grau, C. R. Cottonseed meal for chicks. California Agr. 4:14. 1950.

Grau, C. R. Cottonseed meal for chicks. California Farmer 194: 76. 1951.

19. Boatner, C. H., A. M. Altschul, G. W. Irving, E. F. Pollard, and H. C. Schaefer. The nutritive value of cottonseed for chicks as affected by methods of processing and content of pigment glands. Poultry Sci. 27:315. 1948.

Lillie, R. J., and H. R. Bird. Effect of oral administration of pure gossypol and of pigment glands of cottonseed on mortality and growth of chicks. Poultry Sci. 29:390. 1950.

German, H. L., and J. R. Couch. Effect of methods of processing on the nutritive value of cottonseed meal for chicks. Poultry Sci. 30:913. 1951.

Milligan, J. L., and H. R. Bird. Effect of processing variants on the nutritive value of cottonseed meal for chicks. Poultry Sci. 30:651. 1951.

Morgan, C. L., and C. P. Willimon. Cottonseed meal prepared by different methods for broiler rations. Poultry Sci. 32:917. 1953.

Patrick, H. The effect of processing method and certain supplements on a lysine deficiency in cottonseed meal for chicks. Poultry Sci. 32:942. 1953.

20. Wilgus, H. S., and D. V. Zander. The value of soybean oil meal processed from damaged beans. Poultry Sci. 23:343. 1944.

Card, L. E., and A. V. Nalbandov. The use of field-damaged soybeans in feeding chicks. Poultry Sci. 23:163. 1944.

21. Daniels, A. L., and N. B. Nichols. The nutritive value of the soybean. Jour. Biol. Chem. 32:91. 1917.

22. Kennard, D. C., R. C. Holder, and P. S. White. Poultry fleshing investigations. The utilization of soybean and corn proteins as affected by suitable mineral supplement. Am. Jour. Physiol. 59: 298. 1922.

Kennard, D. C., R. C. Holder, and P. S. White. Mineral supplements to rations for chickens: corn meal and soybean meal. Poultry Sci. 1:65. 1922.

Kennard, D. C., and P. S. White. Mineral mixtures for growth of chickens and egg production. Ohio Monthly Bul. 7(11) :171. 1922.

Card, L. E. Soybean meal as good as meat scrap for chicks. Ill. Rept. 1928:172.

Kennard, D. C. A simple mineral mixture for chickens. Ohio Bimo. Bul. 105 and 106:159. 1924.

Richardson, L. R., A. G. Hogan, and H. L. Kempster. Soybean oil meal as a supplement for baby chicks. Mo. Sta. Res. Bul. 395:19. 1945.

23. Hayward, J. W., and F. H. Hafner. The supplementary effect of cystine and methionine upon the protein of raw and cooked soybeans as determined with chicks and rats. Poultry Sci. 20:139. 1941.

Almquist, H. J., E. Mecchi, F. H. Kratzer, and C. R. Grau. Soybean protein as a source of amino acids for the chick. Jour. Nutr. 24: 385. 1942.

Bird, H. R., and J. P. Mattingly. Addition of dl-methionine to starting and growing mashes. Poultry Sci. 24:29. 1945.

Clandinin, D. R., W. W. Cravens, J. G. Halpin, and E. G. Hart. Supplementary value of methionine, cystine, and choline in a practical soybean oil meal starter ration. Poultry Sci. 25:509. 1946.

Mishler, D. H., C. W. Carrick, and S. M. Hauge. Methionine, choline, betaine, and fish products in a simplified ration. Poultry Sci. 27:677. 1948.

Machlin, L. J., C. A. Denton, and H. R. Bird. Supplementation with vitamin B_{12} and amino acids of chick diets containing soybean or cottonseed meal. Poultry Sci. 31:110. 1952.

24. Christiansen, J. B., H. J. Deobald, J. G. Halpin, and E. B. Hart. Further studies on the nature of the effective supplements for soybean oil meal in chick rations. Poultry Sci. 18:481. 1939.

Carrick, C. W. War-time shifts in poultry rations. Flour and Feed 44(6) :22. 1943.

Berry, E. P., C. W. Carrick, R. E. Roberts, and S. M. Hauge. A deficiency of available choline in soybean oil and soybean oil meal. Poultry Sci. 22:442. 1943.

Marvel, J. A., C. W. Carrick, R. E. Roberts, and S. M. Hauge. The supplementary value of choline and methionine in a corn and soybean oil meal chick ration. Poultry Sci. 23:294. 1944.

Marvel, J. A., C. W. Carrick, R. E. Roberts, and S. M. Hauge. A comparison of soybean oils and soybean oil meals in chick rations

containing distillers' dried solubles. Poultry Sci. 24:46. 1945.
Marvel, J. A., C. W. Carrick, R. E. Roberts, and S. M. Hauge. The value of choline additions to a corn and soybean oil meal chick ration containing distillers' dried solubles. Poultry Sci. 24:181. 1945.
Berry, E. P., C. W. Carrick, R. E. Roberts, and S. M. Hauge. Whey solubles as a source of growth factors in chick rations. Poultry Sci. 22:252. 1943.
Mishler, D. H., C. W. Carrick, R. E. Roberts, and S. M. Hauge. Synthetic and natural vitamin supplements for corn and soybean oil meal chick rations. Poultry Sci. 25:479. 1946.
Patton, A. R., J. P. Marvel, H. G. Petering, and J. Waddell. The nutritional significance of animal protein supplements in the diet of the chick. Jour. Nutr. 31:485. 1946.
Richardson, L. R., and L. G. Blaylock. Vitamin B_{12} and amino acids as supplements to soybean oil meal and cottonseed meal for growing chicks. Jour. Nutr. 40:169. 1950.
Machlin, L. J., C. A. Denton, and H. R. Bird. Supplementation with vitamin B_{12} and amino acids of chick diets containing soybean or cottonseed meal. Poultry Sci. 31:110. 1952.
Savage, J. E., C. W. Turner, H. L. Kempster, and A. G. Hogan. The effects of vitamin B_{12} and thyroprotein on egg production, egg weight, shell quality, and hatchability. Poultry Sci. 31:22. 1952.
25. Kennard, D. C., R. M. Bethke, and V. D. Chamberlin. Supplements to all-plant diet for production of hatchable eggs. Ohio Bul. 705:71. 1951.
Kennard, D. C., and V. D. Chamberlin. Built-up floor litter contains growth factor. Ohio Farm and Home Res. 33, No. 250:21. 1948.
Kennard, D. C., and V. D. Chamberlin. Growth, dietary requirements, and mortality of chickens as affected by management of the floor litter. Poultry Sci. 30:766. 1950.
Kennard, D. C., and V. D. Chamberlin. Built-up litter experiments. Ohio Bul. 705:70. 1951.
Kennard, D. C., and V. D. Chamberlin. All plant diets for growth of chickens and egg production. Poultry Sci. 30:920. 1951.
26. Bethke, R. M., and M. C. Sweet. The comparative value of expeller and toasted solvent soybean oil meals for chicks. Ohio. Bimo. Bul. 199:122.
27. Hayward, J. W., H. Steenbock, and G. Bohstedt. The effect of heat as used in the extraction of soybean oil upon the nutritive value of the protein of soybean oil meal. Jour. Nutr. 11:219. 1936.
Wilgus, H. S., Jr., L. C. Norris, and G. F. Heuser. Effect of heat on nutritive value of soybean oil meals. Indus. Eng. Chem. 28:586. 1936.
Hayward, J. W., J. G. Halpin, J. G. Holmes, C. E. Bohstedt, and E. B. Hart. Soybean oil meal prepared at different temperatures as a feed for poultry. Poultry Sci. 16:3. 1937.
Parsons, H., D. Johnson, A. Marlatt, and V. Rohrer. Oven roasting of soybeans improves their food value. Wis. Bul. 439:21. 1937.
Johnson, L. M., H. T. Parsons, and H. Steenbock. The effect of

heat and solvents on the nutritive value of soybean protein. Jour. Nutr. 18:423. 1939.

Parsons, H., and C. Walliker. Hydrolysis improves quality of soybeans. Wis. Bul. 453:30. 1941.

Hayward, J. W., and F. H. Hafner. The supplementary effect of cystine and methionine upon the protein of raw and cooked soybeans as determined with chicks and rats. Poultry Sci. 20:139. 1941.

Almquist, H. J., E. Mecchi, F. H. Kratzer, and C. R. Grau. Soybean protein as a source of amino acids for the chick. Jour. Nutr. 24: 385. 1942.

Mussehl, F. E. Effect of cooking on nutritive value of soybeans for growing chicks. University of Nebraska Poultry Husb. Leaflet 34. 1942.

Mussehl, F. E. Effect of cooking solvent process soybean flakes on nutritive value for chicks. University of Nebraska Poultry Husb. Leaflet 35. 1942.

Bird, H. R., and G. J. Burkhardt. Factors affecting the nutritive value of soybean oil meals and soybeans for chickens. Md. Bul. No. A27. 1943.

Gerry, R. W., C. W. Carrick, and S. M. Hauge. Untoasted soybean oil meal in a simplified chick ration. Poultry Sci. 27:621. 1948.

Barabas, E. Fott es nyers extrahalt szojadara etetesenek hata a csirkek fejlodesere. Agrartudomany (Hungary) 1:402, 1949.

28. Ackerson, C. W., R. Borchers, and F. E. Mussehl. Trypsin inhibitor. VII. Comparative nutritive value of raw and heated soybean meal for poults. Nebraska Res. Bul. 156. 1948.

Almquist, H. J., and J. B. Merritt. Effect of soybean tryptic inhibitor on experimental arginine deficiency in the chick. Arch. Biochem. & Biophys. 31:454. 1951.

Almquist, H. J., and J. B. Merritt. Effect of soybean antitrypsin on growth of the chick. Archiv. Biochem. & Biophys. 35:352. 1952.

Almquist, H. J., and J. B. Merritt. Effect of raw soybean meal on growth of the chick. Proc. Soc. Exp. Biol. and Med. 79:277. 1952.

Borchers, R. The trypsin inhibitor of soybeans and its effect on chick growth. Poultry Sci. 27:654. 1948.

Borchers, R., C. W. Ackerson, and F. E. Mussehl. Trypsin inhibitor. VI. Effect of various heating periods on the growth promoting value of soybean oil meal for chicks. Poultry Sci. 27:601. 1948.

Ham, W. E., R. M. Sandstedt, and F. E. Mussehl. The proteolytic inhibiting substance in the extract from unheated soybean meal and its effect upon growth in chicks. Jour. Biol. Chem. 161:635. 1945.

29. Bouthilet, R. J., W. L. Hunter, C. A. Luhman, D. Ambrose, and S. Lepkovsky. The metabolism of raw versus heated soybeans in birds with colostomies. Poultry Sci. 29:837. 1950.

Evans, R. J., and J. McGinnis. The influence of autoclaving soybean oil meal on the availability of cystine and methionine for the chick. Jour. Nutr. 31:449. 1946.

Evans, R. J., and J. McGinnis. Cystine and methionine metabolism by chicks receiving raw or autoclaved soybean oil meal. Jour. Nutr. 35:477. 1948.
Evans, R. J., J. McGinnis, and J. L. St. John. The influence of autoclaving soybean meal on the digestibility of the proteins. Jour. Nutr. 33:661. 1946.
Fritz, J. C., E. H. Kramke, and C. A. Reed. Effect of heat treatment on the biological value of soybeans. Poultry Sci. 26:657. 1947.
McGinnis, J., and R. J. Evans. Amino acid deficiencies of raw and overheated soybean oil meal for chicks. Jour. Nutr. 34:725. 1947.
30. Bird, H. R., and G. J. Burkhardt. Factors affecting the nutritive value of soybean oil meals and soybeans for chickens. Maryland Bul. A27. 1943.
Clandinin, D. R., W. W. Cravens, C. A. Elvehjem, and J. G. Halpin. Deficiencies in overheated soybean oil meal. Poultry Sci. 26:150. 1947.
Clandinin, D. R., W. W. Cravens, C. A. Elvehjem, and J. G. Halpin. Too much heat injures soybean oil meal. Wisc. Bul. 472:54. 1947.
Evans, R. J., and H. A. Butts. Studies on the heat inactivation of lysine in soybean oil meal. Jour. Biol. Chem. 175:15. 1948.
Evans, R. J., and J. McGinnis. Cystine and methionine metabolism by chicks receiving raw or autoclaved soybean oil meal. Jour. Nutr. 35:477. 1948.
McGinnis, J., and R. J. Evans. Amino acid deficiencies of raw and overheated soybean oil meal for chicks. Jour. Nutr. 34:725. 1947.
31. Hsu, P. T., W. D. Graham, J. S. Carver, and J. McGinnis. Correlation of nutritive value for chicks of autoclaved soybean oil meal with fluorescence, browning, and sticky droppings. Poultry Sci. 28:780. 1949.
32. Wilgus, H. S., F. X. Gassner, and A. R. Patton. The goitrogenicity of soybeans. Poultry Sci. 19:366. 1940.
Wilgus, H. S., Jr., F. X. Gassner, and A. R. Patton. The goitrogenicity of soybeans. Jour. Nutr. 22:43. 1941.
Wilgus, H. S., Jr., and F. X. Gassner. Effect of soybean oil meal on avian reproduction. Soc. Exp. Biol. and Med. Proc. 46:290. 1941.
33. Glista, W. A., and H. M. Scott. Growth and feed efficiency studies with broilers. 2. Gross water consumption in relation to the level of soybean oil meal in the ration. Poultry Sci. 28:747. 1949.
34. Balloun, S. L., and E. L. Johnson. Underheated soybean oil meal increases blood clotting time of chicks. Poultry Sci. 31:905. 1952.
Balloun, S. L., and E. L. Johnson. Fluorescing properties of expeller soybean oil meals. Poultry Sci. 31:906. 1952.
Balloun, S. L., E. L. Johnson, and L. K. Arnold. Laboratory estimation of the biological value of soybean meal as related to method of preparation. Poultry Sci. 30:906. 1951.
Balloun, S. L., E. L. Johnson, and L. K. Arnold. Laboratory estimation of the nutritive value of soybean oil meals. Poultry Sci. 32:517. 1953.
Bird, H. R., R. V. Boucher, C. D. Caskey, J. W. Hayward, and J. E.

Hunter. Urease activity and other chemical criteria as indicators of inadequate heating of soybean oil meal. Jour. Assn. Off. Agr. Chem. 30:354. 1947.

Ingram, G. R., W. W. Riesen, W. W. Cravens, and C. A. Elvehjem. Evaluating soybean oil meal protein for chick growth by enzymatic release of amino acids. Poultry Sci. 28:898. 1949.

35. Ivey, J. E. Vegetable protein studies. Ala. Rept. 1927:14.

Dougherty, J. E. Animal protein for laying hens. Calif. Rept. 1915:38.

Can soybean oil meal be substituted for tankage? Ind. Rept. 1922:39.

Soybean oil meal can replace tankage. Ind. Rept. 1923:39.

Philips, A. G., and S. M. Hauge. Soybean oil meal in rations for laying pullets. Ind. Bul. 293. 1925.

Lomax, E. B. Some protein foods for poultry. Rept. Fourth World's Poultry Congress. 261. London. 1930.

Macrander, L. Versuche über die Verfütterung von pflanzlichem Eiweiss an Legehennen. Archiv für Geflügelk. 8:161. 1934.

Kempster, H. L. Value of sour milk, beef scrap, cottonseed meal, gluten meal, and oil meal in rations for egg production. Mo. Bul. 236:66. 1926.

Kempster, H. L. Value of sour milk, beef scrap, cottonseed meal, gluten meal, and oil meal in rations for egg production. Mo. Bul. 256:84. 1927.

Kempster, H. L. Value of cottonseed meal, ground soybeans, soybean meal, tankage, meat scrap, and dried buttermilk in rations for egg production. Mo. Bul. 272:78. 1929.

Kempster, H. L. Value of dried buttermilk, meat scrap, cottonseed meal, soybean meal, and ground soybeans in rations for egg production. Mo. Bul. 285:95. 1930.

Comparison of protein foods for table egg production. Harper Adams Utility Poultry Jour. 14:217. 1929.

Parkhurst, R. T., and E. B. Lomax. Comparative value of various protein feeds for laying hens. Harper Adams Agr. Col. Bul. 4:334. 1930.

Kennard, D. C., and P. S. White. Mineral mixtures for growth of chickens and egg production. Ohio Monthly Bul. November-December. 1922:171.

Thompson, R. B. Soybean meal holds promise as vegetable protein for poultry feeds. Okla. Rept. 1930-1932:111.

Robertson, G. S., and R. G. Baskett. The nutritive requirement of poultry. The influence of certain nutritional factors on the size of the egg and the condition of the birds. Scottish Jour. Agr. 11:176. 1928.

Stevenson, G. L. Comparison of protein feeds. S. Dak. Rept. 1926:33.

High protein feeds. S. Dak. Rept. 1928:27.

Suzuki, K., and T. Hatano. Soybean cake as protein supplement of poultry feed. Rept. Fourth World's Poultry Congress. 288. London. 1930.

Soybean oil meal usable as partial source of protein in laying rations. Wis. Bul. 428:46. 1934.
Prentice, J. H., R. G. Baskett, and G. S. Robertson. The nutrition of the chick and its effect on growth, maturity, egg production, and mortality. Rept. Fourth World's Poultry Congress. 242. London. 1930.
Carver, J. S., A. W. Brant, and R. J. Evans. Soybean oil meal in the laying ration. Wash. V. Circ. 15. 1944.
Norris, L. C., and G. F. Heuser. Studies on the amount of animal protein required in poultry rations. Flour and Feed 43(8) :38. 1943.
Heuser, G. F., and L. C. Norris. Soybean oil meal in hen rations. Poultry Sci. 23:371. 1944.
Bird, H. R. Laying mashes containing no animal protein. Flour and Feed 44(5) :16. 1943.
Carver, J. S., J. McGinnis, C. F. McClary, and R. J. Evans. The utilization of raw and heat-treated soybean oil meal for egg production and hatchability. Poultry Sci. 25:399. 1946.
Whitson, D., H. W. Titus, and H. R. Bird. Effect of dietary level of soybean meal on hatchability. Poultry Sci. 25:52. 1946.
Brant, A. W., and J. S. Carver. From one day of age through the first laying year on rations containing soybean oil meal as a protein supplement. Poultry Sci. 26:598. 1947.
Savage, J. E., C. W. Turner, H. L. Kempster, and A. G. Hogan. The effect of vitamin B_{12} and thyroprotein on egg production, egg weight, shell quality, and hatchability. Poultry Sci. 31:22. 1952.

36. Vegetable proteins and mineral supplements for chickens. Ohio Bul. 362:43. 1922.
Philips, A. G., and S. M. Hauge. Soybean oil meal in rations for laying pullets. Ind. Bul. 293. 1925.
Soybean oil meal can replace tankage. Ind. Rept. 1923:39.
Kempster, H. L. The influence of various protein concentrates on egg production. Mo. Bul. 288. 1930.
Kennard, D. C., and P. S. White. Mineral mixtures for growth of chickens and egg production. Ohio Monthly Bul. 7(11) :171. 1922.
Robertson, G. S., and R. G. Baskett. The nutritive requirement of poultry. The influence of certain nutritional factors on the size of the egg and the condition of the bird. Scottish Jour. Agr. 11:176. 1928.
Lomax, E. B. Some protein feeds for poultry. Rept. Fourth World's Poultry Congress. 261. London. 1930.
Suzuki, K., and T. Hatano. Soybean cake as protein supplement of poultry feed. Rept. Fourth World's Poultry Congress. 288. London. 1930.

37. Ivey, J. E. Experiments with poultry at the Alabama Station. Alabama Report 1927:14.
Kempster, H. L. Influence of various protein concentrates on egg production. Mo. Bul. 288. 1930.
Fangauf, R., and O. Brüninghaus. Wie ist die Legetätigkeit der Hühner bei rein pflanzlichem Eiweiss? Archiv für Geflügelk. 10:173. 1936.

Soybean oil meal usable as partial source of protein in laying rations. Wis. Bul. 428:46. 1934.
Soybean oil meal may replace part of the animal protein in poultry rations. Wis. Bul. 435:34. 1936.
Byerly, T. C., H. W. Titus, N. R. Ellis, and R. B. Nestler. Effects of light, soybean, and other diet supplements on seasonal hatchability and egg production. Poultry Sci. 16:322. 1937.
Deobald, H. J., J. G. Halpin, and C. E. Holmes. Learn more about the value of soybean oil meal for poultry. Wis. Bul. 438:56. 1937.
Christiansen, J. B., J. G. Halpin, and E. G. Hart. Studies on the nature of the effective supplements for soybean oil meal in rations for the production of hatching eggs. Poultry Sci. 19:55. 1940.
Heuser, G. F., and L. C. Norris. Soybean oil meal in hen rations. Poultry Sci. 23:371. 1944.
Carver, J. S., J. McGinnis, C. F. McClary, and R. J. Evans. The utilization of raw and heat-treated soybean oil meal for egg production and hatchability. Poultry Sci. 25:399. 1946.
Bird, H. R., M. Rubin, D. Whitson, and S. K. Haynes. Effectiveness of dietary supplements in increasing hatchability of eggs and viability of progeny of hens fed a diet containing a high level of soybean oil meal. Poultry Sci. 25:285. 1946.
Whitson, D., H. W. Titus, and H. R. Bird. Effect of dietary level of soybean meal on hatchability. Poultry Sci. 25:52. 1946.
Savage, J. E., J. W. Turner, H. L. Kempster, and A. G. Hogan. The effects of vitamin B_{12} and thyroprotein on egg production, egg weight, shell quality, and hatchability. Poultry Sci. 31:22. 1952.
38. Ott, W. H. Satisfactory early chick growth on a diet containing no animal protein. Poultry Sci. 23:252. 1944.
Carver, J. S., and R. J. Evans. Animal and vegetable protein combinations in chick starting rations. U. S. Egg and Poultry Mag. 49:468. 1943.
Bearse, G. E., D. Boucher, L. R. Berg, and V. L. Miller. Soybean oil meal in the chick starting ration. U. S. Egg and Poultry Mag. 49:131. 1943.
Carver, J. S., and M. Rhian. Soybean oil meal in the chick starting ration. U. S. Egg and Poultry Mag. 49:131. 1943.
Polk, H. D., and C. E. Barnett. Broiler production with high protein feeds. Miss. Bul. 374. 1943.
Barnett, C. E., and H. D. Polk. Cottonseed meal, shrimp meal, soybean meal, meat scraps, for growing chicks. Miss. Farm Res. June 1942.
Pratt, Jean M. A biological study of the protein and riboflavin content of British Columbia fish meals. Thesis. University of British Columbia. 1942.
Gutowska, M. S., and J. Drescherowna. Porownanie wartosci odzywczej soji krajowej i maczki miesno-kostnej w racjach kurczat. Roczniki Nauk Rolniczych i Lesnych 36:115. 1936.
Card, L. E. Soybean meal as good as meat scrap for chicks. Ill. Rept. 1928:172.
Suzuki, K., and T. Hatano. Soya bean cake as protein supplement

of poultry feed. Rept. Fourth World's Poultry Congress. 288. London. 1930.

Briggs, G. M., E. G. Hill, and M. J. Giles. The practical use of an all-plant ration for starting and broiler chickens. Poultry Sci. 30:750. 1950.

Hammond, J. C., S. K. Haynes, S. J. Marsden, and H. W. Titus. Vegetable protein diets for turkeys. Poultry Sci. 23:105. 1944.

Kempster, H. L., and Q. B. Kinder. The use of vegetable protein concentrates and crystalline riboflavin in practical rations for growing chicks. Mo. Ann. Rept. 1947-48. Bul. 578:42. 1949.

Murphy, R. R., and E. W. Callenbach. Protein for poultry may come from soybean oil meal. Pa. Agr. Sta. Bul. 488:30. 1947.

Thayer, R. H., K. C. Leong, and J. McGinnis. Comparative nutritive value of specific vegetable and animal protein concentrates for chicks. Poultry Sci. 30:782. 1950.

39. Soybean protein satisfactory for growing chicks. Ind. Rept.:53. 1928.

Bethke, R. M., and D. C. Kennard. Protein studies with chicks. Ohio Bul. 446:147. 1930.

40. Draper, C. I., and R. J. Evans. Soybean oil meal in the broiler ration. Wash. V. Circ. 19. 1944.

Hammond, J. C., and H. W. Titus. The use of soybean meal in the diet of growing chicks. Poultry Sci. 23:49. 1944.

Bird, H. R., and G. J. Burkhardt. Factors affecting the nutritive value of soybean oil meals and soybeans for chickens. Md. Bul. A27. 1943.

Almquist, H. J. Summary of reports on minimum levels of animal protein required in supplementation of expeller soybean meal and cereal proteins in poultry mashes. Flour and Feed 44(2) :12. 1943.

Scott, H. H., T. B. Avery, and L. D. Matterson. Conservation of animal protein in chick rations. Flour and Feed 43(12) :32. 1943.

Winter, A. R. Protein feedstuffs for poultry rations. Flour and Feed 43(10) :10. 1943.

Berry, E. P., C. W. Carrick, R. E. Roberts, and S. M. Hauge. Whey solubles as a source of growth factors in chick rations. Poultry Sci. 22:252. 1943.

Heuser, G. F., and L. C. Norris. Soybean oil meal in chick rations. Cornell Bul. 810. 1944.

Norris, L. C., and G. F. Heuser. Studies on the amount of animal protein required in poultry rations. Flour and Feed 43(8) :38. 1943.

Almquist, H. J., E. Mecchi, F. H. Kratzer, and C. R. Grau. Soybean protein as a source of amino acids for the chick. Jour. Nutr. 24: 385. 1942.

Bird, H. R., and A. C. Groschke. Feeds for chick mashes. Flour and Feed 43(5) :7. 1942.

Irwin, M. R., and H. L. Kempster. The value of soybean oil meal in broiler rations. Mo. Bul. 441. 1942.

Sloan, H. J., and L. E. Card. Soybean oil meal found good protein feed for chicks. Ill. Rept. 1937:120.

Philips, A. G., R. H. Carr, and D. C. Kennard. Meat scraps vs. soybean proteins as a supplement to corn for growing chicks. Jour. Agr. Res. 18:391. 1920.
Soybean protein satisfactory for growing chicks. Ind. Rept. 1928: 53.
Roberts, R. E., and C. W. Carrick. Soybean oil meal in broiler rations. Ind. Rept. 1938:81.
Ackerson, C. W., M. J. Blish, and F. E. Mussehl. The utilization of food elements by growing chicks. IV. Meat meal and fish meal compared with meat meal and soybean meal as protein concentrates. Neb. Res. Bul. 97. 1938.
Smetnev, S. New Poultry feeds in poultry breeding. Institute of Poultry Research. Smetnev-Prevo, Moscow.
Hayward, J. W., J. G. Halpin, C. E. Holmes, G. Bohstedt, and E. B. Hart. Soybean oil meal prepared at different temperatures as a feed for poultry. Poultry Sci. 16:3. 1937.
Soybean oil meal proves effective as partial source of protein in poultry ration. Wis. Bul. 425:20. 1933.
Soybean oil meal usable as partial source of protein in laying rations. Wis. Bul. 428:46. 1934.
Christiansen, J. B., H. J. Deobald, J. G. Halpin, and E. B. Hart. Further studies on the nature of the effective supplements for soybean oil meal in chick rations. Poultry Sci. 18:481. 1939.
Christiansen, J. B., H. J. Deobald, J. G. Halpin, and E. B. Hart. Practical supplements for soybean oil meal in chick rations. Poultry Sci. 19:18. 1940.
Halpin, J. G., C. E. Holmes, and W. W. Cravens. Liberal amounts of animal protein help produce early broilers. Wis. Bul. 449:86. 1940.
Halpin, J. G., and C. E. Holmes. Soybean oil meal proves effective as partial source of protein in poultry ration. Wis. Bul. 449:20. 1940.
Halpin, J. G., and W. W. Cravens. What kind of poultry rations in 1942? Wis. Bul. 455:15. 1942.
Hunter, J. E., D. R. Marble, and H. C. Knandel. Vegetable protein in turkey rations. Penn. Ag. Exp. Sta. Bul. 321:13. 1935.
Headley, F. B. The effect of substituting vegetable protein for meat protein in a ration for growing turkeys. Nev. Agr. Exp. Bul. 168. 1944.
Clark, T. B., and C. J. Cunningham. Soybean oil meal in poultry rations. W. Va. Bul. 325:15. 1945.
Heuser, G. F., L. C. Norris, and J. McGinnis. Vegetable protein concentrates fed alone and in combination with soybean oil meal and fish meal as the chief supplementary protein in chick starting rations. Poultry Sci. 25, 1930. 1946.
Brant, A. W., and J. S. Carver. From one day of age through the first laying year on rations containing soybean oil meal as a protein supplement. Poultry Sci. 26:598. 1947.
Bird, H. R., S. J. Marsden, and W. L. Kellogg. Supplements for soybean meal in turkey diets. Poultry Sci. 27:53. 1948.
German, H. L., and R. M. Sherwood. A comparison of soybean oil

meal and cottonseed meal with various protein supplements in chick starter rations. Poultry Sci. 27:663. 1948.

Gerry, R. W., C. W. Carrick, and S. M. Hauge. Vitamin supplements in a soybean meal and mixed grain ration. Poultry Sci. 27: 664. 1948.

Graham, W. D., W. J. Stadelman, E. L. Stephenson, and J. McGinnis. Growth response of chicks fed different soybean oil meals to an animal protein factor concentrate and to fish meal. Poultry Sci. 28:765. 1949.

Richardson, L. R., and L. G. Blaylock. Supplements to soybean and cottonseed meal diets for poults and growing turkeys. Poultry Sci. 29:651. 1950.

Patrick, H. Studies on supplements for high soybean oil meal rations for early poult growth. Poultry Sci. 30:70. 1951.

Slinger, S. J., W. F. Pepper, D. C. Hill, and E. S. Snyder. Supplements to a soybean oil meal-cereal grain broiler diet "adequate" in vitamin B_{12}. Poultry Sci. 31:193. 1952.

Ringrose, R. C., and L. M. Potter. Methionine, vitamin B_{12}, and fish meal as supplements in an all-vegetable chick-starting ration. Poultry Sci. 31:932. 1952.

41. Hammond, J. C. Partial substitutes for soybean meal. Poultry Sci. 23:78. 1944.

42. Berg, L. R., G. E. Bearse, and V. L. Miller. The effect of soybean oil meal on the incidence of "pasting up" in baby chicks. Poultry Sci. 24:122. 1945.

43. Heuser, G. F. Ground raw soybeans not equal to soybean meal for poultry. Farm Research (N. Y., Geneva, Agricultural Experiment Station) 10(4) :4. 1944.

Tomhave, A. E., and C. W. Mumford. Soybeans for baby chicks. Ground soybeans in the ration for laying pullets. Del. Bul. 147:13. 1926.

Tomhave, A. E., and C. W. Mumford. Ground soybeans in the ration for laying pullets. Del. Bul. 152:15. 1927.

Tomhave, A. E., and C. W. Mumford. Utilization of ground soybeans for poultry. Del. Bul. 158:15. 1928.

Tomhave, A. E., and C. W. Mumford. Utilization of ground soybeans for poultry. Del. Bul. 172:23. 1931.

Tomhave, A. E., and C. W. Mumford. Utilization of ground soybeans for poultry. Del. Bul. 179:23. 1932.

Tomhave, A. E., and C. W. Mumford. Ground soybeans as a protein supplement for laying birds. Del. Bul. 197. 1936.

Kempster, H. L. Value of cottonseed meal, ground soybeans, soybean meal, tankage, meat scrap, and dried buttermilk in rations for egg production. Mo. Bul. 272:78. 1929.

Kempster, H. L. Value of dried buttermilk, meat scrap, cottonseed meal, soybean meal, and ground soybeans in rations for egg production. Mo. Bul. 285:95. 1930.

Kempster, H. L. The influence of various protein concentrates on egg production. Mo. Bul. 288. 1930.

Buss, W. J. Rations for laying hens in winter. Ohio Monthly Bul. (1) :324. 1916.

Comparison of high protein feeds. S. Dak. Rept. 1927:29.
High protein feeds. S. Dak. Rept. 1928:27.
Philips, A. G., and S. M. Hauge, Soybean oil meal in rations for laying pullets. Ind. Bul. 293. 1925.
44. Tomhave, A. E., and C. W. Mumford. Utilization of ground soybeans for poultry. Del. Bul. 172:23. 1931.
Tomhave, A. E., and C. W. Mumford. Utilization of ground soybeans for poultry. Del. Bul. 179:23. 1932.
Tomhave, A. E., and C. W. Mumford. Ground soybeans as a protein supplement for growing chicks. Del. Bul. 183. 1933.
Hill, D. C., and H. D. Branion. Failure of vitamin supplementation to improve growth on diets high in raw soybeans. Poultry Sci. 32: 882. 1953.
45. Heuser, G. F. Ground raw soybeans not equal to soybean meal for poultry. Farm Research (N. Y. State Agricultural Experiment Station, Geneva) 10(4) :4. 1944.
46. Mussehl, F. E. Effect of cooking on nutritive value of soybeans for growing chicks. University of Nebraska Poultry Husb. Leaflet 35. 1942.
47. Thayer, R. H. The use of soybeans in fattening rations for broilers and fryers. Proc. Okla. Acad. Sci. 26:27. 1946.
48. Ivey, J. E. Vegetable protein studies. Ala. Rept. 1927:14.
Comparison of vegetable and animal sources of protein for laying hens. Ark. Bul. 203:26. 1926.
Embleton, E. Sources of protein feeds for poultry. Okla. Rept. 1919:50.
Harvey, R. N. Egg-producing values of some Texas feeding stuffs. Tex. Bul. 220. 1917.
The value of peanuts and peanut meal in rations for chickens. Alabama Circ. 80. 1937.
Temperton, H., and F. J. Dudley. Palm kernel and earthnut meals in the rations for laying pullets. Harper Adams Utility Poultry Jour. 25(11). 1940.
Dearstyne, R. S., C. O. Bollinger, and H. P. Brigman. Effect of substituting peanut meal in part for the animal protein in laying mash on egg production, hatchability, and livability of chicks. N. C. Bul. 326. 1940.
Sherwood, R. M., and J. R. Couch. Values of various protein feeds for growing chicks. Tex. Bul. 588. 1940.
Marvel, J. A., C. W. Carrick, R. E. Roberts, and S. M. Hauge. Distillers' dried solubles in chick rations containing corn and vegetable protein supplements. Poultry Sci. 24:252. 1945.
Heuser, G. F., L. C. Norris, and J. McGinnis. Vegetable protein concentrates fed alone and in combination with soybean oil meal and fish meal as the chief supplementary protein in chick starting rations. Poultry Sci. 25:130. 1946.
Altschul, A. M., G. W. Irving, Jr., and W. F. Guilbean. The nutritive value of peanut cake meal protein and nonprotein residue for chicks. Poultry Sci. 27:402. 1948.
49. Feeding demonstrations. From the Sixth Annual Report of the Herts

County Laying Trials. Hertfordshire Institute of Agriculture, Oaklands, St. Albans. The Utility Record. July 1932.
Lomax, E. B. Some protein foods for poultry. Rept. Fourth World's Poultry Congress. 261. London. 1930.
Macrander, L. Versuche über die Verfütterung von pflanzlichem Eiweiss an Legehennen. Archiv für Geflügelk. 8:161. 1934.
Comparison of protein foods for table egg production. Harper Adams Utility Poultry Jour. 14:217. 1929.
Parkhurst, R. T., and E. B. Lomax. Comparative value of various protein feeds for laying hens. Harper Adams Agr. Coll. Bul. No. 4:334. 1930.
Kennard, D. C., and P. S. White. Mineral mixtures for growth of chickens and egg production. Ohio Monthly Bul. November-December:171. 1922.
50. Boughton, D. C., and W. B. Forney. Peanut meal in laying rations. Ga. Bul. June 1939(8) :5. 1939.
Kennard, D. C., and P. S. White. Mineral mixtures for growth of chickens and egg production. Ohio Monthly Bul. November-December:171. 1922.
Goff, O. E., and R. Penquite. Cottonseed meal and peanut meal have a place in baby chick feeds in the South. Okla. Rept. 1930-1932:112.
Bryant, R. L. The use of peanut meal as a source of protein in starting mashes for chicks. Va. Bul. 281. 1931.
Grau, C. R. Protein concentrates as amino acid sources for the chick: Corn gluten meal, cottonseed meal and peanut meal. Jour. Nutr. 32:303. 1946.
Blaylock, L. G., and L. R. Richardson. Peanut meal, mixtures of soybean and cottonseed, and mixtures of soybean and peanut meals as sources of protein for baby chicks. Poultry Sci. 29:656. 1950.
51. The value of peanuts and peanut meal in rations for chickens. Ala. Circ. 80. 1937.
52. Kempster, H. L., and G. W. Hervey. Meat scrap and sour milk for egg production. Mo. Bul. 155. 1918.
Kempster, H. L. Value of sour milk, beef scrap, cottonseed meal, gluten meal, and oil meal in rations for egg production. Mo. Bul. 172:36. 1920.
Lewis, H. R., and W. C. Thompson. Animal vs. vegetable protein. N. J. Rept. 1915:100.
Thompson, R. B. Soybean meal holds promise as vegetable protein for poultry feeds. Okla. Rept. 1930-1932:111.
53. Slinger, S. J., J. H. Pettit, and E. V. Evans. Use of corn gluten feed to replace meat meal in poultry rations. Sci. Agr. 24:234. 1944.
Heuser, G. F., and L. C. Norris. Soybean oil meal in chick rations. Cornell Bul. 810. 1944.
Heuser, G. F., L. C. Norris, and J. McGinnis. Vegetable protein concentrates fed alone and in combination with soybean oil meal and fish meal as the chief supplementary protein in chick starting rations. Poultry Sci. 25:130. 1946.
54. Ringrose, R. C. The nutritive properties of corn gluten meal for poultry. Cornell University Thesis (Ph.D.). 1936.

Ringrose, R. C., L. C. Norris, and G. F. Heuser. The value of corn gluten meal for feeding poultry. Cornell Bul. 752. 1939.
Runnels, T. D., T. B. Clark, and A. H. VanLandingham. Comparison of animal and vegetable protein concentrates singly and combined, in chick rations. Poultry Sci. 19:360. 1940.
Berry, E. P., C. W. Carrick, C. W. Roberts, R. E. Roberts, and S. M. Hauge. Supplementary effect of corn gluten meal with soybean oil meal. Poultry Sci. 25:498. 1946.
Cravens, W. W., W. McGibbon, and J. G. Halpin. "Vegetarian" poultry ration, a possibility. Wisc. Bul. 469:49. 1946.
Mussehl, F. E., C. W. Ackerson, and R. Borchers. Corn gluten meal and soybean meal for growing chicks. Nebraska 60th Ann. Rept. 1947.
55. Grau, C. R. Protein concentrates as amino acid sources for the chick: Corn gluten meal, cottonseed meal, and peanut meal. Jour. Nutr. 32:303. 1946.
Clark, T. B., A. H. VanLandingham, and C. E. Weakley, Jr. Soybean oil meal in poultry rations. II. Soybean oil meal alone and in combination with meat scrap or corn gluten meal. Poultry Sci. 28:521. 1949.
56. Kentucky Agr. Exp. Sta. 62nd Ann. Rept. Corn gluten meal versus soybean meal in animal protein factor studies in laying hens. P. 39. 1949.
57. Hunter, J. E., D. R. Marble, and H. C. Knandel. Vegetable protein in turkey rations. Penn. Agr. Exp. Sta. Bul. 321:13. 1935.
North, M. O. The influence of protein concentrates upon the quality of meat in turkeys. Wyoming Agr. Exp. Sta. Bul. 264. 1943.
58. Draper, C. I. The nutritive value of corn oil meal and feather protein. Iowa Bul. 326. 1944.
59. Bethke, R. M., G. Bohstedt, H. L. Sassaman, D. C. Kennard, and B. H. Edington. The comparative nutritive value of the proteins of linseed meal and cottonseed meal for different animals. Jour. Agr. Res. 36:855. 1928.
Slinger, S. J., J. C. Small, I. Motzok, and F. N. Marcellus. Linseed oil meal replacing meat meal in rations for growing chicks. Sci. Agr. 23:732. 1943.
Ackerson, C. W., M. J. Blish, and F. E. Mussehl. The utilization of food elements by growing chicks. V. A comparison of linseed oil meal and cottonseed meal as portions of the protein concentrate. Neb. Res. Bul. 100. 1938.
Linseed oil meal vs. meat scraps for layers. Ohio. Bul. 417:71. 1928.
Kempster, H. L. Value of sour milk, beef scrap, cottonseed meal, gluten meal, and oil meal in rations for egg production. Mo. Bul. 172:36. 1920.
Sherwood, R. M., and J. R. Couch. Values of various protein feeds for growing chicks. Tex. Bul. 588. 1940.
60. Orr, J. B., G. S. Robertson, A. Kinross, G. Lewis, and H. Newbiggin. Nutritive requirement of poultry. Scottish Jour. Agr. 9:392. 1926.

61. Kratzer, F. H., D. Williams, and Elizabeth Baker. Amino acids required to supplement linseed protein for chick growth. Jour. Nutr. 33:313. 1947.

62. Mani, K. V., N. Nikolaiczuk, and W. A. Maw. Flaxseed mucilage and its effect on the feeding value of linseed oil meal in chick rations. Sci. Agric. (Ottawa) 29:86. 1949.

63. Kratzer, F. H. The treatment of linseed meal to improve its feeding value for chicks. Poultry Sci. 25:541. 1946.

Kratzer, F. H. Effect of duration of water treatment on the nutritive value of linseed meal. Poultry Sci. 26:90. 1947.

Kratzer, F. H. The growth depression of turkey poults caused by linseed oil meal. Poultry Sci. 28:618. 1949.

Kratzer, F. H. Linseed oil meal water-treated or supplemented with pyridoxine satisfactory for poults. California Agric. 4:10. 1950.

MacGregor, H. I., and J. McGinnis. Toxicity of linseed meal for chicks. Poultry Sci. 27:141. 1948.

McGinnis, J., and H. L. Polis. Factors affecting the nutritive value of linseed meal for growing chickens. Poultry Sci. 25:408. 1946.

64. Altschul, A. M., M. L. Karon, and H. C. Schaefer. Note on effect on chick growth of feeding meals prepared from flaxseed and cottonseed treated with ammonia prior to storage. Poultry Sci. 27:408. 1948.

65. Heuser, G. F., and L. C. Norris. Soybean oil meal in chick rations. Cornell Bul. 810. 1944.

Heuser, G. F., L. C. Norris, and J. McGinnis. Vegetable protein concentrates fed alone and in combination with soybean oil meal and fish meal as the chief supplementary protein in chick starting rations. Poultry Sci. 25:130. 1946.

66. Parkhurst, R. T. Results of feeding experiments, 1925-1926. The value of certain vegetable protein feeds supplementing sour skim milk in a ration for laying hens. Idaho Circ. 43:8. 1927.

67. Runnels, T. D., A. E. Tomhave, E. G. Kelly, and M. E. Wall. Growth response of chicks fed diets containing solvent-extracted broccoli meal and soybean oil meal as protein supplements. Poultry Sci. 30:778. 1950.

68. Borchers, R. Castor bean oil meal. I. Destruction of the toxic factor. Poultry Sci. 28:568. 1949.

69. Kistler, P. T., and P. H. Margolf. The effect of various sources of animal protein on the egg production and condition of pullets. Pa. Bul. 196:29. 1925.

70. Serrano, J. A. A comparative study of the effect of copra meal and dried shrimps as supplements in rations for laying hens. Philippine Agr. 17:95. 1928.

Eamilao, D. E. Protein supplements in poultry rations. IX. Studies to determine the best combination of copra meal and fish meal in rations for growing chicks. Philippine Agr. 26:688. 1938.

De Los Santos, A. C. Water-treated copra meal as a protein supplement in a ration for growing chicks. Philippine Agr. 34:174. 1951.

Lioanag, A. M. Copra meal in a ration for growing ducklings. Philippine Agr. 34:236. 1951.

71. Temperton, H., and F. J. Dudley. Research in poultry nutrition in wartime. Empire Jour. Exp. Agr. 36:248. 1941.

72. Brisson, G. J., N. Nikolaiczuk, and W. A. Maw. Feeding value of horsebean (Vicia Faba L.) for chicks. Sci. Agric. (Ottawa) 30:384. 1950.

Mahon, J. H., and R. H. Common. The amino acid composition of the horsebean (Vicia Faba L.) as related to its nutritive value for chicks. Sci. Agric. (Ottawa) 30:43. 1950.

73. Baclig, J. B., and F. M. Fronda. A further study on the influence of ipil-ipil (Leucaena glauca Linn.) seed meal in a ration for growing chicks. Philippine Agric. 32:329. 1948.

Pizarro, P. I. Ipil-ipil (Leucaena glauca Linn.) seed meal in rations for growing chicks. Philippine Agric. 31:73. 1947.

Garcia, P. N., and F. M. Fronda. Water-treated ipil-ipil seed meal in rations for growing chicks. Philippine Agr. 35:143. 1951.

74. Irwin, M. R., and H. L. Kempster. Korean lespedeza seed as a protein supplement in chick rations. Mo. Bul. 462. 1943.

75. Rodriquez, F. L. Protein supplements in poultry rations. 8. Optimum amount of mungo which may be used in a normal ration for growing chicks. Philippine Agr. 25:451. 1936.

76. Milby, T. T. Mung beans as a source of protein for turkey poults. Okla. Acad. Sci. Proc. 25:50. 1945.

Thayer, R. H., and V. G. Heller. Mung beans as a poultry feed. Okla. Bul. 336:1. 1949.

77. Kondra, P. A., and G. C. Hodgson. Mustard seed oil meal in chick starter rations. Poultry Sci. 28:771. 1949.

O'Neil, J. B. Mustard seed oil meal and sunflower seed oil meal in chick starter rations. Sci. Agric. (Ottawa) 28:127. 1948.

78. Squibb, R. L., and Miriam K. Wyld. Effect of corozo palm nut oil meal in the baby chick diet. Poultry Sci. 31:118. 1952.

79. Feeding for egg production. Vegetable vs. animal protein in egg production. Idaho Bul. 117. 1919.

Parkhurst, R. T. Relative value of certain protein feeds for egg production. First year's work, 1920-1921. Idaho Circ. 27. 1922.

Parkhurst, R. T. Value of certain protein feeds for production and quality of eggs. Idaho Bul. 134. 1924.

Parkhurst, R. T. Results of feeding experiments 1925-1926. The value of certain vegetable protein feeds supplementing sour skim milk in a ration for laying hens. Idaho Circ. 43:8. 1927.

Work and progress of the agricultural experiment station. Idaho Bul. 160:27. 1928.

Lampman, C. E. Rations containing peas require animal protein supplements. Idaho Bul. 220:44. 1936.

Peterson, C. F., C. E. Lampman, D. W. Bolin, and O. E. Stamberg. Methionine deficiency of Alaska field peas for chick growth. Poultry Sci. 23:287. 1944.

80. Robertson, E. I., J. S. Carver, and J. W. Cook. Gross value of protein supplements for poultry. Wash. Bul. 388. 1940.

Carver, J. S., B. B. Bohren, and J. W. Cook. The protein value of Alaska pea meal for chickens. *Wash. Bul.* 418. 1942.

Bolin, D. W., C. F. Peterson, C. E. Lampman, and O. E. Stamberg. Chick growth response resulting from methionine additions to various supplements with pea protein. *Poultry Sci.* 25:157. 1946.

81. Fangauf, R., and A. Haensel. Mitteilungen über Roggenkleie, Trockentreber, Malzkeime, und Rapskuchenmehl als Hühnerfutter. *Archiv für Geflügelk.* 12:149. 1938.

Pettit, J. H., S. J. Slinger, E. V. Evans, and F. N. Marcellus. Utilization of sunflower seed oil meal, wheat distillers' dried grains and rapeseed oil meal in poultry rations. *Sci. Agr.* 24:201. 1944.

Olsson, N., Gosta Austrand, and C. Wadne. Protein in chicken rations. *Lantbruksohgskolan Husdjursforsoksanstalten Meddel.* 26:5. 1947.

Blakely, R. M., and R. W. Anderson. Studies with rapeseed oilcake meal. I. The effect of various levels of rapeseed oilcake meal in the diet on the weight of the thyroid glands of turkey poults. *Sci. Agr.* 28:393. 1948.

Kondra, P. A., and G. C. Hodgson. Sunflower seed and rapeseed oil meals in chick starter rations. *Sci. Agric.* (Ottawa) 28:264. 1948.

Turner, C. W. Effect of rapeseed oil meal on the thyroid of the chick. *Poultry Sci.* 27:118. 1948.

Blakely, R. M., H. I. MacGregor, and R. W. Anderson. Rapeseed oilcake meal as a supplement to a fattening diet. *Poultry Sci.* 28: 757. 1949.

MacGregor, H. I., R. M. Blakely, and R. W. Anderson. Toxicity of rapeseed oilcake meal for turkey poults. *Poultry Sci.* 28:774.

Witz, W. M., M. M. Carpenter, and J. W. Hayward. Nutritional studies with rapeseed meal. *Poultry Sci.* 30:786. 1950.

Allen, C. E., and D. S. Dow. The biological assessment of the value of rapeseed oil meal as a dietary component. *Sci. Agr.* 32:403. 1952.

82. Kratzer, F. H., and D. Williams. Safflower seed as an amino acid source for chicks. *Poultry Sci.* 26:623. 1947.

Kratzer, F. H., and D. E. Williams. Safflower oil meal in rations for chicks. *Poultry Sci.* 30:417. 1951.

83. Almquist, H. J., and C. R. Grau. Mutual supplementary effect of the proteins of soybean and sesame meals. *Poultry Sci.* 23:341. 1944.

Grau, C. R., and H. J. Almquist. Sesame protein in chick diets. *Proc. Soc. Exp. Biol. and Med.* 57:187. 1944.

Patrick, H. Deficiencies in a sesame meal type ration for chicks. *Poultry Sci.* 32:744. 1953.

84. Hale, R. W., and W. Bolton. Sesame cake meal as a protein concentrate for laying pullets. *Jour. Agric. Sci.* 38:437. 1948.

Baskett, R. G., J. Houston, R. H. Common, W. Bolton, and S. McConaghy. Poultry nutrition research in Northern Ireland. *World's Poultry Sci. Jour.* 3:162. 1947.

85. Shelton M., and J. R. Couch. Grain sorghum by-product feeds for farm animals. *Tex. Bul.* 743:21. 1951.

Sherwood, R. M., and H. L. German. The value of sorghum gluten meal in all-mash chick starters. *Poultry Sci.* 27:682. 1948.

86. Tabakoff, I. J. Investigation of improved poultry feeding in Bulgaria. Rept. Seventh World's Poultry Congress. 151. 1939.

Alexander, J. C., and D. C. Hill. The effect of heat on the lysine and methionine in sunflower seed oil meal. Jour. Nutr. 48:149. 1952.

Gartley, K. M., S. J. Slinger, and D. C. Hill. Further observations on the use of sunflower seed oil meal in turkey starter rations. Poultry Sci. 29:312. 1950.

Grau, C. R., and H. J. Almquist. Value of sunflower seed protein. Proc. Soc. Exp. Biol. and Med. 60:373. 1945.

Kondra, P. A., and G. C. Hodgson. Sunflower seed and rapeseed oil meals in chick starter rations. Sci. Agric. (Ottawa) 28:264. 1948.

O'Neil, J. B. Mustard seed oil meal and sunflower seed oil meal in chick starter rations. Sci. Agric. (Ottawa) 28:127. 1948.

Pettit, J. H., S. J. Slinger, E. V. Evans, and F. N. Marcellus. Utilization of sunflower seed oil meal, wheat distillers' dried grains, and rapeseed oil meal in poultry rations. Sci. Agr. (Ottawa) 24: 201. 1944.

McGinnis, J., P. T. Hsu, and J. S. Carver. Nutritional deficiencies of sunflower seed oil meal for chicks. Poultry Sci. 27:389. 1948.

Morrison, A. B., D. R. Clandinin, and A. R. Robblee. The supplementary value of sunflower seed oil meal in practical chick starting rations. Poultry Sci. 32:542. 1953.

Slinger, S. J., K. M. Gartley, W. F. Pepper, and D. C. Hill. The influence of animal protein factor supplements and antibiotics on the incidence and severity of white feathers in turkeys. Jour. Nutr. 43:345. 1951.

Slinger, S. J., D. C. Hill, J. M. Gartley, and H. D. Branion. Soybean oil meal and sunflower seed oil meal in rations for Broad Breasted Bronze turkeys. Poultry Sci. 28:534. 1949.

87. Mangold, E. Grundlagen für die Fütterung mit Süsslupinenschrot als Eiweissfutter beim Schwein, Wiederkäuer, und Geflügel. Deutsche Landwirtschafliche Presse 62:77. 1935.

Mangold, E., and H. Damköhler. Süsslupinenschrot als Eiweissfutter für Geflügel; seine Eignung für die Kükenaufzucht. Archiv für Geflügelk. 9:233. 1935.

Mangold, E., and H. Stotz. Süsslupinenschrot als Eiweissfutter für Geflügel; seine Verdaulichkeit bei Hühnern. Archiv für Geflügelk. 9:64. 1935.

Fangauf, R., and A. Haensel. Süsslupinenschrot als Hühnerfutter. Archiv. für Geflügel Kunde 11:161. 1937.

88. Mehrhof, N. R., and G. K. Davis. Value of different protein supplements for chick growth. Florida Annual Rept. 1947:64.

89. Rusoff, L. L., and N. R. Mehrhof. Chick feeding experiments with solvent-extracted tung oil meal. Poultry Sci. 21:451. 1942.

Davis, G. K., N. R. Mehrhof and R. S. McKinney. Effect of tung meal in rations for growing chicks. Poultry Sci. 25:74. 1946.

90. Heuser, G. F., L. C. Norris, and J. McGinnis. Vegetable protein concentrates fed alone and in combination with soybean oil meal

and fish meal as the chief supplementary protein in chick starting rations. Poultry Sci. 25:130. 1946.

Jeppesen, J. H., and C. R. Grau. Whole wheat protein as an amino acid source for chicks. Poultry Sci. 27:588. 1948.

Lewis, E. W. Jr., C. A. Elvehjem and E. B. Hart. Studies on the nature of the nutritional deficiencies of wheat gluten meal. Jour. Nutr. 43:113. 1951.

91. Meteljkow, S. Drojjewanie kormow w ptizewodstwe. Kolchosn, opytnitsch 3:26. 1937. (Ref. Nut. Abstracts 7:1138. 1938.)

92. Weinmiller, L., and K. Mantel. Fütterungsversuch mit Verwendung von Trockenhefe und Magermilch. Archiv für Geflügelk. 11:293. 1937.

93. Fronda, F. M., and M. E. Fronda. Distillery yeast, a possible feed for poultry. Philippine Agric. 31:222. 1943.

94. Couch, J. R., J. R. Reed Jr., R. L. Atkinson, and B. E. Welch. Distillers' grain solubles and dried whey with an APF concentrate in broiler feeds. Proc. 6th Distillers Feed Conf: 47. 1951.

Klose, A. A., and H. L. Fevold. Nutritional value of yeast protein to the rat and the chick. Jour. Nutr. 29:421. 1945.

McGinnis, J. Yeast in poultry diets. Amer. Egg & Poultry Rev. 10:58. 1949.

Ringrose, R. C. Nutritive properties of torula yeast for poultry. Poultry Sci. 28:75. 1949.

95. Evans, R. J., and J. L. St. John. Estimation of the relative nutritive value of vegetable proteins by two chemical methods. Jour. Nutr. 30:209. 1945.

96. Lyman, C. M., W. Y. Chang, and J. R. Couch. Evaluation of protein quality in cottonseed meals by chick growth and by a chemical index method. Jour. Nutr. 49:679. 1953.

CHAPTER 8

POULTRY FEEDS

GREEN FEEDS AND VEGETABLE PRODUCTS

The importance of green food in poultry feeding was first observed because of the response of birds when allowed to range in the spring after being confined during the winter. The resulting spurt in egg production was due probably to the warmer weather and exposure to the sun as well as access to green food. Again, it was observed that production was retarded late in the summer and in the fall when the natural supply of green food became low.

The green growing part of plants has long been recognized as the basis for animal nutrition. The nutritional significane of grass has been pointed out by Elvehjem and Sober.[1] They show that grasses contain appreciable amounts of many of the well-known nutrients and are rich in unknown factors. Assays show them to contain significant amounts of carotene, vitamin C, vitamin E, vitamin K, thiamin, riboflavin, pyridoxine, pantothenic acid, niacin, biotin, and choline. The mineral content is favorable. The protein content may be as high as 30 per cent. Young grass is of higher nutritive value than older herbage since it contains more protein and vitamins (especially riboflavin) and less fiber. Leafy green vegetation[2] and the fresh juice of forage crops have been shown to contain growth factors.

In comparative trials,[3] where green food was furnished during the winter as compared to feeding no green food during that period, often considerable differences in production were secured.

Various reasons have been given to account for the benefits of green food. One of the first explanations given for its value was that it acted as a tonic, stimulant, or invigorator. The specific effect was not designated, but indications were that it had a beneficial effect on the condition of the bird and thus produced more eggs or flesh. It was also believed that green food stimulated the appetite and in that way encouraged greater food consumption and consequently larger production. It promoted activity and was a help to digestion. Sometimes it acts favorably in furnishing additional bulk to the ration. In this respect, it is necessary to distinguish between furnishing the nutritive elements of true green food and mere succulence. In some instances the feed is more palatable in the succulent form as, for example, when feeding germinated or sprouted oats instead of the dry oats.

The health of the hen is influenced also by the feeding of green food. This is shown by greater mortality as well as decreased egg production when green food was not supplied.[4] It has also been reported[5] that the feeding of green food will result in prevention of molt and reduction of summer culling which, with the other factors mentioned, will mean a saving of money.

Greater mortality[6] due to coccidial infections has been found in birds ranged on bare lots than in birds ranged on pastures. Birds on pasture carried heavier worm infections, but were able to withstand heavier parasitic burdens.

The feeding of green food frequently keeps birds busy, and in that way might help to prevent or overcome picking and other forms of cannibalism.

Perhaps the most important fact about green feeds, however, is that they are rich in vitamins. Green feeds, as a group, is the only group which is well supplied with all the vitamins. The other groups of feeds usually are deficient in one or more of the vitamins. The feeding of green food has improved hatchability. This improvement in hatchability is probably due to vitamins.

KINDS OF GREEN FOOD

GRASS RANGE OR PASTURE is the natural method of providing green food, and, where it is supplied abundantly, is probably the best method. Clover and alfalfa ranges are preferred, primarily because the green stuff is available over a longer period of the year. They do not grow up and become tough and unavailable, as grass does. Frequent mowing of grass, however, will help to keep it tender.

For poultry pastures, plants capable of forming a dense, hard-wearing, and lawn-like turf are desirable.[7] Wild white clover and ladino clover are suitable legumes. Grasses suitable for poultry turf are perennial rye grass, meadow grasses, the fescues, creeping bent, and crested dog's-tail. However, poultry does not like the plants after they have become aged and woody and will then only eat them as a last resort. Turkeys[8] prefer ladino clover, but other grasses can be satisfactorily used for grazing.

Crampton and Forshaw[9] presented evidence to show that the

feeding value of the herbage of any single species changes during the growing season. Herbage grown during spring and fall, when plant growing conditions are favorable, has excellent feeding value. Herbage grown during midsummer has lower nutritive value, owing apparently to a reduction in the availability to the animal of the carbohydrate fractions.

A mixture of grasses is usually recommended for poultry pastures. The grasses most commonly used are Kentucky bluegrass, Canada bluegrass, timothy, perennial rye grass, wild white clover, and ladino clover. Regardless of the mixture, the pasture must be mowed frequently so that young grass is kept constantly growing up from the bottom.

Where range is depended upon for green stuff, the units must not be too large or too concentrated. Hens will not range far from the house so that usually the grass adjacent to the house is soon entirely eaten, whereas further away it grows and matures.

Pasture for Growing Birds. The benefits of range rearing may be attributed to improved health due to better nutrition, more sanitary conditions, and more favorable management.

If the chicks are restricted on feed nutrients, either because feed is withheld or because the ration is deficient, they will consume more grass and select those types which will supplement their ration. Thomas[10] fed chicks both high- and low-protein rations and observed that the grass in the run of the low-protein lot was heavily grazed and kept in check, while the herbage in the run of the high-protein lot was untouched. Furthermore, the clover content of the sward in the run of the low-protein lot was reduced to a greater extent than in the run of the high-protein lot. Gutteridge, O'Neil, and Pratt[11] presented evidence to show that the pasture was utilized to an increasing degree on the lower levels of protein. The high animal protein ration (17 per cent) appeared to have been adequate in most respects since the pasture of the group on this ration was only very lightly grazed. There was a suggestion that the vegetable protein groups felt the need of supplementing their ration to a greater degree than the groups fed animal protein through an increased intake of pasture grass.

Chicks on good pasture eat a considerable amount of grass and thus save on the amount of grain and mash required. Reports from poultrymen have indicated feed savings up to 35 per cent. Most of the experimental results, however, do not show savings of this magnitude.[12,16] The feed savings reported range from 5 to 20 per cent. The larger savings were usually obtained when the feeding time was restricted. However, with drastic feed restriction the weights of the pullets usually were lower.

Poultry can utilize fresh, young grass[13] but is unable to deal as effectively with large amounts of it as are the other farm animals. The amount appears to be limited by the capacity of the birds to break down the fiber. Temperton and Dudley, in feeding grass to growing stock, found that when 10 per cent of the mash was replaced by its equivalent in grass on the dry matter basis (representing about 1/3 the gross food intake), much of the grass was found in the droppings in an apparently little altered condition and there was a marked reduction in the rate of growth. However, the grass-reared birds were quicker in maturing. According to a report from Finland, Pihkala concluded that poultry can obtain only 5.5 to 7.0 per cent of its food requirements from pasture. In the feeding of turkeys, Darrow and Morgan reported that the amount of feed saved by the use of range was 9.1 per cent for the Bronze turkey and 3.1 per cent for the Small Whites.

The actual amount of feed saved is not the only benefit of pasture. Perhaps of even greater value is the saving in feed cost since good pasturage permits omission from the ration of ingredients which may be more expensive, such as vitamin carriers, milk by-products, alfalfa meal, and animal protein.[14] In fact, some of the reports indicate that whole grain plus minerals proved to be a satisfactory ration when fed to birds on good pasture.

Variable results have been reported for birds reared on grass.[15,16] However, when compared with rearing on bare ground or in confinement pasture-rearing of pullets has shown some advantages. The birds may be heavier at maturity and usually show deeper pigmentation. Birds on pasture usually consume less food and thus make more economical gains. Mortality, sexual maturity, and subsequent egg production are not influenced much by pasture.

<u>Pasture for Mature Birds.</u> The value of pasture land for mature birds is indicated in experiments conducted in Germany,[17] where a saving of 34.3 per cent of the total cost of feeding Leghorn hens was made, when the birds were kept on open pasturage. Another pasture group required during the summer, when feeding in the open was possible, 32.1 per cent less feed to produce the same weight of eggs than the group without open pasturage.

Reporting on ranges for the laying flock, Berry[18] showed the largest returns over feed cost were received when the laying flock was provided with an alfalfa range. However, the returns were greatest when the flock was allowed access to the range for only 2 hours each day. This short daily period provided sufficient green feed, but the birds did not eat enough green alfalfa to lower egg quality.

The Kentucky Station[19] reported that bare or bluegrass range, in connection with a complete all-mash ration for laying hens, did not influence feed consumption during the summer period after the grass had matured and partly lost its green color. However, the hens consumed 10 to 20 per cent less feed when given access to a bluegrass range during the spring growing season. The bluegrass range during the growing season increased egg production but did not influence weight or hatchability of the eggs, or the health and weight of the hens. Stephenson and Bryant[12] concluded that the use of a sod range during the laying period is preferable to keeping the birds in strict confinement, and that it seems advisable also to keep the birds confined to the house during the fall and winter months unless there is good green pasture available.

Thomas[10] reported that Rhode Island Red layers fed a low protein ration supplemented the protein deficiency by consuming the clover and dandelions instead of the perennial rye grass. Temperton and Dudley[20] showed that the feeding of grass in comparatively large amounts to laying pullets did not have any adverse effects on health but did decrease egg production and produced a very deep-colored egg yolk.

Good pastures for laying hens[21] have generally improved egg production and hatchability, reduced the feed requirements and lowered mortality. However, the yolk color was usually darker. Pastures of oats, Italian rye grass, Japanese mustard, and Kudzu and Bermuda grass have proven of value.

Supplements of green feed have been reported[22] not to affect the interior quality of eggs, as measured by the albumen index, percentage of firm albumen, height of firm albumen, or yolk index. The only marked effect of feeding fresh grass is to increase the quantity of pigment in the yolk. Ovarian hemorrhages[23] leading to the production of blood and meat spots have been reduced by allowing hens access to range.

GREEN CROPS. Alfalfa and clover furnish a good feed when cut green and fed directly to the hens. These feeds are especially desirable for birds closely confined or running on bare yards.

They furnish a good source of green food in summer when second- and third-cutting alfalfa and clover are available. Soybeans and the green cowpea plant have supplied green succulent fodder.[24] Green forage crops have been used as a substitute for three-fourths of the mash for laying hens.[25]

GRAIN PASTURE. For this purpose any of the grains may be used. It is available chiefly in the early spring, its main disadvantage being its temporary nature, inasmuch as most of the shoots soon become old and tough. Rye, sown in the fall, or winter wheat is often used for this purpose.

LAWN CLIPPINGS are usually not available in large quantities but furnish good green food, especially if they contain some clover. Where lawns of any size are maintained in connection with the poultry farm, it is wise to catch the clippings for this purpose.

CABBAGE is a succulent green food. The vitamin content is not so great as in the kinds of green food with thin green leaves. The outer, greener leaves also contain more of the vitamins. It makes an excellent green food although more expensive than some other forms. The small and unmarketable heads may be used to advantage in poultry feeding.

SAUERKRAUT is another form in which cabbage may be fed. It has been fed to young chicks by putting the sauerkraut on a plate and sprinkling feed over it. Mature birds may be fed 3 to 4 pounds a day per 100 hens. The sour taste seems to act as an appetizer. The kraut is made in the usual way, except that a little less salt is used.

RAPE is often used where birds are confined. It is fed much the same as cabbage. Sometimes the birds are given access to the field itself later in the season. Rape gives a very dark color to the yolk of the egg, which, in some cases, has been considered an objectionable feature.

KALE makes a very good green food because of its palatability and productivity. It will yield 20 or more tons of green material per acre. It is used very extensively on the Pacific Coast, where the thousand-headed variety is chiefly grown. It is sown in several plantings in order to give a succession, and in some sections it is thus available the year round. It may also be utilized as shade.

In England,[26] egg production was not satisfactory with the feeding of marrow stem kale to laying pullets. The health of the birds was not influenced and no substantial economy in purchased foodstuffs resulted.

OTHER GREENS, such as lettuce, onions, spinach, beet tops, swiss chard, and the like, may be used to excellent advantage as green food. Waste leaves of cabbage, cauliflower, broccoli, and other plants can be utilized.

SPROUTED GRAINS[27] make it possible to provide green food at any time. The grain sprouter has been referred to as the poultry silo because the sprouted grains are ordinarily used as a winter and early spring source of green food. Oats are the common grain used for sprouting. Sprouted oats also provide a satisfactory way to use oats, since the absorption of water, while not increasing the nutrient, makes the grain more palatable and digestible. One hundred pounds of oats will absorb enough water to make about 350 pounds of the sprouted grain. There is an actual loss of dry matter[28] in sprouting oats so that the advantage of the process is to produce a succulent green food. Sprouted rye[29] was not as satisfactory as sprouted oats.

GERMINATED OATS have been used in place of the sprouted oats. Results of feeding germinated oats to Leghorn pullets at Indiana[30] indicate these things. Germinated oats appeared to increase egg production during the winter months, but they had no significant influence upon egg production during periods of 10 months' duration. No benefit was derived from increased fertility and hatchability of eggs. There was no evidence to indicate that the fiber in the germinated oats was of any particular importance. On the other hand, the Delaware Station[31] reported greater mortality and lower production from pens receiving no germinated oats as compared with ones being fed the same in some tests, and little influence on egg production or mortality in other tests.

Experiments with laying hens in Italy[32] proved that the winter lay was improved by feeding germinated grain. The control birds lost weight, whereas the birds fed the germinated grain gained weight.

SILAGE[33] is frequently suggested as a means of supplying green food. Favorable results have been reported although frequently the value of silage is overestimated.

The West Virginia Station concluded that because of the beneficial effect upon hatchability in the first test and upon egg production in the second, it would seem that, when available, a small amount of corn silage may be fed to laying hens in winter to advantage. On the other hand, there have been some cases of digestive disturbances. They might have been due to the fermentation. As a form of succulence, corn silage has been used satisfactorily by some poultrymen by mixing it in the mash after boiling it.

Grass silage of various types has been given considerable attention. Payne and associates at the Kansas Station[15] reported larger net returns per bird when pullets were fed immature cereal grasses, both in fresh and in ensiled forms. The feeding of oat grass silage resulted in the production of olive-colored egg yolks, commonly classified as "grass eggs." Darker yolk color was observed when hens were fed silage as compared with fresh cereal grasses. Restricting the silage consumption to 2 to 3 pounds daily per 100 hens and feeding a high quality of silage eliminated grass eggs. There was no significant effect of feeding silage upon egg production.

The Tennessee Station[34] concluded that silage feeding as a supplement to the regular rations was a desirable practice. The advantages of silage feeding included greater zest for eating and higher daily feed consumption, increase in weight over poultry not receiving such silage, and better physical condition as determined by appearance, vitality, weight production, egg production, and post-mortem examinations.

The New Jersey Station[35] reported that grass silage fed at the rate of 4 pounds per 100 birds per day prevented the usual drop in hatchability when alfalfa leaf meal and dried buttermilk were removed from the ration. The use of grass silage as a substitute for milk and alfalfa in chick rations up to a month of age was not fully satisfactory because of the inability of the young chick to handle such bulky material.

Temperton and Dudley[36] concluded that, in the feeding of grass silage to laying pullets, the two chief difficulties encountered were in cutting the grass sufficiently short and in getting the birds to eat the silage in sufficient quantity to effect a material saving in mash.

The West Virginia Station[37] concluded that considering the labor involved in making immature silage and the experimental evidence showing little or no beneficial results from feeding the silage to chicks in batteries, to growing pullets and layers confined in pens, poultry rations can be supplemented more efficiently by other vitamin carriers, especially for supplying riboflavin.

A variety of crops can be made into silage. They include alfalfa, the clovers, timothy, redtop, orchard grass, bluegrass, oats, wheat, barley, rye, lawn grass clippings, peas, and soybeans. Good silage has been made with molasses (60 to 80 pounds per ton), phosphoric acid (20 pounds of 70 per cent per ton), or ground grain (150 to 200 pounds per ton).

In the feeding of silage to mature birds the usual recommendation is to feed 4 to 6 pounds to 100 hens daily. They frequently will consume much larger quantities, but this is usually neither necessary nor desirable.

ROOT CROPS AND TUBERS of various kinds have been used in the past to furnish succulence and to take the place of green food. However, their use has declined because it has been found that many of them furnish little, if any, vitamins. Therefore, they do not function as true green foods.

Mangle beets are liked by the fowls but furnish little, of any, vitamins. They would, therefore, furnish only succulence. They are a cheap and easily handled succulent. They can be stored easily in a root cellar or put where they will keep until spring. Mangles are usually fed about midday and given in such amounts that the hens will eat readily the rest of the day.

Carrots, turnips, rutabagas, and other roots may be fed. A good way to feed these types of crops is to shred them. Carrots contain considerable vitamin A. The Michigan Station[38] reported that 4 to 5 pounds of carrots daily per 100 birds provided an adequate amount of vitamin A and that this product was a satisfactory substitute for alfalfa products in the laying ration during the winter feeding period.

Potatoes do not furnish a source of green food. They furnish succulence and may be used, however, after boiling and mixing with mash, but they function the same as grain and ground feed. They can also be fed raw.

The essentials of a good root cellar are protection against freezing, proper ventilation, and drainage.[39]

HAYS[40] have been used in recent years in place of green foods for poultry. The legume hays, particularly, have been fed for this purpose. In 1928 the Ohio Station stated that the best substitute for green food is a high-quality, leafy, immature-cut legume hay. The Washington Station reported that alfalfa hay, chopped into 1-inch lengths, proved an excellent substitute for green food. When it was kept before the birds at all times, they consumed 8 pounds per bird per year. Well-cured, second- or third-cutting alfalfa hay is used. Soybean hay has also been fed with good results. It should be cut when the seeds are just beginning to form in the pods. All the hays are usually cut into ½- to 1-inch lengths and kept available to the hens in wire baskets or containers.

Clover or alfalfa chaff or leaves can be used either in the dry form, giving birds access to it as in the form of hay, or they may be steamed or soaked and mixed with a wet mash.

DRIED GRASSES of various kinds have been fed to poultry with satisfactory results. In general, the dehydrated grasses or those not subjected to too much heat have given the best results. This is probably due to the better retention of their vitamin content, especially vitamin A.[41]

Alfalfa Meal has been the most widely used and has given good results. Ordinary alfalfa meal is of little benefit. Considerable variation[42] is found in the composition and nutritive value of different samples of alfalfa meal. This is particularly true as regards fiber, protein, ash, vitamin A, and riboflavin. Dehydrated alfalfa meals are generally superior to sun-cured meals, especially in regard to the vitamin content. A good alfalfa meal should contain a high percentage of leafy material, have a high protein and ether extract and a low fiber content, and be fragrant and of a bright green color. Usually not over 5 per cent of alfalfa meal is included in the mash.

The South Dakota Station[43] indicated that the optimum percentage of alfalfa meal lies between 10 and 20 per cent and it will substitute for either bran or middlings, but egg production falls off if it is substituted for both. Better results were obtained when it was combined with middlings. The New Mexico Station[44] reported as satisfactory egg production from the birds receiving alfalfa meal as from those on green alfalfa range. The United States Experiment Station in Arizona[45] showed that sun-cured alfalfa meal was a poor substitute for fresh alfalfa, that sun-cured alfalfa leaf meal was more satisfactory than sun-cured alfalfa meal as a substitute for fresh alfalfa, and that whole alfalfa hays were unreliable as substitutes for fresh alfalfa.

The Wisconsin Station[46] reported increased egg production and hatchability by including alfalfa meal in winter rations. Alfalfa meal was better than dried cereal grass, although either one was effective.

The Nebraska Station[47] reported that artificially dried sudangrass meal could replace alfalfa meal in a ration for growing chicks. The Delaware Station[48] concluded that locally produced dehydrated ground clover and perennial grasses could be used in broiler rations in place of western sun-cured alfalfa leaf meal. Experiments reported from South Africa[49] show that cowpea hay meal could replace 8 to 10 per cent of alfalfa meal in chicken rations up to 10 weeks of age.

The Kentucky Station[50] concluded that because of the bulkiness of air-dried bluegrass, due to the high fiber content, it was not a satisfactory ingredient for all-mash rations for growing chicks but that the bluegrass should be fed ad libitum as a succulent feed. Leaf meals of Korean lespedeza, alfalfa, and lespedeza sericea replaced mixed wheat feed, on a basis of equal parts of protein in the feeding of growing chicks, but could not replace wheat feed and either dried skimmilk or meat scrap on a basis of equal quantities of protein.

The Mississippi Station[51] found that kudzu meal and kudzu leaf meal compared favorably in chemical analyses with alfalfa meal and alfalfa leaf meal of good grade.

Other meals which have been fed with satisfactory results are brome grass, crested wheat grass, western wheat grass, brome-alfalfa mixture and sudan grass meals,[52] ladino clover meal,[53] desmodium meal and pigeon pea fodder meal,[54] mangrove leaf meal,[55] ramie meal,[54,56] kikuyu grass meal,[54] and banana leaf meal.[54] Koa haole leaf meal and fresh green koa haole leaves[57] can be fed in moderate quantities. Creeping indigo leaf meal[58] depressed egg production, body weight, and feed consumption of laying birds and growth of chicks.

DRIED VEGETABLE WASTES[59] have been reported as being good sources of protein, carotene, and riboflavin. The Delaware Station concluded that all the wastes used (dried pea vines, lima bean vines, turnip tops, broccoli, and carrot tops) may be fed to broilers or other growing birds at as high a level as 8 per cent in place of alfalfa meal. The broccoli and turnip tops produced a significantly greater degree of pigmentation than the alfalfa meal. All the vegetable wastes were more palatable than the alfalfa meal. When used in a breeder ration cannery by-products[60] have improved a ration containing no alfalfa but was not quite as good.

Semi-solid vegetable wastes[61] have also been reported as being valuable for poultry feeding.

Dried pea vines,[62] high quality bean vine meal,[63] and dehydrated celery tops[64] have been reported to compare favorably with alfalfa meal. Dehydrated flat pea forage[65] was shown to have no value as a protein supplement for growing chicks.

DRIED BEET PRODUCTS.[66] Dried beet pulp as well as similar products, such as dried cabbage, are not relished by fowls and are of questionable value in poultry feeding.

Dehydrated beet leaves[67] have been fed satisfactorily at low levels. At higher levels there was a depressing effect due to the oxolic acid content which could be overcome by increasing the calcium in the ration.

PIMIENTO PEPPER has been fed to poultry by the Georgia Station.[68] It gives a rich yellow color to the shanks, skin, and fat, the amount of color depending on the amount of pimiento fed. The eggs also had higher hatchability.

MISCELLANEOUS GREEN FOODS. It is probable that almost any kind of green plant material can be used in feeding chickens, as well as other animals. Dried nettles have been reported from Italy[69] to be beneficial for both chicks and hens. In California, the spineless cactus has been used as greens for poultry. No injury was apparent in the hen after rhubarb leaves[70] were fed for 30 days as a supplementary feed. Leaves and young shoots of centrosema, ipil-ipil, and sweet potato and ipil-ipil leaf meal have been advantageously fed to ducks.[71]

EPSOM SALTS has sometimes been mentioned as a green food substitute. It is not a substitute for green foods but was used as an alternative for its laxative effect.

COMPARATIVE EXPERIMENTAL RESULTS

In comparing mangels, clover, and sprouted oats as green food, the Kentville (Canada) Experimental Station[72] reports clover as more productive than mangels, which were better than sprouted oats. In studying substitutes for fresh green food, Elford[73] found the value of the various feeds studied to be in the following order: alfalfa meal, sweet clover meal, potatoes, mangels, sprouted oats, Epsom salts.

In a study of root crops at the Fredericton (Canada) Station,[74] it was found that swedes or raw potatoes were superior to mangels, all of which gave better results than Epsom salts.

In a study of the effect of certain green food substitutes (including sprouted oats, yellow mangels, alfalfa leaves, alfalfa leaf meal, and cod liver oil) upon egg production and hatchability at the New Hampshire Station,[75] all substitutes studied were valuable sources of vitamin A, as measured by health and egg production. The cod liver oil pen excelled in egg production. The alfalfa leaf meal pen gave the highest hatchability, followed closely by the pen receiving alfalfa leaves.

In a comparison of chopped alfalfa hay with alfalfa leaf meal at the Ohio Station,[76] the egg production was somewhat better in the lot receiving the chopped alfalfa hay. The hatchability of eggs was practically the same in all lots.

Alfalfa leaf meal, sprouted oats, and germinated oats gave benefits in the order named as regards egg production, per cent hatch, and mortality at the Kansas Station.[77] In this experiment, the basal ration was deficient in vitamin A since white corn was used.

Experiments conducted in Germany[78] indicated that all kinds of green foods and substitutes may be given to laying and breeding hens with good results.

NECESSITY OF GREEN FOOD IN THE RATION

Formerly green food was considered as being necessary or desirable in the poultry ration.[79] Now less emphasis is placed upon it.

Since green foods owe their importance largely to the fact that they are important vitamin carriers, their necessity obviously depends to a large extent upon the ration fed and the conditions under which the birds are kept. With a proper adjustment of the ration, it is possible to minimize the importance of including green foods. At the Cornell Station, there was no apparent benefit in egg production during the winter from adding green food when cod liver oil and milk were included in the ration. They, in part, furnished the same elements which were supplied by green foods. There was some indication, however, that hatchability was benefited by the inclusion of green foods in the ration.

With an increase in our knowledge concerning vitamins, their distribution and functions, we shall probably be able to adjust our rations so as to use little or no green foods and still secure optimum results in all respects. Some reports[80] indicate that normal growth of chicks may be obtained on rations containing no green plant tissue. It has also been shown[81] that green feed is not necessary in rations for good egg production.

In surveys made in connection with pullet management campaigns, it has been noted that there was no difference between the flocks receiving green or succulent feed and those receiving none. It should be noted, however, that the rations fed usually contained some alfalfa and milk.

In an economic study of poultry farming in New York,[82] including surveys from 123 farms, for the year ending September 30, 1930, it was found that, apparently, there was no difference in egg production per bird resulting from the use of green food or germinated oats. "It is believed by some that green feed or germinated oats increase feed intake. At times succulent green feed may serve as an appetizer, but from these data there seems to be some question whether it is worth the trouble required in feeding it."

	No Green Food or Germinated Oats	Green Food Only	Green Food and Germinated Oats	Germinated Oats Only
Number of farms	52	51	5	15
Eggs per hen	142	149	139	143
Number of birds	1542	1265	1640	1507
Per cent lay October December	22	24	19	21
Pounds of feed per bird	82	84	83	80

GROWING GREEN FOOD

The attempt to provide green food from pasture for large numbers of hens has been gradually abandoned. Pasture cannot withstand the attacks of hens and is soon depleted. Instead, green food is grown in separate fields, harvested, and fed to the hens. In some instances severe losses due to ground contamination or predators have also encouraged confinement rearing, with the feeding of freshly cut green food, in place of range rearing.

Another important value of growing green food for chickens is the shade with which it provides them. Furthermore, the growing of crops helps to keep the ranges and yards in sanitary condition. For ranges, crops commonly grown are corn, soybeans, and sunflowers. For the cropping of yards and runs, rye, oats, and rape are usually planted.

POULTRY GREEN FOOD GARDENS AND CALENDARS. As a suggestion for the possible production of different types of green food for poultry, outlines for poultry green food gardens and calendars for the different sections of the country have been suggested.[83]

AMOUNTS OF GREEN FOOD FOR POULTRY

Where poultry is allowed to range, it will gather its green food. Usually it is allowed free range at all times. This is satisfactory where large fields are available and it is not necessary to conserve the feed supply.

Under unlimited range conditions, the birds will usually eat more green food early and late in the day. It was noted in Australia[84] that the pen with free choice (range) consumed more than the pens fed green stuff at noon, and that a considerable portion of it was eaten the last thing before the birds went to roost. The feeding of green stuff after the grain feed at night has resulted in a great improvement in the number of eggs laid. Therefore, on small ranges and when weather conditions are not favorable, the flock is frequently turned out to pasture only for an hour or two each morning or evening. If the flocks are large or the areas small for cropping, poultrymen may keep the birds confined and bring the harvested material to the birds each day.

The amounts of green food that the hens will consume each day varies considerably. One hundred healthy hens will often consume 12 to 15 pounds of green food each day if they have green food in ample supply continually. Also certain kinds are relished and eaten in larger quantities.

There is a question concerning the amounts of green food that are necessary or desirable. There is the possibility that we might, under some conditions, furnish too much green food. That is true because we are furnishing a bulky feed containing 90 per cent or more of water and very small amounts of actual nutrients. Therefore, if we fill up the birds on this bulky feed, it is impossible for them to consume sufficient amounts of grain and mash in order to get enough of the nutrients to give maximum production. The New York Experiment Station[85] concluded that not more than one-third of the total ration can consist of coarse feeds, supplying about 10 per cent of the dry matter, without unprofitably diminishing production. For simple maintenance, much larger proportions can be used. From Finland[86] it has been reported that poultry cannot utilize more than 5.5 to 7 per cent of its annual food from pasture. Halnan[87] indicated limits of food saving for grass as 5 to 10 per cent for fowls, 16 per cent for turkeys, 18 per cent for ducks, and 100 per cent for geese.

Just what the optimum amount of green food is remains to be found out for different rations and different conditions. Favorable results have been obtained where approximately 15 per cent of the total feed was made up of green food. Probably not more than 4 to 6 pounds of fresh green food should be fed a day to one hundred hens.

Where legume hay was used from November to May, the Ohio Station[88] reports a consumption of 6 pounds per bird for that period. The Washington Station[89] indicates that where alfalfa hay, chopped into 1-inch lengths, was kept before the birds at all times they consumed 8 pounds per bird per year. Where succulent green feeds are used, it will require 12 to 15 pounds a year for each hen.

The amount of land necessary to grow the green food crops will depend upon the amount to be fed and the system of feeding.

RECOMMENDATIONS FOR PRACTICE

Some green food or its equivalent should be provided in the ration. Where a good range is available during the spring and early summer, the birds will get all they will need by pasturing. Particular attention, however, needs to be taken during the summer and fall when the grass begins to dry up. That is the time of year when green food is neglected even more than during the winter time. Under those conditions, the birds are outdoors, getting sunshine and exercise, but very little, if any, green food. At that time of the year, fresh-cut clover or alfalfa, rape, or any other green stuff can be fed, or the ration should be changed to supply the equivalent nutrients.

The use of dry products instead of the succulent forms is practised more extensively. This is usually done by feeding clover and alfalfa leaves or chopped green alfalfa hay in wire baskets or containers. Or alfalfa meal is added to the mash.

Since the green foods have an influence on the yolk color, the amounts fed must be limited where the market demand is for pale-yolked eggs. On this account, as well as its effect on palatability, alfalfa meal should be limited to 5 to 10 per cent of the mash. Where milk, yellow corn, some alfalfa hay or meal, cod liver oil, some animal protein, and a combination of the ordinary cereals are used in the ration, it is doubtful whether it is necessary to supply fresh green food, except when it is desired for its physiological effect or to keep the birds active to prevent picking.

When the fresh green foods are used, they are usually fed at noon in such amounts as the birds will eat before night. About 4 to 6 pounds per 100 hens a day are sufficient. When hay is fed, it is kept before the birds at all times in appropriate containers.

REFERENCES

1. Elvehjem, C. A., and H. A. Sober. The nutritional significance of grass. Chromica Botan. 7:301. 1943.
2. Kohler, G. O., and W. R. Graham, Jr. A chick growth factor found in leafy green vegetation. Poultry Sci. 30:484. 1951.
   Hansen, R. G., H. M. Scott, B. L. Larson, T. S. Nelson, and P. Krichevsky. Growth stimulation and growth inhibition of chicks fed forage and forage juice concentrate. Jour. Nutr. 49:453. 1953.
3. Stewart, J. H., and H. Atwood. Poultry experiments. West Va. Bul. 71. 1900.
   Smith, A. C. Value of green feeds in egg production. Rept. Northwest Experiment Sta., Crookston, Minn. 1924:73.
   Kennard, D. C., and R. M. Bethke. Solving the green feed problem. Ohio Bimo. Bul. 12(4). 1927.
4. Legume hay for chickens. Ohio Bul. 402:93. 1926.
5. Schermerhorn, L. G. Green feed for poultry. N. J. Hints 14(7). 1926.
6. Todd, A. C., and B. J. McSpadden. Pastures for chickens and their relation to the parasitic fauna. Poultry Sci. 26:576. 1947.
   Todd, A. C. Pastures for chickens and the parasite fauna. Poultry Sci. 26:646. 1948.
7. Robinson, D. H. Some grass mixtures for poultry purposes. Rept. Fourth International Grassland Congress. 1937.
8. Margolf, P. H., and J. K. Thornton. Turkeys prefer ladino clover but also relish other grasses in pasture tests. Supplement No. 1 to Bul. 488: 8. Pa. 60th Annual Rept. 1948.
   Margolf, P. H., and J. K. Thornton. Turkeys prefer ladino clover but also relish other grasses in pasture tests. World's Poultry Sci. Jour. 3:237. 1947.
9. Crampton, E. W., and R. Forshaw. Pasture Studies. XVI. The nutritive values of Kentucky bluegrass, red top, and brome grass. Jour. Nut. 19:161. 1940.
10. Thomas, J. O. Report of experiments on the feeding of poultry with high, medium, and low protein rations. Welsh Jour. Agr. 13:272. 1937.
11. Gutteridge, H. S., J. B. O'Neil, and J. M. Pratt. Level and so rce of protein in poultry production. I. As related to economical production of growth in pullets. Sci. Agr. 24:164. 1943.
12. Weinmiller, L. Untersuchungen über den Futterwert der Hühnerweide. Rept. Sixth World's Poultry Congress. 363. Germany. 1936.
    Temperton, H., and F. J. Dudley. The control of mash consumption during rearing. Harper Adams Utility Poultry Jour. 26:33. 1941.
    Skoglund, W. C., and J. M. Watkins. Range for chicks. Del. Bul. 238:13. 1942.
    Parker, J. E., and B. J. McSpadden. Pastures for developing pullets and for laying hens. Poultry Sci. 21:475. 1942.
    Davidson, J. A., H. C. Rather, and G. C. Card. Conservation of feedstuffs through turning pullets on pasture. Mich. Quart. Bul. 25(4):324. 1943.

Vondell, J. H. Range utilization by growing chickens. U. S. Egg and Poultry Mag. 49:464. 1943.

Vondell, J. H. Save feed—use the range. Featheredfax. (Mass.) May 10, 1943.

Hoffman, E., and C. E. Phillips. Evaluating ranges for poultry. Del. Rept. 1943:14.

Stephenson, A. B., and R. L. Bryant. The value of a sod range for starting chicks, growing pullets, and laying hens. Va. Bul. 362. 1944.

Parker, J. E., and B. J. McSpadden. Pastures for growing pullets. Tenn. Bul. 188. 1944.

Hoffman, E. Poultry pasture. Delaware Bul. 254. 1945.

Henderson, D. C., H. C. Whelden, Jr., and G. M. Wood. Range and confinement rearing of poultry. Vermont Bul. 568. 1953.

13. Temperton, H., and F. J. Dudley. Feeding grass to growing stock. Harper Adams Utility Poultry Jour. 28:3. 1943.

Pihkala, K. V. Grazing experiments with poultry. Abstract in Herbage Abstracts IV:292. 1934.

Darrow, M. I., and C. L. Morgan. Large vs. small type turkeys. S. C. Bul. 350. 1944.

14. Kennard, D. C., and V. D. Chamberlin. Making the most from pasturage for chickens. Ohio Bimo. Bul. 27:59. 1942.

Kennard, D. C., and V. D. Chamberlin. Good pasturage saves feed and expense for poultry raisers. Ohio Bimo. Bul. 228:183. 1944.

Kennard, D. C., and V. D. Chamberlin. Good range and pasturage pays well in growth of chickens. Ohio Bimo. Bul. 233:76. 1945.

Platt, C. S. Maturing pullets on grass range with exclusive diet of laying mash or grain with oyster shell. Poultry Sci. 23:554. 1944.

Platt, C. S. Maturing pullets on grass range with diets of laying mash or grain with oystershell. Poultry Sci. 24:168. 1945.

Kennard, D. C., and V. D. Chamberlin. A new ration for growing chickens on range and pasturage. Ohio Bimo. Bul. 240:57. 1946.

Kennard, D. C., L. E. Thatcher, and V. D. Chamberlin. Feeding for growth of chickens on pasturage. Ohio Bimo. Bul. 244:22. 1947.

Kennard, D. C., L. E. Thatcher, and V. D. Chamberlin. Ladino clover reduces feed costs for growing chickens. Ohio Agr. Exp. Sta. Bimo. Bul. 246:112. 1947.

Kennard, D. C., L. E. Thatcher, and V. D. Chamberlin. Bare lot, confinement, or legume range for growing chickens. Ohio Farm and Home Research 33 (251):64. 1948.

15. Tomhave, A. E. Protein levels of rations for White Leghorn pullets. Del. Bul. 219:42. 1939.

Gish, C. L., and L. F. Payne. The importance of herbage in poultry management. Poultry Sci. 19:35. 1940.

Gish, C. L., L. F. Payne, and W. J. Peterson. The effect of grass silage on color of egg yolk. Poultry Sci. 19:154. 1940.

Skoglund, W. C., and J. M. Watkins. Range for chicks. Del. Bul. 238:13. 1942.

Payne, L. F., and C. L. Gish. Grass and alfalfa as silage, forage, and meal for poultry. Kans. Bul. 320. 1943.

Stephenson, A. B., and R. L. Bryant. The value of a sod range for starting chicks, growing pullets, and laying hens. Va. Bul. 362. 1944.

Winter, A. R., and K. F. Schlamb. Influence of range versus confinement rearing on growth, feed consumption, egg production, and livability. Poultry Sci. 27:571. 1948.

16. Heuser, G. F., L. C. Norris, and J. H. Bruckner. Pasture experiments with growing pullets. Cornell Bul. 823. 1945.

17. Weinmiller, L. Untersuchungen über den Futterwert der Hühnerweide. Rept. Sixth World's Poultry Congress. 363. Germany. 1936.

18. Berry, L. N. Ranges for the laying flock. N. Mex. Bul. 255. 1938.

19. Buckner, G. D., W. M. Insko, Jr., and A. Harms. Nutritional and economic values of a bluegrass pasture for laying hens. Poultry Sci. 21:466. 1942.

Buckner, G. D., W. M. Insko, Jr., and A. Harms. Spring bluegrass vs. mature bluegrass as pasturage for laying hens. Poultry Sci. 22:248. 1943.

Buckner, G. D., W. M. Insko, Jr., and A. Harms. Influences of spring bluegrass and mature bluegrass pastures on laying hens and on the eggs produced. Poultry Sci. 24:446. 1945.

Kentucky Agricultural Experiment Station. Succulent pasture and bluegrass silage for laying hens. 59th Ann. Rept.:20. 1946.

Kentucky Agricultural Experiment Station. Ladino clover and bluegrass pastures in summer for laying hens. 60th Ann. Rept.:19. 1947.

20. Temperton, H., and F. J. Dudley. Feeding grass to laying pullets. Harper Adams Utility Poultry Jour. 28:7. 1943.

21. Mehrhof, N. R., and G. B. Killinger. Grazing experiments with poultry. Florida Ann. Rept. 1947: 59.

Parker, J. E., and B. J. McSpadden. Pastures for developing pullets and for laying hens. Poultry Sci. 21:475. 1942.

Parker, J. E., and B. J. McSpadden. Pasture studies with laying hens. Tenn. Bul. 185. 1943.

Sipe, G. R., and H. D. Polk. Japanese tendergreen mustard, Italian rye grass and oats as a source of green feed for laying hens. Poultry Sci. 20:406. 1941.

Sturkie, D. G., and J. C. Grimes. Kudzu—its value and use in Alabama. Ala. Circ. 83. 1939.

22. Ringrose, R. C., and C. L. Morgan. A study of the effect of green feed upon interior egg quality. Poultry Sci. 18:125. 1939.

Denton, C. A., and H. W. Titus. Effect of fresh cereal grass on interior quality of eggs. Poultry Sci. 20:188. 1941.

23. Nalbandov, A. V., and L. E. Card. The problem of blood and meat spots in chicken eggs. II. Its importance in poultry flocks and a study of the nutritional factors involved. Poultry Sci. 26:400. 1947.

24. Serfontein, P. J. Cowpeas as a poultry feed. Farming in South Africa, Oct., 1944.

Johnson, W., and Regina Forge. Soybeans as green fodder for poultry. Agric. Gaz. N. W. Wales 60:663. 1949.

25. Goodman, J. G. Green crops as a partial substitute for laying mash. Poultry Sci. 27:665. 1948.
King, D. F. Green feed as a substitute for laying mash for hens. Alabama Progress Rept. Series No. 30. Jan. 1947.
26. Temperton, H., and F. J. Dudley. Feeding marrow stem kale to laying pullets. Harper Adams Utility Poultry Jour. 27:213. 1942.
27. Heuser, G. F. Feeding for egg production. Cornell Bul. 222(Rev.): 25. 1937.
28. Bartlett, J. M. The chemical composition of green sprouted oats. Maine Bul. 266. 1917.
29. Weinmiller, L., and Dr. Mantel. Keimgetreide als Geflügelfutter. Archiv für Geflügelk. 11:356. 1937.
30. Carrick, C. W. Feeding of germinated oats to Leghorn pullets. Poultry Sci. Proc. 1930:91.
31. Tomhave, A. E., and C. W. Mumford. Germinated oats for laying birds. Del. Bul. 179:25. 1932.
Tomhave, A. E., and C. W. Mumford. Germinated oats for laying birds. Del. Bul. 192:24. 1935.
Tomhave, A. E., and C. W. Mumford. Germinated oats for laying pullets. Del. Bul. 205:23. 1936.
Tomhave, A. E., and C. W. Mumford. The value of germinated oats in the laying rations for pullets and breeding hens. Del. Bul. 207: 25. 1937.
32. Mocenni, M. Influenza dell' uso alimentare di embrioni di grano sulla produzione delle galline ovaiole. Rivista di Avicultura 7:2. 1937.
33. Atwood, H. Effect of confinement and green feed on number and hatchability of eggs. W. Va. Bul. 178. 1922.
Die Fütterung von Silage nach dem jetzigen Stand der Erfahrungen. Kalender für Geflügelwirtschaft. June 25, 1933.
Tscherniak, A. Mineral-säuresilage als Geflügelfutter. Archiv für Geflügelk. 9:255. 1935.
Fangauf, R., and A. Haensel. Der Wert von Silage und von frischen Grünfuttergaben bei Hühnern wird überschätzt. Archiv für Geflügelk. 12:265. 1938.
Carbone, E. Silage feeding to laying hens. Rept. Seventh World's Poultry Congress. 202. Cleveland. 1939.
Kentucky Agricultural Experiment Station. Succulent pasture and bluegrass silage for laying hens. 59th Ann. Rept:20. 1946.
Muller, W. Verfütterung von Keimgetreide und Silage an Hühner. Archiv für Geflügelk. 17:16. 1953.
34. Allen, P. W., M. Jacob, N. O. Sjolander, J. A. McBee, and I. H. Smiley. Legume silage as a feed for poultry. Poultry Sci. 18:399. 1939.
Allen, P. W., M. Jacob, N. O. Sjolander, and J. A. McBee. Legume silage as a poultry feed. Tenn. Bul. 172. 1940.
35. What is the value of lawn clippings silage in poultry feeding? N. J. Rept. 1941-1942:30.
Taylor, M. W., W. C. Russell, and C. S. Platt. The value of grass clippings silage for the growing chick. Poultry Sci. 23:213. 1944.

36. Temperton, H., and F. J. Dudley. The feeding of grass silage to laying pullets. Harper Adams Utility Poultry Jour. 27:248. 1942.
37. Clark, T. B., A. H. VanLandingham, and C. E. Weakly, Jr. Young grass-legume silage in the poultry ration. West Va. Bul. 340. 1949.
38. Wells, J. G., Jr., and J. A. Davidson. A comparison of carrots, "Greenmelk," and dehydrated alfalfa leaf meal in the laying ration. Mich. Quart. Bul. 22:199. 1940.
39. Strahan, R. J. Construction and management of root storage cellars. Cornell Ext. Bul. 22. 1917.
40. Cassel, L. W. The value of various proteins and combinations of them for laying pullets. Wash. Bul. 237:42. 1929.
Kennard, D. C., and G. Lingle. Feeding legume hay to chickens. Ohio Bimo. Bul. 13(1). 1928.
Shoup, Mr., and Mrs. G. R. Green feed trials on pullets, 1926-1927. W. Wash. Bul. 10W:24. 1928.
41. Bartlett, S., K. M. Henry, S. K. Kon, L. W. Osborne, S. Y. Thompson, and J. Tinsley. The effect of different methods of drying on the biological value and digestibility of the proteins and on the carotene content of grass. Biochem. Jour. 32:2024. 1938.
Fagan, T. W., and W. M. Ashton. The effect of partial field-drying and artificial drying on the chemical composition of grass. Welsh Jour. Agr. 14:160. 1938.
Smjetnieff, S. J. Artificial drying of grasses of various kinds. Trans. All-Union Inst. Poultry Ind. (Moscow)3(2). 1938.
42. Wilgus, H. S., Jr., L. C. Norris, and G. F. Heuser. The relative vitamin G content of alfalfa meal. Poultry Sci. 15:446. 1936.
43. Stevenson, G. L. Alfalfa for poultry. S. Dak. Rept. 1927:29.
Stevenson, G. L. Alfalfa for poultry. S. Dak. Rept. 1928:28.
44. Berry, L. N. The efficiency of alfalfa leaf meal and alfalfa meal as substitutes for green feed in rations for laying hens. N. Mex. Bul. 203:11. 1932.
45. Heywang, B. W. Alfalfa products as green feed substitutes for layers. Poultry Sci. 12:167. 1933.
46. Halpin, J. G., and C. E. Holmes. Alfalfa meal in winter laying ration increases egg production. Wis. Bul. 438:53. 1937.
Cravens, W. W., J. G. Halpin, S. B. Randle, and C. A. Elvehjem. Hens need vitamin K. Wis. Bul. 451:34. 1941.
Cravens, W. W., and C. E. Holmes. The effect of alfalfa leaf meal and dried cereal grass on hatchability and egg production. Poultry Sci. 20:458. 1941.
Cravens, W. W., and J. G. Halpin. Alfalfa has advantages over dried cereal grass. Wis. Bul. 455:15. 1942.
47. Ackerson, C. W., M. J. Blish, and F. E. Mussehl. The utilization of food elements by growing chicks. VIII. A comparison of alfalfa meal and artificially dried Sudan grass meal in rations for growing chicks. Neb. Bul. 116. 1939.
48. Skoglund, W. C., and A. E. Tomhave. Dehydrated ground clovers and perennial grasses vs. sun-cured alfalfa meal in broiler rations. Del. Circ. 13. 1942.

49. Serfontein, P. J. Cowpea-hay meal in chicken rations. Farming in S. Africa 18:295. 1943.

50. Buckner, G. D., W. M. Insko, Jr., J. H. Martin, and A. Harms. Kentucky bluegrass in all-mash rations. Poultry Sci. 16:426. 1937.

Buckner, G. D., W. M. Insko, Jr., J. H. Martin, and A. Harms. The value of leaf meals of alfalfa, Korean lespedeza and lespedeza sericea in all-mash chick rations. Ky. Circ. 48. 1937.

51. Polk, H. D., and M. Gieger. Kudzu in the ration for growing chicks. Miss. Farm Res. Bul. 414. March 1945.

52. Kohlmeyer, William, A. L. Moxon, and D. G. Jones. The effects of substituting certain dehydrated grass meals for alfalfa meal in chick starting rations and in chicken and turkey breeding rations. Poultry Sci. 26:546. 1947.

53. Culton, T. G., J. R. Smyth, and B. E. Plummer, Jr. Dehydrated ladino clover as a substitute for alfalfa meal in chick starter diets. Maine Bul. 449:438. 1947.

54. Squibb, R. L., and M. K. Wyld. Further studies on the value of desmodium meal in the baby chick diet. Poultry Sci. 29:586. 1950.

Squibb, R. L., A. Falla, J. A. Fuentes, and H. T. Love. Value of desmodium, pigeon pea fodder, and Guatemalan and United States alfalfa meals in rations for baby chicks. Poultry Sci. 29:482. 1950.

Squibb, R. L., M. Guzman, and N. S. Scrimshaw. Dehydrated desmodium, kikuyu grass, ranie, and banana leaf meal forages as supplements of protein, riboflavin, and carotinoids in chick rations. Poultry Sci. 32:1078. 1953.

55. Sokoloff, B., J. B. Redd, and Raymond Dutcher. Nutritive value of mangrove leaves (Rhizophora mangle L.) Quart. Jour. Florida Acad. Sci. 12:191. 1949.

56. Davis, G. K., N. R. Mehrhof, C. L. Comar, L. Singer, and K. Boney. Ramie meal—a new feed. Florida Exp. Sta. Ann Rept. 1947: 63.

57. Quisenberry, H. J., and C. I. Draper. Koa haole leaf meal as alfalfa meal substitute. Hawaii Biennial Report 1944-1946.

Palafox, A. L. The use of fresh green koa haole leaves in chick rations. Poultry Sci. 27:558. 1948.

58. Rosenberg, M. M., and A. L. Palafox. The effect of creeping indigo (Indigofera endecaphylla) when fed to growing chickens. World's Poultry Sci. Jour. 6:284. 1950.

Rosenberg, M. M., and A. L. Palafox. The effect of creeping indigo (Indigofera endecaphylla) on laying chickens. World's Poultry Sci. Jour. 7:9. 1951.

59. Kelley, E. G., M. E. Wall, and J. J. Willaman. Vegetable wastes as animal feedstuffs. Feedstuffs 15(26):18. 1943.

Tomhave, A. E., E. Hoffman, E. G. Kelly, M. E. Wall, and D. A. Colker. A preliminary investigation on the use of certain dried vegetable wastes as poultry feeds. Del. Bul. 247. 1944.

Willaman, J. J., R. K. Eskew, R. H. Morris, 3rd, E. G. Kelley, D. A. Colker, N. C. Aceto, M. E. Wall, A. E. Tomhave, and E.

Hoffman. Preparation and use of leaf meals from vegetable wastes. U. S. Dept. Agric. Tech. Bul. 958. 1948.

Skoglund, W. C., A. E. Tomhave, and A. F. Kish. Dehydrated vegetable wastes in poultry feeds. Delaware Bul. 271:11. 1948.

Runnels, T. D., E. F. Waller, E. G. Kelley, and S. Krulick. Growth promotion and pigmentation properties of dehydrated broccoli leaf meal in a practical broiler diet. Poultry Sci. 30:930. 1951.

60. Halpin, J. G., W. W. Cravens, and W. H. McGibbon. Cannery refuse may be used in poultry rations. Wisc. Bul. 472:54. 1947.

61. Lillie, R. J., and G. M. Briggs. A preliminary investigation on the use of semi-solid vegetable wastes in poultry rations. Poultry Sci. 27:7. 1948.

62. Bird, H. R. Dehydrated pea vines and starfish meal in poultry feeds. Poultry Sci. 23:76. 1944.

63. Driggers, J. C., R. A. Dennison, G. K. Davis, and N. R. Mehrhof. Bean vine meal in chick rations. Fla. Cir. S-30. 1951.

64. Davis, G. K., N. R. Mehrhof, J. C. Driggers, and R. A. Dennison. Dehydrated celery tops in chick rations. Fla. Cir. S-37. 1951.

65. Miller, V. L., G. E. Bearse, and L. R. Berg. Ground dehydrated flat pea forage as a protein supplement for chicks. Poultry Sci. 27:282. 1948.

66. Atwood, H. Effect of confinement and green feed on number and hatchability of eggs. W. Va. Bul. 178. 1922.

67. Robertson, E. I., M. Brin, and L. C. Norris. The use of dehydrated beet leaves in chick rations. Poultry Sci. 26:582. 1947.

Wilgus, H. S., H. P. H. Johnson, A. L. Esplin, and P. B. Smith. Beet leaves for poultry. Colo. Sci. Series Paper. 289.

68. Brown, W. L. Some effects of pimiento pepper on poultry. Ga. Bul. 160. 1930.

Brown, W. L. The quantitative relation of egg yolk pigmentation to pimiento feeds. Ga. Bul. 183. 1934.

69. Mollo, A. Observations on the employment of nettles in chick feeding. Rept. Second World's Poultry Congress. 157. Spain. 1924.

Marracino, R. L'ortica nell' alimentazione dei polli. Quad. Nutrizone 3:480. 1936.

Marracino, R. L'ortica nell' alimentazione dei polli. Quad. Nutrizone 6:1. 1939.

70. Schneider, H. Feeding experiments with rhubarb leaves with rabbits, sheep, goats, and hens. Biedermanns Zentralblatt für Agrikulturchemie und rationellen Landwirtschaftsbetrieb. Abt. A64: 371. 1935.

71. Burgos, C. X., and M. Rufino. Studies on ipil-ipil leaf meal as a protein feed for chicks. Bur. An. Ind. (Philippines) Recorder 12 (No. 5):27. 1950.

Dingayan, A. B., and F. M. Frouda. A comparative study of the influence of the leaves and young shoots of centrosema, ipil-ipil, and sweet potato as green feed on the growth of chicks. Philippine Agric. 34:110. 1950.

72. Mangels, clover, and sprouted oats as green feed. Canada Exp. Farms (Kentville, N. S.) Rept. 1923:69.

73. Elford, F. C. The comparative value of grainless, gritless, and green-feed-lacking rations for egg production. Rept. Poultry Husbandman Dominion Exp. Farms (Canada) 1928:43.
74. Turnips vs. mangels vs. potatoes for green feed. Exp. Sta. Rept. (Fredericton, Canada, N. B.) 1929:54.
75. Stuart, H. O. Effect of certain green feed substitutes upon egg production and hatchability. Poultry Sci. 8:354. 1929.
76. Alfalfa hay chopped vs. leaf alfalfa meal for layers. Ohio Bul. 417: 72. 1927.
77. The effect of an inadequate ration on the production and hatchability of eggs. Kans. Rept. 1926-1928:103.
78. Lang, H. Green foods and their substitutes with regard to laying and breeding hens. Rept. Sixth World's Poultry Congress. 37. Germany. 1936.

Fangauf, R., and A. Haensel. Süsslupinenschrot als Hühnerfutter. Archiv für Geflügelk. 11:161. 1937.

79. Thompson, W. C. Report of the Department of Poultry Husbandry. N. J. Rept. 1929:281.
80. Smith, R. M., and S. R. Johnson. The effect of green feed supplement on chick growth. Poultry Sci. 20:473. 1941.
81. Miller, M. W. The value of succulence in poultry rations. Poultry Sci. 16:351. 1937.
82. Misner, E. G. Economic studies of poultry farming in New York. III. Department of Agricultural Economics, N. Y. State College of Agriculture. Stencil. September 1931.
83. Sanborn, W. Florida pasture and green feed for 100 hens. Fla. Bul. 21. 1919.

Kennard, D. C. A garden for chickens. Ohio Bimo. Bul. 13(2). 1928.

Thompson, R. B., and R. Penquite. Shade and green feed for chickens. Okla. Circ. 69. 1928.

Schoth, H. A. Green feed and pasture for poultry. Ore. Circ. 85. 1928.

Thayer, R. H. Planning a year-round poultry green feed program for Oklahoma. Okla. Circ. C 120. 1946.

84. Poultry farming. (Green stuff after the grain feed at night.) Dept. Agr. (Victoria, Australia) Bul. 54. 1924.
85. Wheeler, W. P. Feeding experiments with poultry. N. Y. (Geneva) Rept. 1928:24.
86. Pihkala, K. V. Grazing experiments with poultry. Laiduntamiskokeita Kanoilla. Suom. Laiduntalous 6:57. 1934.
87. Halnan, E. T. Poultry as converters of vegetable food for human use. Chem. and Ind. No. 12:189. 1948.
88. Kennard, D. C., and R. M. Bethke. Solving the green feed problem. Ohio Bimo. Bul. 12 (4) 1927.
89. Cassel, L. W. The value of various proteins and combinations of them for laying pullets. Wash. Bul. 237:42. 1929.

CHAPTER 9

FACTORS IN MAKING A POULTRY RATION

In formulating rations there are many factors which must be considered, and the final result must be the best balance of all these factors. The best results cannot be obtained unless the ration is complete. In order to make a ration complete, it must meet certain requirements. The results obtained will be in proportion to its completeness.

ESSENTIALS OF A RATION

PROTEIN. The ration must contain suitable protein, both as to amount that is present and as to its nature or quality. It is essential that a certain minimum amount be present in the ration. Quantities can be larger without actual harm to the bird, but large quantities are not economical since the protein feeds are relatively expensive.

The protein must also be of correct quality. The proteins of various feeds differ because all do not contain the same amino acids, or where they contain the same ones they are not present in the same proportions. It is these differences that account for variations in quality of proteins. Furthermore, some of these amino acids seem to be more important than others.

The requirement for protein varies for different purposes. The growing animal needs more than the mature bird. Also the egg producer requires more than the nonproducer. The growing chick needs more protein in early life, when it is growing rapidly, than it does later on when relative growth slows down.

With our increase in knowledge, the requirements of a ration will be considered from the standpoint of amino acids, rather than from the standpoint of the more complex proteins, because it is really the deficiency or lack of any one of them which will limit results. Sometimes an increase in the percentage of total protein has resulted in improvement, not because the animal needed more total protein but because, by increasing the total protein, the amount of a certain amino acid which was deficient in the smaller quantity was also increased. The same improvement could have been obtained without increasing total protein, but by making adjustments in feeds so as to bring the amount of that particular amino acid up to the necessary level. Until such time when we shall have more definite information on this subject, the safe practice is to use a reasonable variety of feeds in our rations, including animal protein feeds.

ENERGY. We must also supply an abundance of energy or fuel to keep the animal working properly, that is, to furnish energy to keep up body temperature and supply the body processes. This energy is often expressed as calories. It really is in part a matter of total food consumption. It is an important factor, since very often results in production, even with a balanced ration, are limited by a lack of food intake. The art of feeding consists in getting the birds to eat sufficient feed daily.

This energy is furnished usually in the form of carbohydrates and fat, which are considered the energy portion of feeds and are most economical for that purpose. Protein can be used for this purpose when fed in excess, but it is too expensive to use for energy. Besides furnishing energy, some of the fatty acids are also essential as such.

MINERALS. The ration must contain a suitable inorganic content. The practical poultryman must consider only the ones that might probably be deficient in his ration. When using a good ration, including natural feeding stuffs, the deficiencies are not many, being probably only sodium, chlorine, calcium, phosphorus, manganese, and iodine.

The sodium and chlorine are furnished by common salt. Calcium for eggshell formation is best supplied in the carbonate form. Oystershells and limestone will supply calcium. Where wheat by-products, meat scrap, and milk are used, there will usually be enough phosphorus. If phosphorus is determined to be necessary, bone meal or other phosphorus carriers are usually fed. Manganese is added as a manganese compound, and iodine as iodized salt.

Where minerals are necessary, they need to be added in only comparatively small quantities. It is possible to add too much of some. For instance, too much calcium will depress growth and increase mortality in chicks. Too much magnesium will upset the birds. An excess of fluorine is also detrimental. We also find in the body certain minerals balanced by others, so that excesses of any of them might so use up the others as to cause deficiencies that would not occur without such excesses.

Thus it is necessary to show judgment and precaution in respect to minerals as much as in handling other parts of the ration. The attitude of some persons, namely, that the addition of minerals will do no harm, even if they do no good, is not sound. Furthermore, the opinion sometimes encountered that if a small amount of minerals is good a large amount should be better is entirely unjustified.

VITAMINS. The ration must contain sufficient vitamins. The quantity of any of the different vitamins required by poultry varies with age and condition. Chicks and laying hens have a larger vitamin requirement than nonproducers. In this instance, however, molting hens should not be classified as nonproducers. Renewal of feathers should be classified as production, in the same way as growth and the laying of eggs, and it makes necessary the feeding of a liberal supply of vitamins.

WATER, AIR, LIGHT, AND SUNSHINE. The ration must contain an abundance of these factors.

Water. Very often the water supply is neglected. Water is just as essential as feed. It is probably more necessary to keep in mind the importance of water for poultry than for other animals because of the drinking habits of poultry. Poultry needs to have water available practically constantly, because it partakes of only small amounts at a time. The larger farm animals can be watered once or twice a day, at which time they can drink sufficient amounts to carry them through the rest of the day.

Water is necessary for all animals in order for them to carry on the various body activities. Water softens the food in digestion, aids in its assimilation, and is very important as a carrier in the distribution of the nutrients to the various parts of the body. It also functions in the various body secretions, and it helps to equalize body temperature.

Water makes up a large part of the body of the fowl itself. Probably around 55 to 60 per cent or more of the fowl's body is made up of water. The egg also has a very large water content; roughly about 65 per cent or two-thirds of the egg. A dozen eggs contain over a pint of water. Our ordinary feeds, such as grain and mash, which constitute the biggest part of the feed of the bird, are very low in water content, running usually somewhere around 10 to 15 per cent.

If water is not available, digestion and assimilation will be hindered. Secretions and excretions will be limited, the blood thickened, the body temperature raised, and finally death will result. An individual can live a longer period of time if only water, rather than food, is available. The body tissues will be drawn upon for a supply of energy. If water is restricted, death will occur comparatively rapidly. A decrease in the supply or a restriction of water to poultry will decrease egg production and finally stop it. Egg production can be stopped almost entirely in the course of 48 to 60 hours by taking away all water.

Water should be available at all times. The hen drinks little at a time, but very frequently. It is necessary to have water available whenever there is feed available. With our present system of dry mash feeding, this means whenever the birds are off the roost. This might prove to be a very important factor during freezing weather and where artificial illumination is used.

The amounts of water that are consumed by birds are influenced by several factors. More water is consumed during hot weather. When the birds are producing more heavily under the same conditions of temperature, there is a higher consumption of water.

As far as actual water consumption is concerned, the following figures might be of interest in showing the amounts consumed daily by one hundred Single Comb White Leghorns.

November	11 quarts	May	20 quarts
December	11	June	22
January	13	July	20
February	15	August	16
March	17	September	14
April	19	October	13

Frequently the question is asked concerning the necessary temperature of the water. It should not be too cold in winter or too warm in summer. The chill should be taken off in the winter because, if the water is too cold, it does not encourage the hens to consume what is necessary. Oregon[1] reports that pullets drank 25.4 per cent more warmed water than cold water during freezing weather. Results at Idaho[2] indicate that hens in pens receiving water warmed to 40 to 50° F. consumed 20 per cent more water and gave an egg production decidedly in favor of the pens receiving the warm water.

Fresh Air. Sufficient fresh air must be supplied to furnish the oxygen for combustion or burning the feed and to carry off harmful waste products. The amounts of oxygen that are necessary depend upon the amount of food that needs to be broken down and metabolized, the amount of work that the individual does, and to some extent upon the temperature of the environment. The rate of metabolism determines the amount of oxygen that is required. The problem of providing air in the poultry house is to remove moisture rather than to furnish enough oxygen.

Light and Sunshine. Light and sunshine are two of nature's beneficial factors. These factors are not only the ultraviolet rays supplying vitamin D but some of the other rays of sunshine as well, which are being shown to be necessary for the well-being of the animal.

PROPER MECHANICAL OR PHYSICAL CONDITION. This factor has a bearing upon food consumption. The capacity of the fowl for food is limited and must be used to the best advantage if high production is desired. It is necessary to obtain adequate food consumption, which will not be accomplished unless the ration is palatable. This factor must, therefore, be kept in mind, since it is possible to have feeds with correct analysis that are not consumed in sufficient quantities. Consequently, we should avoid, or at least greatly restrict the amount of, such feeds.

Palatability depends to some extent upon the mechanical condition of the feed. Such characteristics as hardness of kernel, size of particle, stickiness when mixed with water, and bulkiness must be considered. Fowls do not like a very hard kernel. The particles should not be too large. When mixed with water, the ration should be crumbly. Thus large amounts of sticky feeds should not be fed.

As regards bulk, the ration should be reasonably filling and yet be able to pass readily through the body. A certain amount of bulk is necessary, especially with a concentrated diet, to enable the digestive juices to act readily. Furthermore, Sheehy[3] concludes that a feed mixture which, in addition to being complete, contains the proper amount of bulk and fiber, that is, is satisfactory from the mechanical aspect, controls feather plucking. The retention, by feed, of much water in the alimentary tube and the appearance in the lower gut of bulky, semi-liquid material, rather than dry dense residues, give a feeling of satiety which inhibits the development of cannibalistic tendencies. The birds must have a feeling of being comfortably filled. The perverted appetites of birds are frequently an attempted corrective against concentrated rations. On the other hand, too much fiber should be avoided, as the fowls have to grind everything taken into the body even though they digest little, if any, of the fiber. The fiber should be kept as low as possible. It should not go much beyond 5 per cent for the whole ration. Hence too much oats, buckwheat, ground oats, wheat bran, alfalfa meal, and the like should not be fed. Too much fiber might cause constipation and inflammation of the digestive tract.

Shaw and Fisher[4] state that bulk or cubic content of a food is one of the first considerations in making a poultry ration meet feeding standards. Halnan[5] indicates the following:

> In trials with adult fowls it was found that the maximum amount of food they would eat as a mash was 290 cubic centimeters. The volumes of a certain number of foods were measured [Table 15] and variations from 33 c.c. to 185 c.c. per ounce were obtained according to the foods and their mechanical condition. Thus, one ounce of wheat measured 39 c.c. as grain and 50 c.c. as meal. One ounce of broad bran measured 185 c.c. dry and 140 c.c. wet.
>
> If it be assumed that the food capacity of an adult bird is 290 c.c. it would eat just over 2 ounces of wet bran daily, or 5.8 ounces of wheat meal. Any feeding standard based on a daily consumption of 4 ounces of food would, therefore, not work in practice if the volume of the food exceeded 73 c.c. per ounce. Actual cases of failure of egg production attributed to this cause have been brought to notice; the food was perfectly balanced and adequate for egg production on the assumption of a 4-ounce daily consumption, but failed because it was bulky, owing to the presence of excessive fiber, so that the bird was unable to consume the whole 4 ounces considered necessary. In constructing rations for any given purpose it is, therefore, essential to pay strict attention to the volume or bulkiness of the food.

Sheehy and Sheil[6] report that food consumption figures indicate an effort on the part of the group receiving a ration of low concentration to compensate for the comparative poverty of the ration by eating an excess of it, that the rate of growth increased progressively as the concentration of the mash was raised, and that the more concentrated mash conduced to greater egg production in the prewinter period. In an experiment conducted at Cornell in which three pens received the same ration, except that one contained 20 per cent of bran, another 20 per cent of standard wheat middlings, and the third 20 per cent of red dog flour, the average food consumed by the birds was in relation to the bulk of the ration. It required more grams of feed to produce an egg on the bran ration than on the middlings ration, which in turn required more feed than the red dog flour ration.

The ration must not be too coarse or too fine,[7,9] since texture will affect food consumption. In general, oats and barley should be fine ground, whereas corn and wheat should be ground coarse. Dusty feed is disliked. Medium to coarse rations have generally given better results than very fine or very coarse rations. More feed is wasted in the drinking water when birds are fed finely ground feed.

TABLE 15. WEIGHTS AND BULKINESS OF FEEDS*

Feed	Weight per Bushel, lb.	Bulkiness, cc. per oz.	
		Dry	Wet
Alfalfa meal	. .	75	. .
Barley			
Whole	48	43	. .
Meal	. .	48	. .
Blood meal	. .	33	. .
Buckwheat			
Whole	48	50	. .
Meal	. .	45	. .
Corn			
Whole	56	41	. .
Meal	48-50	49	. .
Dried buttermilk	. .	45	. .
Dari			
Whole	56	40	. .
Meal	. .	50	. .
Peanut meal	. .	46	. .
Fish meal	. .	43	. .
Gluten feed	. .	57	. .
Meat meal	. .	45	. .
Millet			
Whole	50	37	. .
Meal	. .	52	. .
Dried skimmilk	. .	48	. .
Oats			
Whole	32	53	. .
Fine-ground	. .	74	. .
Peas			
Whole	60	36	. .
Meal	. .	55	. .
Rye	56	. .	. .
Soybean meal	. .	52	. .
Wheat (hard)			
Whole	60	39	. .
Meal	. .	50	. .
Wheat (soft)			
Whole	60	40	. .
Meal	. .	47	. .
Wheat bran	20	185	140
Wheat middling (fine)	. .	52	50
Wheat middling (coarse)	. .	79	70

*Ministry of Agriculture and Fisheries, Great Britain, Bul.-7.

A condition called pressure necrosis[8,9] is attributed to the fine consistency of the ration fed. This condition is apparently due to a combination of factors. Birds closely confined in a brooder battery and fed finely ground food might eat the dry mash without taking sufficient drink to keep the mouth clean of adhering food material. The calcareous-like mass of accumulated food material in the mouth results in the pressure necrosis, causing the loss of either the upper or the lower mandible. The incidence of curled or deformed tongue[10] in turkeys was reported greater on fine mash than on coarse mash or pellets.

ABSENCE OF FACTORS HAVING UNFAVORABLE PHYSIOLOGICAL EFFECTS. It is necessary that nothing be present to cause the individual to function abnormally, since the best results can be obtained only when the individual approaches normality. It is entirely possible to meet all the conditions already stipulated and yet overcome their favorable influence by the presence of a toxic or poisonous substance.

Injury wrought by microorganisms in the alimentary tract would prevent the hen from making the best use of the feed. In fact, any condition of disease would to a greater or lesser degree cause pathological functioning.

We might also have such undesirable physiological effects as constipation or looseness of the bowels, caused by the inclusion of too much of certain ingredients in the ration. Some feeds, as oil meal, wheat bran, molasses, and dried whey, are laxative, whereas others, like cottonseed feed, are constipating.

FACTORS IN SELECTING THE RATION

Besides the essentials of a ration the following factors should be considered.

ADAPTABILITY. It is necessary to consider the purpose of the ration, that is, its adaptability for the purpose. The ration needs to be changed to meet the requirements of the particular purpose. Sometimes it means a change in the ration itself, that is, a change in the mixture or the ingredients of the ration. Sometimes it may mean a change in the method of feeding or the management of the birds. By adapting it to the purpose, we consider whether we are feeding for egg production, for growth, for fattening, for the handling of broody hens, the care of setting hens, or management of the birds during the molting period. It may mean the care of pullets for egg production under various conditions or at different times of the year, or it may mean the management of breeders. Furthermore, we might be concerned with the feeding of other kinds of poultry such as ducks, geese, turkeys, pigeons, or game birds. Each of these conditions or purposes has some specific or definite considerations that need to be met.

NUTRITIVE RATIO OR BALANCE. Another factor to be considered is the nutritive ratio or the balance of proteins to carbohydrates and fat. This factor is important because the protein is necessary to build up the parts that are nitrogenous and because the protein cannot be replaced by the carbohydrates and fat. The carbohydrates and fat can be replaced to some extent by the protein, in that protein can furnish energy.

We must keep in mind the fact that the hen usually will not produce an egg unless that egg can be complete. Therefore, the quantity of production will be limited by the part of the ration that is present in lowest proportions. For example, if wheat alone is fed, as far as the protein is concerned, the hen would be able to lay one egg every 3 days; as far as the lime is concerned, she could produce one egg every 12 days; and as far as the carbohydrates and fat are concerned, she could lay 3 eggs every day. Another comparison which brings balance out quite clearly is the rating of feeds in terms of potential yolks and whites which different feeds can form. This method was used by Quisenberry.[11] For example, he estimated that 100 pounds of corn would be capable of producing 255 yolks and 134 whites, because corn is a wide feed containing more carbohydrates and fat. If corn alone was fed, there could be used only enough of the yolk material to produce 134 eggs, since the protein is a limiting factor. The remainder would not be used for that purpose. It might be stored as body fat, but most of the excess would not be used. It would be wasted. On the other hand, in meat scrap there are enough carbohydrates and fat in 100 pounds to produce 106 yolks and enough protein to form 1100 whites. Thus most of the protein could not be used. Hence a balance is needed in order to get as nearly as we can a combination of feeds which will supply a sufficient quantity of these various nutrients in proper proportions, so that there will not be an excess of any part to be wasted.

What will be the probable results if an unbalanced ration is fed? The ration might be unbalanced in being too wide, containing too much of the carbohydrates and fats. If that is true, there will be failure to produce growth in young stock because we are limiting the muscle builder. At first, we would get a storage of fat, because some of the excess carbohydrates and fat would be stored in fatty tissue;, but this would not go on indefinitely, and some would be wasted. In mature birds egg laying would be retarded for lack of the protein to furnish the albumen or whites of the eggs. Again, we would probably get some storage of fat, but that also would probably be accompanied by a softness or flabbiness of the muscles of the birds. Such birds would be more subject to disease and internal hemorrhages.

On the other hand, we might have a ration that is too narrow, furnishing more protein. This is a more costly practice because of the higher price of the protein part of the ration. There would be incomplete digestion and probably indigestion of some kind. The kidneys and liver might be overtaxed because they would need to get rid of the excess nitrogen waste. Uric acid poisoning might develop under those conditions.

The question might be asked whether it is possible to overfeed a balanced ration. The answer to that is only one of opinion; but it is probable, if we have a proper mechanical condition of the ration, that the birds would not overfeed on a balanced ration.

DIETARY REQUIREMENTS. There must be a sufficient quantity of feed and a sufficient quantity of the different nutrients to furnish the necessary material for the production of the product. Dietary requirements are available for some of the nutrients. The National Research Council[12] has issued recommended nutrient allowances for poultry. These furnish a good guide for the calculation of rations. However, the final measure will be the results obtained in feeding the rations.

VARIETY. Variety in the ration stimulates the appetite and increases the consumption of food. Of the same or similar breeds or varieties of chickens, the large eaters are the best layers. The birds that consume the most food have more material to make eggs or meat and are likely to lay more or to grow more. In fact, there is a distinct relation between the amount of food consumed and the number of eggs laid, where birds of the same size and variety are compared.

Furthermore, until such time when we know the exact make-up of feeds in respect to all its different parts, and until we know more about the quantitative requirements of poultry, it will be a safer practice not to limit the poultry ration to a very few feeds.

It is desirable that the mash mixture contain five or more ingredients, one being a source of animal protein food. The grain mixture should contain at least two grains.

There is also the possibility that there are still unknown factors in poultry feeding which might be supplied by using a variety of feeds. On the other hand, it is not necessary to go to the other extreme and include fifteen to twenty-five ingredients in the poultry ration. Variety should be reasonable in amount, particularly since it usually can be provided without increasing the cost.

COST AND AVAILABILITY. Naturally the ration should be modified to fit the local market and farm conditions. Home-grown grains should be fed just so far as is economical. The particular value of each feed must be considered. For example, it is economy to use the feeds which give profitable results in feeding practice. The value of the feeds should also be computed on the amount of available nutrients, for it is the digestible part that is of use to the bird; it is the digestible portion that becomes available and is made into eggs or flesh. It must be borne in mind, however, that the feed in question may be rendered more or less valuable than indicated by its total digestible nutriment by such other factors as the nature of the feed, the quality of the nutrients, palatability, and fiber content.

FACTORS IN SELECTING FEEDS FOR A RATION

Composition or chemical analysis is not the only thing to be considered in selecting feeds. Other factors must be thought of when one is making a choice.

PALATABILITY. Palatability is an important factor because the birds must consume large amounts of feed. In general, we can say that the more feed the bird consumes, the greater will be the returns in production. This is true both for eggs and for growth. The birds soon learn to pick out the feeds that they like and to eat quantities of them. The factor of palatability varies sometimes with the same feed, depending upon its condition. For example, dry oats are not so palatable as germinated oats, sprouted oats, or even just soaked oats. The palatability of individual feeds necessarily has its effect upon the mixtures in which they are used. It is not impossible to use, in a mixture, feeds that are unpalatable, but it is not wise to include too large quantities of them in the mixture for fear it might affect the palatability of the mixture.

Palatability of a food is dependent on the effect of such food on the senses of smell, taste, touch, and sight. Chickens select feed by shape, size, color, and surface conditions of the feed.[13] Chickens do not have a keen sense of taste. Hence taste sense has little importance during the act of feeding. The hen can distinguish three tastes: sour, salty, and bitter. Wheat-form kernels of grain are preferred, and the larger kernels are usually eaten first. Color does not play an important part. In the case of grits one report has shown a marked preference for light-colored grit (grey, white) as compared with dark-colored ones (blue, green, brown, black).

There is a difference in the palatability of feeds.[14] In practically every case reported, wheat is eaten in the largest amounts and might easily be considered the most palatable feed for poultry. Next in order of palatability are corn, kafir, barley, oats, sunflower seeds, peas, and rye. Rough rice also is very palatable. Buckwheat is not eaten readily. In testing the liking of chicks for certain seeds, Newbiggin and Linton[15] conclude that color, size, dullness or shininess, and chemical composition have no influence upon choice. The grains eaten in largest quantities were those offered in their natural state, that is, neither decorticated nor kibbled. They conclude, therefore, that "natural" foods may be selected in preference to "treated" foods. Hens also seem to prefer the softer kernels of grain.

Of the ground feeds, corn meal is eaten in largest amounts. Wheat standard middlings and wheat bran are next in order. The meat products and milk usually rate good. The flaked buttermilk is eaten more readily than the powdered.[16] Semi-solid buttermilk is usually well liked. Red dog flour, flour middlings, oil meal, blood meal, ground oats, and alfalfa meal are not so palatable. Unpalatable feeds decrease food consumption of a mixture in which they are used unless the amounts used are small and are balanced by the great palatability of such feed as corn meal. Palatability of ground feeds seems to be closely linked with their physical condition. Feeds that are sticky, bulky, or fibrous are not liked. Granular feeds are attractive.

DIGESTIBILITY. Another factor to keep in mind is the digestibility of the feeds. Naturally this factor is important because the digestible part of the feed is the valuable part, the part the bird utilizes in metabolism. Digestibility, to some extent, is associated with palatability. Palatability probably stimulates the secretions of digestive juices (for example, when foods are palatable to man, we say that our mouths water).

Feeds that are low in fiber and high in protein and nitrogen-free extract are usually highly digestible. The reverse would also be true, that the ones high in fiber and low in protein are less digestible. The nutrients of succulent feeds are probably a little more digestible than those in a nonsucculent condition.

The addition of salt to the ration does not affect the digestibility of the feeds. The addition of salt might increase the quantity of feed that is eaten. In that way, we might make available to the birds a larger amount of nutrients by a greater feed consumption.

The grinding of the feed may or may not increase digestibility. It is thought that grinding of the feeds for poultry slightly decreases digestibility. If feed is furnished in the whole form, such as grain, the hen has to grind the feed so that it stays in the digestive tract for a longer period and the digestive juices have more time to act. The amount of feed actually digested probably depends upon the amount of digestive juices, as well as the length of time the feed is exposed to the digestive process. In feeds that are passed rapidly through the digestive tract we find low digestibility. This seems to be true when comparing corn meal with cracked corn. The low digestibility of such feed as wheat middlings, which is slightly laxative, compared with other feeds of similar composition, is probably due to rapid passage through the digestive tract. Any feeds that stay longer in the digestive tract probably have a larger proportion digested.

In general, we might say that cooking feeds lowers the digestibility of protein, but increases the digestibility of starch. As far as we know, the age of the individual or the breed does not affect the actual digestibility of the feed. This is also true of the frequency of feeding or the amount of feed that is given.

Assuming that we do not have factors entering in that will cause a more rapid passage of the feed through the digestive tract, digestibility is affected by environmental and external conditions. The flow of the digestive juices is very readily checked by fright and other disturbances.

As a general rule, we can say that the most palatable feeds are also the most digestible, probably because a favorable and vigorous activity is promoted in the digestive tract.

WHOLESOMENESS. Another factor to be considered is the wholesomeness or quality of feeds. In poultry feeding, this quality is quite important. The hen has a very dull taste perception. Very little saliva is secreted, and taste organs are not present to the extent that they are in other farm animals. That means that it is quite possible to get substances not entirely wholesome into the body of the hen. One of the first indications that this is happening is loss of appetite and diarrhea. Besides, we have certain other specific conditions. In the case of moldy feed or litter, we frequently get infection from the aspergillus mold, causing aspergillosis. Very often when we have that condition, we say that the birds are going light. Where birds have access to putrid meat, we might have cases of limber neck or ptomaine poisoning. We must be sure, therefore, that both the feed and the litter are of good quality. It does not pay in poultry feeding to take a chance on either one of them.

EFFECT ON THE QUALITY OF THE PRODUCT. The quality of the product might be affected by the feed. Some feeds do have an effect upon the color, flavor, odor, and other characteristics.

Effect on Color. The origin of the coloring matter in the yolk of the egg and the body of the fowl is the food of the hen.[17] The bulk of the coloring matter in hens' egg yolk is xanthophyll. Xanthophyll is the general term used to describe carotenoids of the formula $C_{40}H_{56}O_2$. The hen has the ability to store xanthophylls but practically no carotene, the cow assimilates carotene but practically no xanthophyll. Chicks raised on rations almost devoid of carotenoids produced hens normal in all respects, except for the lack of yellow color. The yolks of the eggs produced were devoid of pigment. The effect of feeds depends upon the amount of coloring matter present.

Effect on Body Color. In one trial,[18] where white corn meal was substituted for the yellow and no green food was fed, the yellow pigment gradually faded from the shanks, beak, and skin and at the end of 6 weeks the yellow pigment was left only in the toes. Heiman and Tighe[19] reported that increasing the pigment intake of chicks resulted in the proportional increase in the concentration of the pigment in the shanks, that the pigment accumulated in the shanks in an essentially linear proportion in relation to time, and that, where the pigment was withdrawn from the ration, there was a steady loss of pigment from the shanks until they were practically colorless.

Certain common poultry feeding stuffs, such as meat scraps, fish meal, fish oil, and soybean oil meal, contain a factor, or factors, which inhibit the deposition of yellow pigment[20] in the shanks of growing chicks. Bird further showed that with mashes designed to produce rapid pigmentation, a 10-day period was sufficient to change the shanks of Barred Rock X New Hampshire crossbred chicks from cream color to a deep yellow.

Effect on Yolk Color. The yolks of eggs are particularly affected by the coloring matter of the feed.[21] However, Bohren, Thompson, and Carrick[22] have shown that the yolk might obtain small but persistent amounts of pigment from some other source, probably from body tissues. Green feed and yellow corn are rich in xanthophyll and produce highly colored egg yolks; red corn and hemp seed produce slightly colored yolks; wheat, wheat bran, oats, barley, cottonseed meal, rape seed, meat scrap, and blood meal have little effect on the color of the yolk. Large quantities of the coloring matter found in egg yolk are found in grass and also nearly all kinds of yellow flowers.[23]

The feeding of ground, dried, ripe, pimiento peppers[24] produced eggs that were orange colored, as compared with light lemon-yellow eggs for the control pen. Rations containing pimientos also imparted a rich yellow color to the shanks, skin, and fat, the amount of color depending upon the amount of pimiento fed. Experiments carried out in Hungary[25] proved that the feeding of paprika caused a much darker color in the yolk, the color being four times deeper than at first, within 3 weeks' time.

In a study of seasonal variations in yolk color, Parker concludes that the most important factor in yolk color is the amount of greens actually eaten by the birds.[26] Birds having an unlimited supply of green feed produced eggs with dark-colored yolks. Kale at the rate of 5 pounds per 100 birds a day or alfalfa leaves to the amount of 5 per cent of the mash gave yolks of a desirable color.

Because alfalfa meal is known to be a valuable ingredient in poultry rations, levels that are too high have sometimes been used. There is a close association between the amount of alfalfa fed and the depth of yolk color. However, no unfavorable reactions are experienced where approximately 5 per cent of alfalfa meal is used in the mash.

Carver and Heiman[26] found that Argentine corn (flint) produced eggs with deeper-colored yolks than domestic corn (dent). The groups fed higher proportions of pigment-bearing foods produced eggs with deeper-colored yolks, but the amount of pigmentation deposited in the egg yolks was not proportionate to the amount of pigment in the ration. The color changes induced by the rations fed began to take effect after the fourth or fifth day of feeding. It took about 13 days to reach maximum pigmentation. When pigmented foods were withdrawn, it required about 26 days for the pigmentation to become stabilized. An index of 12 – 13 is satisfactory. This index will be produced by 20–30 per cent of Argentine corn, 8 per cent of dehydrated alfalfa, or 4 per cent of dehydrated alfalfa plus 10 per cent of Argentine corn.

Frequently discoloration of new-laid eggs is reported, due to the consumption of certain materials. Olive-colored egg yolks[27] are reported to be produced by shepherd's purse and penny cress, weeds belonging to the mustard family. Thompson of the Oklahoma Station has also reported the development of eggs with orange-colored yolks from a ration containing 12 per cent of kafir smut. The feeding of cottonseed meal frequently causes the appearance of cottonseed spots on the yolks of the eggs or olive yolks.[28] (See also Chap. 7.)

Olsen[29] reported production of eggs with olive-colored yolks from diets containing whole acorns, ground acorns, ground acorn meats, or ground acorn hulls. Temperton[27] reports the production of eggs with greenish-brown yolks only when the acorns were germinated.

Peterson[30] and coworkers found that hens fed an all-mash ration containing 10 per cent of lobster shell produced highly colored orange-red yolks, which they attributed to the effect of the tetraoxycarotenoid astacin present in lobster shells.

It is possible to color artificially the yolks of eggs and body fat by means of dyes.[31] Rogers reports that fowls fed Sudan III produce eggs with yolks of a bright red color. The forming of the coloring matter in the yolk takes place in the shape of concentric rings or layers. Rhodamine Red colors the yolk slightly. Auramine Yellow and Saffranine Red act in much the same way as the Rhodamine Red. In testing a large number of dyes, Denton states that the water-soluble dyes were not deposited in any part of the egg, while seven of the alcohol-soluble dyes were deposited in the yolk, producing slight green, green, pink, magenta, blue, and red yolks. Hexyl blue dye was withdrawn from the body fat depots and deposited in the yolk. The Rhodamine Red colors the albumen strongly, giving a pink color. It also colors the body muscles, the feathers, which are being grown when the dye is in the blood, and the shell and albumen of the egg.

Effect on Feather Color. The yellow and red lipochrome colors originate in the food. If food not containing these colors is given, the feathers[32] fade completely. Dyes other than carotenoids are not absorbed by the feathers. Carotene causes a yellow color in the feathers, and paprika-containing food causes an orange color.

Effect on Eye Color.[33] Feed has a significant effect on eye color. A ration lacking the yellow pigments prevents the deposition of such pigments in the iris of Single Comb White Leghorns. Since both the diet and the vascular system of the iris play an important role in determining eye color, caution must be exercised in the culling of Single Comb White Leghorns on the basis of eye color alone.

Effect on Taste. In general, feed has little effect on taste.[34] The hen puts the feeds that it consumes through an effective refining process. However, certain feeds have been reported as affecting the flavor of the egg or flesh. Certain feeds, if given in large quantities, might affect the flavor to a slight extent. For example, rape, turnips, cabbage, and fish have been reported as affecting flavor. The feeding of fresh onions very quickly develops a distinct taste in the eggs. The Oklahoma Station[35] reports that hens fed 5 grams of garlic pod daily produced in 5 days egg yolks with a distinct flavor. The flavor was not found in the albumen until after 30 days of garlic feeding. At no time was an odor found in any part of the egg, either raw or cooked. Feeding 5 grams of dried onions produced no changes in flavor, odor, or appearance.

Cod liver oil, as usually fed, has not been reported as affecting the flavor of the egg. The feeding of two number three capsules[36] of cod liver oil daily, however, produced a very distinct fishy flavor in the yolk in 30 days, but no flavor in the albumen. The flavor was found in eggs after 6 months of storage.

Off-flavor in the meat of chicks and turkeys has been reported.[36] This has been traced to the feeding of cod liver oil or large amounts of fish meal, especially meals with a high fat content. Fish oil and fish meal should be discontinued in the ration fed market turkeys at least 8 weeks before they are dressed. Carrick and Hauge report that feeding 2 per cent of cod liver oil imparted a "fishy" taste to the flesh of chickens and that it took about 2 weeks for them to lose the "fishy" taste; that the taste on this amount was not apparent when the chicken was warm but seemed to be intensified when eaten cold; that the degree of "fishy" flavor was affected by the method of cooking; and that 4 per cent of oil gave a decided flavor to the flesh. Apparently, the amount of oil is a factor. One per cent or less of oil in the ration usually does not impart any flavor; but to eliminate any possible effect, the recommendation is frequently made, especially with broilers, to eliminate the oil for a week or 10 days before selling.

Certain feeding practices have been followed to affect the flavor of the flesh. For example, the feeding of celery is thought to impart a flavor. The characteristic gamey flavor in wild birds is produced to some extent by the food which the birds are eating.

In reporting the effect of feeds upon the quality of meat in turkeys, North[37] reported a more intense flavor and aroma of oat-fed roasted birds, as compared with those fed corn, wheat, barley, or rye. Corn-fed birds were more tender after roasting. Dry skimmilk produced a less intense aroma in the breast meat of the roasted birds. The least desirable flavor was found in birds which had been fed cottonseed meal. When a feed, 60 per cent of the protein concentrate of which was cottonseed meal, was fed, the juice was found to have a poorer quality than when the other supplements were fed (soybean oil meal and corn gluten meal). Corn gluten meal produced juice of a better quality than any of the other concentrates.

Payne[27] reports that eggs of an olive color, caused by the birds feeding on shepherd's purse, have a strong flavor. The Kansas Station[38] also reports a trend for dark-colored yolks to have a slightly higher flavor score (more objectionable), although the differences probably would not be readily detected by the average consumer.

Effect on Body Composition. The nature of the carcass fat[39] has been shown to be affected by the kind of dietary fat.

Effect on Egg Size. Many factors affect egg weight in the domestic fowl, such as age, sexual maturity, body weight, time of day the egg is laid, position in the clutch, and breeding, as well as deficiencies in the ration.[40] Feeding has a very definite influence on the size of eggs. Idaho[41] indicates that the highest percentage of small eggs is obtained where no protein feed was given. Results in Northern Ireland[42] also indicate, for a period of 2 years, the production of 44 per cent of second-grade eggs on a ration of cereals only, as compared with 23 to 26 per cent on rations having protein concentrate additions. The feeding of grain only showed lower egg weight in trials at Oklahoma[43] and 12 per cent reduction in egg weight at West Virginia.[44] Eggs produced on low-protein rations are smaller than those produced on rations of higher protein content.[45]

The egg was larger when certain animal protein feeds were added to the ration.[41, 46, 47] Idaho reported the following egg size when comparing pea meal and sour skimmilk. It has also been reported by several stations that milk, especially sour skimmilk,

Egg Size	Percentage of Eggs	
	Pea Meal	Sour Skimmilk
Up to 22 oz. per dozen	38	21
22-24	43	37
24-28	19	42

was superior to other animal protein concentrates in the effect it had on the weight of the egg produced.[41, 48-50]

The proportion of second-grade eggs, as reported by Robertson and Baskett,[42] decreased from 44 per cent to 27 per cent by the addition of minerals to a basal ration made up of cereals. They conclude that the evidence is strong that the weight of the egg is a function of the mineral portion of the ration. Kentucky[50] reports that in the absence of a calcium carbonate supplement the eggs became smaller.

With inadequate amounts of vitamin D, the average egg weight was materially reduced.[47, 51] Graham[51] reports that adding cod liver oil to the ration of laying pullets brought a slight increase in egg weight from February to July.

Parkhurst[47] also reports that green feed proved of value in increasing egg size. Smith[52] states that germinated oats caused a consistent increase in the average weight of eggs.

A well-balanced ration has been reported to give larger eggs and less variability than a poorly balanced ration.[48, 53] Parkhurst[48] and Atwood and Clark[54] indicate that rations which tend to increase or decrease production tend to have a similar influence on egg weight. Atwood and Clark also report that a physiological disturbance produced by the drug kamala caused a decrease in production, with an attendant decrease in egg weight. The altered physiological condition of the birds caused a fluctuation in the weight of the eggs, owing to materially decreased secretion of albumen. It was also observed at Cornell that egg weight was lowered during an attack of infectious laryngotracheitis.

Effect on Eggshells. The lack of sufficient amounts of vitamin D will decrease the amount of lime in the shell, decrease the percentage of eggshell, and produce thin and soft-shelled eggs.[51, 55-58]

Morgan and coworkers[59] report that feeding cod liver oil to pullets on range, under climatic conditions of South Carolina, tends to increase the breaking strength of shells of eggs, the percentage of shell, and the percentage of calcium carbonate in the shells, but the increase is slight.

A lack of an adequate calcium supply, in chemical combination available to the hen for the manufacture of eggshell, will tend to produce smaller and thin-shelled eggs.[50, 57, 60]

Experiments reported from Cornell[61] and Arkansas[62] show that the breaking strength of eggs is related to the quantity of manganese in the diet. The ash content of the eggshells was also found to increase with an increase in the manganese content of the diet.

Effect on Storage Quality of Eggs. The feeding of cottonseed meal, even when showing no discoloration of yolk or white when newly laid, caused eggs in cold storage to show discolored yolks and in some cases discolored whites. Eggs from hens fed cottonseed meal, crude cottonseed oil, partially refined cottonseed oil, and ether extract of cottonseed oil deteriorate in storage (see also Chap. 7).

The California Station[63] reports that in every case the fat of those plants belonging to the family of which cottonseed is a member gave a positive reaction to the Halphen test. Cheeseweed and California windbreak seeds were included in the diet of laying birds, and the eggs reacted to the test. They developed "pink white" on storage as did eggs from birds fed cottonseed. However, the deterioration of eggs resulting from cottonseed meal is caused by two distinct substances. Gossypol gives the yolk an olive-green color and a gelatinous consistency; the Halphen substance causes an abnormal enlargement of the yolk and a reddish color of the yolk and albumen to develop in storage.

Swensen, Fieger, and Upp[64] report that the olive-colored yolks are due to chemical combination of gossypol with ferric iron released from the egg protein of the yolk during storage. Addition of soluble ferric salts to the ration prevented the formation of olive yolks.

Effect on Interior Egg Quality. As far as the albumen of the egg is concerned, in general, feeds have not influenced interior egg quality[65, 66] as much as other factors, such as breeding and handling.

Illinois[67] reports that the feeding of high proportions of the common grains, corn, wheat, or oats, did not influence the percentage of thick white enough to result in eggs of distinctly inferior quality, but that there was some indication that the proportion of thick white may be influenced by the ration fed. The further addition of mineral supplements or a decided increase in the potential alkalinity of the ration had no noticeable effect on the percentage of thick white.

A report from Wyoming[68] indicates that hens fed rye produced eggs with a lower ratio of thick white to thin white and a lower yolk index, causing the eggs to appear aged in spite of their being strictly fresh. Barley also showed a slight tendency to produce a lower ratio of thick white.

The New Mexico Station[69] showed that the index of quality of eggs produced by hens receiving green feed was less than that of eggs from hens receiving no green feed, and that the eggs produced on green feed depreciated in quality more rapidly with increased age. The Oklahoma Station[35] indicated that in all instances eggs from the pens receiving green feed had a thin and more liquid albumen than eggs from pens receiving no green feed.

In general, variation in the percentage of thick albumen or other characteristics of interior quality was not definitely attributed to the amount or kind of protein fed.[65, 70] However, Heiman, Carver, and St. John[70] found that the level of protein apparently affected albumen quality, in that they obtained a significant difference in albumen index between hens fed 12 to 13 per cent protein from plant sources only and those fed higher percentages of protein from both plant and animal sources.

Experiments at Cornell indicated that such nutritive factors as proteins, carbohydrates, fats, minerals, vitamins, and water had little if any effect upon the percentage of thick albumen. The Colorado[71] Station reported that egg albumen quality does not appear to be related to the content of vitamin A, carotene, nicotinic acid, folic acid, and apparent pyridoxine.

EFFECT ON VITAMIN CONTENT OF EGGS. The vitamin content of the feed has an effect upon the vitamin content of the egg. Experiments at the Ohio Station[72] indicate that access to bluegrass or feeding 2 per cent of cod liver oil increased the vitamin A potency of the egg yolk five times. Alfalfa hay also tended to increase the vitamin A content.

The vitamin D[55, 72, 73] content of the eggs is also influenced by feeding or exposure to ultraviolet rays. Hart and associates report the antirachitic potency of egg yolks from irradiated hens as being about ten times that of yolks from nonirradiated hens. The Ohio Station indicates that egg yolks from birds fed cod liver oil or irradiated ergosterol, or exposed to sunlight, had five to ten times as much vitamin D as egg yolks from birds confined behind window glass. Branion, Drake, and Tisdall increased the number of Steenbock units of vitamin D from 4 to 30 by adding 2 per cent of cod liver oil and as high as 18,000 units by the addition of highly potent viosterol. Kentucky reports that the yolks of eggs produced in the spring and stored until fall and winter were found to have a higher content of vitamin D than the yolks of eggs produced in the fall and winter under like conditions. Work done at Cornell would indicate that egg yolks produced by hens receiving direct sunlight were more potent in vitamin D than egg yolks from hens receiving cod liver oil or ultraviolet light.

The content of the water soluble vitamins of eggs has been influenced by the ration.[74] The Ohio Station reported that attempts to increase the pantothenic acid content of eggs by feeding hens feeds high in this factor have given negative results. On the other hand, Bauernfeind and Norris showed that hens receiving a heated experimental diet deposited less pantothenic acid in their eggs than hens fed a normal diet. Snell and coworkers also reported that eggs from hens maintained on a diet low in pantothenic acid showed markedly lowered pantothenic acid content, and that within the limits of the experiment the pantothenic acid content of the egg is directly proportional to that of the diet. Gillis, Norris, and Heuser showed that the pantothenic acid content of the egg varied directly with the content of the diet and reached levels much higher than present in the blood.

Norris and Bauernfeind report the average riboflavin content of fresh eggs produced by hens fed egg mashes to be approximately 2.07 micrograms per gram of edible substances (105 micrograms per egg) and that of the eggs produced by hens fed breeder mashes to be 2.48 micrograms per gram (125 micrograms per egg). The lowest riboflavin value obtained experimentally was approximately 0.82 microgram per gram of edible substance (40 micrograms per egg), and the highest value was 3.26 micrograms per gram (165 micrograms per egg). In these studies it was found that the riboflavin content of fresh eggs could be increased approximately 1.9 micrograms per gram above that of the eggs laid by hens fed the basal diet (the riboflavin content of the eggs produced on the basal diet was 0.82 microgram per gram in one experiment and 1.40 micrograms per gram in two other experiments). The time required to attain maximum riboflavin storage in eggs and that required to deplete to the basal levels varied from about 2 to 4 weeks. In general, the riboflavin content of egg white changed more rapidly than that of egg yolk.

Experiments at Cornell showed that the vitamin B_{12} content of the egg is influenced by the amount of this vitamin in the diet and that the vitamin B_{12} in the diet is related to hatchability.

EFFECT ON MINERAL CONTENT OF THE EGG. Experiments[75] show that both the iron and copper content of eggs can be affected by feeding.

It has also been shown that the iodine content of eggs is affected by the iodine content of the ration.[76] An increase as great as 450 times the original content has been reported by the feeding of iodine preparations.

Experiments conducted at Cornell[61] and Kentucky[77] indicate that the manganese content of eggs from a low-manganese group was smaller than from high-manganese groups and that the breaking strength of eggs increases as the quantity of manganese in the diet increases.

EFFECT ON COMPOSITION OF THE EGG. As far as total composition is concerned, there is very little effect of the feeds on the chemical composition of the egg. The composition of the various parts of the egg (white, yolk, shell) varies greatly, but these variations are independent of the system of feeding.[78] In comparing the composition of eggs produced on a nitrogenous as compared with a carbonaceous ration, one finds very little difference in the protein, fat, and water content of the yolk. The white of the egg might show slightly more protein on the nitrogenous diet. This might be true because the white of the egg is a secretion. The Wisconsin Station[55] reported that irradiation with ultraviolet light did not affect the calcium and phosphorus content of the whites and yolks. Kentucky workers[79] reported that, as long as the economy of the hens permitted the formation of an eggshell, the contents of the egg remained reasonably constant, thereby permitting an average supply of calcium, magnesium, and phosphorus for the proper development of the embryo of the chick, and that the presence or absence of oystershell in the diet had no appreciable effect upon the percentages of protein and of calcium in the white and yolk. The hen endeavors to keep a steady chemical condition of her egg and will do so even at the expense of her body.

U.S.D.A. workers[80] indicated some effects of diet upon composition, although the effects were usually small. The yolks appeared to be more readily affected than the whites. The most consistent differences were observed in the percentage of protein in the dry matter of the yolk of eggs. The various N or protein determinations showed little or no difference. McFarlane, Fulmer, and Jukes[81] found no significant difference in the composition of the proteins of eggs of poor hatchability, so far as the total nitrogen, total amino-nitrogen, tyrosine, tryptophan, and cystine content were concerned, as compared to the composition of the proteins of eggs of high hatchability. There was no clear evidence that the diet of the hen had any influence on these values.

Pollard and Carr[82] report great differences in the proteins of eggs from pigeons fed different cereals, especially wheat, rye, oats, and corn, which contained high tryptophan.

Dietary fat has been reported as having some effect upon type of egg fat[83] of the hen.

EFFECT ON OTHER EGG CHARACTERISTICS. Atwood and Weakley[84] report that their results would indicate that the presence of a considerable amount of animal protein in the ration for laying hens tends to weaken the vitelline membrane. Ovarian hemorrhages, resulting in blood and meat spots[85] in eggs, have been reported as being reduced substantially by allowing the hens thus affected access to range or by feeding them Cerogras. Anderson[86] indicates that evidence available strongly suggests that diet may influence to a very considerable degree the bacterial flora and the normal bacteriostatic properties of the eggs produced.

REFERENCES

1. Kable, G. W., and F. E. Fox. Electric water heaters for poultry. Ore. Sta. Circ. 81. 1927.
2. Beresford, H. Stock tank and poultry water heaters. Agr. Eng. 11 (8). 1930.
3. Sheehy, E. J. Effect of fiber and bulk in the diet of chickens on their growth and on the prevention of feather picking and cannibalism. Rept. Seventh World's Poultry Congress. 205. Cleveland. 1939.

   Sheehy, E. J., and E. M. Burke. The effect of fiber and "bulk" in the diet on the progress of chickens and prevention of feather picking and cannibalism. Irish Free State Dept. Agr. Jour. 37:42. 1940.
4. Shaw, T., and E. A. Fisher. Bulkiness of food as a factor in poultry feeding. Jour. Ministry Agr. (Great Britain) 40:327. 1933.
5. Halnan, E. T. The scientific principles of poultry feeding. Ministry Agr. and Fisheries Bul. 7. London. 1930.
6. Sheehy, E. J., and K. Sheil. The optimum concentration (starch equivalent) of the meal mixture for chickens and growing pullets fed on all-mash diet. Rept. Fourth World's Poultry Congress. 277. London. 1930.
7. Berg, L. R., and G. E. Bearse. Granulation of ingredients in poultry mashes. Wash. Bul. 470:135. 1945.

   Berg, L. R., and G. E. Bearse. Studies of the granulation of chicken laying mashes. Poultry Sci. 27:653. 1948; Wash. Bul. 522, 1951.

   Berg, L. R., and G. E. Bearse. The effect of the size and the shape of feed particles on the development of growing poults. Poultry Sci. 26:532. 1947.

Coburn, D. R., and R. B. Nestler. Food particle size and quality in relation to disease in artificially propagated quail chicks. Jour. Am. Vet. Med. Assn. 110(838):30. 1947.

Davis, R. L., G. M. Briggs, and H. J. Sloan. The modulus of ground corn in a corn-soybean oil meal chick starting ration. Poultry Sci. 31:745. 1952.

Davis, R. L., E. G. Hill, H. J. Sloan, and G. M. Briggs. Detrimental effect of corn of coarse particle size in rations for chicks. Poultry Sci. 30:325. 1951.

Eley, C. P., and E. Hoffman. Feed particle size as a factor in water consumption and elimination. Poultry Sci. 28:215. 1949.

Kennard, D. C., and L. B. Nettleton. Palatability of poultry feeds. Ohio Bimo. Bul. 128:161. 1927.

Kennard, D. C. Poultry. Coarse vs. fine mash. Ohio Sta. Special Circ. 28:15. 1930.

Nikolaiczuk, N. The adverse effect of texture upon the feeding value of linseed oil meal for chicks. Poultry Sci. 30:773. 1950.

8. Conklin, R. L., and W. A. Maw. Pressure necrosis—A battery brooder feed problem. Proc. Twenty-first Annual Meeting Poultry Sci. Assn. 1929. Bul. Ala. Poly. Inst. XXV(1):35. 1930.

Blakely, R. M. The effect of the granulation of single cereal grains on the incidence of pressure necrosis in poult starter mashes. Sci. Agric. 28:554. 1948.

Nikolaiczuk, N. The adverse effect of texture upon the feeding value of linseed oil meal for chicks. Poultry Sci. 30:773. 1950.

9. Poley, W. E. The utilization of wheat and wheat by-products in feeding young chickens. I. The effect of the fineness of grinding wheat. Poultry Sci. 17:331. 1938.

Roberts, R. E., and C. W. Carrick. Fine, medium, and coarse cracked corn. Ind. Rept. 1938:80.

10. Bragg, D. D. An attempt to determine the cause of curled tongue in young Beltsville turkeys. Poultry Sci. 32:294. 1953.

11. Quisenberry, T. E. "The balanced ration" for egg production. Mo. State Board Agr. Year Book 1915:478.

12. National Research Council. Recommended nutrient requirements for domestic animals. No. 1. Nutrient requirements for poultry. Washington, D. C. Revised Jan. 1954. Pub. 301.

13. Engelmann, C. Vom Geschmacksinn des Huhnes. Forschung und Fortschritt 13:425. 1937.

Engelmann, C. Wählt das Huhn seine Nahrung nach dem Geschmack. Umschau 44:828. 1940.

Engelmann, C. Über den Geschmackssinn des Huhnes. Forschungsdienst 13:363. 1942.

Römer, R. Geruchs-, Farben-, Form- und Geschmackssinn beim Huhn. Geflügelhof.; May 27, 1949:339.

14. Banta, L. What judgment does a hen use in selecting her food? Poultry Sci. 11:365. 1932.

Funk, E. M. Can the chick balance its ration? Poultry Sci. 11:94. 1932.

Jackson, H. W. Characteristics of hens. Pa. Rept.:228. 1911-1912.

Kempster, H. L. Food selection by laying hens. Jour. Am. Assn. Instructors and Investigators in Poultry Husb. 3:26. 1917.

Kempster, H. L., and E. M. Funk. Will chicks balance their own ration? Mo. Bul. 310. Annual Rept. 1932:49.

Kennard, D. C., and L. B. Nettleton. Palatability of poultry feeds. Ohio Bimo. Bul. 12(5):161. 1927.

Poultry farming. Dept. Agr. (Victoria, Australia) Bul. 54. N.S. 1924.

Tomhave, A. E., and C. W. Mumford. Self selection of feeds by hens. Del. Bul. 174. 1931.

Tuason, N. A., and F. M. Fronda. Studies on Philippine poultry feeds. I. Availability and palatability. Philippine Agr. XII:459. 1924.

Winter, A. R., E. L. Dakan, and A. Bayes. Protein levels for finishing pullets. Poultry Sci. 11:30. 1932.

15. Newbiggin, H. F., and R. G. Linton. The palatability of certain seeds to chicks. Scottish Jour. Agr. 10:422. 1927.

16. Pearl, R., and T. E. Fairchild. Studies on the physiology of reproduction in the domestic fowl. XIX. Influence of free choice of food material on winter egg production and body weight. Am. Jour. Hygiene 1:253. 1921.

17. Carver, J. S., and V. Heiman. The effect on yolk color of Argentine corn, domestic corn and dehydrated alfalfa. Poultry Sci. 14:299. 1935.

Heiman, V., and L. A. Wilhelm. The transmission of xanthophylls in feeds to the yolk of the hen's egg. Poultry Sci. 16:400. 1937.

Kempster, H. L. The relation of carotinoid pigments to poultry. Proc. First World's Poultry Congress. 120. Holland. 1921.

Mattikow, M. A critical review of the literature on the coloring matter in egg yolk. Poultry Sci. 11:83. 1932.

Palmer, L. S., and H. L. Kempster. Relation of plant carotinoids to growth. Fecundity and reproduction of fowls. Jour. Biol. Chem. 39:299. 1919.

Palmer, L. S., and H. L. Kempster. The influence of specific feeds and certain pigments on the color of the egg yolk and body fat of fowls. Jour. Biol. Chem. 39:331. 1919.

Parker, S. L., S. S. Gossman, and W. A. Lippincott. Studies on egg quality. I. Introductory note on variations in yolk color. Poultry Sci. 5:131. 1926.

Sjollema, B., and W. F. Donath. Over het gehalte aan vitamine A, carotine en xanthophyll in dooiers van kippeneieren. Voeding 1: 133. 1939.

18. Pigmentation and food. Some experimental work on the S.P.B.A. farm. Rudgwick, Sussex, England. 1930.

19. Heiman, V., and L. W. Tighe. Observations on the shank pigmentation of chicks. Poultry Sci. 22:102. 1943.

20. Bird, H. R. Increasing yellow pigmentation in shanks of chickens. Poultry Sci. 22:205. 1943.

Culton, T. G., and H. R. Bird. Effect of certain protein supplements in inhibiting pigment deposition in growing chicks. Poultry Sci. 20:432. 1941.

Hammond, J. C., and H. M. Harshaw. Some factors influencing shank and skin color in the growing chicken. Poultry Sci. 20:437. 1941.

Hammond, J. C., D. Miller, and D. Whitson. Effect of the diet of the hen on the shank color of her day-old chicks. Poultry Sci. 21:525. 1942.

Nilson, H. W., and R. S. Schayer. Feeding fish meals to pullets. Comm. Fish. Rev. 8(9):1. 1946.

21. Bilek, F. Experimental changes of the pigments in the yolk with reference to the contents of vitamins. Rept. Sixth World's Congress. 29. Germany. 1936.

Graner, E. A. A influencia dos pigmentos amarelo-larauja varios alimentos na coloracao da gema de ovo de galinha. An. Escola Agric. "Luiz de Quiroz" 4:372. 1947.

Grzimek, B. Alles was wir über die Dotterfarbe wissen. Geflügel-Börse 6. 1933.

Henderson, E. W., and H. L. Wilcke. Effect of ration on yolk color. Poultry Sci. 12:266. 1933.

Hughes, J. S., and L. F. Payne. The relation of the carotenoid pigment of feed to the carotenoid pigments of egg yolk. Poultry Sci. 16:135. 1937.

Kuchler, H. Ist die blase Farbe des Dotters von Farmeiern durch die Fütterung bzw. durch Zusätze zum Futter zu bessern? Tierärtzliche Rundschau 39:289. 1933.

Kupsch, W Die Veränderung und Wertbestimmung der Eidotterfarbe. Archiv für Geflügelk. 8:97. 1934.

Payne, L. F., and L. A. Wilhelm. Egg yolk color as affected by certain xanthophyll bearing feeds. Poultry Sci.12:330. 1933.

Roemmele, O. Die Beeinflüssung der Dotterfarbe durch die Fütterung und ihre Bedeutung für die Ernährung und Zucht. Zeitschrift für Fleischhygiene und Milchhygiene 44:147. 1934.

Titus, H. W., J. C. Fritz, and W. R. Kauffman. Some observations on egg yolk color. Poultry Sci. 17:38. 1938.

Wilhelm, L. A., and V. Heiman. The effect on yolk color of various ingredients of poultry feeds. Poultry Sci. 16:416. 1937.

22. Bohren, B. B., C. R. Thompson, and C. W. Carrick. The transfer of carotenoid pigments to the egg yolk. Poultry Sci. 24:356. 1945.

23. Yellow color of egg yolk from grass. Land. Tuin-en Meerhof. 15. November 1930.

24. Morgan, W. A., and J. G. Woodruff. Waste pimiento pepper for coloring egg yolks. Ga. Bul. 147. 1927.

Brown, W. L. Some effects of pimiento pepper on poultry. Ga. Bul. 160. 1930.

Brown, W. L. The quantitative relation of egg yolk pigmentation to pimiento feeds. Ga. Bul. 183. 1934.

Brown, W. L. The influence of pimiento pigments on the color of the egg yolk of fowls. Jour. Biol. Chem. 122:655. 1938.

25. Benedek, L. The color of yolks. Internationale Eierbörse. Dec. 16, 1937.

26. Parker, S. L. Studies on egg quality. II. Seasonal variations in yolk color. Poultry Sci. 6:259. 1927.

Effect of feed on egg yolk color. Ore. Sta. Rept. 1928-1930:110.
Influence of alfalfa on yolk color. Idaho Sta. Bul. 170:25. 1930.
Carver, J. S., and V. Heiman. The effect on yolk color of Argentine corn, domestic corn, and dehydrated alfalfa. Poultry Sci. 14:299. 1935.

27. Payne, L. F. The cause of olive-colored egg yolks. Poultry Sci. 4: 102. 1925.
Temperton, H. Some nutritional causes of discolorations in the internal contents of eggs. Harper Adams Utility Poultry Jour. 28: 71. 1943.
Temperton, H. The feeding of acorns to laying pullets and ducks. Empire Jour. Exp. Agr. 11:43. 1943.

28. Thompson, R. B., W. P. Albright, E. E. Schnetzler, and V. G. Heller. Feeds and their relation to egg quality. Okla. Rept. 1930-1932: 128.
Upp, C. W. Storage studies of Louisiana eggs. La. Bul. 229. 1932.
Upp, C. W. Will Louisiana eggs keep? La. Circ. 13. 1934.
Schaible, P. J., L. A. Moore, and J. M. Moore. Gossypol, a cause of discoloration in egg yolks. Science 79:372. 1934.
Albright, W. P., and R. B. Thompson. Variations of egg yolk color and characteristics produced by feeding and environment. Poultry Sci. 14:373. 1935.
Smith, R. M. The influence of some factors on the storage quality of eggs. Ark. Bul. 341. 1937.

29. Olsen, M. W. Acorns one cause of olive-colored yolks. Poultry Sci. 211:497. 1942.

30. Peterson, W. J., J. S. Hughes, L. F. Payne, and W. M. Prondfit. The xanthophylls of olive-colored yolks. Proc. Am. Chem. Soc., Abst. B., 3. 1939.

31. Rogers, C. A. Feeding color—an aid in studying physiological development. International Assn. Instructors and Investigators Poultry Husb. 1:77. 1909.
Grossfeld, J., and H. R. Kanitz. Versuche über Künstliche Färbung von Hühnereidottern durch Fütterung. Zeitschrift für Untersuchungen der Lebensmittel 74:471. 1937.
Denton, C. A. Some observations on feeding dyes to laying chickens. Poultry Sci. 19:281. 1940.

32. Giersberg, H., and R. Stadie. Zur Entstehung der Gelben und Roten Gefieder Farben der Vogel. Zeitschrift für Vergleichende Physiologie 18:696. 1933.
Brockman, H., and O. Volker. The yellow feather coloring matter of canaries (Serinus canaria canaria L.) and the occurrence of carotenoids in birds. Hoppe-Seyle Zeitschrift für physiologische Chemie 224:193. 1935.

33. Ball, R. F. The effect of the ration upon iris color of Single Comb White Leghorns. Poultry Sci. 23:377. 1944.
Nelson, N. M. Feed influence on eye color in White Leghorn chickens. Poultry Sci. 23:541. 1944.

34. Vondell, J. H., and J. N. Putnam. The effect of certain feedstuffs on the flavor, albumen condition, and yolk color of eggs. Poultry Sci. 24:284. 1945.

35. Albright, W. P., and R. B. Thompson. Variations of egg yolk color and characteristics produced by feeding and environment. Poultry Sci. 14:373. 1935.

Thompson, R. B., W. P. Albright, E. E. Schnetzler, and V. G. Heller. Feeds and their relation to egg quality. Okla. Rept. 1930-1932: 128.

36. Carrick, C. W., and S. M. Hauge. The effect of cod-liver oil upon flavor in poultry meat. Poultry Sci. 5:213. 1926.

The off-flavored turkey problem. U. S. Egg and Poultry Mag. 43: 362. 1937.

Marble, D. R., J. E. Hunter, H. C. Knandel, and R. A. Dutcher. Fishy flavor and odor in turkeys. The effect of cod liver oil (not U.S.P.) and white fish meal. Poultry Sci. 16:363. 1937.

Marble, D. R., J. E. Hunter, H. C. Knandel, and R. A. Dutcher. Fishy flavor and odor in turkey meat. Poultry Sci. 17:49. 1938.

Asmundson, V. S., T. H. Jukes, H. M. Fyler, and M. L. Maxwell. The effect of certain fish meals and fish oils in the ration on the flavor of the turkey. Poultry Sci. 17:147. 1938.

Schaible, P. J., R. Griswold, J. A. Davidson, and E. J. Miller. Progress report upon the investigation of off-flavored turkeys. Mich. Sta. Quart. Bul. 20(3):127. 1938.

Bryant, R. L., and G. T. Stevenson. Fishy flavor in turkey meat caused by feeding menhaden fish meal. Va. Bul. 321. 1939.

Cruikshank, E. M. The effect of cod-liver oil and fish meal on the flavor of poultry products. Rept. Seventh World's Poultry Congress. 539. Cleveland. 1939.

Olsson, N. Forsok rorande fiskprodukternas tillvaratagande och anvandbarhet som foder for hons och Kycklingar. Lantbrukshogskolan Husdjursförsoksanstalten Meddel. 7:1. 1942.

37. North, M. O. The influence of cereal grains upon the quality of meat in turkeys. Wyo. Bul. 248. 1941.

North, M. O. The influence of protein concentrates upon the quality of meat in turkeys. Wyo. Bul. 264. 1943.

38. McCammon, R. B., M. S. Pittman, and L. A. Wilhelm. The odor and flavor of eggs. Poultry Sci. 13:95. 1934.

39. Chu, T. K., and F. A. Kummerow. The deposition of linolenic acid in chickens fed linseed oil. Poultry Sci. 29:846. 1950.

Davis, H. J., and C. W. Upp. Studies on the fat requirements of the domestic fowl. Poultry Sci. 20:459. 1941.

Halnan, E. T., and E. M. Cruickshank. Some aspects of fat metabolism in fowls and their practical significance. Proc. Fifth World's Poultry Congress (Rome) 2:612. 1933.

Klose, A. A., E. P. Mecchi, G. A. Behman, and H. Lineweaver. Chemical characteristics of turkey carcass fat as a function of dietary fat. Poultry Sci. 31:354. 1952.

40. Funk, E. M., and H. L. Kempster. Egg weight in the domestic fowl. Mo. Bul. 332. 1934.

41. Moore, P. Annual report for year ending June 30, 1916. Idaho Bul. 92:28. 1916.

Parkhurst, R. T. The value of certain protein feeds for production and quality in eggs. Idaho Bul. 134. 1924.

42. Robertson, G. S., and R. G. Baskett. The nutritive requirement of poultry. The influence of certain nutritional factors on the size of the egg and the condition of the bird. Scottish Jour. Agr. 11:176. 1928.

Robertson, G. S., and R. G. Baskett. The feeding of poultry. Jour. Agr. N. Ireland 2:22. 1929.

43. Thompson, R. B., and R. Penquite. Forcing doesn't injure breeding hens. Okla. Rept. 1926-1930:118.

44. Atwood, H. Some factors affecting the weight of eggs. W. Va. Sta. Bul. 201. 1926.

45. Heuser, G. F. The protein requirements of laying hens. Rept. Fourth World's Poultry Congress. 276. Germany. 1936.

46. Parkhurst, R. T., and E. B. Lomax. The comparative value of various protein feeds for laying hens. National Institute of Poultry Husbandry. Harper Adams Agr. Col. Bul. No. 4. April 1930.

Roemer, R. Poultry feeding in Germany. Proc. Third World's Poultry Congress. 239. Canada. 1927.

Berry, L. N. Relative value of cottonseed meal and tankage for egg production. N. Mex. Bul. 183. 1930.

47. Parkhurst, R. T. Some factors affecting egg weight in the domestic fowl. Poultry Sci. 12:97. 1933.

48. Parkhurst, R. T. The influence of certain feeds on the weight of eggs. Harper Adams Utility Poultry Jour. 13:478. 1927-1928.

49. Work and progress of the Agricultural Experimental Station for the year 1923. Idaho Bul. 133:13.

Work and progress of the Agr. Exp. Sta. for the year 1925. Idaho Bul. 142:20.

Parkhurst, R. T. Summarized report of 1925-1926 poultry feeding experimental work. Idaho Circ. 43. March 1927.

Kistler, P. T., T. B. Charles, and H. C. Knandel. Effect of various sources of animal protein on the egg production and condition of S.C.W.L. pullets. Pa. Sta. Bul. 206. 1926.

50. Buckner, G. D., and J. H. Martin. Effect of calcium on the composition of the eggs of laying hens. Jour. Biol. Chem. 41:195. 1920.

Buckner, G. D., J. H. Martin, and A. M. Peter. Calcium metabolism in the laying hen. Ky. Bul. 250. 1923.

Buckner, G. D., J. H. Martin, and A. M. Peter. Calcium metabolism in the laying hen. III. Calcium carbonate and hatchability. Ky. Bul. 291. 1929.

Evans, R. J., J. S. Carver, and A. W. Brant. The influence of dietary factors on egg shell quality. II. Calcium. Poultry Sci. 23: 36. 1944.

51. Carver, J. S., E. I. Robertson, D. Brazie, R. H. Johnson, and J. L. St. John. The vitamin D requirements of chickens. Wash. Bul. 299. 1934.

Graham, W. R., Jr. Some factors affecting the weight of egg in domestic fowl. Sci. Agr. 12:427. 1932.

52. Smith, R. M. The influence of certain supplements on the production, hatchability, fertility, and weight of eggs. Ark. Bul. 293. 1933.

53. Atwood, H. Certain correlations in the weight and number of eggs and the weight of fowls. W. Va. Sta. Bul. 182. 1923.
54. Atwood, H., and T. Clark. Further studies on factors influencing the weight of eggs. Poultry Sci. 8:193. 1929.
55. Hart, E. B., H. Steenbock, S. Lepkovsky, S. W. F. Kletzien, J. G. Halpin, and O. N. Johnson. The nutritional requirement of the chicken. V. The influence of ultraviolet light on the production, hatchability, and fertility of the egg. Jour. Biol. Chem. 65:579. 1925.
56. Hughes, J. S., L. F. Payne, and W. L. Latshaw. The influence of ultraviolet light on leg weakness in growing chicks and on egg production. Poultry Sci. 9:151. 1925.
57. Martin, J. H., S. E. Erickson, and W. M. Insko. Effect of vitamin D supplements on laying hens. Ky. Bul. 304. 1930.
Taylor, L. W., and J. H. Martin. Factors influencing thickness of egg shell. Poultry Sci. 8:39. 1928.
58. Hendricks, W. A., A. R. Lee, and A. B. Godfrey. Effects of cod-liver oil and ultra-violet irradiation, as influenced by oyster shell, in the diet of confined laying hens. Jour. Agr. Res. 43: 517. 1931.
59. Morgan, C. L., J. H. Mitchell, and D. S. Roderick. Effect of cod-liver oil on the quality of egg shells. Proc. Twenty-second Annual Meeting Poultry Sci. 39. 1930.
60. Deobald, H. J., E. J. Lease, and E. B. Hart. Studies on the calcium metabolism of laying hens. Poultry Sci. 15:179. 1936.
61. Gallup, W. D., and L. C. Norris. Studies on the importance of manganese in the nutrition of poultry. Poultry Sci. 16:351. 1937.
Caskey, D. C., and L. C. Norris. Further studies on the role of manganese in poultry nutrition. Poultry Sci. 17:433. 1938.
Gallup, W. D., and L. C. Norris. The effect of a deficiency of manganese in the diet of the hen. Poultry Sci. 18:83. 1939.
Wilgus, H. S., L. C. Norris, and G. F. Heuser. The role of manganese in poultry nutrition. Rept. Seventh World's Poultry Congress. 171. Cleveland. 1939.
62. Lyons, M. Some effects of manganese on eggshell quality. Ark. Bul. 374. 1939.
63. Almquist, H. J., and F. W. Lorenz. Some possible causes of pink egg white. U. S. Egg and Poultry Mag. 38:48. 1932.
Almquist, H. J., and F. W. Lorenz. "Pink whites" in stored eggs. U. S. Egg and Poultry Mag. 39:28. 1933.
Lorenz, F. W., and H. J. Almquist. Effect of malvaceous seeds on stored-egg quality. Indus. Eng. Chem. 26:1311. 1934.
Lorenz, F. W. Egg deterioration due to ingestion by hens of malvaceous materials. Poultry Sci. 18:295. 1939.
64. Swensen, A. D., E. A. Fieger, and C. W. Upp. The nature of egg yolk discoloration produced by cottonseed meal. Poultry Sci. 21: 374. 1942.
65. Perry, F. D. Influences of rations and storage on the physical characteristics of eggs. Iowa Res. Bul. 192. 1936.
Parker, J. E., Relation of type of ration to the interior quality of hen's eggs. N. Dakota Bul. 8:3. 1946.

66. Ringrose, R. C., and C. L. Morgan. A study of the effect of green feed upon interior egg quality. Poultry Sci. 18:125. 1939.
Wilcke, H. L. External measures of egg viscocity. Iowa Bul. 194. 1936.
67. Card, L. E., and H. J. Sloan. The effect of different diets on interior egg quality. Poultry Sci. 13:313. 1934.
Card, L. E., and H. J. Sloan. The effect of mineral supplements on interior egg quality. Poultry Sci. 14:300. 1935.
68. North, M. O. Poultry feeding, housing, and lighting experiments at the Wyoming Experiment Station. Wyo. Bul. 203. 1934.
69. Walker, A. L., L. N. Berry, and P. W. Cockerill. Factors affecting the market qualities of New Mexico eggs. N. Mex. Bul. 224. 1934.
70. Sowell, D. F., and C. L. Morgan. The relationship of protein supplement to interior egg quality. Poultry Sci. 15:219. 1936.
Miller, M. W., and G. Bearse. Protein supplements for laying hens. Wash. Bul. 347. 1937.
Heiman, V., J. S. Carver, and J. L. St. John. The protein requirements of laying hens. Wash. Bul. 331. 1936.
71. Charkey, L. W., E. Dyar, and H. S. Wilgus, Jr. The nutrient content of high and low quality fresh eggs. II. Vitamins. Poultry Sci. 26: 632. 1947.
72. Fat-soluble vitamin content of hens' eggs. Ohio Bul. 402:92. 1927.
Bethke, R. M., D. C. Kennard, and H. L. Sassaman. Fat-soluble vitamin content of hens' egg yolk as affected by the ration and management of the layers. Jour. Biol. Chem. 72:695. 1927.
Bethke, R. M., and W. Hosack. Antirachitic properties of egg yolks. Forty-eighth Annual Rept. for 1928-1929. Ohio Bul. 446. 1930.
73. Hughes, J. S., L. F. Payne, R. W. Titus, and J. M. Moore. Relation between the amount of ultraviolet light received by hens and the amount of antirachitic vitamin in the eggs produced. Jour. Biol. Chem. 66:595. 1925.
Branion, H. D., T. G. H. Drake, and F. F. Tisdall. Vitamin D content of egg yolk. U. S. Egg and Poultry Mag. 40:20. 1934.
Antirachitic value of egg yolks. Ky. Rept. 1929:32.
Bryant, R. L. Means of influencing the vitamin content of egg yolk. Cornell University Thesis. 1926.
74. Bauernfeind, J. C., and L. C. Norris. The antidermatosis vitamin required for reproduction in the domestic fowl. Science 89:416. 1939.
Bethke, R. M., and W. Wilder. Relative antineuritic and antipellagric vitamin content of fresh eggs. Ohio Sta. Bul. 470:185. 1934.
Bethke, R. M., P. R. Record, and D. C. Kennard. The relation of the vitamin G complex to hatchability and nutritive value of the eggs. Poultry Sci. 12:332. 1933.
Bethke, R. M., P. R. Record, and F. W. Wilder. The effect of the ration of the hen on the vitamin G content of eggs with observations on the distribution of vitamin B and G in normal eggs. Jour. Nutr. 12:309. 1936.
Ellis, N. R., D. Miller, H. W. Titus, and T. C. Byerly. Effect of diet on egg composition. III. The relation of diet to the vitamin B

and the vitamin G content of eggs, together with observations on the vitamin A content. Jour. Nutr. 6:243. 1933.
Engel, W. R., P. H. Philips, and J. G. Halpin. The effect of a riboflavin deficiency in the hen upon embryonic development. Poultry Sci. 19:135. 1940.
Gillis, M. B., G. F. Heuser, and L. C. Norris. Pantothenic acid in the nutrition of the hen. Jour. Nutr. 35:351. 1948.
Halpin, J. G., H. R. Bird, O. L. Kline, and C. A. Elvehjem. Vitamins B and G in eggs increased by special ration. Wis. Bul. 428: 46. 1934.
Heiman, V., and L. C. Norris. The relative vitamin G content of milk sugar feed (dried whey) and dried skimmilk. Poultry Sci. 12:332. 1933.
Heiman, V. The relative vitamin G content of dried whey and dried skimmilk. Poultry Sci. 14:137. 1935.
Norris, L. C., H. S. Wilgus, A. T. Ringrose, V. Heiman, and G. F. Heuser. The vitamin G requirement of poultry. Cornell Bul. 660. 1936.
Norris, L. C., and J. C. Bauernfeind. Effect of the level of dietary riboflavin upon the quantity stored in eggs and the rate of storage. Food Res. 5:521. 1940.
Snell, E. E., E. Aline, J. R. Couch, and P. B. Pearson. The effect of diet on the pantothenic acid content of eggs. Jour. Nutr. 21:201. 1940.
Yacowitz, H., R. F. Miller, L. C. Norris, and G. F. Heuser, Vitamin B_{12} studies with the hen. Poultry Sci. 31:89. 1952.
75. Erikson, S. E., R. E. Boyden, J. H. Martin, and W. M. Insko, Jr. The iron and copper content of egg yolks. Ky. Res. Bul. 342. 1933.
Lesne, E., P. Zizine, and S. Briskas. Le taux du Fer et du Cuivre dans l'oeuf; les variations de ces deux metaux suivant l'age de la poule. Comptes Rendus Societe Biologie. 128:935. 1938.
76. Almquist, H. J., and J. W. Givens. Effects of common feed ingredients on the iodine content of hen's eggs. Poultry Sci. 14:182. 1935.
Freund, L. Jodeier. Münchener Tierärtzliche Wochenschrift 315. 1935.
Jaschik, A., and J. Kieselbach. Iodine in eggs. Zeitschrift für Untersuchung der Lebensmittel 62:572. 1931.
Müller-Lehnhartz, and Wendt. Mineralstoffe und Vitamine in der Ernährung des Huhnes. Zeitschrift für Fleischhygiene und Milchhygiene 18:364.
Scharrer, K., and W. Schropp. Feeding of iodine to chickens. Biedermanns Zentr. B. Tierernähr. 4:249. 1932.
Schmidt, J. The feeding of iodine to poultry. Deutsche Tierärtzliche Wochenschrift 662. 1931.
Viollier, R., and E. Iselin. Über Jodeier. Mitteilungen Geb. Lebensmittal. Hyg. 26:62. 1935.
Straub, J. Über den Jodgehalt von Jodeiern. Zeitschrift für Untersuchung der Lebensmittel. 65:97. 1933.
Vezzani, V., T. Devalle, E. Meynier, and R. Simonetti-Cuizza. The production of eggs impregnated with iodine and their uses in the

treatment of children's ailments. Rept. Sixth World's Poultry Congress. 47. Germany. 1936.

Salvatore Terranova Leone. Production of iodized eggs. Boll. Chimfarm. 75:303. 1936.

Sumita, E., A. Kawabata, and Y. Fujioka. The influence of kelp meal feed on the iodine contents of the hen's eggs. Rept. Sixth World's Poultry Congress. 44. Germany. 1936.

Simpson, B. W., and R. Strand. Feeding iodine to poultry. New Zealand Jour. Agr. 40:403. 1930.

Wilder, O. H., R. M. Bethke, and P. R. Record. Iodine content of hen's eggs as affected by the ration. Jour. Nutr. 6:407. 1933.

77. Lyons, M., and W. M. Insko, Jr. Chondrodystrophy in the chick embryo produced by a mineral deficiency in the diet of the hen. Poultry Sci. 16:365. 1937.

78. Terroine and Belin. Influence de l'alimentation sur la composition quantitative de l'oeuf de poule. Bul. de la Societe de Chimie Biologique: 1074. 1927.

79. Buckner, G. D., and J. H. Martin. Effect of calcium on the composition of the eggs and carcass of laying hens. Jour. Biol. Chem. 41:195. 1920.

Buckner, G. D., J. H. Martin, and A. M. Peter. Effect of a calcium carbonate supplement in the diet of hens, on the weight, protein content, and calcium content of the white and yolk of their eggs. Am. Jour. Phys. 72:458. 1925.

80. Calvery, H. O., and H. W. Titus. The composition of the proteins of eggs from hens on different diets. Jour. Biol. Chem. 105:683. 1934.

Titus, H. W., T. C. Byerly, and N. R. Ellis. Effect of diet on egg composition. I. Partial chemical analysis of eggs produced by pullets on different diets. Jour. Nutr. 6:127. 1933.

81. McFarlane, W. D., H. L. Fulmer, and T. H. Jukes. Studies in embryonic mortality in the chick. I. The effect of diet upon the nitrogen, amino-nitrogen, tyrosine, tryptophane, cystine, and iron content of the proteins and on the total copper of the hen's egg. Biochem. Jour. 24:1611. 1930.

82. Pollard, C. B., and R. H. Carr. Cereal values as determined by number, fertility, and composition of eggs. Science, N.S. 59:22. 1924.

83. Cruickshank, E. M., J. Houston, and T. Moore. The effect of the dietary fat on the body fat and egg fat of the hen. Biochem. Jour. 33:1630. 1939.

Buckner, G. D., W. M. Insko, Jr., A. H. Henry, and E. F. Wachs. Effect of four all-mash rations on laying hens. Kentucky Bul. 495. 1947.

Davis, H. J., and C. W. Upp. Studies on the fat requirements of the domestic fowl. Poultry Sci. 20:459. 1941.

Halnan, E. T., and E. M. Cruickshank. Some aspects of fat metabolism in fowls and their practical significance. Proc. Fifth World's Poultry Congress (Rome) 2:612. 1933.

Reiser, R. Fatty acid changes in egg yolk of hens on a fat-free and a cottonseed oil ration. Jour. Nutr. 40:429. 1950.

Reiser, R. The biochemical conversions of conjugated dienoic and trienoic fatty acids. Arch. Biochem. & Biophys. 32:113. 1951.

Reiser, R. The syntheses and interconversions of polyunsaturated fatty acids by the laying hen. Jour. Nutr. 44:159. 1951.

84. Atwood, H., and C. E. Weakley, Jr. Certain characteristics of hen eggs. W. Va. Sta. Bul. 166. 1917.

85. Nalbandov, A. V., and L. E. Card. The problem of blood and meat spots in chicken eggs. II. Its importance in poultry flocks and a study of the nutritional factors involved. Poultry Sci. 26:400. 1947.

86. Anderson, C. F. Experiments at Parafield Poultry Station. Jour. Dept. of Agr. of South Australia. 42:584. 1939.

CHAPTER 10

FEEDING SYSTEMS AND PRACTICES

Considerable variation in feeding systems and practices is met with in recommendations for and actual feeding of poultry. Methods of feeding have long been given serious attention by poultrymen. Still there is no standard uniform method of feeding universally practiced by poultrymen. This lack of uniformity, no doubt, is an indication that the make-up of the ration and food intake are more important than the method of feeding. It has been pointed out repeatedly that food consumption and egg production follow each other closely. Hewitt[1] reports a very close relationship between egg yields and food consumption in 20 years of poultry feeding experiments.

Several types of rations or systems of feeding have been evolved and used. They range from the mashless, or all-grain, rations to the grainless, or all-mash, rations, with the combination or grain-mash rations ranging between the two extremes. Also various modifications or combinations of these systems are used. Each system has its advantages and disadvantages.

WHOLE-GRAIN METHOD

This was the original method of feeding poultry. When the flocks were small and the hens ranged over the farm, they picked up seeds and grains. When necessary to supplement this feeding, extra grain was fed in the barnyard. Later, when large numbers of birds were kept and were more closely confined, the grain was supplemented with some animal protein feed to take the place of bugs and worms. The first practice was to feed beef scrap dry in hoppers. The results[2-4] of early experiments were not entirely satisfactory in all cases, and this practice was superseded by combination rations.

Later experiments[5] have reported as good production and in some cases better production from feeding grain plus an abundant supply of liquid skimmilk or condensed buttermilk. It is possible to feed grains in various combinations. In the main, it is better not to limit the grain to one cereal. Average grain consumption was 73 pounds a year per hen and average milk consumption 13 gallons in the Kentucky trials. Excellent and economical egg production was obtained at the Washington Station by feeding unground grain mixtures (wheat and oats; wheat, barley, and oats; wheat, corn, and oats), supplemented with sour skimmilk. An average yearly production of approximately 250 eggs per pullet was obtained from all the pens in one series. About 55 pounds of dry feed and 185 pounds of milk per year were consumed by each Leghorn pullet.

Because of restricted milling, making wheat by-products unavailable, and because of transport difficulties, many Australian poultry farmers during World War II resorted to the feeding of soaked grain.[1] Wheat, being most plentiful, was the common choice of grain. Highly satisfactory results were obtained by feeding whole grain supplemented by meat meal.

ALL GRAIN FOR CHICKS. The feeding of all grain and beef scrap to chicks at Cornell[6] showed variable results, depending upon meat intake and food consumption.

In recent years the feeding of grain to chicks for the first 2 or 3 days has been recommended in order to prevent "pasting up." Peterson[7] reported that feeding chicks cracked grains as the only feed for the first 2 days had a protective value against "pasting up," where the first week brooder temperature was above or below 98° F. However, at the end of 3 weeks there was no significant difference in the average net gain, number of chicks "pasted up," or average feed consumption for either system of feeding. In groups brooded at low temperatures, the mortality was somewhat less where grain was given as the only feed for the first 2 days, as compared with those fed the all-mash ration.

POINTERS ON FEEDING ALL GRAIN. In connection with using home-grown laying rations, Carver[8] suggested that no one should feed a whole-grain plus milk ration without a regular daily supply of skimmilk or buttermilk. The whole grain should be limited to 16 pounds, and the milk supply should be at least 40 pounds per day per 100 birds.

MERITS OF THE ALL-GRAIN METHOD. Some of the advantages of the whole-grain system of feeding are:

1. Making possible easy use of large amounts of home-grown grains.
2. Saving expense and trouble of grinding.
3. Easy determination of quality of ingredients.

4. No loss of any part of the grain, such as the germ, when whole grains are used.

WHOLE-GRAIN AND GROUND-GRAIN OR COMBINATION SCRATCH-MASH METHOD

One of the early developments in poultry feeding was the use of ground feeds or mashes in connection with grain. In 1895 the New York Experiment Station at Geneva[9] reported that a pen of Leghorns, 37 per cent of whose food consisted or ground and moistened grain, produced eggs at a greater profit than did a pen of hens fed whole grain. Furthermore, two lots of laying hens of large and small breeds having their grain food whole only and dry, ate more food at a greater cost per fowl and for live weight.

ADVANTAGES OF THE SCRATCH-MASH SYSTEM. Some of the reasons or advantages of mash feeding are:

1. Less grinding for the gizzard. Less food needed.
2. Use of valuable by-products (milling, slaughter-house, etc.)
3. Convenient way to include animal protein feeds.
4. Higher protein ration possible.
5. Possibility to make variations to meet varying requirements.
6. Ease of balancing mineral and protein and vitamin deficiency of grains.

DISADVANTAGES OF THE SCRATCH-MASH SYSTEM. The chief disadvantage seems to be the difficulty of knowing the proportions of grain and mash which a hen consumes. Also, it is easy to throw the ration out of balance by a variation in the proportion of grain to mash consumed. This is particularly true where the birds eat heavily of grain, because there is likely to be a protein and mineral deficiency. Consuming too much mash also disturbs the balance, but in this case there is an excess of these nutrients and it is not so serious since the hens can care for a considerable excess. However, the cost is increased because of the higher-priced protein feeds.

GROUND-GRAIN OR ALL-MASH METHOD

The New York (Geneva) Experiment Station[10] reported, in 1897, that a ration consisting mostly of the ordinary ground-grain foods and containing no whole grain was more profitably fed to chicks than another ration consisting mostly of whole grain and containing no ground grain. More food was eaten when the ground grain was fed than when the whole grain was fed, and the chicks made more rapid gains.

In 1903 Stewart and Atwood[2] concluded that "with young White Leghorn fowls a large proportion, if not all, of the ration can be composed of ground food without diminishing either the egg production, decreasing the hatchability of the eggs, or injuring the health of the fowls."

Satisfactory gains were secured at Cornell[6] with chicks up to 6 and 8 weeks on rations that were fed in the ground form.

Wisconsin,[11] in 1924, reported the successful rearing of 6,000 birds on an all-mash ration. This ration consisted of 80 parts of ground yellow corn, 20 parts of wheat middlings, 5 parts of raw bone, 5 parts of pearl grits, and 1 part of salt. Skimmed milk was given ad libitum as a drink and no water. Since then there has been a renewed interest in all-mash feeding.

The all-mash system of feeding ignores the exercise theory of feeding scratch grain. It is believed, by its advocates, that the birds secure enough exercise in the ordinary activity of feeding and walking about the pen.

ALL MASH FOR HENS. Buss of the Ohio Experiment Station[4] reported no difference in the number of eggs produced per hen in 2 years from hens receiving all-mash and hens receiving grain-mash rations. Since that time many experiments have reported practically no difference between the two methods[12] from the standpoint of amount of feed, number of eggs, size of eggs, weight of hens, mortality, health, fertility, and hatchability. A few trials indicated more uniform results with the all-mash ration. In some instances the grinding of feeds for the all-mash ration made it uneconomical.

Many experiments[13] report better results with rations containing both mash and scratch grain as compared with all-mash rations. Some trials report a tendency for birds to gain more weight on grain-mash rations. Also yolks were more variable in color in the grain-mash lots than in the all-mash lots.

In experiments conducted at Cornell, the difference in egg production, especially for pullets, has usually been in favor of the grain-mash rations, as shown in Table 16.

The Western Washington Station[14] concluded that the all-mash ration proved satisfactory where skimmilk was available as a drink.

During World War II, because of the scarcity of grain, British poultry producers were forced to feed an all-mash diet. The

TABLE 16. EGG PRODUCTION ON ALL-MASH AND GRAIN-MASH RATIONS AT CORNELL

Year	All Mash	Grain and Mash
	Pullets	
1927	173 ± 5.4	188 ± 3.7
1928	195 ± 4.3	205 ± 4.7
	179 ± 5.3	194 ± 4.5
	189 ± 4.7	200 ± 6.2
1929	203 ± 6.2	218 ± 5.5
1930	194 ± 5.6	226 ± 4.6
1931	210 ± 3.8	220 ± 5.7
Av.	191.6 ± 1.99	207.4 ± 1.84
	Hens	
1930	170 ± 3.9	184 ± 3.4
1931	176 ± 2.5	175 ± 4.5

results were sufficiently favorable to raise the question as to whether they would return to grain feeding when the war was over. Some authorities think not because they believe that feeding mash is cheaper.

High energy all-mash rations have proven very satisfactory. The development of mechanical feeders[15] has also favored the all-mash ration by raising total feed consumption.

ALL MASH FOR CHICKS. This method of feeding has proved very popular for chick feeding. The Ohio Experiment Station[12, 16] has used it successfully for many years. A Colorado report showed that the all-mash ration gave greater uniformity of growth, less death loss, and was more economical. The South Dakota Station[17] indicated all mash was satisfactory for chicks and simplified feeding. Feed consumption was reported less in the all-mash lot. However, after 6 to 8 weeks the scratch and mash ration was considered more successful. Reports from England[18] indicate no difference in weight at 20 weeks, cost of feeding, and quality of pullets produced on the all-mash as compared with the grain-mash system. Experience at Cornell also shows this condition. Other experiment stations indicate the all-mash method to be preferable for chicks.

ALL MASH FOR FATTENING. A review of fattening practices indicates almost universal agreement in using ground feeds almost exclusively for this purpose.

ADVANTAGES OF THE ALL-MASH SYSTEM. Some of the favorable points of this system might be listed as follows:

1. More sanitary. The feed does not have a chance to become

contaminated by damp and filthy litter. (This would also apply where grain is hopper-fed.)

2. Simplicity. Fewer mixtures need be considered, and routine is simplified.

3. Less skill required in feeding. Superior results will probably be secured in the hands of the unskilled feeder.

4. Less labor required.

5. No change of feed. A mash mixture is fed throughout the period.

6. A definite ration. There is no guesswork or confusion about what proportion of scratch grain to feed.

7. More uniform food intake. Each individual gets all the ingredients of the ration in the same proportion. This advantage makes the system particularly adaptable to experimental work.

8. Uniformity of growth.

9. Uniformity of yolk color.

10. Adaptable to mechanical feeders.

DISADVANTAGES OF THE ALL-MASH SYSTEM.

1. Less flexible. Proportions of grain to mash cannot be varied to meet changing needs of the birds. This might necessitate frequent changing of the all-mash mixture or supplementation.

2. More and better feeding appliances needed.

3. Ground grains are slightly more expensive.

4. It is more difficult to teach chicks to eat mash.

ALL-MASH FEEDING PRACTICE. The all-mash rations usually contain a larger amount of cereals and one-half the amount of protein concentrates that are used in mashes to be fed with grain. The mixture should not be too fine; otherwise food consumption will be discouraged. Feeding fresh mash at least once a day (prefereably in the afternoon) will also encourage consumption. Sufficient hopper space must be furnished, and the hopper must be of the type that will not clog. The National Institute of Poultry Husbandry in England gives the following specifications for feeding space when all-mash rations are used:

1-4 weeks	6 feet per 100
4-10 weeks	12-14 feet per 100
10-20 weeks	16-20 feet per 100
Mature	24 feet per 100

With all-mash mixtures there is less stirring over of the litter. The litter is likely to become matted and wet. In this respect, proper sanitation is more difficult in the all-mash pens and necessitates more frequent cleaning.

If the mature birds are to be fed an all-mash ration, it is best to feed an all-mash ration to the chicks.

In making up all-mash rations, one must be sure that they are complete and that the mixture is one that can be eaten in sufficient quantity. In some instances, difficulty was encountered in developing all-mash rations. These rations were adapted from combination laying mashes in common use, with the result that they were too bulky because of a high content of fiber-rich feeds. It is not possible for a hen to eat as much of such a mash during a day as of a heavier, more concentrated mash. Bulkiness in a mash is not a serious fault, however, when a mash possessing this characteristic is fed along with a scratch mixture consisting mainly of cracked corn and wheat. But when a bulky mash is fed as an all-mash ration and it is not possible to get satisfactory results, the tendency is to blame the all-mash system of feeding. This blame, however, is unwarranted. The blame must be laid to the bulky nature of the mash, which makes it impossible for the birds to eat as much feed as those fed a ration consisting of both scratch and mash mixtures. In other words, the all-mash ration was incomplete. Its nutritive value was low because of too high a content of fiber-rich feeds. High energy mashes have overcome this difficulty.

PELLETS OR CUBED FEEDS

This system of feeding is really a modification or adaptation of the all-mash system. It consists of mechanically pressing the mash into hard dry pellets or "artificial grains."

Dairy farmers and feeders of other forms of livestock in Europe have long been accustomed to feed balanced rations in the form of nuts or cubes. The idea has also been applied to a considerable extent to poultry feeding.

PELLETS FOR HENS. The National Institute of Poultry Husbandry[19] in England, in one report, indicates that pellets have given satisfactory results and compare favorably with all-mash feeding. In another trial, one of the B vitamins was destroyed in the pelleting process, which adversely affected hatchability of the eggs and growth of the chicks, with loss of chicks showing symptoms of vitamin B deficiency.

At Cornell a pen of pullets fed pellets laid 175 eggs, whereas the all-mash pen laid 189 eggs per bird. Other reports[20] show favorable results for pellets when fed to hens. Some observations on pellet feed were better maintenance of body weight and greater tendency toward cannibalism. A report from Germany[21] indicates that hens prefer grain to pellets, that better production was secured by feeding the birds mash and grain, and that the feeding of pellets was not economical. In these experiments it was clearly shown that the birds distinguished between differently shaped pellets and nuts.

Pelleting high fiber feeds[22] such as oat hulls, alfalfa meal, and feed screenings increased the effectiveness of these feeds as compared with them in non-pelleted form.

PELLETS FOR YOUNG STOCK.[23] From the point of view of growth and food consumption per unit of gain, a ration in pellet form has been reported as good or superior to one supplied as dry mash. The mash-fed chicks usually consume more feed as well as feed per unit of gain than the pellet-fed chicks. The pellet-fed chicks usually gain more and consume more water. A greater incidence and severity of feather picking is likely to occur with pellet-fed birds, especially when the chicks are confined. At Cornell pelleting a medium-energy chick ration improved the same so as to make it comparable to a high-energy ration. The increase in growth, due to pelleting, is more marked as the fiber in the ration is increased.

In comparing pellets versus mash for table duck production, Tallent[24] secured slightly greater weights for the ducklings fed the mash. The ducklings did not eat the dry pellets readily till they were 5 weeks old. On the other hand, McMurray[25] observed no difficulty in this respect and obtained better growth with pellets. At Cornell[26] feeding pellets to ducklings resulted in best growth when compared with other methods of feeding. Serfontein[27] found no difference in weight between lots receiving whole dry pellets and those being fed ground pellets in a wet form. Feeding the dry whole pellets resulted in less feed wastage, saved labor and hopper space, and was more hygienic.

Pellets have also been fed satisfactorily to turkeys.[28] There seems to be some advantage in offering a choice of coarse and fine particles at the start. Pelleting enables a satisfactory use of higher levels of dehydrated green feeds.

ADVANTAGES OF PELLET FEEDING. The advocates of this system of feeding advance the following points in its favor:

1. No waste. There is little billing of feed out of the hoppers, and when knocked out of the feed hopper the pellets are often picked up again.

2. No clogging of hoppers.
3. No selection of ingredients.
4. Every kernel is balanced.
5. Less storage space required, as the bulk of the feed is reduced by compression.
6. Greater convenience in feeding.
7. More sanitary, especially when fed in hoppers.
8. More palatable. Hens naturally prefer a granular feed. This may mean increased consumption.
9. Time and labor saved in feeding.
10. Feeding simplified. (Can be fed like grain or mash or both.)
11. Less feed required.
12. Less feeding space required.

DISADVANTAGES OF PELLET FEEDING.

1. Cost of manufacture.
2. Less flexibility.
3. Camouflaging of the ingredients.
4. More vices. Owing to less exercise and the fact that a bird can fill up quickly on pellets, there may be more toe picking, cannibalism, and feather pulling.
5. Crumbling of pellets.
6. Vitamin content of ration may be affected. This is true if the feeds are subjected to high temperatures.

Pellets are produced in varying sizes to meet the needs of the size of the birds. To adults usually the pellets 1/8 to 3/16 inch in diameter are fed. They may be fed as an all-in-one ration, may be used in connection with scratch feed, or may be used as a supplement to either. They can be fed in combination with an all-mash ration without upsetting the balance. They may be fed either in hoppers or in the litter for extra exercise. They can be used as a supplement in place of wet-mash feeding. Sometimes difficulty is experienced in getting sufficient pellet consumption during the short days of winter. In that case it may be necessary to litter-feed some pellets and even moisten and feed them.

The feeding of pellets, either alone or in connection with mash, has proved satisfactory for birds kept in batteries or cages.

KERNELS

Kernels constitute an all-mash ration made in granular form so that it cannot be "unscrambled" by the birds. They are produced by compressing dry, finely ground foods into hard or granular form by means of tremendous pressure. Except for form, they are similar in many respects to pellets. The advantages indicated for pellets also, in the main, hold for kernels. Some improvement in growth rate has been reported from the feeding of granules to chicks.[29]

FREE-CHOICE OR CAFETERIA SYSTEM

In this method of feeding the bird is given a chance to select its own feeds since the individual feeds are made available separately. This system is advocated by some on the grounds that individuality is the basic biological factor. The individual needs of the hen vary, depending upon its weight, production, and condition. It is believed by some feeders that the hen will balance her own ration if given an opportunity, owing to an instinctive ability of animals to choose the proper food constituents when given free choice of diet. This ability to balance their ration has been shown to a surprising extent by some farm animals. Of man it has been stated that, in ordinary life, appetite is a fairly reliable guide to the quantity of fuel food required (the more work the larger the appetite), but it is no guide to the right kind of food. Likes and dislikes are not a reliable guide, especially among an abundance of artificial foods. As a result of a study of individuality in the nutritive instincts and of the causes and effects of variations in the selection of food, Dove[30] states that the expressions of the nutritive instincts vary from individual to individual. Some individuals appear wise and others unwise (less wise) in their choice of food. This fact contraindicates the group technique of free-choice feeding.

In discussing how animals choose their food, Harris[31] states that the power of picking out the particular food is possible only under certain quite special circumstances and by no means always. Animals chose the right food if it "made them feel better" almost immediately after they had eaten it, and they could then associate their rapid recovery with the particular food that they had just eaten. If a "reward" follows the eating of a particular food and if there is something about the smell or taste or looks of the food by which the animal is able to recognize the food again and distinguish it from other foods, he will learn to take it quite easily. (This is a matter of experience and not instinct.) Rats may actually die from protein starvation when offered pure protein, fats, etc., because of delayed effect. Reactions to vitamin B and salt are immediate. The effect of cod liver oil is not immediate.

Jukes[32] showed that the choice of food by chicks was the same when the sugar content was varied, even when the amount of sugar was as high as 20 per cent. Marked preference was shown when the salt content was above 2 per cent, the quinine content above 0.03 per cent, or the citric acid above 2 per cent. Tests to determine whether the taste factor (sugar content) was important in the chicks' choice of food in vitamin G and A deficient diets were negative.

Price[33] concluded that chicks have the ability to select the proper feeds. This ability was shown in their selection of butters high in a factor that increased the blood calcium and phosphorus and prolonged life. When given free choice of samples of butter that could not be distinguished by man, the chicks selected and ate two and one-half times as much of the butter containing a large amount of the active factor as they did of the butter containing a small amount of it.

It has been reported by workers in Germany[34] that the appetite of poultry is not only dependent on physiologic conditions but that it is also strongly influenced psychologically by various outside influences. The manner in which food is given influences consumption. More is eaten from large than from small piles. The approach of one or more hungry hens is of influence. More is eaten when the birds are fed together than when they are fed separately. A hen that had to watch two other birds eat first took 42 per cent more food than normally. More food is eaten from a soft surface than from a hard surface. Large grains are preferred to small. Less is eaten in semi-darkness, in green light, and in blue light than in red or yellow light. Chicks picked at all kinds of objects which were clearly distinguishable from the subsoil or background if the objects could be taken in the beak. However, they swallowed only that which was really nutritive.

The hen can distinguish three tastes—salt, sour, and bitter. However, the taste sense is not important since chickens select feed more by shape, size, color, and surface condition.[35]

De Bocarmé[36] observed that poultry eat a certain amount of such substances as dry leaves, beech twigs, pebbles, glass, splinters, but that these are consumed in an attempt to furnish the necessary mineral salts. Therefore, if the feed is completely adequate, the animals will automatically cease to devour substances other than feed.

Food consumption is also influenced by the condition of the feed. Alder[37] reported that coarse mashes are more desirable for laying hens than finely ground mashes and resulted in higher egg production and lower mortality.

It has been shown[38] that there is variation in the kinds and proportions of the ingredients that individuals will select. They also vary as regards the efficiency with which they utilize food. The amounts of the different foods varied with the condition of the birds; that is, whether they were laying or not. The greatest changes, while laying, were in beef scrap and shell consumption. The laying ration was narrower.

Graham[39] states that chicks do not grow faster or have less mortality on a free-choice diet, but the free-choice chickens, on the whole, were much more contented than the check lots and were much less inclined to feather pulling.

Funk[40] states that chicks were able to select a balanced ration and grow normally to 8 weeks if the necessary ingredients were accessible. Results from the Minnesota[41] Station indicate that chicks are able to select their correct protein level only when a high-protein mash is fed with the grain.

In a comparison of free choice of grain and mash mixtures, Amon[42] reported no appreciable difference in weight at 24 weeks, in mortality, or in rate of maturity.

The results with hens have been variable. Some reports[43-45] indicate satisfactory production with free-choice feeding as compared with controlled feeding. Other experiments[42, 46] favor the controlled feeding.

Graham[47] reports considerable variation in the intake of whole corn, whole oats, and mash when hens are allowed free choice. The intake by an individual also varies from day to day and week to week.

A report from South Africa[48] shows that, with three groups of laying pullets fed mashes low, medium, and high in protein, there was a tendency for the three groups to adjust the protein to a common level by varying the relative amounts of mash and grain consumed.

Since birds fed free-choice usually consume a larger proportion of grain, mash concentrates, or mixtures containing higher amounts of protein, have been suggested for use with hopper feeding of grain. However, Kennard and Chamberlin[49] show that, whereas flocks varied greatly in the proportion of whole corn, wheat, or oats they consumed, the proportion of total grain to mash was comparatively constant and in proportion to the protein content of the mash. With free choice of grain, many feeders prefer the higher protein mash because of the natural tendency for the birds to consume grain and hence less risk of a protein deficiency. Tomhave and Skoglund[50] report excellent production with New Hampshire pullets when given free choice of a 32 per cent protein concentrate and a mixture of corn, wheat, and oats. With Barred Rock pullets fed free-choice grain and 21 per cent protein mash, egg production was low and mortality high. In this case, the birds consumed too much grain.

Davidson and associates[51] report approximately 6 per cent of the deaths in White Leghorn pullets due to cannibalism under the all-mash system and approximately 36 per cent where mash and grain were fed by the "cafeteria" system. Von Ebbell,[52] reporting on cannibalism in laying hens, states that all remedies recommended failed to subdue the vice once started, with the exception of a change in feeding practice from free-choice feeding of grain and mash (which results in higher grain consumption) to rationed grain feeding. Kennard and Chamberlin[53] reported that feather picking and cannibalism became so firmly established in 6 groups of 70 Rhode Island Red pullets each, fed on low-protein (15 to 17 per cent) rations and whole grains, that it was necessary in controlling them to remove the upper beak by a special tearing process.

In all trials, it is noted that certain feeds are not consumed in quantities. Palatability is an important factor in the free-choice system. The feeds must be readily eaten by the birds. Probably, too, as in the case of continuous hopper feeding, regulation of some feeds at certain times may be necessary.

HOPPER FEEDING

Mash, grit, shell, and charcoal are usually hopper fed. Grain may be hand fed in the litter or hopper fed. The chief reason advanced for feeding grain in litter has been to induce the birds to exercise. The hopper feeding of grain is based on the assumption that laying hens do not need to scratch in litter, but get enough exercise in their regular activities. However, the feeding of at least part of the grain in litter helps to keep the litter in better condition than feeding all the grain in hoppers or troughs. With hopper feeding of grain, the hens can eat the feed quickly. This may be an advantage in winter. It might also assure hens going to roost with full crops. The free choice of grain usually results in a greater consumption of grain. Hopper feeding favors the saving of labor and ensures more correct feeding where the poultryman is either inexperienced or cannot afford the time for regular hand feeding.

HOPPER FEEDING OF GRAIN TO HENS. Rice[3] reported no difference in egg production between two pens receiving grain plus beef scrap, one of which was hand fed the grain and the other hopper fed. Similarly, reports from other stations[4, 54, 55] show no difference in egg production where the grain is fed in litter or where it is hopper fed.

In Australia[56] an average production of 179 eggs, where grain was always before the birds, was obtained as compared with 164 eggs, where it was fed in the litter.

Other experiments[42, 55, 57] show better results where the grain is limited as in litter feeding. Free-choice feeding of grain and mash in these instances resulted in lower egg production, higher cannibalism mortality, and greater feed cost per dozen eggs. Greater variability in yolk color was produced by the free-choice feeding of grain. The difference was greater for Leghorns than for the heavier breeds.

In experiments conducted at Cornell there was no difference between feeding the grain in the litter or in hoppers in the case of hens. With pullets there was no difference in some trials, with a slight favor for the litter feeding in others (Table 17).

TABLE 17. EGG PRODUCTION OF HENS WITH HOPPER FEEDING GRAIN AT CORNELL

Year	Grain in Litter	Grain in Hopper
	Pullets	
1928	194 ± 4.5	193 ± 4.4
	200 ± 6.2	189 ± 4.4
1929	218 ± 5.5	217 ± 4.9
1930	226 ± 4.6	207 ± 5.5
1931	220 ± 5.7	214 ± 4.3
	211.3 ± 2.3	203.5 ± 2.2
	Hens	
1930	184 ± 3.4	184 ± 3.7
1931	159 ± 4.6	159 ± 3.9

In comparing hopper feeding of grain, with the hoppers open all the time, as contrasted to that with the hoppers open only at night, the New Hampshire Station[58] concludes that either system is satisfactory and that the birds adjust their feed intake to their requirements. In this trial the birds ate almost as much mash as grain.

In experiments conducted at Cornell comparing hopper feeding of grain at night only with grain available in hoppers all the time, the egg production was:

Year	Night Grain Only	Grain Available All the Time	Regulated Grain Available
1929	217 ± 4.9	215 ± 5.0	
	210 ± 3.5 216 ± 4.8	213 ± 4.8	
1930	207 ± 5.5	190 ± 6.5	
1931	214 ± 4.3		209 ± 4.7

The first year there was no difference in results. The next year the production was lower for those birds that had the grain available all the time. A study of the records, however, indicated that there were only a few times during the year when the production was not equal to that of the other pen and during those periods the birds consumed much more grain than mash. Consequently, the next year the birds were allowed constant access to grain, except when they ate too large a proportion of grain (more than 2 parts of grain to 1 of mash), in which case the hoppers were closed during the forenoon. This practice avoided the slumps with the result that there was little difference in the average yearly production.

Higher grain and lower mash consumption by the birds on free-choice grain emphasized the need of a mash with a higher content of vitamins and protein than is necessary for best results with the standard program.[58] Continuous hopper feeding of grain has been reported more successful when fed with a high-protein concentrate mash.[59] The Ohio Station[60] suggests the free choice of whole-grain and mash concentrate for layers primarily for farm poultry keepers, who produce their grains and who desire a minimum additional expense in balancing their poultry rations. Skoglund[61] suggests that the concentrate system is not as well suited to Leghorns as to the heavier breeds. Hays[62] concluded that with free-choice feeding of grain a high-protein mash was desirable for high-producing layers.

AUTOMATIC GRAIN FEEDERS

The feeding of grain by means of automatic feeders is similar in effect to the hopper feeding of grain constantly. The early automatic grain feeders were planned to give the birds more exercise by dropping grain in small amounts into the litter. Automatic feeders were serviceable for people with irregular hours, since most people appreciated the advisability of regular routine in caring for flocks. The limitations of the automatic feeders are that they cannot exercise judgment in the balance of grain and mash, and do not enable or encourage close observation of the condition of the flock.

MECHANICAL FEEDERS. Mechanical feeders have been developed recently to automatically feed mash and pellets or grain to large flocks. These consist of a central hopper or feed supply from which run troughs to carry the feed through the house. The feed is moved through the troughs by means of a chain or similar contrivance. The movement of feed can be controlled so as to be continuous or intermittent. These automatic feeders are adapted to large flock operations of young or mature birds. They save time and labor in feeding and in many instances feed wastage. The mechanically fed groups eat more than corresponding hand-fed groups.

Reported trials[15] have shown no significant difference in egg production, body weight, or mortality for the mechanically fed lots as compared with hand-fed groups.

Both all-mash and grain-mash rations have been used with automatic feeders. All-mash high-energy rations have been preferred. It has been suggested that for maximum production it is necessary to supplement the all-mash mixture with pellets.[63]

WET VS. DRY MASH

The feeding of wet mash was one of the first supplements used in connection with grain feeding of poultry. It was usually fed one or more times a day, and the birds were given all they would eat. The dry-mash system, in which the dry mash is kept before the birds for a certain part or all of the day, came into use about 1900.

EXPERIMENTS WITH HENS. In 1907 Rice[3] reported an egg production of 129 eggs for hens having dry mash available all day and being hand fed grain twice a day, as compared with 121 eggs for hens being fed wet mash at noon and hand fed grain twice a day. Buss[4] also reported approximately the same production over a period of 2 years for hens fed the mash dry in hoppers or fed moist mash once daily in a trough.

Reports from Australia[56, 64] show an advantage in egg production in feeding supplemental wet mash. Results from England[65] show the lowest production when feeding wet mash only and improvement when the dry mash is supplemented with wet mash. The combination of the two proved particularly advantageous during the winter months. Body weights were also maintained more satisfactorily.

A report from South Africa[66] indicated more eggs from birds receiving dry mash than from birds getting a wet mash. In one experiment at Cornell, feeding wet mash only at noon gave a lower yearly egg production (141 eggs) than where dry mash only was available all the time (161 eggs). We find, however, in this case that most of the difference is traceable to one period, when feeders were changed and the birds consumed less food. When a wet mash was fed as a supplement to the dry mash, the results were not always consistent. Usually there is a small increase, especially during the fall and winter months (Table 18).

TABLE 18. WET-MASH FEEDING AT CORNELL

Method of Feeding	No Wet Mash	Plus Supplemental Wet Mash
All mash	179 ± 5.3	189 ± 4.7
Trough-fed grain + dry mash	193 ± 4.4	189 ± 4.7
	212	{ 232 216
Litter-fed grain + dry mash	194 ± 4.5	200 ± 6.2
	136 ± 3.1	127 ± 3.3

The supplemental wet mash should be fed toward the middle of the day and preferably before the night feeding of grain, unless it is desired to increase the proportion of grain consumed. Where the supplemental wet mash was fed after the night grain, the birds consumed 49 per cent of the total feed in the form of grain, as compared with 44 per cent of the total feed in the form of grain where the supplemental wet mash was fed before the night grain or at noon.

Results from North Dakota[67] indicated that the feeding of a moist fleshing mash made little difference in the rate of egg production, percentage gain in weight, or mortality of either Rhode Island Red or White Leghorn pullets. The use of the moist fleshing mash materially decreased the consumption of whole grains and decreased somewhat the consumption of dry mash. Heavy feeding of grains was equally as effective as a moist fleshing mash in increasing the body weight of laying pullets, and, since egg production and mortality were not affected, it was concluded that the producer receives no extra return for the time spent in making and feeding a moist fleshing mash.

The North Carolina Station[68] reported benefits from feeding yeast-fermented mash as compared with wet mash. The yeast-fermented mash, when fed both to White Leghorns and to Rhode Island Reds, stimulated the appetite and led to higher feed consumption and higher egg production. The birds also came into production more rapidly. In one test the mortality rate was also lower.

A survey of poultry farms in 1926, by E. G. Misner of the Department of Agricultural Economics at Cornell, indicated a greater production on those farms that fed wet mash the year round. These results were not confirmed, however, in a subsequent survey of 123 poultry farms for the year ended September 30, 1930. His conclusions from the latter survey are:

> Rations now contain more dried milk products than a few years ago. They are more palatable. Illumination and the use of cod liver oil are more general. The advantage of using wet mash does not appear as great as when a study was made in 1926. Still, poultrymen using wet mash obtain three-fourths of a dozen eggs more than those feeding no wet mash.

	Number of Farms	Eggs per Hen	Per Cent Lay, October-December
No wet mash	28	140	20
Wet mash irregularly	51	149	21
Wet mash year round	44	147	26

In summarizing reports from pullet management campaigns in New York State, no difference in annual production was reported from farms feeding wet mash as compared with those using dry mash only. This might lead one to conclude that the use of wet mash does not help in sustaining high egg production. However, a flock that is vigorous and healthy and well housed can maintain good production without resort to wet mash or other encouragements to greater mash consumption. Very often it is only after a flock has failed to produce satisfactorily that the owner resorts to wet-mash feeding, hoping for improvement. Hence it may be to the credit of wet-mash feeding that results in such flocks are as good as they are.

EXPERIMENTS WITH YOUNG STOCK. In the production of table poultry conducted in England,[69] dry mash as a rearing ration gave better results than wet mash, but there was no difference between a dry mash and a combination of wet and dry mash. Other experiments[70] show no significant difference between dry-mash and wet-mash feeding for growing chicks.

ADVANTAGES OF DRY-MASH FEEDING. Some of the points in favor of the dry-mash system are:

1. Less labor.
2. Large flocks possible. All the birds have an equal chance for feeding.
3. No freezing in winter.
4. No must, mold, or sourness in summer.
5. Less apparatus required. Where large quantities of wet mash are used, mixers are necessary.

ADVANTAGES OF WET-MASH FEEDING.

1. More palatable if properly used. Stimulates food consumption, although this may be only temporary.
2. Less sorting and wasting.
3. Swollen feed.
4. Waste meat, table scraps, etc., readily included.

MASH FEEDING PRACTICE. The generally accepted practice is to keep the dry mash in front of the birds all the time as the main source of mash. The dry mash is then supplemented with a wet mash or pellets when it is necessary to maintain or increase food intake. (The regular laying mash can be used as satisfactorily as a special fattening mash.) Feeding a wet mash is not necessary all the time or when the birds are consuming enough food in the dry form. Feeding extra milk or increasing food consumption in other ways will have the same effect as feeding a wet mash.

High-protein mashes are often used. Davidson[71] reports slightly less total feed with such a supplement. Home-grown grains can be used to better advantage by using a high-protein mash. However, this increases the problem of supplying the vitamins.

FORM IN WHICH TO FEED GRAIN

Grain is frequently fed in the bundle, and corn is fed on the cob. They are fed so with the idea of saving threshing or shelling, or to give the hens more exercise. It is possible to accomplish these things, but we need to keep in mind that by so doing we may not know exactly how much grain we are feeding. The tendency is to underfeed on grain rather than to overfeed. Besides, there is a rapid accumulation of straw or cobs which needs to be taken care of. Straw probably will need to be removed more frequently than is necessary for sanitary purposes.

Shall the corn be fed whole or cracked? Feeding whole corn has certain advantages, such as decreasing the danger of spoiling, avoiding the loss of part of the grain in cracking, and more readily determining the quality. As long as the kernels are not too large, it can be fed. If whole corn is to be fed to the hens, it is advisable to begin feeding the same to the pullets on range. The basis for feeding cracked corn is to produce a larger number of particles and induce the hen to greater activity, that is, to give her more exercise. Activity is necessary to make the hens healthier, to strengthen the muscles, to make them eat more, and to produce heat and body activity, which is essential for production. The feeding of finer particles probably depends upon whether or not the bird gets enough exercise in its ordinary activities. Some think that a hen will eat more whole corn because it can be picked up quickly. This, however, does not necessarily hold true. Often the hens will eat more of the cracked corn, in which case it might be an advantage to feed it.

Soaking grain in milk or water has also been practiced.[72] Hadlington reports that a flock of 150 pullets fed for 3 months on soaked wheat showed higher return over cost of feeding than the flock fed on the ordinary ration. Newman states that the soaking of grain for 24 hours is an economic proposition, resulting in improved health, better production, and a slight reduction in the amount of food consumed.

In a study of palatability of grains, Newbigin and Linton[73] state that "one fact stands out clearly in this experiment, and that is that the first four foods selected by the chicks, namely, millet, canary seed, dari, and hemp, are the only grains (with the exception of linseed) offered to the chicks in their natural state, i.e., neither decorticated nor kibbled. It may, therefore, be that the deciding factor in the natural selection of food by young chicks is the condition in which they are offered, 'natural' foods being selected in preference to 'treated' foods."

PRACTICES IN CONNECTION WITH FEEDING LIQUIDS

Is it necessary to feed both water and milk when we are using liquid milk as our source of animal protein feed? That will depend to quite an extent upon the season of the year and the extent to which it is necessary to have the birds consume the liquid product. It will depend upon whether milk is being supplied as a food or drink or both. If the birds are not getting any meat scraps in their mash, it will be necessary to restrict and sometimes entirely eliminate the water in order to get them to consume sufficient quantities of milk. On the other hand, if we restrict the water or eliminate it, we need to use the milk as their drink also. Under those conditions, they are likely to consume larger amounts of the liquid milk than are necessary. This would not be economical. Where the birds get meat scrap in their mash, usually a combination of water and milk is used. Both are kept available or the milk is fed alone until consumed, at which time water is supplied.

The question is often asked whether it is necessary to warm the water in the winter.[74] If the water is too cold, it will not stimulate consumption, and we need to get a considerable water consumption in order to have the birds function properly. Records from Oregon indicate that pullets drank 25.4 per cent more warmed water than cold water during freezing weather and that water consumption was increased 5 per cent per pullet and 4.2 per cent per 100 eggs laid by warming it during average western Oregon winter weather, in which the temperatures were above freezing 90 per cent of the time. Beresford, reporting results obtained in Idaho, states that the pens receiving 40 to 50 F. degree water gave an egg production record decidedly in favor of the pens receiving the warm water. In these pens also 20 per cent more water was consumed.

Frequently hot water is used to mix a wet mash during cold weather because some think that a warm mash is more appetizing.

Therefore, it is advisable at least to take off the chill from the water in cold weather. Where heating appliances are used to keep the water from freezing, this is automatically taken care of. Otherwise, warm water can be furnished two or three times a day.

On the other hand, a cool drink in the summer is also relished by the hen. Anything that will increase the contentment of the birds will probably have its effect on production.

COOKING FEEDS

A number of years ago it was quite common to cook feeds for poultry. With the increase in the size of flocks, this practice has very largely disappeared. Certain feeds, such as beans and potatoes, seem to be improved for poultry by cooking. Cooking involves extra equipment, expense, and labor, which it is doubtful are repaid in results.

RANGE VS. CONFINEMENT

The question of range as compared with confinement resolves itself into whether or not the birds are getting what is necessary for them. The favorable results previously obtained by free range, as compared with confinement, are due probably not so much to the fact that the birds had free range as to the fact that they were getting nutrients under free-range conditions, which they were not getting when they were kept confined. It is possible to restrict birds to comparatively small areas and get just as good results if they are getting the same nutrients as birds on free range. Access to outdoors, for exercise and sunshine, and provision for green feed will give just as good results as running on the range. Poor results from confinement are due to a deficiency in the ration rather than to the fact that the birds did not have a chance to range. With the development of commercial poultry keeping the practice is for greater confinement of both growing chicks and laying stock. In addition, many poultrymen are now keeping their chicks for the first few weeks of life in battery brooders, where the amount of space provided is much more limited than in ordinary confinement.

These changed practices in management, as well as new developments in methods of feeding, have brought the manner of feeding strongly to the attention of poultrymen and have led to the belief on the part of some that the newer systems of feeding might be responsible, in some unknown manner, for certain of the difficulties occurring frequently in poultry. The belief, however, is not well founded. It should be remembered that the confinement of poultry has brought about restriction of exercise and a change in the nature of the ration. As long as unlimited range was provided, hens were to some extent independent of the ration supplied, for they were able to supplement this ration with succulent green food, bugs and worms, and other poultry titbits, the food value of which, except for the green feed, is little known. Furthermore, restriction of exercise and confinement to the neighborhood of the feed hoppers has caused greater feed consumption, which in turn has stimulated growth and egg production.

Confinement has given better control of sanitation and other conditions. However, a complete ration and more exact feeding and management are required to prevent vices and troubles.

FEED RESTRICTION

Heywang[75] showed that restricting the amount of diet intake to 75 per cent and 87½ per cent of the amount consumed by the group fed on an ad libitum basis caused a decrease in the total average number of eggs produced but did not affect the average size of the egg laid by the fowls in the different groups or the average body weight of the fowls.

Burmester and Card[76] report the effect of restricted feeding time when feeding an all-mash ration and pellets to Leghorn-Rhode Island crossbreds kept in individual laying cages. With the all-mash ration, body weight and egg production declined rapidly when hens were restricted to less than 6 hours of feeding time each day. The mash-fed hens, when restricted to short feeding periods, would eat continuously for more than an hour, when feed was offered, in an effort to get sufficient total food. Hens fed pellets could eat a given quantity of feed in a much shorter time and hence were able to maintain their weight and to continue to lay while on feeding schedules as short as 2 hours daily in one continuous period, or 20 minutes every 12 hours.

Temperton and Dudley[77] found that restriction of food of laying pullets, under a system of dry-mash feeding, resulted in lower egg production and lower final body weight, as compared with birds fed ad libitum. Where pullets had access to mash on only 6 days of each week, there was little difference in egg production; final body weights were slightly in favor of the unrestricted birds; there was a 6 per cent saving of feed in favor of the restricted feeding. Taylor[78] found production not as good where hoppers were closed 2 hours a day as where they were open all the time and a decided decrease in production where the hoppers were closed one day a week.

Fangauf and Haensel[79] report that, when hens have free access to mash, the restriction of the amount of grain fed will cause an increase in mash consumption so that there is not much difference in total food intake.

Kennard and Chamberlin,[80] in comparing various rations and methods of feeding layers, conclude that any of the methods may be safely recommended with the possible exception of the one which provided a 32 per cent protein mash and restricted the free choice of corn and oats to 2 hours daily.

Restricted feeding of pullets[82] has been reported as retarding growth and delaying sexual maturity but having no material effect on subsequent performance.

Temperton[81] restricted the mash consumption of pullets on

range by limiting the time during which the birds could obtain mash. There was a much greater consumption of grain in those groups to which the mash was restricted so that the net saving in feed was 5.6 per cent, with only a small difference in body weight at the end of the rearing period. Temperton and Dudley[83] reported that the general result of restricting feeding during the rearing period to 80 and 90 per cent of the amount consumed under unrestricted feeding has been a lower final weight at the end of rearing for the restricted groups. There appear to be no important after effects of the rearing restrictions in the subsequent laying period of pullets reared on restricted rations but with unrestricted rations during the laying period. With pullets reared on restricted rations and with the restriction of mash during laying, there is a tendency for egg production, or body weight, or both, to be below the corresponding characteristics for birds fed "ad lib." Quicke and Kellerman[84] report that after 10 weeks of age weekly 48-hour fasts had no apparent detrimental effect on the growth and mortality of cockerels during a test period of 24 weeks with a saving of 17 per cent in food consumption. The pullets, however, were affected detrimentally especially during the laying period. Feeding small amounts of green feed during the fasting periods proved advantageous.

Edgar and Herrick[85] tested the susceptibility of chickens to coccidiosis when they had access to feed at all times or were not fed until after 7:00 A.M. In every instance the chickens that had access to feed at all times were more resistant to coccidiosis. The difference in susceptibility was believed to be sufficiently great to justify recommending that poultrymen keep feed before chickens at all times.

In observations on ad libitum and restricted feeding, in chickens a day to 12 months old, Novikoff and Biely[86] found that the restricted feeding involved a greater amount of labor and resulted in somewhat lower rate of growth and egg production, with no significant differences in the pathology of the two groups of birds.

SUDDEN FEED CHANGES

Sipe and Polk[87] report that suddenly changing the feed of laying birds did not reduce egg production during the first month after the change or cause the birds to molt. Berg and Bearse[88] reported that suddenly changing the texture of the mash or changing from mash to pellets and vice versa did not affect the rate of lay. O'Neil[89] concluded that sudden feed changes had a deleterious effect on production and that changes in the color of the mash may be an influencing factor.

Platt[90] reports on emergency changing of the ration during the winter. Removing the mash but feeding grain ad libitum did not affect egg production adversely unless continued for more than 6 days. Removing the grain resulted in a marked drop in production.

Whether or not sudden feed changes will affect production appears to depend on the way in which the change influences total feed intake and restriction of the necessary nutrients.

GENERAL SUMMARY

A review of the different systems and practices would seem to indicate that the method or system does not appear to be the important thing. The important factor seems to be whether the birds consume as much feed under one condition as another and whether, under that method of feeding, they are getting a proper balance of nutrients in their feeds. Hence, it probably comes down to a matter of balance of the ration combined with palatability so as to get sufficient feed consumption. Method in itself is not the important factor.[91]

If frequent minor variations are disregarded, there is one method much more commonly used than any other. It may be called the scratch-mash system of feeding. In this system, poultry is given two feed mixtures, one consisting of whole and cracked grains and the other of ground ingredients. Several years ago a decided variation from the scratch-mash system of feeding, called the all-mash method, was developed. A combination of these two systems of feeding has come into extensive use for rearing chicks. In this system, an all-mash ration is fed during the first month or two after hatching, and a ration consisting of a scratch mixture and a growing mash thereafter to maturity.

Acceleration in growth and increase in egg production have put greater strain on the body of the bird and therefore greater demands on the ration fed. Therefore, if the system of feeding practiced makes it possible to get sufficient daily feed consumption, emphasis should be laid not on manner of feeding but on the nature of the ration used. Any difficulties not caused by disease or inherited weaknesses are in all probability due to the use of rations partially deficient in one or more of the essential nutrients.

Rations for feeding poultry should be complete in all nutritive factors. When birds are confined, it becomes more difficult, but not impossible, to meet this requirement because succulent green feed of the proper type and bugs and worms have been automatically removed from their ration. Many nutritive factors needed by hens, but still undiscovered, may be contained in these natural food materials picked from the range. The way out of such a situation is to make use of the so-called protective feedstuffs, such as milk, green feeds, and vitamin-rich feeds, in building poultry rations.

Wide variations in feeding methods are possible as long as they do not make it impossible to get sufficient daily food consumption, or interfere with the building of a ration complete in all essential nutritive factors With these limitations in mind, there is no one best way of feeding poultry.

REFERENCES

1. Hewitt, A. C. T. Poultry feeding experiments. The Poultry Farmer (N. S. W., Australia) 10(9):17. 1942.
   Pederick, W. O., and A. G. Clark. Poultry Feeding Tests. The Poultry Farmer. (N. S. W., Australia) August 1944.
2. Stewart, J. H., and H. W. Atwood. Poultry experiments. W. Va. Bul. 88. 1903.
3. Rice, J. E. Comparison of four methods of feeding early hatched pullets. Cornell Bul. 249. 1907.
4. Buss, W. J. Feeding experiments with laying hens. Ohio Bul. 322. 1918.
   Kennard, D. C., and V. D. Chamberlin. Rations and methods of feeding layers. Ohio Bimo. Bul. 210:129. 1941.
5. Cassel, L. W. Feeding experiments with Leghorns. Wash. Bul. 210. 1927.
   Martin, J. H. Grain and sour skimmilk as a laying ration. Poultry Sci. 1:50. 1921-22.
   Martin, J. H. Mashless rations. Poultry Sci. 4:26. 1924.
   Martin, J. H. Sources of animal protein for laying hens. Kentucky Bul. 260. 1925.
   Schlamb, K. F., and R. L. Bryant. Skimmilk and grain for laying hens. N. Dakota Bimo. Bul. 13:104. 1951.
   Walker, A. L. The relative feeding value and cost of milk in egg production. N. Mex. Bul. 150. 1925.
   Willham, O. S. Grain and skimmilk versus grain and mash for egg production. Okla. (Panhandle) Bul. 52. 1933.
6. Rice, J. E., and C. Nixon. Seven methods of feeding young chickens. Cornell Bul. 282. 1910.
   Nixon, C. Methods of chick feeding. Cornell Bul. 327. 1913.

7. Peterson, L. I. The starting of chicks on grain and its effect in preventing "pasting up" at various temperatures. Poultry Sci. 23:101. 1944.
8. Carver, J. S. Washington home grown laying rations. Wash. Poultry Pointers 4. 1931.
9. Wheeler, W. P. Feeding experiments with laying hens. N. Y. (Geneva) Bul. 90. 1895.
Wheeler, W. P. Feeding experiments with laying hens. The relative efficiency of whole and ground grains. N. Y. (Geneva) Bul. 106. 1896.
10. Wheeler, W. P. Feeding experiments with chicks and capons. N. Y. (Geneva) Bul. 126. 1897.
11. Hart, E. B., H. Steenbock, J. G. Halpin, and O. N. Johnson. New chick feeding facts. Wis. Bul. 371. 1924.
12. Bobby, F. C. The all-mash method of feeding chickens. Jour. Min. of Agr. (England) 35:950. 1929.
Cassel, L. W. Feeding experiments with Leghorns. Wash. Bul. 210. 1927.
Kennard, D. C. Ground grain vs. whole grain for chickens. Ohio Bimo. Bul. X(7 and 8):120. 1925.
Kennard, D. C., and R. M. Bethke. The all-mash method of feeding chicks and pullets. Ohio Bimo. Bul. XI(I):7. 1926.
Kennard, D. C., and R. M. Bethke. All-mash method of feeding chickens. Ohio Bimo. Bul. XI(4):181. 1926.
Kennard, D. C., and R. M. Bethke. Ground grain versus grain for layers. Poultry Sci. 5:128. 1926.
Kennard, D. C., and R. M. Bethke. The all-mash method of feeding chickens. Proc. Third World's Poultry Congress. 194. 1927.
Poultry feeding experiment. Repts. Ohio County Exp. Farms. 1928.
Martin, J. H., and W. M. Insko. Feeding trials with laying hens. Ky. Bul. 294. 1929.
Morgan, C. L. All-mash method of feeding laying hens. S. C. Rept. 1930:93.
Morton, G. E. Poultry Experiments. Colo. Rept. 1927:18.
North, M. O. Feeding systems for laying hens. Wyo. Bul. 230. 1938.
Thompson, R. B. All-mash or mash and grain good. Okla. Rept. 1926:96.
Thompson, R. B., and R. Penquite. All-mash vs. grain and mash. Okla. Rept. 1930:137.
Less feed with all-mash. Internat. Baby Chick News. Mar. 1, 1931: 9.
Is scratch grain necessary? Ind. Rept. 1926:37.
Is the all-mash method practical for layers? Ind. Rept. 1928:54.
Rhys, I. W. All-mash method of feeding poultry. Harper Adams Utility Poultry Jour. 15:673. 1930.
Rhys, I. W. All-mash method of feeding poultry. National Institute of Poultry Husbandry, England. Leaflet 17. 1930.
13. Card, L. E. Box feeding of grain does not cut egg yields. Ill. Rept. 1926—1927:134.
Stevenson, G. L. All-mash ration for layers. S. Dak. Rept. 1927: 28.

Stevenson, G. L. Feeding all-mash rations. S. Dak. Rept. 1928:26.
Stevenson, G. L. Results of poultry feeding experiments. S. Dak. Bul. 242. 1929.
Fangauf, R., and O. Brüninghaus. Bringt die Körnerlose Fütterungsmethode Vorteile? Archiv für Geflügelk. 8:305. 1934.
Weinmiller, L., and K. Mantel. Geflügelfütterung ganz ohne Getreide. Archiv für Geflügelk. 12:245. 1938.
Carver, J. S. Methods of feeding Leghorn hens. Wash. Bul. 254. 1931.
Robertson, E. I., J. S. Carver, and J. W. Cook. Methods of feeding laying hens. Wash. Bul. 381.
North, M. O. Poultry feeding, housing, and lighting experiments at the Wyoming Experiment Station. Wyo. Bul. 203. 1934.
Lee, C. E., S. W. Hamilton, C. L. Henry, and M. E. Callanan. The effect of substituting an all-mash and pellet ration for grain, mash, and pellets on flock production, costs, and returns. Poultry Sci. 18:375. 1939.

14. Shoup, Mr. and Mrs. G. R. Feeding trial. Western Wash. Bul. 10-W:32. 1928.
15. Bressler, G. O., D. C. Sprague, and A. S. Mowery. Can mechanical methods of feeding poultry replace hand methods? Poultry Sci. 29:176. 1950.
Callenbach, E. W. Feeding chickens by machine. Poultry Improvement Board of New York. Yearbook 1949-50:16.
Lee, C. E. New facts on automatic units simplify feeding practices. Everybody's Poultry Magazine. Jan. 1952.
16. Kennard, D. C., and R. M. Bethke. The all-mash method of feeding chickens. Proc. Third World's Poultry Congress: 194. Canada, 1927.
17. Stevenson, G. L. Feeding all-mash rations. S. Dak. Rept. 1928:26.
18. Rhys, I. W. All-mash method of feeding poultry. National Institute of Poultry Husb. (England) Leaflet 17. 1930.
19. Molyneux, H. M. Pellet and all-mash experiments. Nat. Inst. Poultry Husb. (England) Leaflet 16. 1930.
Molyneux, H. New systems of poultry feeding. Jour. Ministry Agr. (Great Britain). 38:903. 1931.
Molyneux, H. M. Management problems. Harper Adams Utility Poultry Jour. 17:528. 1931.
20. Berg, L. R., and G. E. Bearse. Studies of the granulation of chicken laying mashes. Wash. Bul. 522. 1951.
Carver, J. S. Methods of feeding Leghorn hens. Wash. Bul. 254. 1931.
Morgan, R. B., and B. W. Heywang. A comparison of a pelleted and unpelleted all-mash diet for laying chickens. Poultry Sci. 20:62. 1941.
Morris, L. Pelleted versus unpelleted mash for laying hens. Wyoming Agr. Exp. Station Mimeograph Release, July 1947.
Morris, L. Pelleted and unpelleted mash for laying hens. Poultry Sci. 26:122. 1947.
Ponsignon, M. The use of pellets in feeding poultry. Vie a la campagne 3:376. 1934.
21. Fangauf, R., and A. Haensel. Die Verfütterung von Körnerkraftfutter. Archiv für Geflügelk. 10:353. 1936.

22. Biely, J., D. Cooper, and B. March. Pelleted feed screenings as scratch feed in a poultry ration. Poultry Sci. 30:778. 1951.
Jensen, L. S., and J. McGinnis. A comparison of feeding pelleted and unpelleted diets containing different levels of alfalfa to laying hens. Poultry Sci. 31:307. 1952.
Lillie, R. J., S. K. Haynes, and H. R. Bird. Effect of fiber in non-pelleted and pelleted mash upon egg production and feed efficiency. Poultry Sci. 30:922. 1951.
23. Bearse, G. E., L. R. Berg, C. F. McClary, and V. L. Miller. The effect on chick growth and feed efficiency of pelleting rations of different fiber levels. Poultry Sci. 31:907. 1952.
Bearse, G. E., L. R. Berg, C. F. McClary, and V. L. Miller. The effect of pelleting chicken rations on the incidence of cannibalism. Poultry Sci. 28:756. 1949.
Heywang, B. W., and R. B. Morgan. A comparison of a pelleted and unpelleted all-mash diet for growing chickens. Poultry Sci. 23: 16. 1944.
Patton, J. W., and L. A. Rauls. Pellet versus mash forms of chick feed. Feedstuffs 10(40):12. 1938.
Patton, J. W., H. H. Buskirk, and L. A. Rauls. A study of the relative merits of pellets and mash poultry feeds. Vet. Med. 32:423. 1937.
Ponsignon, M. The use of pellets in feeding poultry. Vie a la campagne 3:376. 1934.
Stewart, W. I., and C. W. Upp. The effect of form of feed on growth and feed efficiency, pellets versus mash versus granules for broilers. Poultry Sci. 30:63. 1951.
24. Tallent, V. K. Pellets versus mash for table duck production. Harper Adams Utility Poultry Jour. 17:539. 1931.
25. McMurray, M. Table poultry experiment, 1935. Table ducklings (pellets versus wet mash). Harper Adams Utility Poultry Jour. 20:498. 1934.
26. Heuser, G. F., and M. L. Scott. Studies in duck nutrition. I. Methods of feeding. Poultry Sci. 30:161. 1951.
27. Serfontein, P. J. The value of pellets in the feeding of ducks. Poultry Bulletin, South Africa 15, 168:9. 1951.
28. Carver, J. S., and L. A. Wilhelm. The physiological response of turkeys to mash and pellet feeds. Wash. Bul. 354. 1937.
Carver, J. S., L. A. Wilhelm, and J. W. Cook. Methods of feeding turkeys. Wash. Bul. 356. 1938.
Payne, L. F., T. B. Avery, and D. C. Warren. Mash versus pellets for feeding growing turkeys. Kansas 13th Biennial Rept. 1946:53.
Slinger, S. J., K. M. Gartley, and E. V. Evans. Pelleted and unpelleted diets high in dehydrated green feeds for turkeys grown in confinement. Poultry Sci. 28:556. 1949.
Ziegenhagen, E. H., L. B. Corman, and J. W. Hayward. Feed particle size as a factor affecting performance of turkey poults. Poultry Sci. 26:212. 1947.
29. Mussehl, F. E., C. W. Ackerson, and R. L. Borchers. A comparison of mash and granules for chicks. Nebraska Rept. 1950:121.
30. Dove, W. F. A study of individuality in the nutritive instincts and

of the causes and effects of variations in the selection of food. Am. Naturalist 69:469. 1935.

31. Harris, L. J. Vitamins in theory and practice. Macmillan. 1935.
32. Jukes, C. L. Selection of diet in chicks as influenced by vitamins and other factors. Jour. Comp. Psychology 26:135. 1938.
33. Price, W. E. The role of a new vitamin-like activator in the control of dental caries. Jour. Am. Dental Assn. 30:888. 1943.
34. Gallus, Beck. Neue Beiträge zur Zwei-Komponenten-Theorie des Hungers. Versuche mit Hühnern. Zeitschrift für Psychologie 283. 1930.
    Baege, M. H. Hunger und Appetit bei Hühnern. Geflügel-Börse 56. 1934.
35. Anderson, J. O., and G. M. Briggs. Chickens' preference for feed as influenced by its color. Poultry Sci. 27:651. 1948.
    Engelmann, C. Über den Geschmakssinn des Huhnes. Forschungsdienst 13:363. 1942.
    Römer, R. Geruchs-, Farben-, Form-, und Geschmackssinn beim Huhn. Geflügelhof, May 27: 339. 1949.
36. De Bocarmé, Ph. Visart. Influence of natural instincts upon the devouring of substances other than feed. Rept. Sixth World's Poultry Congress. 236. Germany. 1936.
37. Alder, B. Coarse mashes more desirable for laying hens. Farm and Home Science (Utah) 2(3). 1941.
38. Jackson, H. W. Individual characteristics of hens. Pa. Rept. 1911: 228.
    Kempster, H. L. Food selection by laying hens. Jour. Am. Assn. Instructors and Investigators in Poultry Husb. 3:26. 1917.
    Banta, L. What judgment does a hen use in selecting her food? Poultry Sci. 11:364. 1932.
39. Graham, W. R. Can we learn anything from a free choice of feeds as expressed by chickens? Sci. Agr. 13:203. 1932.
40. Funk, E. M. Can the chick balance its ration? Poultry Sci. 11:94. 1932.
41. Briggs, G. M., M. H. Swanson, E. G. Hill, and H. J. Sloan. Self selection of diet by chicks. I. Choice of mash and grain. Poultry Sci. 28:758. 1949.
42. Amon, V. G. Studies on the influence of free choice of feed in poultry feeding. Philippine Agr. 19:445. 1930.
43. Pearl, R., and T. E. Fairchild. Studies on the physiology of reproduction in the domestic fowl. XIX. On the influence of free choice of feed material on winter egg production and body weight. Am. Jour. Hygiene I:258. 1921.
44. Charles, T. B., and H. O. Stuart. Poultry thrives on cafeteria system. N. H. Bul. 256:18. 1931.
45. Platt, C. S., and V. Darago. Cafeteria feeding of Leghorn pullets. N. J. Hints 29(1). 1941.
46. Tomhave, A. E., and C. W. Mumford. Self selection of feeds by hens. Del. Bul. 174. 1931.
47. Graham, J. C. Individuality of pullets in balancing the ration. Poultry Sci. 13:34. 1934.
48. Rhodes, C. C., L. H. Bartel, and P. E. F. Jooste. The effects of

varying amounts of animal protein fed to White Leghorn pullets 1. The influence of low, medium, and high protein diets on the weight and number of eggs. Empire Jour. Exp. Agr. 3:215. Also in Farming in S. Africa 10:347. 1935.

49. Kennard, D. C., and V. D. Chamberlin. The ration as affected by free-choice feeding of whole grain and mash. Ohio Bul. 592:100. 1938.

Kennard, D. C., and V. D. Chamberlin. Rations and methods of feeding White Leghorn pullet layers. Ohio Bimo. Bul. 214:10. 1942.

Kennard, D. C., and V. D. Chamberlin. Rations and methods of feeding Rhode Island Red pullets. Ohio Bimo. Bul. 219:165. 1942.

50. Tomhave, A. E., and W. C. Skoglund. Rations and methods of feeding. Del. Bul. 238:13. 1942.

51. Davidson, J. A., P. J. Schaible, A. W. Brant, and C. G. Card. Cannibalism in White Leghorn pullets in the laying house. Poultry Sci. 20:458. 1941.

52. Von Ebbell, H. Ueber den Kannibalismus bei Legehennen. Archiv für Geflügelk. 13:357. 1939.

53. Kennard, D. C., and V. D. Chamberlin. An experience with feather picking and cannibalism of pullet layers. Ohio Bimo. Bul. 229: 215. 1944.

54. Amon, V. G. Studies on the influence of free choice of feed in poultry feeding. Philippine Agr. 19:445. 1930.

Card, L. E. Box feeding of grain does not cut egg yields. Ill. Rept. 1926-1927:134.

Carver, J. S. Methods of feeding Leghorn hens. Wash. Bul. 254. 1931.

Hicks, W. H. Feeding laying pullets. Rept. Supt. Exp. Farm. Agassiz. B. C., Canada. 1928:35.

Mehrhof, N. R., E. F. Stanton, and D. F. Sowell. Methods of feeding grain to laying pullets. Fla. Bul. 380. 1942.

Sloan, H. J. Free-choice grain feeding wins approval. Minn. Farm & Home Sci. 2 (No. 3):8. 1945.

55. Fangauf, R., and A. Haensel. Körnerfutter zu beliebiger Aufnahme. Archiv für Geflügelk. 10:137. 1936.

Hübner, O., and W. Liebscher. Versuch über die Wahlfütterung der Küken und Legehühner. Rept. Sixth World's Poultry Congress. 279. Germany. 1936.

Lauprecht, E. Beitrag zur Frage der Zuteilung des Körnerfutters und der Wirkung des Futterwechsels bei Legehennen. Archiv für Geflügelk. 11:19. 1937.

56. Rugg, W. C. Poultry farming. Dept. Agr. Victoria, Australia, Bul. 54:36. 1925.

Hadlington, E. Feeding experiments at Hawkesbury Agricultural College. Poultry Notes. Department of Agriculture, N. S. Wales, August 1931.

57. Carver, J. S. Methods of feeding Leghorn hens. Wash. Bul. 254. 1931.

Carver, J. S., E. I. Robertson, J. W. Cook, and J. L. St. John. Protein requirements of laying hens. Wash. Bul. 368. 1938.

Carrick, C. W. Research solves farm problems. Ind. Report. 1941:95.

Charles, T. B., and H. O. Stuart. Hopper-feeding grain. N. H. Circ. 33. 1930.

Davidson, J. A. Continuous hopper feeding of corn and oats to laying pullets. Mich. Quart. Bul. 19(1):3. 1936.

Davidson, J. A. Hopper feeding grain to laying pullets: A comparison of continuous hopper feeding of grain with daily hand feeding. Mich. Quart. Bul. 20(2):94. 1937.

Lee, C. E., J. C. Scholes, and C. L. Henry. The effect of "free-choice" grain feeding on egg production, feed consumption, body weight, and egg quality. Poultry Sci. 23:360. 1944.

Lee, C. E., J. C. Scholes, and C. L. Henry. The effect of "free-choice" grain feeding on egg production and feed consumption. Poultry Sci. 28:10. 1949.

McClary, C. F., G. E. Bearse, and V. L. Miller. A study of feeding methods for laying hens. Western Wash. Rept. 1942:57.

58. Charles, T. B., and H. O. Stuart. Hopper feeding grain. N. H. Circ. 23. 1930.

Wilson, W. O. Corn, wheat, and barley for chickens. S. Dak. Bul. 376.

59. Carver, J. S. Methods of feeding Leghorn hens. Wash. Bul. 254. 1931.

Carver, J. S., E. I. Robertson, J. W. Cook, and J. L. St. John. Protein requirements of laying hens. Wash. Bul. 368. 1938.

Kempster, H. L., and Q. B. Kinder. The use of laying concentrates for egg production. Mo. Bul. 528:43. 1949.

Robertson, E. I., J. S. Carver, and J. W. Cook. Methods of feeding laying hens. Wash. Bul. 381. 1939.

60. Kennard, D. C., and V. D. Chamberlin. Free choice of whole grain and mash concentrate for layers. Ohio Bimo. Bul. 157:154. 1932.

61. Skoglund, W. C. Methods of feeding laying hens. Delaware Bul. 271:12. 1947.

62. Hays, F. A. Free-choice feeding of high producing layers. Poultry Comment 8 (No. 6) Dec. 1951.

63. Lee, C. E., O. A. Rowoth, C. L. Henry, and J. Presto. The effect of supplementary all-mash pellets in the all-mash feeding program for layers using automatic feeders. Poultry Sci. 32:429. 1953.

64. Hadlington, E. Feeding experiments at Hawkesbury Agricultural College. Poultry Notes. Dept. of Agr. N. S. Wales. August 1931.

Hall, M. D., and A. G. Clark. Werribee 1947-48 poultry feeding tests. The Poultry Farmer (Australia) Oct. 9, 1948: 9.

McArdle, A. A. Dry vs. wet mash for poultry feeding trial at Parafield Poultry Station. The Poultry Farmer (Australia) 15 (17):38. 1947.

McArdle, A. A. Five years of poultry feeding and housing trials. The Poultry Farmer (Australia) 17(32):10. 1950.

Rugg, W. C., and W. P. Pederick. Poultry feeding experiment. Jour. of the Dept. of Agr. (Victoria) 22:420. 1924.

65. Temperton, H., and F. J. Dudley. The effect of systems of feeding on growth and egg production. V. A comparison of controlled and

unrestricted dry mash, wet mash, and pellet feeding for laying pullets. Harper Adams Utility Poultry Jour. 33:37. 1948.

Rhynehart, J. G. A comparison of wet mash, dry mash, and a combination of both in the feeding of laying pullets. Eggs. Aug. 12-19, 1931.

Rhys, I. W. All-mash method of feeding poultry. Harper Adams Utility Poultry Jour. 15:673. 1930.

66. Owen-John, A. Poultry feeding. Union of South Africa Dept. of Agr. Jour. 6:176. 1923.

67. Goodearl, G. P. Feeding for winter egg production. N. Dak. Bimo. Bul. 1(1):7. 1938.

Goodearl, G. P. Fleshing mash vs. heavy feeding of grain for winter egg production. N. Dak. Bul. 301. 1941.

68. Dearstyne, R. S., and C. O. Bollinger. Some effects of feeding yeast-fermented mash to laying pullets. N. C. Bul. 55. 1938.

69. Experiments in table poultry production. Ministry Agr. and Fisheries (Great Britain) Bul. 91. 1935.

70. Jourdain, W. L. Dry mash versus wet mash. For feeding of chicks in brooder. New Zealand Jour. Agr. 52:233. 1936.

Torres, A. diP. Agriculturaalgumas observacoes no escola superior de Agricultura "Luiz de Queiroz." Rev. Agric. (Piracicaba) 23:87. 1948.

71. Davidson, J. A. The use of high-protein laying mashes. Mich. Quart. Bul. 22(2):87. 1939.

72. Hadlington, E. Soaked wheat feeding experiments. Hawkesbury Agricultural College. Nov. 7, 1936.

Newman, T. Soaked grain—A year of discovery on the S.P.B.A. Experimental Farm. Eggs. Oct. 23, 1935.

73. Newbigin, H. F., and R. R. Linton. Palatability of certain seeds to chicks. Scottish Jour. Agr. 10:422. 1927.

74. Kable, G. W., and F. E. Fox. Electric water heaters for poultry. Ore. Circ. 81. 1927.

Beresford, H. Stock tank and poultry water heaters. Agr. Eng. 11. (8) 1930.

75. Heywang, B. W. The effect of restricted feed intake on egg weight, egg production, and body weight. Poultry Sci. 19:29. 1940.

76. Burmester, B. R., and L. E. Card. The effect of restricted feeding time on food intake, body weight, and egg production. Poultry Sci. 18:402. 1939.

77. Temperton, H., and F. J. Dudley. Controlled feeding of laying pullets. Harper Adams Utility Poultry Jour. 27:73. 1942.

Temperton, H., and F. J. Dudley. Further note on restricting the food supply to laying pullets. Harper Adams Utility Poultry Jour. 27:215. 1942.

78. Taylor, M. W. P.A.G.B. feeding experiments. Modern Poultry Keeping (England) LV:270. 1946.

79. Fangauf, R., and A. Haensel. Die Herabsetzung der Körnergabe bei Hühnern. Archiv für Geflügelk. 13:192. 1939.

80. Kennard, D. C., and V. D. Chamberlin. Rations and methods of feeding layers. Ohio Bimo. Bul. 201:149. 1939.

81. Temperton, H. The control of mash consumption during rearing. Harper Adams Utility Poultry Jour. 26:33. 1941.

82. Fronda, F. M., and I. M. Cruz. The influence of restricted feeding on pullets from 12 to 24 weeks old. Philippine Agr. 35:90. 1951.

Milby, T. T., and D. H. Sherwood. The effect of restricted feeding on growth and subsequent production of pullets. Poultry Sci. 32: 916. 1953.

83. Temperton, H., and F. J. Dudley. The restriction of food to growing and laying stock. I. Restriction of mash supply for pullets during rearing. Harper Adams Utility Poultry Jour. 29:15. 1944.

Temperton, H., and F. J. Dudley. The restriction of food to growing and laying stock. II. The egg production of pullets reared on restricted rations but with unrestricted rations during the laying period. Harper Adams Utility Poultry Jour. 29:19. 1944.

Temperton, H., and F. J. Dudley. The restriction of food to growing and laying stock. III. The effect of limiting the laying rations of pullets reared on restricted rations. Harper Adams Utility Poultry Jour. 29:24. 1944.

Temperton, H., and F. J. Dudley. The restriction of food to growing and laying stock. IV. The effect of limiting the available energy in rations for laying hens. Harper Adams Utility Poultry Journal 30:28. 1945.

84. Quicke, G. V., and J. H. Kellermann. Studies on intermittent inanition in the feeding of poultry. Science Bul. 282, Agr. Res. Series No. 11. Union of S. Africa 1947-48.

85. Edgar, S. A., and C. A. Herrick. Feeding habits in relation to the severity of cecal coccidiosis, Eimeria tenella. Poultry Sci. 23:30. 1944.

86. Novikoff, M., and J. Biely. Observations on two methods of feeding chickens from one day old to twelve months of age. Poultry Sci. 24:245. 1945.

87. Sipe, G. R., and H. D. Polk. The response of laying hens to sudden feed changes. Poultry Sci. 18:394. 1939.

88. Berg, L. R., and G. E. Bearse. Studies on the granulation of chicken laying mashes. Washington Bul. 522. 1951.

89. O'Neil, J. B. The effect of sudden changes of feed upon production. Poultry Sci. 25:83. 1946.

90. Platt, C. S. Emergency substitutions for laying mash in the diet of White Leghorn pullets. Poultry Sci. 23:126. 1944.

Platt, C. S. Sprouted soybeans, mash, and grains for emergency feeding of White Leghorn pullets. Poultry Sci. 24:505. 1945.

91. Callenbach, E. W., and R. R. Murphy. Feeding systems for laying hens. Pa. Bul. 425. 1942.

Temperton, H., and F. J. Dudley. The effects of systems of feeding on growth and egg production. Harper Adams Utility Poultry Jour. 31:13. 1946.

Temperton, H., and F. J. Dudley. The effects of systems of feeding on growth and egg production. 2. The effects in the pullet year of dry versus wet mash feeding during brooding and rearing. Harper Adams Utility Poultry Jour. 31:39. 1946.

Temperton, H., and F. J. Dudley. The effects of systems of feeding on growth and egg production. 3. Dry mash vs. wet mash for laying pullets. Harper Adams Utility Poultry Jour. 31:35. 1946.

Temperton, H., and F. J. Dudley. The effect of systems of feeding on growth and egg production. IV. A comparison of dry mash, wet mash, and pellet feeding for growing pullets. Harper Adams Utility Poultry Jour. 33:1. 1948.

Vondell, J. H. Methods of feeding layers and breeders. Poultry Sci. 27:531. 1948.

CHAPTER 11

HEALTH FEEDING

In order to keep in a healthy and productive condition, an animal must be furnished a ration complete in all respects. If there is something lacking in the feed, production or health, or both, will suffer. The so-called nutritional diseases are the best examples of a deficiency condition. They are due chiefly to a lack of vitamins or minerals in the ration. For example, if vitamin D is not supplied, the bird will suffer from rickets. Perosis may result if the chick does not get enough manganese. These specific nutritional diseases or deficiencies are discussed in detail in Chap. 3 dealing with vitamins and minerals.

RELATION OF THE DIET TO HEALTH

We must always keep in mind the fact that the ration may have an effect upon the health of the animal and the incidence of disease, particularly in middle and old age. In comparing a rat colony on a good diet with one on an ill-balanced diet, it was found that the well-nourished animals showed no illness, no death from natural causes, and no infant mortality, whereas the poorly nourished animals showed indications of a number of diseases and disorders.[1] Apparently, diet is important in the preservation of healthy cells and tissues with consequent normal function.

The Iowa Experiment Station[2] reported that the ration might have an effect upon the incidence of so-called range paralysis. A report from Northern Ireland[3] has shown that the addition of supplements of limestone flour to a complete rearing ration impaired the health of the birds and increased the mortality due to coccidiosis. Other experience also indicates that an excess of calcium in the chick ration will depress growth. (See Chap. 3 on minerals.)

One report indicates gout as being caused in chickens that were fed too richly with lime.[4] Besides too large a quantity of lime, other causes have been given for the development of gout.[5] It is usually influenced by many months of one-sided feeding and confinement. It is also looked upon as a disease connected with metabolism.

One of the benefits of milk feeding is attributed to its development of the aciduric or lactic acid bacillus group of bacteria in the intestines. They are favorable bacteria. On the other hand, meat and other high-protein diets increase the indo-producing bacteria and other organisms of the so-called putrefactive type.[6]

The severity of coccidiosis has been influenced by the type of ration fed.[7-12]

An adequate supply of the various nutrients is essential for resistance to disease. Boari[13] reported that chicks on a vitamin-deficient diet infected with *B. avisepticus* acquired immunity with much more difficulty. Seeler and Ott[14] reported more severe avian malaria infections in chicks when the diet was deficient in folic acid, protein, and unidentified factors.

Diet has a relation to the development of internal parasites. Results from the Kansas Station[15] showed that the resistance of chickens to parasitism was affected by vitamin A and vitamin B. The inclusion of liquid skimmilk and meat meal as supplements in the diet increased the growth rate and the resistance in the chicken to the nematode *Ascaridia lineata* but that the plant diet produced the slowest growth rate and the least potent resistance in the chicken to the growth of the nematode. In the case of chicks infected with *Eimeria tenella*, it has been reported that vitamin K in their food showed a mortality of only 10 per cent in comparison to 70 per cent mortality in the unprotected group.[16] Chickens receiving a diet deficient in calcium and phosphorus were less resistant to infestation with the nematode *Heterakis gallinae* than were those receiving the same diet to which adequate amounts of calcium and phosphorus compounds were added.[17]

POISONS IN FEED

The health of the animal may also be affected if the feed contains some harmful substance or if the animal consumes some material which is detrimental. When the poultryman suffers losses, one of his first reactions is to blame the feed and to suspect that it contained something poisonous.

A number of years ago the American Feed Manufacturers Association issued a publication entitled Was It the Feed? In this publication are presented the replies of state representatives of the Association of American Feed Control Officials who were asked for résumés of actual cases of suspected feed toxicity which were referred to them for investigation. The following observations are representative of the replies.

Dr. H. R. Kraybill of the Indiana State Agricultural Experiment Station reported as follows:

> Recently I have summarized the results of the examination of 689 samples that have been submitted during the last 10 years. Only 4 of these samples showed the presence of harmful ingredients. In one of these cases, powdered arsenate of lead was accidentally spilled into the feed. In another case, through accident in mixing, 37 per cent of salt was present. In some instances, animals that have died were submitted with the samples of feed. These animals were autopsied by the Department of Veterinary Science, and, in practically every case, disease was found to be present which would account for the death of the animal.

Mr. Leas, in charge of the feed inspection work in Ohio, wrote as follows:

> Every year we have around 150 such cases. They write that they are sending the feed that [they think] has killed their chickens and want to know whether or not the feed has been responsible. Our chemist gives them a microscopical examination, analyses of protein, fat, fiber, etc., and then we feed them to guinea pigs and obtain the starting weight and final weight of the guinea pig. In only 1 case out of over 1000 samples received have we found any poisonous effects of the feed.

In Maryland, of 61 samples of feed suspected of having killed chickens, some of which were accused of killing birds by the score, not a single one was found to kill healthy birds even though the possible deleterious effects were greatly magnified by giving the feed as the entire ration after a starvation period. The Nebraska Station pointed out the typical complaint as this: "We used this feed and lost a lot of chicks. Please analyze and tell us what is in it that is killing them." In their experience, in testing feeds over a period of years, they state that in one case the ration submitted was unusually laxative because of too much molasses, but losses were not excessive. In all other cases, no abnormal losses were observed.

In most cases, it has been shown that the feed did not contain any poison or harmful material. In a small number of cases, losses have been attributed to the presence of poison, usually lead arsenate or Paris green. This might have become available to the stock either through malicious intent or through carelessness. In one case, it was found that the feed was contaminated with arsenic dusting powder in the warehouse. In another case, an old paint barrel was used for molasses. Sometimes it might be traced to letting the stock have access to certain materials about the premises, such as empty paint cans. Or they might have eaten decayed animal matter, secured from dead animals.

Losses may also be attributed to faulty management, such as maintaining insanitary conditions and improper changes in feed, but more frequently the cause of losses is traced to the presence of disease. One feed control official pointed out that during the baby chick season a sudden wet, cold spell of weather is very likely to be followed by an influx of complaints of feed that is suspected of being poisonous.

LOSSES DUE TO INSECTS

Chickens on range may consume considerable amounts of animal life, such as insects and worms. In general, they can do this without harm. However, it has been reported that chickens, ducklings, goslings, and young turkeys may be killed by eating rose chafers.[18] Healthy chicks, usually between the ages of 2 and 14 weeks, may suddenly act sleepy and listless and die on range with full crops. On examination, the crop may be found to contain rose bugs or chafers in large numbers. The rose chafer has in it a poison that affects the nervous system. Hens usually are not killed by eating these insects.

Mortality in turkeys has been reported due to the feeding of grasshoppers.[19] Enteritis due to injury from the legs of the insects which even punctured the intestines, was observed. One precaution suggested was the feeding of a liberal quantity of mash in the morning.

Mortality in pigeons due to the pea beetle (*Bruchus pisorum L.*)[20] has also been accompanied by inflamed and swollen intestinal lining.

POSSIBLE LOSSES TRACEABLE TO GRAINS

In the feeding of moldy corn, Gibbs[21] reported that severe intestinal reactions occurred in all the chickens when first placed on the moldy corn ration and one died of enteritis. After feeding on moldy corn continuously for 4 weeks, the chickens apparently developed a tolerance and did not show any further ill effects. Ronk and Carrick[22] fed moldy corn to laying hens for 30 days with no ill effects. Chicks receiving 20 per cent of moldy corn and 30 per cent of good corn grew as rapidly as those receiving

50 per cent of good corn. The chicks receiving 30 per cent and 40 per cent of moldy corn, however, grew less rapidly. No apparent deleterious effects resulted when chicks received moldy corn that was infected with species of penicillium, diplodia, fusarium, mucor or rhizopus, aspergillus, and undetermined organisms, including yellow bacteria. There were no apparent mortalities due to the feeding of moldy corn, except possibly one due to aspergillosis. Borchers and Peltier[23] added 10 per cent of a moldy foodstuff, consisting of a mixture of wheat bran, corn, and soybean meal prepared under controlled conditions with selected mold isolates, to a chick starting ration without any apparent deleterious effect.

The feeding of scabby barley or wheat to chicks, growing chickens, or laying birds has had no apparent effect upon rate of growth, mortality, or production.[24, 25] The Maryland Station[26] has reported on the use of field-damaged wheat for poultry. No detrimental results were noted in the feeding of it to hens for a period of 6 weeks. The wheat was highly discolored, with a large percentage of the grain sprouted and slightly moldy. However, in using such wheat, they recommend the following: "Use only as a part of the ration and if fed heavily use each alternate month. If possible run the wheat through a fanning mill to blow out dirt and mold. If the wheat is molded badly, heat in an oven to kill the mold spores. Feed only during good weather and when diseases are not prevalent."

The feeding of new wheat to chickens has been reported as favoring the development of blue comb disease.[27] Feeds associated with this condition have been reported to be high in bacterial floras. On the other hand, heavy feeding of new wheat is reported by the Ohio Station[25] as being not detrimental when fed to growing birds or laying pullets.

The question frequently arises as to the use of wheat or other grains which have been treated for the control of plant diseases. The reports seem to indicate that grain treated with eosin[28] or mercury compounds are quite harmless when treated in the ordinary way and fed in regular quantities. On the other hand, unfavorable results have been obtained with grains treated with certain compounds. It would appear desirable to feed any treated grain to a small number of birds before using it generally or in large amounts.

The question also frequently arises as to the possibility of using for the feeding of poultry grain which is affected by smut. Horvath[29] reported that 4 per cent of corn smut added to the diet for 3 months was not injurious to hens and did not affect their chemical blood composition or egg-laying capacity. The Oklahoma Station[30] gathered the sorghum heads from a field in which 70 per cent of the heads were infested with a kernel smut, determined the number of damaged kernels, and estimated the amount of smut. The spores of the smut were fed to young and grown chicks without any apparent effects on growth, egg production, or hatchability. The Oklahoma Station[31] also indicated that the feeding of 12 per cent of kafir smut mixed in the mash, or smutty wheat used in the mash, did not decrease egg production, fertility, and hatchability, where the ration was otherwise adequate. The Maryland Station[32] used wheat damaged with stinking smut as a poultry food with reasonably satisfactory results from the standpoint of palatability and the absence of deleterious effects, although its feeding value appeared somewhat reduced owing to the destructive action of the smut.

Caution is usually advised in connection with the feeding of grain affected with ergot, since it has been reported that the presence of this fungus would cause diarrhea. Lobl[33] reported poisoning by ergot. He stated that the chickens hopped about like sparrows. The toes of some of them were mummified, and of others swollen and soft. In some cases, the skin broke loose from the sole.

Aspergillosis[34] is a disease caused by the aspergillus mold, the mold which grows on damp feed. It produces spores that blow about when the feed becomes dry. If these spores are inhaled, the disease results.

It has been reported that young chicks fed on barley died in a few days. Examination showed that coarse barley hulls cut the intestines to ribbons. Irritation of the eyes caused by barley barbs from the litter has also been observed in chicks.

LOSSES DUE TO TOXIC PLANTS

Hart[35] reported that seeds of *Araujia sericifera* proved to be toxic to fowls in three feeding experiments with White Leghorn roosters. The toxic principle caused enteritis, incoordination of movement, and loss of balance and of muscular control. Toxicity increased with maturation of the seeds. Five grams of ripe seeds proved lethal.

In the feeding of cocoa wastes to poultry, Temperton and Dudley[36] reported that death occurred even when only 10 per cent of this food was included in the daily ration. The theobromine content of this ration was 1.9 per cent. They suggested that the only satisfactory method of avoiding risk is to use only cocoa bean products from which the theobromine has been removed, but the cost of this would make the price too high. The bird appears perfectly healthy and may even be in the act of consuming food when it suddenly becomes rigid for a few seconds, falls back contorted with muscular spasms, and dies. After death, the limbs are fixed and the joints immovable for a few minutes, but later the whole body becomes limp and rigor mortis follows after the normal interval. Upon post-mortem, no obvious cause of death can be found.

The seeds of corn cockle (*Agrostemma githago L.*) have been shown to be toxic to chickens,[37] as well as to other animals. The poisonous principle is a glucoside found in all parts of the plant, but mainly in the seed. Birds affected with cockle poisoning present a generally listless or sleepy and unkempt appearance, with rough feathering and diarrhea. Characteristic lesions of cheesy material in the mouth and under the tongue have been reported. Cockle poisoning decreases the respiratory rate and heart rate of the bird. The resistance of the bird to coccidiosis, paralysis, fowl pox, and diphtheria has been reported decreased, even when sublethal doses have been fed. In the case of chicks, lesions were observed even when very small amounts of ground cockle were added to the feed, but weight was not affected until more than 2 per cent of ground cockle was added. Larger amounts finally resulted also in mortality. Larger amounts of the ground cockle are necessary to secure like results in older birds. Older birds seem to have developed a tolerance to the poison. Whole cockle is unpalatable and, when fed in that form, usually will not be consumed in large amounts. But whole cockle can be consumed in large quantities without any very serious detrimental effects.

Certain species of crotalaria seed[38] have been shown to be toxic for chickens, quail, and doves. The seeds are not relished and will not be eaten in large quantities, except under unnatural conditions, such as close confinement with constant access to the seed.

Daubentonia seed poisoning in poultry has been reported by the Florida Station.[39] The seed is highly toxic to poultry, and death occurred soon after the seeds were consumed.

The toxicity of *Glottidium vesicarium* Harper seeds for fowls has been reported by the Florida Station.[40] Well-fed birds usually refuse to eat the seeds voluntarily. Semi-starved birds will eat some of the seeds but usually not enough to prove fatal. However, a number of cases of natural poisoning by the seeds have been observed.

It has been reported that hedge mustard (*Erysimum crepidifolium*)[41] is readily eaten by geese and has often killed off a whole flock in a few hours. The whorled milkweed has been reported as a poisonous plant for poultry[42] and for turkeys.[43] The top parts of the plant are more toxic than the roots. The birds show inability to stand, together with spasmodic twitchings of the limbs and head. Immature tender plants appear more toxic than the more mature weed. The birds will not consume much of the weed if they are provided with sufficient wholesome green feed.

Losses have been reported from the consumption of mustard seed and also from plants which produce hydrocyanic acid in the intestinal tract.[44]

Parsley[45] is a very potent herb which should rightly be considered more as a medicinal plant than as a poultry green feed to be used freely. The whole parsley is a poisonous plant. Most varieties of cultivated or wild parsley are fairly toxic for fowls, and the roots are even more so than the leaves.

Potato or solanin poisoning[46] has been reported in ducks which have been fed on cooked sprouted potatoes. The green sprouts of potatoes contain a considerable amount of the solanin. It has been suggested that one should never use the water in which potatoes have been boiled for mixing a wet mash, particularly when the potatoes have commenced to sprout.

Tar weed seed,[47] which has been shown to be toxic for swine, horses, and calves, has been reported as not being toxic for poultry, when occurring in the usual amounts in unscreened western wheat.

A number of other plants have been reported as being poisonous to poultry. They include the leaves of white snake root, black night shade,[48] particularly the green berries, leaves of lily of the valley, sprouts of cocklebur, and pokeberry and Jimson weed seeds, seeds of the lead plant,[49] and some vetch seeds.[50]

Whole wheat frequently gives better results, especially in fattening, than wheat by-products. In some cases, this may be explained by the fact that the by-products contain some of the injurious seeds, such as cockle, ergot, and darnel.[51]

LOSSES DUE TO CHEMICALS

A case of poisoning by acetic acid has been reported for fifteen chicks in a house, the floor of which was covered with beechwood sawdust on which the sun was shining. This was thought to be a case of poisoning by inhalation.[52] Sodium bicarbonate and boric acid have been reported injurious to chicks.[53]

Arsenical poisoning has been reported in the fowl.[54] Arsenical preparations, among the most useful insecticides, are used in dips against ticks, internally against worms, as a spray, and as bait for locusts. It has been shown that when arsenic is administered in small quantities such as in poison bait for grasshoppers, or in spray for fruit trees, the domestic fowl can tolerate comparatively large doses over a long period without any visible ill effects.[55]

Copper compounds are toxic for domesticated birds.[56] Copper sulphate poisoning has been reported as due to the feeding of wheat treated with copper sulphate for mildew or to giving a copper sulphate solution as drinking water.[57] Copper sulphate poisoning commences clinically with blue-green diarrhea, falling out of plumage, loss of appetite, and vomiting. Death is accompanied by cramp. Copper sulphate solutions are frequently used for the prevention and control of certain diseases. Water containing more than 0.25 per cent (1–400) copper sulphate was found to be deleterious to the health of turkeys when given as the only source of drinking water.[58]

Fluorine toxicosis has been reported to inhibit egg production. Since fluorine is a cumulative poison, caution must be exercised in the use of mineral supplements containing fluorine in poultry feeding.[59] Similarly, other common minerals present in feeds may be harmful when fed in excess (see Chap. 3, p. 25).

Nicotine is frequently used in the control of round worms in chickens. However, high levels of nicotine must be avoided since they will affect the growth of the chicks and increase mortality.[60]

Poisons used in vermin extermination have been the source of poisoning.[61] The most characteristic symptoms of thallium poisoning in chickens are bluish discoloration of the comb and wattle, paralysis of the legs, diarrhea, and loss of feathers. Young chickens appear to have a greater power of resistance against thallium poisoning than older birds. Zinc phosphide and sodium fluoroacetate have also been reported as being toxic. Toxicity symptoms have also been shown after the administration of DDT.

Carbide poisoning in hens,[62] colchicin[63] poisoning in ducks, and naphthalene[64] poisoning in hens have also been reported.

The general symptoms of poisoning are depression, ruffled feathers, general debility and unthriftiness, purple comb, diarrhea, and inflammation of the intestinal tract.

In general, toxins act qualitatively in the same manner on birds as on mammals. Quantitatively, there are great differences between birds and other animals. Birds are very sensitive to a few poisons, such as cyanide and carbon monoxide, alcohol, and nicotine. On the other hand, they are less sensitive than mammals to other poisons, such as urea, arsenic, and nerve poisons.[65]

SALT POISONING

Too much salt is toxic.[66] The symptoms of salt intoxication are inability to stand, intense thirst, pronounced muscular weakness, and convulsive movements just before death. A viscous discharge from the beak has also been noted, as well as symptoms of paralysis and blue comb. Post-mortem examination reveals edema and lesions in many organs, but particularly hemorrhages and severe congestion in the gastro-intestinal tract, muscles, liver, kidneys, and lungs.

The toxicity of salt seems to depend to some extent upon the manner in which it is administered, the presence of water, the age of the birds, and the resistance which has been developed toward it. The minimum lethal dose seems to be about 4 grams per kilogram of body weight or 0.4 per cent of the body weight. Young stock can assimilate greater quantities of salt than adult birds. Concentrations between 0.5 per cent and 0.9 per cent salt in the drinking water produced extreme thirst, short rapid breathing, and edematous swelling within a few days. Ducks have been reported to be more susceptible to salt poisoning than chickens.[67]

POSSIBLE HARM FROM DRUGS AND HORMONES

Considerable attention has been devoted in the past few years to hormones and their effects on the animal. Caution must be used in the application of hormones to feeding, since they might have deterimental effects. For example, thyroid, when given in excess, will retard the rate of growth or even cause a loss of body weight.

A number of sulfa drugs have been used for the prevention and control of poultry diseases. It is necessary to exercise precaution in their use and feed according to directions, since large dosages may be harmful.[68]

LOSSES FROM CANNIBALISM

Management and environment are important factors in avoiding or controlling losses from cannibalism and feather picking. However, it is also recognized that the ration and feeding management might have an influence in this respect. Malnutrition[69] due to a deficiency of protein, minerals, or other factors might of itself result in an increase in cannibalism and feather picking.

POULTRY FEEDING FROM THE PATHOLOGICAL STANDPOINT

Much can be done to maintain the health of the flock by proper attention to feeding management. One program along this line is given by Axworthy,[70] in which he suggests that the following be avoided. (1) Excess fiber in the mash or poor quality meals of a fibrous nature. They might result in infection of the gizzard, inflammation of the intestinal tract (mechanical enteritis), and inflammation of the kidneys (secondary). (2) Lack of fiber. This might result in pasted beaks and impacted crops. It is likely to be accompanied by loose, bad-smelling diarrhea, intestines filled with a mucoid pasty mass, and an atonic condition of the intestinal tract. (3) Excess protein. This may be accompanied by enlarged and inflamed kidneys (nephritis) and ureters distended with urates. (4) Unpalatable mash. This might result in depraved appetite, causing the eating of litter, and a mechanical enteritis. (5) Stale or moldy food. This might result in the development of aspergillosis. (6) Overfatness. The hens are likely to be more susceptible to disease such as egg peritonitis. (7) Sharp flinty substances. They may cause laceration and inflammation of the intestinal tract.

REFERENCES

1. Heiser, V. G. The influence of nutrition on the diseases of middle and old age. Sci. Monthly. Oct., 1939:304.
2. Wilcke, H. L., F. D. Patterson, E. W. Henderson, and C. Murray. The effect of the ration upon the incidence of so-called range paralysis. Poultry Sci. 12:226. 1933.
3. Prentice, J. H. The relation of the calcium content of the ration to mortality in the chicken. Jour. Ministry Agr. N. Ireland 6:69. 1938.
4. Pallaske. Über eine eigenartige Kalkdiathese (Kalkgicht) beim Huhn. Tierärztliche Rundschau. 1933:255.
5. Hartwick, H. Über das Vorkommen der Viszeralgicht (Eingeweidegicht) bei Junghühnern und Hühnerkücken. Tierärztliche Rundschau 46:812.

   Mayall, G. Visceral gout in poultry. Vet. Jour. 1929:230.
6. Hull, T. G., and L. Rettger. Influence of milk and carbohydrate feeding on the character of the intestinal flora. Jour. Bact. 2:47. 1917.
7. Beach, J. R., and D. E. Davis. The influence of feeding lactose or dry skimmilk on artificial infection of chicks with Eimeria avium. Hilgardia 1:167. 1925.
8. Becker, E. R. Dietary control in experimental coccidiosis. Science 86:403. 1937.

   Becker, E. R., and P. C. Waters. The influence of the ration on mortality from caecal coccidiosis in chicks. Iowa Jour. Sci. 12: 405. 1938.
9. Herrick, C. A., C. E. Holmes, and S. H. Waxler. Steamed bone meal favors coccidiosis. Wis. Bul. 453:5. 1941.
10. Heuser, G. F. Influence of vitamins on growth and resistance to coccidiosis. Reliable Poultry Jour. April 1924:226.
11. Jones, E. Elizabeth. The effect of diet on the course of experimental coccidiosis in the chicken. Jour. Am. Vet. Med. Ass'n. 38:193. 1934.
12. Mann, T. B. Chick rearing. X. Roughage and protein as dietary factors influencing coccidiosis in chicks, with notes on the limitation of sulphamezathine in the control of coccidiosis. Jour. Agric. Sci. 37:145. 1947.
13. Boari, D. Avitaminiosis. Its effect on immunity. Giornale di clinica medicina 17 (1936) Nov., Pediatria No. 4:367. 1937.
14. Seeler, O. A., and W. H. Ott. Studies on nutrition and avian malaria. Jour. Infect. Diseases 77:82, 181. 1945.
15. Ackert, J. E., and T. D. Beach. Resistance of chickens to the nematode Ascaridia lineata affected by dietary supplements. Am. Micros. Soc. Trans. 52:51. 1933.

    Ackert, J. E., and L. O. Nolf. Resistance of chickens to parasitism by vitamin B. Am. Jour. Hygiene 13:337. 1931.

    Ackert, J. E., M. F. McIlvaine, and N. Z. Crawford. Resistance of chickens to parasitism affected by vitamin A. Am. Jour. Hygiene 13:320, 1931.

16. Baldwin, F. M., O. B. Wiswell, and H. A. Jankiewicz. Hemorrhage control in chicks infected with Eimeria tenella when protected by antihemorrhagic factor, vitamin K. Proc. Soc. Exp. Biol. & Med. 48:278. 1941.
17. Clapham, Phyllis A. The effect of dietary deficiency on infestation of chickens with the nematode Heterakis gallinae. Jour. of Helminthology 12:123. 1934.
18. Allen, W. H. Why chicks die? N. J. Hints 12(7). 1924.
Lamson, G. H., Jr. The rose chafer as a cause of death of chickens. Conn. Bul. 110. 1922.
19. Heller, V. G., and L. Morris. Grasshoppers in turkey feeding. Okla. Exp. Sta. Rept. 1934-36: 77. 1936.
Wickware, A. B. Grasshoppers. A potential danger to turkeys. Canad. Jour. Comp. Med. & Vet. Sci. 9:80. 1945.
20. Grzimek, B. Mortality in pigeons. Krankes Geflügel (Berlin) 1944:172.
21. Gibbs, C. S. Moldy corn. Mass. Bul. 280:242. 1931.
22. Ronk, S. E., and C. W. Carrick. Feeding moldy corn to chickens. Poultry Sci. 10:236. 1931.
23. Borchers, R., and G. L. Peltier. Molded foodstuffs. I. Supplementary value in chick starting rations. Poultry Sci. 26:194. 1946.
24. Titus, H. W., and A. B. Godfrey. Comparison of scabbed barley, normal barley, and yellow corn in diets for laying chickens. U.S.D.A. Tech. Bul. 435. 1934.
Is scab infested barley harmful to chickens? Ind. Rept. 1929:60.
25. Winter, A. R., and C. M. Ferguson. Feeding new scabby wheat to chickens. Feedstuffs 15(52):20. 1943.
26. Waite, R. H. Field damaged wheat for poultry. Md. Bul. 231. 1919.
27. Gordon, R. F., and J. B. Blaxland. The occurrence in England of outbreaks of disease in poultry resembling the "so-called pullet disease" of America. Vet. Jour. 101:3. 1945.
Petty, M. A., and G. D. Quigley. The microflora of wheat feeds as related to the incidence of blue comb in chickens. Poultry Sci. 26:7. 1947.
Quigley, G. D. The effect of wheat upon the incidence of pullet disease or blue comb. Poultry Sci. 23:386. 1944.
Quigley, G. D. Further studies with wheat and pullet disease. Poultry Sci. 27:647. 1948.
28. Gilch, H. Fütterungsversuche an Hühnern mit Getreide das mit quecksilberhaltigen Mitteln gebeizt ist. Dissertation, Pharmacological Institute. University Leipzig. 1932.
Honcamp. Die Denaturierung von Getreide mit Eosin zu Fütterungszwecken und die Verfütterung von Eosinierten Weizen an Geflügel. Biedermanns Zentralblatt 5:87. 1933.
Hopfengärtner. Beinflusst Eosin-Weizenfütterung der Hühner die Konservierungsfähigkeit der Eier? Münchener Tierärztliche Wochenschrift 87:397. 1936.
Reghi, M. Effetti dell eosina e del blu di metilene usati come denaturanti delle granaglie. Rivista di Avicultura 5:533. 1935.
Roemer, R., and J. Jaeger. Fütterungsversuche mit Eosinierten

Weizen bei Legehennen und Masthähnchen. Die Tierernährung 5:108. 1933.

Wagner, F. Gesundheitsshädigungen nach Verfütterung von Eosinweizen. Süddtsch. landw. Tierzucht 27:401. 1933.

29. Horvath, A. A. Studies in blood composition of animal under pathological conditions. III. Feeding hens with corn smut. Poultry Sci. 9:313. 1930.
30. Sorghum smuts prove harmless. Okla. Rept. 1927-1930:180.
31. Penquite, R., and V. G. Heller. Effect of sorghum and wheat smuts on chickens. Okla. Rept. 1930-1932:120.
32. Quigley, G. D., and R. H. Waite. Miscellaneous feeding trials with poultry. Md. Bul. 325. 1931.
33. Lobl, J. Poisoning by ergot. Dreptul nostru 11:20. 1935. (Reference in Berliner Tierärztliche Wochenschrift 1935:424.)
34. Brunett, E. L. Poultry diseases. Cornell Bul. 337:51. 1935.
35. Hart, L. Poisonous to fowls: seeds of Araujia sericifera. Agr. Gazette (N. S. Wales) 51:472. 1940.
36. Temperton, H., and F. J. Dudley. A note on the feeding of a cocoa waste to poultry. Harper Adams Utility Poultry Jour. 28:12. 1943.
37. Corn cockle. Jour. Board Agr. Great Britain 17:38. 1910.

Bayon, H. P. Corn cockle seeds in poultry feeds. Chanticleer. Nov., 1933.

Chestnut, V. K. Thirty poisonous plants. U.S.D.A. Farmers' Bul. 86. 1898.

Heuser, G. F., and A. E. Schumacher. The feeding of corn cockle to chickens. Poultry Sci. 21:86. 1942.

Kornauth, C., and C. Arche. The physiological effect of corn cockle when fed to swine. Landwirtschaftlichen Versuchs-Stationen 40: 177. 1892.

Quigley, G. D., and R. H. Waite. Miscellaneous feeding trials with poultry. Md. Bul. 325:343. 1931.

Schneider, Dr. Saponinvergiftung durch Verfütterung von Eosiniertem Weizen. Deutsche Landwirtschaftliche Geflügelzeitung. Sept. 22, 1932.

Schneider, Dr. Kornradevergiftung beim Geflügel und ihre Einwirkung auf die Legeleistung. Archiv für Geflügelk. 7:121. 1933.

Theret, M. Intoxication des volailles par la nielle des bles. Rec. Vet. Ecole d'Alfort 122:125. 1946.

38. Emmel, M. W. The pathology of Crotalaria spectabilis Roth seed poisoning in the domestic fowl. Jour. Am. Vet. Med. Assn. 90: 627. 1937.

Emmel, M. W. The toxicity of crotalaria retura L. seeds for the domestic fowl. Jour. Am. Vet. Med. Assn. 91:205. 1937.

Piercy, P. L., and L. L. Rusoff. Crotelaria spectabilis poisoning in Louisiana livestock. Jour. Am. Vet. Med. Ass'n. 108:69. 1946.

Thomas, E. F. The effect of feeding crotalaria seed to chickens and other birds. Fla. Rept. 1932:57.

Thomas, E. F. The toxicity of certain species of crotalaria seed for the chicken, quail, turkey and dove. Jour. Am. Vet. Med. Assn. 85:617. 1934.

39. Shealy, A. L., and E. F. Thomas. *Daubentonia* seed poisoning of poultry. *Fla. Bul.* 196. 1928.
40. Emmel, M. W. The toxicity of *Glottidium vesicarium* (Jacg.) Harper seeds for the fowl. *Jour. Am. Vet. Med. Assn.* 87:13. 1935.
41. Lerche. Vergiftungen von Gänsen durch Schotendotter. *Deutsche Landwirtschaftliche Geflügelzeitung* 1933:877.
Völker, R. Die Giftwirkung des Bitterstoffe Erysimupikron. *Berliner Tierärztliche Wochenschrift* 1934:232.
42. Campbell, H. W. The whorled milkweed as a poisonous plant for poultry. *Calif. Dept. of Agr. Monthly Bul.* Vol. XX(8):577. 1931.
Campbell, H. W. Poisoning in chickens with whorled milkweed. *Jour. Am. Vet. Med. Assn.* 79:102. 1931.
43. Stiles, G. W. Poisoning of turkey poults from whorled milkweed. *Poultry Sci.* 21:263. 1942.
44. Couch, J. F. Poisoning of livestock by plants that produce hydrocyanic acid. *U.S.D.A. Leaflet* 88. 1932.
45. Kay, N. D. Parsley. *Poultry (Australia).* Oct. 14, 1933.
46. Brown, F. C. Utility poultry keeping. *New Zealand Dept. Agr. Bul.* 66:23. 1922.
Salomon, S. Kartoffelvergiftung bei Enten. *Berliner Tierärztliche Wochenschrift* 51:85. 1935.
47. McCulloch, E. C. The use of grain containing tarweed seed as poultry feed. *Jour. Am. Vet. Med. Assn.* 101:481. 1942.
48. Harvey, R. B., A. H. Larson, R. H. Landon, W. L. Boyd, and L. C. Erickson. Weeds poisonous to livestock. *Minn. Bul.* 388:8. 1945.
49. Eveleth, D. F., A. I. Goldsby, and O. A. Stevens. Tests on the seed of lead plant as a feed for chickens and pheasants. *N. Dak. Bimo. Bul.* 11:129. 1949.
50. Horvath, A. A. Toxicity of vetch seed for chickens. *Poultry Sci.* 24:291. 1945.
51. Aleinikov, A. N. The substitution of wheat offals (screenings) for whole grain in fattening poultry. *Trans. All-Union Inst. Poultry Industries (Moscow)* 3:149. 1938.
52. Kesko, N. Poisoning by acetic acid. *Jugoslovenski Veterinarski Glasnig* 12:274. 1932.
53. Wegner, M. I., W. W. Cravens, and J. G. Halpin. Boric acid injures chickens. *Wisc. Bul.* 449:91. 1940.
Witter, J. F. A preliminary report on the injurious effect of sodium bicarbonate in chicks. *Poultry Sci.* 15:256. 1936.
54. Tocuason, W. K., and R. F. Gordon. Acute arsenical poisoning in fowls. *Vet. Record* 1938:403.
55. Chorley, J. K., and R. McChlery. Experiments on the toxicity to fowls of arsenite of soda and poisoned locusts. *Rhodesia Agr. Jour.* 32:322. 1935.
Thomas, E. F., and A. L. Shealy. Lead arsenate poisoning in chickens. *Jour. Agr. Res.* 45:317. 1932.
VanZyl, J. P. On the toxicity of arsenic to fowls. *South African Poultry Mag.* Nov., 1930.

Effect of arsenic on chickens. Poultry Tribune. Feb., 1937.
56. Pullar, E. M. Toxicity of various copper compounds and mixtures for domesticated birds. Australian Vet. Jour. 16:147. 1940.
57. Döhler. Is stain poisonous? Thesis. Leipzig. 1936.
58. Hinshaw, W. R., and W. E. Lloyd. Studies on the use of copper sulphate for turkeys. Poultry Sci. 10:392. 1931.
59. Phillips, P. H., J. G. Halpin, and E. B. Hart. The influence of chronic fluorine toxicosis in laying hens upon the fluorine content of the egg and its relation to the lipoid content of the egg yolk. Jour. Nutr. 10:93. 1935.
60. Grzimek, B. Die Wirkung von Nikontinsulfat auf Hühner. Tierärztliche Rundschau 41:1935.
Hunter, J. E., D. E. Haley, and H. C. Knandel. Effect of concentrations of nicotine on growth and development. II. Growth and development of chicks as influenced by the addition of ground tobacco to the ration. Poultry Sci. 13:91. 1934.
61. Blaxland, J. D., and R. F. Gordon. Zinc phosphide poisoning in poultry. Vet. Jour. 101:108. 1945.
Cottral, G. E., G. D. Dibble, and B. Winton. The effect of sodium fluoroacetate ("1080" rodenticide) on White Leghorn chickens. Poultry Sci. 26:610. 1947.
Landauer, W. Influence of thallium salts on the moulting mechanism of fowls. Jour. Agr. Res. 43:67. 1931.
Marsden, S. J., and H. R. Bird. Effects of DDT on growing turkeys. Poultry Sci. 26:3. 1947.
Nelson, A. A., J. H. Draize, G. Woodard, O. G. Fitzhugh, R. B. Smith, and H. O. Calvery. Histopathological changes following administration of DDT to several species of animals. Public Health Rept. 59 (31):1009. 1944.
Plazikowski, V., and S. Svensson. Experimental thallium poisoning of dog and fowl. Skandinavisk veterinär-tidskrift 26:68. 1936.
Robertson, A., J. G. Campbell, and D. N. Graves. Experimental zinc phosphide poisoning in fowl. Jour. Compar. Pathol. & Ther. 55:290. 1945.
Rubin, M., H. R. Bird, N. Green, and R. H. Carter. Toxicity of DDT to laying hens. Poultry Sci. 26:410. 1947.
Salisbury, R. M. The toxicity of DDT for poultry. Australian Vet. Jour. 23:361. 1947.
Schneider, Dr. Vergiftung durch Zeliokörner beim Geflügel. Deutsche Tierärztliche Wochenschrift 1933:403.
62. Kuscher, A. Karbidvergiftung bei Hühnern. Tierärztliche Monatsschrift 25:692. 1938.
63. Entenmann, E. Colchicinvergiftung bei Enten. Thesis. Munich. 1937.
64. Napthalene poisoning. Poultry Tribune. March 1937.
Hudson, C. B. Napthalene poisoning in poultry. Jour. Am. Vet. Med. Ass'n. 89:219. 1936.
65. Forchheimer, L. Über die Wirkung verschiedener Gifte auf Vogel. Tierärztliche Rundschau 1931:624.
66. Blaxland, J. D. The toxicity of sodium chloride for fowls. Vet. Jour. 102:157. 1946.

Blaxland, J. D. Salt poisoning in poultry. Modern Poultry Keeping 54 (25):489. June 19, 1946.
Bressler, G. O., S. Gordeuk, E. W. Callenbach, and G. H. Pritham. The effect of salt and carbolineum in producing ascites in turkey poults. Poultry Sci. 30:738. 1951.
Doll, E. R., F. E. Hull, and W. M. Insko, Jr. Toxicity of sodium chloride solution for baby chicks. Vet. Med. 41:361. 1946.
Erich, A. Investigations concerning the operation of foods containing herring pickle and bits of herring for fowls; a contribution to the question of kitchen salt poisoning in poultry. Thesis, Tiersuchteninstitut der Universität Leipzig. 1935.
Kare, M. R., and J. Biely. The toxicity of sodium chloride and its relation to water intake in baby chicks. Poultry Sci. 27:751. 1948.
Krakower, C. A., and M. Goettsch. Effect of excessive ingestion of sodium chloride on the chick, with particular reference to renal changes. Arch. Pathol. 40:209. 1945.
Krakower, C. A., and H. E. Heino. Relationship of growth and nutrition to cardiorenal changes induced in birds by a high salt intake. Arch. Pathol. 44:143. 1947.
Matterson, L. D., H. M. Scott, and E. Jungherr. Salt tolerance of turkeys. Poultry Sci. 25:539. 1946.
Mitchell, H. H., L. E. Card, and C. G. Carman. The toxicity of salt for chickens. Ill. Bul. 279. 1926.
Quigley, G. D., and R. H. Waite. Salt tolerance of baby chicks. Md. Bul. 340. 1932.
Scrivner, L. H. Experimental edema and ascites (water belly) in poults. Jour. Am. Vet. Med. Assoc. 108:27. 1946.
Selye, H. Production of nephrosclerosis in the fowl by sodium chloride. Jour. Am. Vet. Med. Assn. 103:140. 1943.
Too much salt in ration may kill young chicks. Penn. Agr. Exp. Sta. 60th Ann. Rept:29. 1947.
67. Torrey, J. P., and R. Graham. A note on experimental salt poisoning in ducks. Cornell Veterinarian 25:50. 1935.
68. Bankowski, R. A. A decrease in egg production following sulfamerazine and sulfamethazine medication. Jour. Am. Vet. Med. Assn. 113;49. 1948.
Riedel, B. B. The effect of sulfamerazine upon egg production and hatchability. Poultry Sci. 29:621. 1950.
Singsen, E. P., H. M. Scott, and L. D. Matterson. The effect of sulfaquinoxaline on growth rate and feed efficiency of chicks. Poultry Sci. 27:627. 1948.
69. Schaible, P. J., J. A. Davidson, and S. L. Bandemer. Cannibalism and feather picking in chicks as influenced by certain changes in a specific ration. Poultry Sci. 26:651. 1947.
70. Axworthy, R. H. Poultry feeding from the pathological standpoint. Rept. Poultry Path. Res. Lab. Reading (Eng.) June 1931.

CHAPTER 12

FEEDING AND MANAGEMENT OF YOUNG CHICKENS

The object to be accomplished in the feeding of young chickens is to grow strong, well-matured, normal individuals with little or no mortality, at a cost that is consistent with good results.

CHANGES IN WEIGHT DURING GROWTH

One of the purposes of a chick ration is to produce normal growth. Normal growth refers to the weights, limited by inheritance, which the chicks should attain when kept under favorable conditions. It is necessary to keep in mind, however, that the rate of growth is subject to variation, depending upon breeding, management, and environmental conditions. Hence there are definite standards for each variety or strain which has a different weight at maturity.

The actual weights of chicks, and especially the weights during the early growth period, have improved owing to advances in breeding, feeding, and management. Weights and feed consumption representative of earlier results[1] have been bettered by more recent figures shown in Tables 19 and 20.

There is very little difference in the growth of chickens that are reared indoors or on range when they are fed equivalent rations. However, Kentucky[2] reported that the pullets and cockerels reared indoors and without direct sunshine were not so vigorous and active or so healthy in appearance as those reared outdoors.

The time of hatching does have an influence upon growth. The general tendency is for early hatched chicks to grow faster than late-hatched chicks.[3] However, Kempster[4] also reports that these differences may be explained on the basis of high temperatures during the growing season. The type of growth curve, therefore, varies, depending on the date the chicks are hatched and the temperatures that prevail during the growing season.

The energy of the young stock is thrown into growth and motion. If either growth or activity is stopped for any period of

TABLE 19. GROWTH AND FEED CONSUMPTION OF CHICKS

Age in Weeks	Body Weight Per Bird, lb. Cockerels and Pullets 50-50 (except as noted)		lb. Feed per lb. Body Weight to Age Shown	
	Leghorns	Heavy Breeds	Leghorns	Heavies
1	.15	.19	.8	.8
2	.25	.33	1.4	1.3
3	.36	.51	1.6	1.5
4	.55	.77	1.9	1.8
5	.78	1.2	2.2	2.0
6	1.2	1.5	2.5	2.2
7	1.4	1.9	2.6	2.3
8	1.7	2.2	2.7	2.5
9	2.0	2.4	2.8	2.7
	Pullets Only		Pullets Only	
10	1.9	2.5	3.3	2.9
11	2.1	2.9	3.4	3.1
12	2.3	3.3	3.6	3.3
13	2.5	3.6	3.9	3.6
14	2.7	3.9	4.2	3.8
15	2.9	4.3	4.4	4.0
16	3.1	4.6	4.7	4.1
17	3.2	4.9	5.1	4.2
18	3.3	5.2	5.6	4.3
19	3.4	5.4	5.8	4.4
20	3.5	5.7	6.1	4.7

Reproduced by permission from Profitable Poultry Management, 20th Edition, 1952, by Clarence E. Lee. Copyrighted by the Beacon Milling Co. Inc., Cayuga, New York.

TABLE 20. GROWTH AND FEED CONSUMPTION OF S.C.W. LEGHORN FEMALES AT CORNELL UNIVERSITY

Age in Weeks	Average Weight, lb.	Total Feed Consumed, lb.
2	0.28	0.49
4	0.64	1.55
6	1.10	2.91
8	1.30	4.06
12	2.14	9.36
16	2.77	13.84
20	3.36	18.86
23	3.73	23.16

time, the results will not be favorable. Both must continue steadily according to the laws of growth. Growth represents increases in tissues, such as bones, muscle, skin, feathers, and nerves. Besides water, these increases are chiefly in protein and minerals.

GROWTH RELATIONS

Before we can consider chick feeding intelligently, it is necessary to be familiar with the way the chick grows. With poultry in general, we have very rapid growth early in life. This growth is more rapid than in any other farm animal. Although the average chick will double its weight in about a week to 10 days, it is not unusual to find individual chicks doing this in a week. It is unlikely, however, that it will again double its weight within a like period of time.

RATE OF GROWTH. The mode of growth or percentage rate of increase[5] varies with age. Average weekly gains are greatest during the first month or 6 weeks. During the next month or 6 weeks, the average rate of gain will be cut in half, after which time there is usually a steady decrease in the rate of growth until no more gains are made.

Since there is more danger of trouble when the growth is relatively rapid, it is usually agreed that the greatest possibilities of trouble occur during the first period. If the chicks can be successfully reared to 2 months of age, the danger periods are generally passed.

ACTUAL GAINS. As far as actual gains are concerned, there will be some variation from period to period. There is a tendency, however, for the actual gains to increase until the chicks are about 3 months of age, after which time there is a general decrease.

FEED RELATIONS. The amount of food consumed increases with the increase in the size of the bird. Since the rate of growth is also rapid at the start, the gains per unit of food are larger

Period, Weeks	Pounds of Feed to Produce One Pound of Gain
0—4	2.42
4—8	3.80
9—12	6.30
13—16	7.10
17—20	8.51

early in life. A larger proportion of the food goes into growth. Hence more economical gains are made when the chicks are growing rapidly, as shown by the accompanying figures, which indicate, for a typical group of birds, the amounts of feed required to produce 1 pound of gain in Leghorn pullets at different ages.

EARLY HANDICAPS. A number of reports[5-7] have shown that depressed growth in earlier periods was compensated for later by more rapid growth, when the nutrient level became adequate. Where there is a partial deficiency, early growth may be slow. However, this growth may be made up in later periods so that, with the same breeding, the final mature weight of such chicks will be approximately the same as that of chicks which grew faster at the start, in which case later growth is relatively not so rapid. There is, however, also probably some level for the various nutrients below which one cannot safely feed because the resulting severe stunting can never be entirely overcome.

Parker[8] showed that a variety of early handicaps, including poisons, starvation, and high and low temperatures, failed to alter markedly the course of yolk absorption in baby chicks and also failed to produce permanent effects in body weights.

Mayhew[9] reported that chickens severely infected with coccidiosis at 12 or 13 weeks of age do not recover their loss in weight; that is, they do not become equal in weight to the controls during the following 9 to 10 weeks.

Several workers[10-12] concluded that retarding the growth of chicks resulted in a definite delaying of sexual maturity with variable effects upon body weight and egg production of the mature birds. Retarding of growth and maturity did not appear to be a sound economic practice, but it could be followed if desired without fear of permanent injury to the birds.

There are many advantages of securing early rapid growth (which is the normal condition), such as maintained vitality and body reserve, earlier broiler marketing, and sufficient weight of pullets at time of laying to produce good production and egg size. Titus and Jull[6] point out that, in the lots receiving skimmilk (and growing rapidly early), the point of inflection of the growth curve occurred earlier than in the lots not receiving it. This suggested to them that the more nearly a "perfect" condition of nutrition is approached, the more nearly will the whole of the growth curve approach the curve of diminishing increment, which they believe most nearly to fit the growth data of chickens developing normally. Hendricks, Jull, and Titus[13] further suggest that the curve of diminishing increment may be of value in determining the suitability of a given feed for growth.

FEED REQUIREMENTS

An analysis of the bodies of chicks at various stages of growth will help to understand feed needs. The data in Table 21 are given by Halnan:[14]

TABLE 21. ANALYSIS OF CHICKS AT VARIOUS AGES

Age in Weeks	Ash, Grams	Protein, Grams	Energy, 100 Calories
1	1.04	6.9	0.7
3	3.02	17.2	1.7
7	9.53	45.4	3.4
11	17.3	84.0	6.2
15	45.5	223.5	14.8
20	64.8	282.8	20.5
24	90.0	338.0	24.4
28	94.0	376.0	32.1

AMOUNT OF FOOD. During the early stages, the rate of growth of the chick is limited by its capacity to consume food. Titus and Hendricks[15] conclude that if chicks are fed at different levels of feed intake (with a complete ration) up to about one pound, the average live weight of the chicks in all the pens could be considered as a function of feed consumption alone. A possible explanation of this is that the maintenance requirement of the young growing chick is only a small fraction of the total amount of feed consumed.

There is probably little possibility of overfeeding a chick in its early stages of growth if the ration is properly compounded. In order to get maximum food consumption, it is important to provide sufficient and proper feeding space. The Nutrition Council of the American Feed Manufacturers recommends the following feeding space as being satisfactory for 100 chicks:

Age in weeks	
1 day— 2 weeks	100 linear inches
3— 6 weeks	175 linear inches
7—12 weeks	300 linear inches

The following drinking space is suggested:

1 day— 2 weeks	20 linear inches or two 1-gallon fountains
3—12 weeks	40 linear inches or two 3-gallon fountains

From the results obtained in various rearing experiments Axelsson[16] has calculated the total food requirements for maintenance and growth of "light," "medium," and "heavy" chicks at different ages (Table 22).

TABLE 22. FOOD REQUIREMENTS OF THE GROWING FOWL (POUNDS PER DAY PER 100 BIRDS)

Month of Life	Light Breeds		Medium Breeds		Heavy Breeds	
	Females	Males	Females	Males	Females	Males
1	4.4	4.7	4.7	4.9	4.9	5.1
2	8.6	9.3	9.1	10.0	9.8	10.7
3	12.6	13.8	14.2	15.6	15.4	16.8
4	16.1	17.7	17.9	20.3	20.0	22.4
5	18.2	20.3	21.0	23.5	24.0	26.3
6	18.9	21.4	21.9	25.4	24.9	29.1
7	18.6	21.0	22.4	26.1	27.5	30.5
8	....	....	21.7	25.6	27.5	30.5
9	....	....	....	....	26.6	29.6

For additional information on the amount of food for young stock, see Chap. 19, "Economics of Feeding."

The best growth is induced by a ration having a balance of the essential nutrients. Any deficiency or defect in the diet which prevents normal development will also increase the variability in growth.[17]

PROTEIN. It has been pointed out by various investigators that the protein requirements of different species of animals are more or less proportionate to the rate of growth.

Bunge[18] also shows that the rate of growth is proportional to the protein in the natural food (milk), as indicated by the length of time required to double the initial weight (Table 23).

It has also been pointed out by various authorities that the protein requirements of chicks are greater than the protein needs of laying hens. The unabsorbed yolk material, present in the chick at the time of hatching, contains a large amount of protein. It has been stated that this ratio of protein to the other parts is about 1:1.4. When we consider the wild birds, we note that the young are fed very largely on grubs and worms, which are primarily protein.

Growth in chicks and the accompanying protein requirements

TABLE 23. RELATION IN MAMMALS OF GROWTH RATE TO PROTEIN OF MILK

Time for Newborn Animal to Double Its Weight		Milk Per Cent Protein	Milk Nutritive Ratio
Man	180 days	1.6	1:8.6
Horse	60	2.0	1:4.2
Cow	47	3.5	1:3.8
Goat	22	3.7	1:3.6
Sheep	15	4.9	1:3.4
Hog	14	6.1	1:3.0
Dog	9	9.7	1:2.5
Rabbit	6	15.5	1:1.5

may be divided into three periods. The first period, calling for rapid growth and a high protein level, includes approximately the first 6 weeks. The second period, during which growth is less rapid and the protein level can be decreased, extends from the end of the first period to about 3 months. The third period, during which growth is further decelerated and the protein level can be again decreased to some extent, continues from the end of the second period until the end of the growing period.

Funk[19] reports that when chicks were given free choice of food they selected a ration containing 18 to 19 per cent protein.

Most of the experimental results[20-30] indicate that the early rate of growth of chicks is increased as the protein level is increased to about 20 per cent, that lots receiving low-protein rations weigh less practically throughout, that mortality is usually increased in the low-protein lots, and that the protein can be decreased in the later periods. Some reports indicate higher levels[31] as being desirable or satisfactory from the standpoint of the health and well-being of the animal. Some trials[32] show that heavier breeds made more satisfactory gains when a higher level of protein was used.

ing, and cannibalism developing in low-protein pens as early as the second and third week. Feather eating and pick-outs were also observed in low-protein pens at Cornell. Tomhave[29] indicates a direct relationship between the number of bare-breasted birds and the level of protein. Gericke and Platt[33] indicated that feather development over the entire body showed a significant increase in direct relation to the amount of protein in the ration (10.4 to 15.4 per cent), and the development of each feather tract was of the same order. Carver and associates[20] and Zuzuki and

Hatano[24] report no influence of the protein level upon the development of liver, kidney, spleen, pancreas, heart, adrenal body, pituitary body, thymus gland, and testicles.

In work with experimental coccidiosis, Jones[34] states that chickens on high-protein diets maintained their weight at a level nearer that of their uninfected controls than chickens on a low-protein diet. High-protein diets may thus be considered to furnish a reserve that prevents undue loss of weight as a result of coccidial infection. Luttermoser and Allen[35] report that young chickens fed a diet containing 13 per cent protein and experimentally infected with the tapeworm (*Raillietina cesticillus*) gained less weight than their uninfected controls throughout the duration of a 6-week period, whereas the young chickens fed a diet containing 26 per cent protein and infected with the same number of cysticeroids did not differ markedly in weight from their uninfected controls.

Titus[36] reported that chicks made the greatest gain per pound of feed when the diet contained 21 per cent protein. On the basis of this level, the 20 per cent protein ration showed an efficiency of 99.7 per cent; the 19 per cent protein ration, 98.7 per cent; the 18 per cent protein ration, 97.2 per cent; and the 17 per cent protein ration, 94.6 per cent. The rations containing less than 17 per cent protein decreased very rapidly in efficiency. The level of protein intake, so long as it is not less than about 13 per cent, has little effect on the maximum live weight ultimately attained. However, the time required to reach the maximum live weight is greatly increased as the level of protein intake decreases from 21 to 13 per cent.

The Delaware,[29] New Jersey,[37] and Washington[20] stations indicate that decreasing amounts of protein in the growing rations will meet the requirements which change with age.

Titus[36] concludes that even though the optimum level of protein intake is, from the physiological standpoint, about 21 per cent, from the standpoint of economy it may be only 18 or 19 per cent, because the efficiency of feed utilization for growth is only slightly less at these levels. The difference in cost will be an important factor in determining the most economical level. He has found it a good practice to feed a diet that contains 20 to 21 per cent of protein until the chickens are about 12 weeks old and then gradually decrease the protein content to 16 or 17 per cent by the time the pullets are ready to lay.

The results of all trials at Cornell[26] indicate that to obtain early rapid growth the ration should contain approximately 20 per cent protein during the first month. This amount can be reduced 2 per cent for each succeeding month. The indications also are that the ration should never contain much less than 15 per cent protein.

AMINO ACID REQUIREMENTS. Some of the amino acids are essential and must be present in the ration. Others can be synthesized by the chick. The essential amino acids can be supplied in minimum amounts only when there are sufficient dispensable amino acids present so that the essential ones are not used for their synthesis.

Considerable research has been reported concerning the quantitative amino acid requirements[38] of chickens. These requirements may be summarized as follows: arginine 1.2 per cent; glycine 1.0–1.5 per cent; isoleucine 0.5 per cent; leucine 1.5 per cent; lysine 0.67 to 1.0 per cent; methionine (with cystine present) 0.28 to 0.42 per cent; sulfur-bearing amino acids (methionine + cystine) 0.7 to 1.0 per cent; phenylalanine 1.6 per cent; threonine 0.45 to 0.6 per cent; tryptophan 0.18 to 0.5 per cent; valine 0.7 per cent.

FAT. It is not necessary to include fat in the ration for chicks since they can utilize carbohydrates for fat formation. However, there is some evidence that certain unsaturated fatty acids are needed in the diet.[39] Davis and Upp[40] reported that chicks fed a fat-free ration grew somewhat more slowly than the chicks receiving fat, but that the slight difference was overcome by the time the pullets reached maturity. Russell, Taylor, and Polskin[41] reported that the growth rate of chicks to 14 weeks of age fed a low-fat diet (0.1 per cent) was not significantly below that of chicks fed a normal ration (4.1 per cent fat). Chicks on the low-fat diet utilized crystalline carotene despite the very low level of fat intake.

In studying the tolerance of growing chicks for soybean oil in their ration, Henderson and Irwin[42] found that the mean weight of chicks at 8 weeks did not vary significantly until the ration contained 10 per cent of oil, after which a significant decrease in weight was obtained.

MINERALS. Calcium and phosphorus are the minerals of chief importance in chick rations. The result of research indicates that the minimum calcium requirement of chicks is 0.6 to 0.7 per cent of the ration in the presence of sufficient vitamin D. The minimum requirement for phosphorus[43] is 0.6 per cent of which 0.4 should be in the inorganic form. There is some indication that somewhat less is required for growth than for bone calcification. The requirement also decreases somewhat with age.

Furthermore, the evidence indicates that these elements should be present in a satisfactory ratio and that they have an interrelationship with vitamin D.[44] The calcium-phosphorus ratio of the blood and bones is about 2 of calcium to 1 of phosphorus. In the chick ration it appears possible to extend this over a range of 1.0:1 to 2.5:1 without any striking upset in the normal blood picture or any marked retardation in growth. A ratio of about 1.5:1 seems preferable.

There is little experimental evidence to show exactly what are the upper levels of calcium and phosphorus, beyond which it is unsafe to go. However, it would appear that 1.8 to 2.0 per cent of calcium and 0.9 to 1.0 per cent of phosphorus are probably the maximum levels it is wise to use in chick rations.

In order to prevent perosis, the ration should contain a minimum amount of 35 to 50 parts per million of manganese.[45] For an average ration the addition of 1/4 pound of manganese sulphate per ton will supply this amount.

The sodium and potassium requirements,[46] which vary with growth rate, have been reported as being 0.10 – 0.30 per cent for sodium and 0.23 – 0.40 per cent for potassium. The requirement for chloride is probably less than 0.6 per cent.

The iodine requirement[47] has been reported between 30 and 150 parts per billion; and the magnesium requirement[48] as 40 milligrams per 100 grams of feed.

Salt is usually added to most chick rations. One quarter to one-half per cent is the most common recommendation.

VITAMINS. The vitamin A requirement[49] of the chick ration has been reported as ranging from 150 to 350 International units of vitamin A per 100 grams of feed. The usual amounts of cod liver oil, 25 to 30 per cent of yellow corn, or green food will furnish this amount.

The vitamin B_1 requirement[50] of chicks has been reported as being 130 to 150 micrograms per 100 grams of feed. If the ration is made up of 30 per cent cereals, sufficient thiamine will be supplied.

If the birds are not exposed to direct sunshine, it will be necessary to feed them cod liver oil or some other vitamin D carrier. Twenty to twenty-five units per 100 grams of feed have been reported to prevent rickets, but approximately twice that amount are needed to give satisfactory growth.[51]

The amount of riboflavin needed by the chick will depend upon its age.[52] The first two weeks it will be 300 to 350 micrograms per 100 grams of feed, which will decrease to 100 micrograms per 100 grams after 2 months of age. When fed a constant amount, chicks needed approximately 290 micrograms per 100 grams of feed in order to attain normal weight at 8 weeks of age. Less riboflavin is needed to prevent curled-toe paralysis than for growth.

The pantothenic acid requirement[53-55] of chicks has been reported as ranging from 500 to 550 micrograms of pantothenic acid per 100 grams of diet. Less is needed for the prevention of dermatosis than for maximum growth. Rhode Island Reds were found less susceptible to pantothenic acid deficiency than Leghorns. Usually there will not be a pantothenic acid deficiency in practice since normal, commercial chick diets were shown to contain 1300 to 1700 micrograms of pantothenic acid per 100 grams.

The amount of vitamin B_6 (pyridoxine)[56-58] required by baby chicks has been variously reported as being 200 to 500 micrograms per 100 grams of ration.

Biotin has also been found necessary in the chick ration to prevent a typical dermatitis and promote growth in chicks. Hegsted and coworkers[59] report that the biotin requirement of the chick is at least 7 to 10 micrograms per 100 grams of the ration.

The choline[60] requirement of diets for chicks has been reported as being 0.1 per cent. This amount, however, may be influenced to some extent by the amount of methionine and betaine in the ration.

The niacin[61] requirement of chicks has been reported as being 8 to 13.5 milligrams per 100 grams. The variation can be accounted for in part by the tryptophan in the diet since this amino acid can be converted to niacin. The requirement for older chicks is considerably lower.[62]

The folic acid requirement of chicks as reported from Cornell[63] is indicated as 25 micrograms per 100 grams of diet for survival, 45 micrograms for growth and hemoglobin formation, and 55 micrograms for good feathering.

The vitamin B_{12}[64] requirement of the chick has been variously reported as ranging from 0.15 to 2.7 micrograms per 100 grams of ration. This great variation can be largely accounted for by the store of vitamin B_{12} in the chick at hatching. The higher values will apply to chicks hatched from eggs produced by hens on a diet deficient in vitamin B_{12}.

Normal blood-clotting time[65] was obtained by adding 1 per cent of alfalfa meal or 5 milligrams of menadione (vitamin K) per kilogram.

Other vitamins have been reported as being essential for normal chick growth, but information is lacking concerning quantitative requirements or the values of feeds in respect to them.

FIBER. Because fiber is not digestible, it is usually felt that the fiber content of chick rations should not be too high, especially since the bulk may decrease available food nutrients and particularly energy. Good results have been obtained with rations containing widely varying amounts of fiber. As an example, the Oklahoma Station[66] reports no effect on the growth or health of the chicks, up to 20 weeks of age, that could be attributed to the amount of fiber in rations containing 3.84 to 10.29 of fiber. Feather picking was worse in the low-fiber lots. Increasing amounts of fiber results in poorer gain and poorer efficiency of the feed. On the other hand, the Kentucky Station[67] concluded that maximum growth was obtained on rations containing approximately 5 per cent or less fiber from any source.

Increasing the amount of such ingredients[68] as oats, barley, wheat middlings, and wheat bran has depressed growth and efficiency of feed utilization.

A requirement for chicks of 800–850 calories of available energy per pound of diet has been reported.[69–71] On the other hand, Hill and Dansky[72] found that Red-Rock crossbred chicks grew well on a ration containing 510 calories. However, their feed intake was greatly increased, and the greatest fat deposition was obtained on the ration containing 985 calories per pound. It appears that the available energy requirement for growth can be stated to be about 850–1000 calories per pound.

STANDARDS. Until recently very little information was available concerning standards for requirements for young stock. The standard, as given by W. P. Wheeler of the New York (Geneva) Experiment Station, was an early attempt to indicate the digestible nutrients required per day for each 100 pounds of live weight (Table 24).

SUMMARY OF NUTRIENT REQUIREMENTS FOR CHICKS

Having considered all the evidence to date, the Committee on Animal Nutrition of the National Research Council[73] suggests the amounts given in the table on page 362 as desirable standards

TABLE 24. WHEELER'S STANDARDS FOR RATIONS FOR CHICKS

	Total Dry Matter	Ash	Protein	Carbohydrates	Fats	Fuel Value	Nutritive Ratio
For the first two weeks	10.1	0.5	2.0	7.2	0.4	18,800	1:4.1
At 2 to 4 weeks of age	9.6	0.7	2.2	6.2	0.5	17,730	1:3.4
At 4 to 6 weeks of age	8.6	0.6	2.0	5.6	0.4	15,640	1:3.3
At 6 to 8 weeks of age	7.4	0.5	1.6	4.9	0.4	13,780	1:3.7
At 8 to 10 weeks of age	6.4	0.5	1.2	4.4	0.3	11,680	1:4.3
At 10 to 12 weeks of age	5.4	0.4	1.0	3.7	0.3	10,000	1:4.4

for the probable dietary requirements of growing chicks. The figures do not include margins of safety to compensate for possible losses of vitamins during feed processing, transportation, and storage and for variations in feed composition and in environment. In earlier reports the National Research Council suggested allowances which included margins of safety of 66 per cent for vitamin A, 50 per cent for vitamin D, and 20 per cent for the water-soluble vitamins.

THE RATION

The successful rations are made up of a combination of cereals and animal protein concentrates. Quality of protein is supplied by the use of milk, meat scraps, fish products, and soybean oil meal.

For chick growth and well-being, the ration must supply the necessary vitamins. Vitamin A is supplied mainly in the yellow corn and alfalfa meal, and in fish oil when fed. Vitamin B occurs in the various cereals. Vitamin D is provided by fish oils and activated animal sterol, or exposure to sunshine. Riboflavin is furnished by milk products and fermentation by-products. Vitamin B_{12} is supplied by feeds of animal origin and fermentation by-products.

Calcium and phosphorus are the minerals needed in largest amounts. Where reasonable amounts of animal protein feeds are used, sufficient phosphorus is present. Calcium, however, is usually low and is provided by adding some calcium carrier such as pulverized limestone or oystershells.

Those feeds which are processed the least and which represent more nearly the whole product are safest to use. The feed

REQUIREMENTS* OF YOUNG CHICKENS

	Starting Chickens, 0–8 weeks	Growing Chickens, 8–18 weeks
Total protein, %	20	16
Vitamins		
Vitamin A activity (U.S.P. units)†	1200	1200
Vitamin D, (I.C.U.)‡	90	90
Thiamine chloride hydrochloride, mg.	0.8	?
Riboflavin, mg.	1.3	0.8
Pantothenic acid, mg.	4.2	4.2
Niacin, mg.	12.0	?
Pyridoxine, mg.	1.3	?
Biotin, mg.	0.04	?
Choline chloride, mg.	600	?
Folacin, mg.	0.25	?
Minerals		
Calcium, per cent	1.0	1.0
Phosphorus, per cent§	0.6	0.6
Salt, per cent ‖	0.5	0.5
Potassium, per cent	0.2	0.16
Manganese, mg.	25	?
Iodine, mg.	0.5	0.2
Magnesium, mg.	220	?
Amino acids, %		
Arginine	1.2	—
Lysine	0.9	—
Histidine	0.15	—
Methionine	0.8	—
or		
Methionine¶	0.45	—
Cystine	0.35	—
Tryptophan	0.2	—
Glycine**	1.0	—
Phenylalanine	1.6	—
or		
Phenylalanine††	0.9	—
Tyrosine	0.7	—
Leucine	1.4	—
Isoleucine	0.6	—
Threonine	0.6	—
Valine	0.8	—

* In percentage or amount per pound of feed.

† May be fish oil vitamin A or pro-vitamin A from vegetable sources.

‡ International chick units.

§ At least 0.45 per cent of the total feed of starting chickens should be inorganic phosphorus. All the phosphorus of non-vegetable feed ingredients is considered to be inorganic. Approximately 30 per cent of the phosphorus of vegetable products is nonphytin phosphorus and may must not be too bulky, or the actual food intake will be restricted, depressing growth.

It is not necessary to use very complex rations for satisfactory results.[74] On the other hand, it is not safe to restrict the ration to too few feeds. The Nebraska Experiment Station[75] reports a significantly greater rate of gain in weight and retention of nitrogen, calcium, and phosphorus on a mixed concentrate consisting of meat scraps, fish meal, and dried buttermilk than on a single supplement of meat scraps.

To meet the requirements for chick rations the suggested formula patterns are tabulated on the next page.

FEEDING MANAGEMENT

TIME OF FIRST FEED. When should chicks receive their first feed? It was noted early that the chick absorbed the unused yolk just before hatching time. The unused part of the egg, as reported by Tangl,[76] represents 48 per cent of the original energy in the egg. It is found largely in the abdomen of the chick and is absorbed during the early days of life. This energy is sufficient to maintain the body temperature of chicks for 72

---

be considered as part of the inorganic phosphorus required. A portion of the phosphorus requirement of growing chickens must also be supplied in inorganic form. For these birds the requirement for inorganic phosphorus is lower and not as well defined as in the case of starting chickens.

|| This figure represents added salt or sodium chloride added as such or in marine or fermentation products of high sodium chloride content.

¶ Cystine will replace methionine as long as the ration contains not less than 0.45 per cent methionine.

** The chick can synthesize glycine, but the synthesis does not proceed at a rate sufficient for maximum growth.

†† Tyrosine will replace phenylalanine as long as the ration contains not less than 0.9 per cent phenylalanine.

TENTATIVE REQUIREMENTS FOR CERTAIN VITAMINS AND MINERALS, 0–8 WEEKS

	mg. per lb.
Vitamin B_{12}	0.004
Vitamin K	0.18
Iron	9.0
Copper	0.9

hours or more. It was, therefore, believed that chicks should not be fed before this time, since the introduction of food would prevent or delay the absorption of the yolk and cause trouble by overloading the digestive system. However, it was shown later that the assimilation of the yolk is a fairly stable and regular process from day to day, influenced only slightly by feeding.[8, 77]

The next question is whether there is any advantage in feeding early or late. The yolk is not largely absorbed until the chicks

RECOMMENDED FORMULA PATTERNS FOR CHICK MASHES

Ingredients	Starter (all-mash)	Growers (with grain) Confinement	Pasture
	lb./ton	lb./ton	lb./ton
High-energy grain products (corn, wheat, wheat red dog flour, milo, oatmeal)	900 +	700 +	500 +
Medium- and low-energy grain products (oats, barley, wheat flour middlings, standard middlings, bran)	0-400	0-600	0-800
Vegetable proteins (soybean meal, corn gluten meal, peanut meal)	300-400	350-450	400-500
Animal proteins; minimum levels (fish meal, fish solubles, meat scraps)	50-100	50-100	—
Other B-vitamin carriers (dried milk products, dried yeast, dried distillers' solubles, fermentation solubles)	100	100	—
Dehydrated alfalfa meal	50-100	100	—
Additional riboflavin* (if needed)	+	+	—
Additional vitamin B_{12}* (if needed)	+	+	—
Additional vitamin A* (if needed)	+	+	—
Vitamin D_3 (feeding oils or D-activated animal sterols)	+	+	—
Calcium and phosphorus supplements (steamed bone meal, dicalcium phosphate, defluorinated phosphate, limestone)	30-50	60-80	80-100
Salt	5	10	20
Manganese sulfate (65% feeding grade)	0.4	0.5	0.5
Antibiotic feed supplement	+	±	±

* Refers to the use of riboflavin supplements, vitamin B_{12} supplements, and vitamin A sources of guaranteed vitamin content or other vitamin-rich feedstuffs when the formula is otherwise deficient in any of these nutrients.

REQUIRED COMPOSITION OF CHICK MASHES

Nutrient	Starter (all-mash)	Growers (with grain) Confinement	Pasture
Protein, %	20	20	20
Calcium, %	1-1.4	1.5-2*	1.5-2*
Phosphorus			
Total %	0.6	0.9	0.9
Available %	0.4	0.7	0.7
Vitamin A,† I.U./lb.	2000	4000	—
Vitamin D, I.C.U./lb.	135	270	—
Riboflavin, mg./lb.	1.6	1.3	—
Vitamin B_{12},‡ mg./lb.	1.5-2	1.5-2	—

* Free choice feeding of oystershell or other calcium supplement recommended since this level of calcium will not meet full requirements.

† If corn constitutes half of scratch grain mixture for growing chicks the level of vitamin A in the mash can be reduced by 1000 I.U./lb.

‡ Refers to vitamin B_{12} supplied by fish products, meat scrap and vitamin B_{12} supplements.

are about a week old. Deaths from starvation begin in about 5 days. It has been shown by many workers[8, 77, 78] that early feeding is not harmful. Some of these tests indicate that early mortality is greater in the lots where feed is withheld, the rate of mortality increasing as feeding time is delayed. Later mortality does not seem to be affected. Too great periods of starvation will cause the chicks to pick up litter to satisfy the hunger craving, with resultant impaction in the crop.

It is probably safe to say that the chicks can have food as soon as they want it, a problem of feeding not to be confused with brooding management. For example, some authorities recommend removing chicks from the incubator and confining them in chick boxes for 24 hours or more, not to keep the chicks from eating but to insure against their getting chilled or overheated during this critical period. If the chicks are placed in the brooder houses, they should be kept near the hover and should have feed and drink available. Frequently milk is given as a drink for the first day or two. It serves both as drink and food.

In general, it would seem that chicks may be fed as soon after hatching as they care to eat, with no harmful results upon weight or mortality. Furthermore, it is well to feed them not later than 36 to 48 hours after hatching.[79] The fact that chicks will go for much longer periods before receiving their first feed should be looked upon as a fortunate curcumstance, which permits shipping chicks long distances, rather than as the correct time to feed them.

FEEDING METHODS. During recent years there has been a general tendency to feed chicks all-mash rations. They are also fed grain-mash rations and modified rations, in which the all-mash is used as a starting mash and later grain is fed. About equally favorable results can be obtained from grain-mash rations, all-mash rations, and modifications of the two systems, if the nutrients are properly provided (Table 25).

TABLE 25. GROWTH OF CHICKENS BY DIFFERENT METHODS OF FEEDING AND RESULTING PRODUCTION DURING THE FIRST LAYING YEAR (CORNELL EXPERIMENT STATION)

	Lot 1	Lot 2	Lot 3
	All Mash to 8 Weeks. Grain and Mash After 8 Weeks	Grain and Mash from the Start	All Mash to 26 Weeks
Av. wt. of pullets			
4 weeks	178 grams	162 grams	177 grams
8	496	463	492
12	777	764	782
24	1526	1519	1495
Feed per bird to 26 weeks	23.4 lb.	23.1 lb.	23.8 lb.
Date of first egg	Aug. 31	Aug. 30	Aug. 19
Eggs: Aug.	. . .	. . .	0.2
Sept.	3.0	3.5	2.4
to Oct. 6	1.2	1.7	1.0
	4.2	5.2	3.6

Pullets were placed in laying houses at 26 weeks and put on a grain-mash ration.

	Lot 1	Lot 2	Lot 3
Number at start	32	44	49
Died during year	7 (22%)	10 (23%)	8 (16%)
Culled during year	4	2	1
Completed year	21 (66%)	32 (73%)	40 (82%)
Average first year egg production	231	225	233

Up to six weeks Lot 3 was fed the same ration as Lot 1. For 6 to 12 weeks 10% meat scrap and 5% milk were used (5% meat scrap being omitted). After 12 weeks 5% milk and 5% meat scrap were fed. All received the Cornell Laying Ration after 26 weeks.

As already indicated, the growth of the chick varies with age. During the early periods, when growth is rapid, there is a greater requirement for protein, minerals, and vitamins. Excesses may or may not be detrimental but are usually not economical. Therefore, when all-mash or grain-mash rations are fed, it is desirable, if not necessary, to have two or three different mixtures to cover the growing period.

The modified system, such as the Cornell ration, permits a single mixture for both a starting and growing mash. The mash is fed as an all-mash ration for about 4 to 8 weeks. At that time grain is introduced and is consumed by the birds in increasing quantities, thus automatically reducing the protein of the ration in the later periods.

FEEDING GROWING PULLETS. The pullets must not suffer any setbacks during the summer. Some of the things to be watched are the green food supply, water, and amounts of grain consumed. They must have an adequate and complete ration at all times.

FEEDING COCKERELS. Cockerels that are kept for future breeders should be given exactly the same care and attention as the pullets. Put them on a separate range, where they will get the same opportunities for range and outdoor conditions, the same feeds, and the same methods as the pullets.

FEEDING BROILERS. The terms "broiler" and "fryer" are now used synonymously and refer to a 10- to 12-week old chicken weighing 3 to 4 pounds (Table 26). In broiler production it is necessary to take advantage of the early rapid growth of

TABLE 26. GROWTH RATE AND FEED CONSUMPTION OF HEAVY BREED BROILERS AT CORNELL UNIVERSITY

Age in Weeks	Average Weight, lb.	Total Feed Consumed, lb.
1	.19	.17
2	.37	.50
3	.60	.99
4	.91	1.68
5	1.23	2.52
6	1.61	3.50
7	2.01	4.63
8	2.44	5.78
9	2.87	7.22
10	3.29	8.66
12	3.99	11.96

chicks. This produces tender meat and efficient feed utilization.

Rapid growth can best be obtained on rations containing higher levels of protein.[80] Most of the experimental results indicate a level of 20 – 21% of protein as being satisfactory. Almquist and Asmundson[81] report that Single Comb White Leghorn cockerels grew more rapidly during the first week on a 30 per cent protein mash, as compared with a 20 per cent mash, and maintained their advantage in weight up to 8 weeks of age. Receipts over feed cost per bird were increased by starting the broilers on the high-protein mash when the high-protein mash was fed for not more than 4 weeks. Other reports,[82] however, show no advantage of starting chicks on high-protein diets provided they contain all the necessary amino acids, vitamins, and other nutrients in sufficient amount and in proper balance.

Antibiotics have been shown to stimulate early growth and to improve feed efficiency. The growth response of supplementary methionine[83] has been variable, but it has generally improved feed efficiency. The various nutrients as indicated for growth must also be supplied.

Since the efficiency of a ration is related to its energy value, emphasis has been placed on high-energy rations for boiler production. Hence the ration must be made up of cereal grains and grain products of high-productive energy value. High-energy rations will produce birds with a high-quality carcass carrying a sufficiently high-fat content for good finish and pigmentation. High-energy rations have also been reported as producing birds that will lose less weight in transit to market.[84] High-energy ration fed stock has also yielded higher weight returns in cooked form with both the fast- and the slow-cooking methods.[85]

All-mash rations are generally used for broilers. However, it is possible to feed some grain with these rations during the final 2 or 3 weeks of the broiler production period. The Arkansas Station[86] reported the best gains for broilers where the starter mash was fed throughout a period of 12 weeks but where the chicks had access to a scratch ration of whole wheat and medium corn chops during the last 6 weeks.

The use of artificial illumination to provide a 14-hour day and the feeding of wet mash or pellets are means of speeding up growth by increasing food consumption.

Since appearance is an important consideration in marketing broilers, it is advisable to include feeds in the broiler rations which will produce deeper pigmentation, such as yellow corn, corn gluten meal, and alfalfa meal.

Cod liver oil should not be used in the broiler ration the last 2 weeks before marketing, as the flesh might be tainted with a fishy odor or taste.

To meet the requirements for broiler rations the tabulated formula patterns are suggested on p. 370.

COCCIDIOSIS RATION. A common former recommendation for the treatment of coccidiosis was the so-called milk flush. The milk-sugar, changing to acid in the chicks' intestines, and the excessive amount of water consumed seemed to clear the chicks' digestive tracts quite effectively.

At the present time coccidiosis is more commonly controlled by the means of sulfa drugs which are fed both prophylactically and therapeutically.

FALL MANAGEMENT OF PULLETS. Pullets should be well developed in body before they start to lay. It is important that pullets be in good condition with a surplus of body fat when they commence to lay if they are to withstand the demands of heavy laying. To do this a common practice is to feed heavily on grain in the fall. It is a mistake, however, to feed pullets wholly on grain as they approach maturity unless special adjustment has been made, for this slows up complete development. Mash should always be fed along with scratch grain, as the mash is more complete in protein, minerals, and vitamins than the scratch grain. The combination of the two furnishes the birds a more complete assortment of food elements at the time they are finishing their development.

Some poultrymen have a very definite impression that the time at which the birds begin to lay can be decidedly regulated by the amount of protein, and particularly animal protein, furnished to the pullets the last month or 6 weeks, and in come cases only 2 or 3 weeks, before those birds come into production. It is doubtful whether one can influence the age of sexual maturity of pullets unless one feeds below the necessary amount of protein, in which case growth is delayed.

Results at Washington[20] indicate that the higher protein levels affect the rate of sexual maturity. The difference between the extremes was about 40 days. The slower-maturing pullets on the low-protein levels also laid the larger eggs. This is probably true because egg size is closely correlated with age. On the other hand, a number of stations[21-24, 26, 87, 88] indicate that liberal protein feeding during growth did not materially affect age of sexual maturity. The Oklahoma Station[25] states that more time is required to reach sexual maturity with rations under 16

RECOMMENDED FORMULA PATTERNS FOR BROILER MASHES

Ingredients	Broiler Starter, lb./ton	All-Mash grower, lb./ton	Mash-Grain* grower lb./ton
High energy grain products (corn, wheat, red dog flour, milo)	900 +	1000 +	900 +
Medium energy grain products (oats, barley, wheat flour middlings)	0-300†	0-300†	0-300†
Vegetable proteins (soybean meal, corn gluten meal, peanut meal)	400-550	300-450	400-550
Animal proteins: minimum levels (fish meal, fish solubles, meat scraps)	50-100	50-100	50-100
Other B-vitamin carriers (Dried milk products, distillers' dried solubles, fermentation solubles, dried yeast)	100	50	100
Alfalfa meal (minimum 17% protein)	50	50	50
‡ Additional riboflavin (if needed)	+	+	+
‡ Additional vitamin B_{12} (if needed)	+	+	+
‡ Additional vitamin A (if needed)	+	+	+
Vitamin D_3 (feeding oils or D-activated animal sterols)	+	+	+
Calcium and phosphorus supplements (steamed bonemeal, dicalcium phosphate, defluorinated phosphate, limestone)	20-60	20-60	30-60
Salt	5	5	10
Manganese sulfate (70% feeding grade)	0.5	0.5	1
Antibiotic feed supplement	+	+	+
Required nutrient levels of mash mixtures:§			
Protein, %	20	17.5	21
Calcium, %	1-1.4†	1-1.4†	1.6-2.0†
Phosphorus, total %	0.6-0.8†	0.6-0.8†	0.9-1.1†
Phosphorus, available %	0.4	0.4	0.7
Vitamin A, USP units/lb.	2000	2000	4000
Vitamin D, I.C.U./lb.	135	135	270
Riboflavin, mg/lb.	1.6	1.6	2.7
Vitamin B_{12}, μg/lb.	2	2	4
Niacin, mg/lb.	12	?	?
Pantothenic acid, mg/lb.	4.5	?	?
Productive energy, cal/lb.	850	900	800

* Formulated for use with feeding rates 60% mash and 40% grain.

† Higher figure is maximum recommended level.

‡ Refers to the use of riboflavin supplements, vitamin B_{12} supplements, and vitamin A sources of guaranteed vitamin content or other

per cent protein but that there is no difference in weight at maturity (10 months of age). Results at the Iowa Station[89] suggest that egg weight may be dependent on size or capacity of body or oviduct instead of body weight. In that event the most rapid attainment of maximum egg size by pullets in the autumn might be expected from rations which stimulate rapid growth of body framework, and hence "fattening" rations may delay the attainment of maximum egg size.

If the age at which birds come into production is to be influenced to any extent, it can be done only by reducing the protein 2 months or more before the birds begin to lay, in which case growth will be materially delayed. This is a questionable practice.

It is not advisable to "hold back" pullets in the fall. Early laying is an inherited factor controlled primarily by breeding. Time of laying can be influenced only a few weeks by feeding. The best all-round results are obtained when the birds are so managed that they can be kept growing continually and come into production normally.

In general, one can say that a considerable range in the protein level of the growing ration is possible and still obtain satisfactory growth. Egg size is related to some extent to body weight but to a greater degree to age of sexual maturity. With a sufficiency of the various nutritive factors, higher protein rations are not harmful and are to be preferred to low-protein rations which will retard growth. Since both breeding and feeding have an influence upon growth, sexual maturity, and egg size, it is necessary to consider the effect of both and to synchronize the breeding and feeding factors. For example, birds that have been bred to lay at 5 months should be fed to produce body growth as rapidly as possible in order to have them ready to lay at that time, rather than to try to hold back their development in the hope that sexual maturity can be delayed.

For those pullets that are still immature, owing to late hatching, slow development, or unfavorable rearing, the growing rations will need to be continued. It might even be necessary to introduce wet mashes or other measures to increase food consumption. If the short days still find them unprepared for pro-

---

vitamin-rich feedstuffs when the formula is otherwise deficient in any of these nutrients.

§ Estimates of required nutrient levels are based largely on the recommendations of the National Research Council Committee on Animal Nutrition.

duction, the days can well be lengthened by the use of artificial illumination.

CONFINEMENT AND BATTERY REARING. Where the chicks are reared in confinement and in batteries, it is especially essential that the ration be complete and correct in all respects since the chicks must depend entirely upon the feed given them. Chicks on range can succeed on rations that are not complete since they can supplement them with sunshine, green plant material, and other protective and nutritious substances.

CHICK RATIONS

It is possible to formulate many chick rations that will meet the requirements and hence be satisfactory. A number of recommended rations for growing chickens will be found in the Appendix. (See page 528.)

REFERENCES

1. Heuser, G. F., and F. E. Andrews. Weight changes in chickens. Cornell Ext. Bul. 240. 1932. (Reprinted March 1934.)
2. Buckner, G. D., J. H. Martin, and W. M. Insko, Jr. The effect of confinement brooding on growth and egg production. Ky. Res. Bul. 346. 1934.
   Buckner, G. D., J. H. Martin, and W. M. Insko, Jr. The growth of White Leghorn chicks. Poultry Sci. 13:110. 1934.
3. Kempster, H. L., and E. M. Funk. Influence of time of hatching on rate of growth. Mo. Bul. 310:50. 1932.
4. Kempster, H. L. The influence of summer temperatures on the rate of growth of chickens. Poultry Sci. 17:259. 1938.
   Kempster, H. L. The normal growth of chickens. Mo. Bul. 423. 1941.
5. Heuser, G. F., and L. C. Norris. The influence of the protein level on the rate of growth in chickens. Rept. Fourth World's Poultry Congress. 328. London. 1930.
6. Titus, H. W., and M. A. Jull. The growth of Rhode Island Reds and the effect of feeding skimmilk on the constants of their growth curves. Jour. Agr. Res. 36:515. 1928.
7. Jordan, W. H. The feeding of farm animals. Macmillan. 1905.
8. Parker, S. L. Effects of early handicaps on chickens as measured by yolk absorption and body weight to twenty weeks of age. Hilgardia 4:1. 1929.

9. Mayhew, R. L. Studies on coccidiosis. II. The effects of coccidiosis upon the weights of chickens artificially inoculated during the 13th and 14th weeks. Poultry Sci. 11:102. 1932.

10. Atwood, H. The influence of rations fed to growing chickens on the later egg production of the females. Preliminary report. Poultry Sci. 1:176. 1922.

Atwood, H. Influence of rations fed to growing chickens on the characteristics of the adult females. W. Va. Bul. 179. 1923.

11. Platt, C. S., and H. W. Stover, Jr. Sexual maturity, adult mortality, and egg production of White Leghorn pullets in relationship to their diet during the growing period. New Jersey Bul. 716. 1945.

12. Prentice, J. H., R. G. Baskett, and G. S. Robertson. The nutrition of the chick and its effect on growth, maturity, egg production, and mortality. Rept. Fourth World's Poultry Congress. 242. London, 1930.

13. Hendricks, W. A., M. A. Jull, and H. W. Titus. The utilization of feed by chickens. I. The requirements for growth. Poultry Sci. 11:74. 1932.

14. Halnan, E. T. The scientific principles of poultry feeding. Ministry Agr. and Fisheries London Bul. 7. 1930.

15. Titus, H. W., and W. A. Hendricks. The early growth of chickens as a function of feed consumption rather than of time. Rept. Fourth World's Poultry Congress. 307. London. 1930.

16. Axelsson, J. The general nutritive value (energy value) of foods for poultry. Harper Adams Utility Jour. 23:43. 1937-1938.

17. Hammond, J. C., and H. R. Bird. Effects of nutrition on variability in the growth of chickens. Poultry Sci. 21:230. 1942.

18. Bunge, G. V. Lehrbuch der Physiologie des Menschen. Leipzig. Vol. II. 2nd ed. 1905.

19. Funk, E. M. Can the chick balance its ration? Poultry Sci. 11:94. 1932.

20. Carver, J. S., L. W. Cassel, and T. E. Aspinwall. Protein requirements for growing chicks. Wash. Bul. 245:51. 1930.

St. John, J. L., J. S. Carver, J. P. Helphrey, W. Miller, and L. W. Cassel. The effect on growth of various protein levels of dry skimmilk in a chick mash. Poultry Sci. 9:320. 1930.

Carver, J. S., D. Brazie, and S. A. Moore. Protein requirements of growing chicks. Wash. Bul. 260:50. 1931.

St. John, J. L., O. Johnson, C. Kempf, and V. Hefty. Poultry Nutrition. Wash. Bul. 275:24. 1932.

Carver, J. S., J. L. St. John, T. E. Aspinwall, and I. V. Flor. Protein requirements of chickens. Poultry Sci. 11:45. 1932.

St. John, J. L., J. S. Carver, O. Johnson, and D. Brazie. Optimum protein levels for chickens. Proc. Fifth World's Poultry Congress. 567. Rome. 1933.

St. John, J. L., J. S. Carver, O. Johnson, S. A. Moore, and H. Gerritz. The biological value of rations containing fish meal. Jour. Nutr. 7:13. 1934.

Carver, J. S., J. L. St. John, M. W. Miller, and G. E. Bearse. The comparative efficiency of various proteins for growing chicks. Wash. Bul. 321. 1935.

Carver, J. S., and V. Heiman. The protein requirements of chicks. Wash. Bul. 342:54. 1936.

Carver, J. S., V. Heiman, E. I. Robertson, and J. W. Cook. Protein requirements of chicks. Rept. Seventh World's Poultry Congress. 141. Cleveland. 1939.

Carver, J. S., V. Heiman, J. W. Cook, and J. L. St. John. The protein requirements of White Leghorn pullets. Wash. Bul. 383. 1939.

21. Rept. Agr. Exp. Sta. Univ. Calif. 1930:88.

22. Dearstyne, R. S., C. O. Bollinger, G. K. Jones, and H. P. Brigman. The influence of certain protein levels on the growth of pullets. N. C. Bul. 304. 1936.

23. Tepper, A. E., H. O. Stuart, and T. B. Charles. Added proteins boost gains. N. H. Bul. 262:25. 1932.

Tepper, A. E., T. B. Charles, and F. D. Reed. Protein levels in battery brooding chicks. N. H. Circ. 40. 1933.

Tepper, A. E., R. C. Durgin, and T. B. Charles. Protein requirements of chickens at various stages of growth and development. N. H. Bul. 312. 1939.

Tepper, A. E., R. C. Durgin, T. B. Charles, S. R. Shimer, and H. A. Davis. Protein requirements of chickens at various stages of growth and development II. N. H. Bul. 335. 1941.

Ringrose, R. C., T. B. Charles, S. R. Shimer, and H. A. Davis. Protein requirements of chickens at various stages of growth and development. N. H. Bul. 351:49. 1943.

24. Zuzuki, K., and T. Hatano. The protein requirement of growing chickens. Jour. Agr. Chem. Japan.

25. Morris, L., R. B. Thompson, and V. G. Heller. The effect of varying the amounts of protein in the poultry ration on growth and subsequent egg production. Poultry Sci. 11:364. 1932.

Penquite, R. Protein requirement highest during first eight weeks. Okla. Rept. 1938-1940:149.

Heller, V. G., and R. Penquite. The optimum protein level for chickens as influenced by sex. Poultry Sci. 24:465. 1945.

26. Heuser, G. F., and L. C. Norris. The influence of the protein level on the rate of growth in chickens. Rept. Fourth World's Poultry Congress. 328. London. 1930.

Norris, L. C., and G. F. Heuser. The relation of the protein requirement of chicks to the rate of growth. I. The quantity of protein required by chicks during early growth. Poultry Sci. 9:378. 1930.

Heuser, G. F., and L. C. Norris. The influence of the protein level on the growth of chickens and its relation to subsequent behavior. Proc. Fifth World's Poultry Congress. 551. Rome. 1933.

27. Embleton, H. Poultry feeding experiments. Ariz. Bul. 143:97. 1933.

Embleton, H. Poultry feeding experiments. Ariz. Bul. 177. 1941.

Herner, M. C. Hatching, brooding, rearing, and feeding chicks. Manitoba Ext. Bul. 101. 1934.

Gutteridge, H. S., J. B. O'Neil, and J. M. Pratt. Level and source of protein in poultry production, Sci. Agr. 24:4. 1943.

Animal protein studies with chicks. Ind. Rept. 1927:48.
Protein requirements for growing pullets. Ind. Rept. 1928:54.
Roberts, R. E. Protein requirements of growing pullets. Poultry Sci. 9:19. 1929.
Roberts, R. E. Liquid and condensed milk for chicks. Poultry Sci. 11:226. 1932.
Roberts, R. E., and C. W. Carrick. Amounts of protein supplements in rations for broilers. Ind. Bul. 425. 1937.
Roberts, R. E., and C. W. Carrick. Influence of starting rations upon subsequent growth. Poultry Sci. 21:476. 1942.
Kempster, H. L., and E. M. Funk. Protein concentrates in chick rations. Mo. Bul. 310:47. 1932.
Brody, S., E. M. Funk, and H. L. Kempster. Age changes in the heat production of chickens as measured by a graphic method. Poultry Sci. 11:133. 1932.
Mussehl, F. E. Nutrient requirements of growing chicks. Neb. Res. Bul. 38. 1926.
Ackerson, C. W., M. J. Blish, and F. E. Mussehl. The utilization of food elements by growing chicks. VI. The influence of the protein level of the ration on the growth of chicks. Neb. Res. Bul. 108. 1939.
Morris, L. High and low protein rations tested. In "Research leads to farm progress." Okla. Rept. 1926-1930:99.
Morris, L., and V. G. Heller. One-fifth protein correct amount in chick ration. Okla. Rept. 1930-1932:122.
Heiman, V. Chicks need proteins of high quality. American Feed and Grain Dealers. 31 (5):6. 1947.

28. Charles, T. B., P. H. Margolf, R. J. Miller, and R. P. Tittsler. The effect of various protein-carbohydrate ratios upon the mortality, growth and condition of Single Comb White Leghorn chicks. Pa. Bul. 230:37. 1928.
Margolf, P. H. The effect of various protein-carbohydrate ratios upon the mortality, growth, and condition of Single Comb White Leghorn chicks. Pa. Bul. 243:28. 1929.
Swift, R. W., A. Black, L. Voris, and E. M. Funk. The optimum protein content of rations for growing chicks. Poultry Sci. 10:288. 1931.

29. Tomhave, A. E., and C. W. Mumford. Protein levels of rations in growing chicks. Del. Bul. 192:24. 1935.
Tomhave, A. E., and C. W. Mumford. Protein levels of rations in growing chicks. Del. Bul. 205:22. 1936.
Tomhave, A. E., and C. W. Mumford. Protein levels of rations in growing chicks. Del. Bul. 207:24. 1937.
Tomhave, A. E. Protein levels of rations in growing chicks. Del. Bul. 214:15. 1938.
Tomhave, A. E. Protein levels of rations for White Leghorn pullets. Del. Bul. 219. 1939.

30. Thomas, J. O. Report of experiments on the feeding of poultry with high, medium and low protein rations. Welsh Jour. Agr. 13:272. 1937.

Macdonald, A. J. The protein requirements of poultry. Harper Adams Utility Jour. 22:487. 1937.
Prevo, A. A., and T. M. Polivanowa. The differentiation of protein amounts in the diet of chicks according to growing periods. Trans. All-Union Inst. Poultry Industries. Moscow, U.S.S.R. 3(2). 1938.
Hammond, J. C., W. A. Hendricks, and H. W. Titus. Effect of percentage of protein in the diet on growth and feed utilization of male chickens. Jour. Agr. Res. 56:791. 1938.
31. Heywang, B. W., H. R. Bird, and A. R. Kemmerer. The level of protein in the diet of growing New Hampshire chickens during hot weather. Poultry Sci. 32:781. 1953.
McConachie, J. D., W. R. Graham, and H. D. Branion. A study of the protein requirements of growing chicks. Sci. Agr. 15:754. 1935.
Milne, H. I. Protein requirements of growing chicks. Sci. Agr. 12:604. 1932.
32. Chicken raising experiments. Queensland Agr. Jour. 44:425. 1935.
33. Gericke, A. M. M., and C. S. Platt. Feather development in Barred Plymouth Rock chicks. N. J. Bul. 543. 1932.
34. Jones, E. E. The effect of diet on the course of experimental coccidiosis infection in the chicken. Jour. Am. Vet. Med. Assn. 85: 193. 1934.
35. Luttermoser, G. W., and R. W. Allen. The influence of diets high and low in protein on the growth rate of chickens infected with the tapeworm, Raillietina cesticillus. Poultry Sci. 21:111. 1942.
36. Titus, H. W. Practical nutritive requirements of poultry. U. S. Dept. Agr. Food and Life. Yearbook Agr. 1939:811.
37. Platt, C. S. Protein requirements of growing pullets. N. J. Hints 30(3). 1943.
38. Almquist, H. J. Amino acid requirements of chickens and turkeys —A review. Poultry Sci. 31:966. 1952.
Almquist, H. J., and E. Mecchi. Tryptophane requirement of the chick. Proc. Soc. Exp. Biol. & Med. 48:526. 1941.
Almquist, H. J., and E. Mecchi. Lysine requirement of the chick. Proc. Soc. Exp. Biol. & Med. 49:174. 1942.
Almquist, H. J., and E. Mecchi. Glycine requirement of the chick. Proc. Soc. Exp. Biol. & Med. 49:541. 1942.
Almquist, H. J., and J. B. Merritt. Protein and arginine levels in chick diets. Proc. Soc. Exp. Biol. & Med. 73:136. 1950.
Bird, F. H. The lysine requirement of eight-week-old chickens. Poultry Sci. 32:10. 1953.
Glista, W. A., H. H. Mitchell, and H. M. Scott. The amino acid requirements of the chick. Poultry Sci. 30:915. 1951.
Grau, C. R. The threonine requirement of the chick. Jour. Nutr. 37:105. 1949.
Grau, C. R., and H. J. Almquist. Requirement of tryptophane by the chick. Jour. Nutr. 28:263. 1944.
Grau, C. R., and D. W. Peterson. The isoleucine, leucine, and valine requirements of the chick. Jour. Nutr. 32:181. 1946.
Klose, A. A., and H. J. Almquist. Methionine in the diet of the chick. Jour. Biol. Chem. 138:467. 1941.

Milligan, J. L., L. J. Machlin, H. R. Bird, and B. W. Heywang. Lysine and methionine requirement of chicks fed practical diets. Poultry Sci. 30:578. 1951.

West, J. W., C. W. Carrick, S. M. Hauge, and E. T. Mertz. The relationship of choline and cystine to the methionine requirement of young chickens. Poultry Sci. 30:880. 1951.

Wilkening, M. C., B. S. Schweigert, P. B. Pearson, and R. M. Sherwood. Studies on the requirement of the chick for tryptophane. Jour. Nutr. 34:701. 1947.

39. Carver, D. S., and E. L. Johnson. Unidentified growth factors for the chick in vegetable oils and fatty acid concentrates. Poultry Sci. 32:701. 1953.

Reiser, R. The essential role of fatty acids in rations for growing chicks. Jour. Nutr. 42:319. 1950.

Reiser, R. The metabolism of polyunsaturated fatty acids in growing chicks. Jour. Nutr. 42:325. 1950.

Reiser, R., and J. R. Couch. The essential role of fat in the rations of growing chicks. Poultry Sci. 28:781. 1949.

40. Davis, H. J., and C. W. Upp. Studies on the fat requirements of the domestic fowl. Poultry Sci. 20:459. 1941.

41. Russell, W. C., M. W. Taylor, and L. J. Polskin. Fat requirements of the growing chick. Jour. Nutr. 19:555. 1940.

42. Henderson, E. W., and W. E. Irwin. The tolerance of growing chicks for soybean oil in their ration. Poultry Sci. 19:389. 1940.

43. Fisher, H., E. P. Singsen, and L. D. Matterson. The influence of feed efficiency on the phosphorus requirement for growth and bone calcification in the chick. Poultry Sci. 32:749. 1953.

Gillis, M. B., L. C. Norris, and G. F. Heuser. The effect of phytin on the phosphorus requirement of the chick. Poultry Sci. 28:283. 1949.

O'Rourke, W. F., P. H. Phillips, and W. W. Cravens. The phosphorus requirements of growing chickens as related to age. Poultry Sci. 31:930. 1952.

Singsen, E. P. The phosphorus requirement of the chicken. Storrs Agr. Exp. Sta. Bul. 260. 1948.

44. Carver, J. S., R. J. Evans, and J. McGinnis. Calcium, phosphorus, and vitamin D interrelationships in the nutrition of the growing chick. Poultry Sci. 25:294. 1946.

45. Gallup, W. D., and L. C. Norris. The amount of manganese required to prevent perosis in the chick. Poultry Sci. 18:76. 1939.

Insko, W. M., Jr., M. Lyons, and J. H. Martin. Quantitative requirement of the growing chick for manganese. Jour. Nutr. 15; 621. 1938.

Wilgus, H. S., Jr., L. C. Norris, and G. F. Heuser. The role of manganese and certain other trace elements in the prevention of perosis. Jour. Nutr. 14:155. 1937.

Wilgus, H. S., L. C. Norris, and G. F. Heuser. The role of manganese in poultry nutrition. Proc. Seventh World's Poultry Congress. 171. 1939.

46. Burns, C. H., W. W. Cravens, and P. H. Phillips. The sodium and potassium requirements of the chick and their interrelationship. Jour. Nutr. 50:317. 1953.

47. Godfrey, P. R., C. W. Carrick, and F. W. Quackenbush. Iodine nutrition of chicks. Poultry Sci. 32:394. 1953.
48. Almquist, H. J. Magnesium requirement of the chick. Proc. Soc. Exp. Biol. and Med. 49:544. 1942.
49. Johnson, E. L., C. W. Carrick, and S. M. Hauge. The vitamin A requirements of young chickens. Poultry Sci. 27:308. 1948.
Record, P. R., R. M. Bethke, and O. H. M. Wilder. Vitamin A requirements of growing chickens. Poultry Sci. 14:297. 1935.
Ringrose, R. C., and L. C. Norris. A study of the vitamin A requirement of the chick during early life. Poultry Sci. 15:390. 1936.
Sherwood, R. M. Vitamin A requirements of poultry. Seventh World's Poultry Congress Report. 123. 1939.
Sherwood, R. M., and G. S. Fraps. Requirements of chickens for vitamin A when fed as carotene. Texas Bul. 583. 1940.
Taylor, M. W., and W. C. Russell. The provitamin A requirement of growing chickens. Poultry Sci. 26:234. 1946.
Wilson, W. O., C. H. Schroeder, and W. A. Higgins. Further studies on the vitamin requirements of chicks. Poultry Sci. 15: 426. 1936.
50. Jukes, T. H., and H. Heitman, Jr. Biological assay of thiamin with chicks. Jour. Nutr. 19:21. 1940.
51. Baird, F. D.. and D. J. Greene. The comparative vitamin D requirements of growing chicks, turkeys and pheasants. Poultry Sci. 14:70. 1935.
Carver, J. S., E. I. Robertson, D. Brazie, R. H. Johnson, and J. L. St. John. The vitamin D requirements of chickens. Wash. Bul. 299. 1934.
Heiman, V., and L. W. Tighe. Comparative vitamin D requirements of White Leghorn and crossbred chicks. Poultry Sci. 21:511. 1942.
Lachat, L. L., and H. A. Halvorson. Studies relative to the estimation of vitamin D. VI. Comparative vitamin D requirement of the chick for sardine (pilchard), concentrated, and cod liver oils, irradiated yeast, irradiated ergosterol, and irradiated cholesterol. Assn. Off. Agr. Chem. Jour. 19:637. 1936.
Murphy, R. R., J. E. Hunter, and H. C. Knandel. The vitamin D requirements of growing chicks and laying hens. Pa. Bul. 334. 1936.
Olsson, N. Investigations on the vitamin D requirements of chicks, poults, ducklings, and goslings. Annals of the Royal Agr. Coll. of Sweden. Vol. 16. 1949.
Roberts, R. E., and C. W. Carrick. Levels of phosphorus and vitamin D in broiler starting rations. Ind. Agr. Exp. Sta. 58th Ann. Rept. 78. 1945.
52. Heuser, G. F., H. S. Wilgus, and L. C. Norris. The quantitative vitamin G requirement of chicks. Poultry Sci. 17:105. 1938.
Norris, L. C., H. S. Wilgus, Jr., A. T. Ringrose, V. Heiman, and G. F. Heuser. The vitamin G requirement of poultry. Cornell Bul. 660. 1936.
Baskett, R. G., J. Houston, R. H. Common, W. Bolton, and S.

McConaghy. Poultry nutrition research in Northern Ireland. World's Poultry Sci. Jour. 3:162. 1947.

Bird, F. H., V. S. Asmundson, F. H. Kratzer, and S. Lepkovsky. The comparative requirements of chicks and turkey poults for riboflavin. Poultry Sci. 25:47. 1946.

53. Bauernfeind, J. C., L. C. Norris, and G. F. Heuser. The pantothenic acid requirement of chicks. Poultry Sci. 21:142. 1942.

Heuser, G. F., M. B. Gillis, and L. C. Norris. The pantothenic acid requirement of poultry. Rept. 8th World's Poultry Congress. 1948:114. Copenhagen.

54. Waisman, H. A., R. C. Mills, and C. A. Elvehjem. Factors required by chicks maintained on a heated diet. Jour. Nutr. 24:187. 1942.

55. Hegsted, D. M., and T. R. Riggs. The pantothenic acid requirement of chicks receiving a purified diet. Jour. Nutr. 37:361. 1949.

56. Hogan, A. G., L. R. Richardson, H. Patrick, B. L. O'Dell, and H. L. Kempster. Vitamin B_6 and chick nutrition. Poultry Sci. 19:352. 1940.

Hogan, A. G., L. R. Richardson, H. Patrick, B. L. O'Dell, and H. L. Kempster. Vitamin B_6 and chick nutrition. Poultry Sci. 20:180. 1941.

57. Briggs, G. M., Jr., R. C. Mills, D. M. Hegsted, C. A. Elvehjem, and E. B. Hart. The vitamin B_6 requirement of the chick. Poultry Sci. 21:379. 1942.

58. Kratzer, F. H., F. H. Bird, V. S. Asmundson, and S. Lepkovsky. The comparative pyridoxine requirements of chicks and turkey poults. Poultry Sci. 26:453. 1947.

59. Hegsted, D. M., R. C. Mills, G. M. Briggs, C. A. Elvehjem, and E. B. Hart. Biotin in chick nutrition. Jour. Nutr. 23:175. 1942.

60. Hegsted, D. M., R. C. Mills, C. A. Elvehjem, and E. B. Hart. Choline in the nutrition of chicks. Jour. Biol. Chem. 138:459. 1941.

Jukes, T. H. The effect of certain organic compounds and other dietary supplements on perosis. Jour. Nutr. 22:315. 1941.

McKittrick, D. S. The interrelations of choline and methionine in growth and the action of betaine in replacing them. Arch. Biochem. 15:133. 1947.

61. Briggs, G. M. Jr., R. C. Mills, C. A. Elvehjem, and E. B. Hart. Nicotinic acid in chick nutrition. Proc. Soc. Exp. Biol. & Med. 51:59. 1942.

Childs, G. R., C. W. Carrick, and S. M. Hauge. The niacin requirement of young chickens. Poultry Sci. 31:551. 1952.

West, J. W., C. W. Carrick, S. M. Hauge, and E. T. Mertz. The tryptophan requirement of young chickens as influenced by niacin. Poultry Sci. 31:479. 1952.

62. Sunde, M. L. The niacin requirements of chickens from 6 to 11 weeks. Poultry Sci. 32:926.

63. Robertson, E. I., L. J. Daniel, F. A. Farmer, L. C. Norris, and G. F. Heuser. The folic acid requirement of chicks for growth, feathering, and hemoglobin formation. Proc. Soc. Exp. Biol. & Med. 62:97. 1946.

Robertson, E. I., L. J. Daniel, F. A. Farmer, L. C. Norris, and G. F. Heuser. Folic acid requirement of growing chicks. Poultry Sci. 25:411. 1946.

64. Briggs, G. M., E. G. Hill, and M. J. Giles. Vitamin B_{12} in all-plant rations for chicks and sparing activity of methionine and choline. Poultry Sci. 29:723. 1950.

Davis, R. L., and G. M. Briggs. The vitamin B_{12} requirement of the chick. Poultry Sci. 30:628. 1951.

Norris, L. C., R. F. Miller, and H. Yacowitz. Studies on the vitamin B_{12} requirements of poultry. Proc. 1950 Cornell Nutr. Conf.: 53. 1950.

Ott, W. H. Further studies of the activity of crystalline vitamin B_{12} for chick growth. Poultry Sci. 30:86. 1951.

65. Griminger, P., H. Fisher, W. D. Morrison, J. M. Snyder, and H. M. Scott. The influence of different levels of alfalfa meal added to a corn-soybean meal type of ration on blood-clotting time. Poultry Sci. 32:902. 1953.

66. Morris, L. Fiber in ration tested. Okla. Rept. 1926-1930:151.

Morris, L., R. B. Thompson, and V. G. Heller. Crude fiber in chicken rations. Poultry Sci. 11:219. 1932.

Morris, L., V. G. Heller, and R. B. Thompson. Nine percent of fiber good in the baby chick ration. Okla. Rept. 1930-1932:124.

Penquite, R. Tests of fiber in ration continued. Okla. Rept. 1938-1940:149.

67. Insko, W. M., Jr., and T. G. Culton. Fiber in chick starting rations. Poultry Sci. 28:769. 1949.

68. Heuser, G. F., L. C. Norris, H. T. Peeler, and M. L. Scott. Further studies on the apparent effect of digestibility upon growth, weight maintenance, and egg production. Poultry Sci. 24:142. 1945.

Mishler, D. H., C. W. Carrick, and S. M. Hauge. Vitamin supplementation of chick rations as affected by grain products. Poultry Sci. 30:886. 1951.

Scott, H. M., L. D. Matterson, and E. P. Singsen. Nutritional factors influencing growth and efficiency of feed utilization. I. The effect of the source of carbohydrate. Poultry Sci. 26:554. 1947.

69. Robertson, E. I., R. F. Miller, and G. F. Heuser. The relation of energy to fiber in chick rations. Poultry Sci. 27:736. 1948.

70. Panda, J. N., and G. F. Combs. Studies on the energy requirement of the chick for rapid growth. Poultry Sci. 29:774. 1950.

71. Hill, F. W. Energy requirements of chickens. Proc. Cornell Nutr. Conf. for Feed Mfgrs.:26. 1952.

72. Hill, F. W., and L. M. Dansky. The influence of diet on the body composition of growing chicks. Proc. Cornell Nutr. Conf. for Feed Mfgrs.:27. 1951.

73. Recommended nutrient allowances for domestic animals. Number 1. Recommended nutrient allowances for poultry. Rept. Com. Animal Nutr. National Research Council, Washington. June 1944. Revised March, 1950.

Nutrient requirements for domestic animals. Number 1. Nutrient requirements of poultry. Rept. Comm. Animal Nutrition, National Research Council, Washington, D. C., 1954. Pub. 301.

74. King, D. F., and G. A. Trollope. Simplified rations for farm chickens. Ala. Circ. 66. 1934.
Musseh1, F. E., R. Hill, and C. W. Ackerson. Simple or complex chick rations. Poultry Sci. 8:198. 1929.
Musseh1, F. E., and C. W. Ackerson. Utilization of protein concentrates by the growing chick. Poultry Sci. 16:119. 1935.
Newbiggin, H. F., and R. G. Linton. Chick feeding experiments. Scottish Jour. Agr. 14:186. 1931.
75. Ackerson, C. W., M. J. Blish, and F. E. Musseh1. The utilization of food elements by growing chicks. II. A comparison of protein concentrates from single and multiple sources. Neb. Res. Bul. 94. 1937.
76. Lusk, G. The elements of the science of nutrition. W. B. Saunders Co. 1917.
77. Heywang, B. W., and M. A. Jull. The influence of starving and feeding mash and scratch grain, respectively at different times on yolk absorption in chicks. Poultry Sci. 9:291. 1930.
78. Elford, F. C. Rept. Dominion (Canada) Poultry Husbandman for the Year 1926:10.
Time of first feed for chicks. Ore Rept. 1928-1930:110.
Roberts, R. E. When should chicks be given first feed? Poultry Sci. 7:220. 1928.
Safe to feed chicks as soon as hatched. Buckeye-Newtown Hatchery Helper 5(3). November 1929.
79. Smith, A. C. The best age for the chicks' first feed. Minn. Rept. 1932:33.
Fronda, F. M., T. B. Felipe, and G. A. Monegas. The influence of withholding feeds from newly hatched chicks. Philippine Agric. 25:770. 1937.
80. Tomhave, A. E. Broiler feeding experiments. Del. Bul. 210. 1938.
Halpin, J. G., C. E. Holmes, and W. W. Cravens. Liberal amounts of animal protein help produce early broilers. Wis. Bul. 449:86. 1940.
Halpin, J. G., and C. E. Holmes. Wisconsin No. 45 is a good broiler ration. Wis. Bul. 451:35. 1941.
Singsen, E. P., and L. D. Matterson. Experiments with high efficiency broiler rations. Proc. 7th Distillers' Feed Conf. 1952: 34.
Melass, V. H., and R. M. Sherwood. Riboflavin and protein studies with broilers. Texas Agr. Exp. Sta. Progress Report 969. 1945.
81. Almquist, H. J., and V. S. Asmundson. High protein mashes for broilers. Poultry Sci. 23:67. 1944.
82. Singsen, E. P. Nutritional factors influencing growth and efficiency of feed utilization. Poultry Sci. 26:555. 1947.
Singsen, E. P., and L. D. Matterson. The Connecticut broiler ration and recommended high energy rations. Conn. Progress Rept. Feb. 1, 1949.
83. Matterson, L. D., L. Decker, E. P. Singsen, A. Kozeff, J. Waddell, C. J. Hasbrouck, H. R. Bird, H. Menge, and T. D. Runnels. The value of supplemental methionine in practical chick starter and broiler rations. Poultry Sci. 32:817. 1953.

Menge, H., C. A. Denton, H. R. Bird, and G. F. Combs. Effect of supplemental DL-methionine and varying protein levels on growth and feed requirements of broiler chickens. Poultry Sci. 32:827. 1953.

84. King, R. A. Why hauling shrinks vary. U. S. Egg & Poultry Mag. 56:14. 1950.

85. Maw, W. A., N. Nikolaiczuk, and W. W. Johnson. High-efficiency broiler rations and cooking losses. Poultry Sci. 30:770. 1950.

86. Johnson, S. R., and R. M. Smith. Feeding methods reflect profits in broilers. Ark. Bul. 443:11. 1944.

87. Bethke, R. M., P. R. Record, and D. C. Kennard. The protein requirements of growing pullets. Ohio Spec. Circ. 28:9. 1930.

Winter, A. R., E. L. Dakan, and A. Bayes. Protein levels for finishing pullets. Poultry Sci. 11:30. 1932.

88. Callenbach, E. W., J. E. Nicholas, and P. H. Margolf. Poultry brooding systems. Pa. Bul. 340. 1937.

Callenbach, E. W., and J. E. Nicholas. Effect of rearing environment on sexual development of fowls. Pa. Bul. 368. 1938.

89. Henderson, E. W. Monthly weight changes of White Leghorn pullets in relation to concurrent egg weight and rations. Poultry Sci. 16:347. 1939.

Henderson, E. W. Monthly weight changes of White Leghorn pullets in relation to concurrent egg weight and rations. Growth 2:267. 1938.

CHAPTER 13

FEEDING AND MANAGEMENT FOR EGG PRODUCTION

Considerable variation is found in the rations that are used for egg production and the methods of feeding them. However, there are certain requirements that are met by all successful rations. Even though many apparent changes in feeding practices have occurred during the past few years, the principles have not changed to any extent.[1]

FEED REQUIREMENTS FOR EGG PRODUCTION

The amount of feed required by fowls is dependent upon the size of the bird, the number of eggs laid, the size of the eggs, increase in weight, and variations in maintenance needs, as influenced by activity, temperature, and the like.

PROTEIN. Satisfactory production cannot be obtained unless additional protein, besides that found in grains, is supplied.[2]

Halnan[3] made the accompanying estimates of the protein and energy requirements of a laying hen.

Hens in production require a continuous supply of protein since the nitrogen required for egg production is largely, if not

FOR GROWTH AND MAINTENANCE (PULLETS)
PER BIRD PER DAY

Weight of Bird (in lb.)	Digestible Protein (in grams)	Starch Equivalent (in grams)
3	6.5	51.7
4	7.4	58.1
5	8.3	64.1
6	9.2	69.7
7	10.1	75.0
8	11.0	80.0
For the Production of a 2-oz.* Egg		
	15.0	40.0

* (28.35 grams = 1 oz.)

entirely, drawn from the food.[4] An insufficient amount of protein will result in decreased egg production, lower body weight, and smaller egg size. A shortage of albumin in the ration has been reported as resulting in pickouts which ceased directly after albumin had been fed.[5]

Where birds were given the opportunity of balancing their own ration,[6, 7] some birds laid well and gained on a 12 to 13 per cent protein level while others wanted or required a higher level. Non-laying birds thrived and prepared to lay on an 11 per cent protein ration. In general, egg production was in accordance with the protein level, but the highest levels were not always the most economical.

Experimental results[8-15] generally show that a ration containing 12 per cent protein was not sufficient for satisfactory egg production, body weight, or egg size; that the 14 per cent protein ration gave satisfactory egg production but did not maintain body weight at all times and was not conducive to best egg size: that the 16 per cent protein ration was satisfactory in all respects.

Workers in the United States Department of Agriculture[16] report that increasing the percentage of protein in the diet, within the limits of 11.2 per cent and 23.6 per cent by the use of protein supplements of different origin, augmented egg production (1) by increasing intensity of production, (2) by increasing egg weight through direct effect on yolk weight, and (3) indirectly by increasing body weight and yolk weight, thereby increasing albumen weight. Increasing the protein level, within the limits stated, increased the quantity of egg produced per unit weight of feed eaten. Increasing the protein content decreased the efficiency of protein for egg production.

In studying the relationship of ruptured yolk to fowl paralysis, Moore[17] reports that results over a period of 3 years indicate higher mortality from a flock receiving a 13.5 per cent protein ration than from one receiving an 18.5 per cent protein diet. Bronkhorst[18] reports higher mortality due to prolapse from pullets on a basal mash containing 10 per cent of meat meal than from pullets fed mixtures containing 15 and 20 per cent of meat meal. Prolapse was frequently followed by cannibalism and did not appear to be influenced by egg size, egg yield, or age at sexual maturity.

Byerly[19] suggests, as a result of food requirement studies, that possibly smaller birds require a higher percentage of crude protein in the diet than larger birds, for the same degree of production.

The question might arise concerning a possibility of feeding an excess of protein. The Western Washington Station[20] states that all-mash rations containing 30 per cent of a protein concentrate did not produce a high percentage of organic trouble. It would appear from this, as well as from the experience of others, that hens can tolerate a fairly high protein ration if other conditions are favorable.

As a general summary, it would seem that in order to promote satisfactory production, maintain body weight, and secure good egg size, the ration should contain 15 to 16 per cent of protein. Part of this should come from animal source. If the birds are on good range, favorable results can be obtained with a lower amount of protein in the ration.

AMINO ACID REQUIREMENTS.[21] The requirements of some of the essential amino acids for laying hens have been reported as follows: tryptophan, 0.15 per cent; lysine, 0.52 per cent; leucine, 1.35 per cent; sulfur-bearing amino acids, 0.53 to 0.63 per cent with a minimum of 0.28 per cent for methionine.

FAT. It has been shown that fat, as such, in the diet is not essential since it can be synthesized from the carbohydrates of the ration. Russell and coworkers[22] concluded that the reduction of the fat content of the ration to 1.56 per cent of fat was not deleterious to the performance of laying and breeding flocks. Although the hen on a low-fat ration was not able to absorb carotene as efficiently as on a normal ration, vitamin A was absorbed equally well on a normal or on a low-fat ration.

Heywang and Titus[23] found no difference in egg production, yolk weight, or live weight between pullets being fed a diet of low fat content and pullets being fed diets containing 4 per cent of coconut oil, palm oil, peanut oil, cottonseed oil, soybean oil, or hempseed oil. Heywang[24] reported slightly lowered egg production from pullets receiving 8 per cent of corn oil in their diet. The pullets receiving 2, 4, or 8 per cent of corn oil in their diet maintained a heavier average weight than those receiving the basal diet of low fat content. No statistically significant differences in hatchability that could be attributed to the differences in fat content of the diets were observed.

MINERALS. Calcium and phosphorus[25] are the two minerals needed in largest amounts. Both egg production and shell strength are decreased by deficiencies of calcium and vitamin D. Experiments at Cornell indicated 1.65 per cent of calcium as being sufficient. The minimum phosphorus requirement is 0.6 per cent of which 0.4 to 0.45 per cent should be inorganic.

The manganese[26] requirement for egg production is very low. More is required for hatchability. Forty to fifty parts per million of the feed will satisfy both needs.

VITAMINS. From the results reported on vitamin A[27] requirements it would appear that a ration containing a minimum of 2000 to 2250 International units of vitamin A per pound will give normal results. A ration containing 35 per cent of yellow corn and 2½ per cent of alfalfa will supply this amount.

If the birds do not get the benefit of direct sunshine, it will be necessary to supply vitamin D in the ration. About 250 International units of vitamin D per pound of feed are essential.[28] It can be furnished by the use of fish oils or activated animal sterols.

The riboflavin[29] requirement for layers is relatively low, being less than 130 micrograms per 100 grams of feed. The amounts found in ordinary rations seem to be sufficient. However, higher levels[30] appear to be required for hens in batteries.

The pantothenic acid[31] requirement for hens for satisfactory egg production and weight maintenance is not more than 150 micrograms per 100 grams of ration.

The folic acid[32] requirement for egg production is not as large as that for hatchability. It appears to be approximately 25 micrograms per 100 grams of ration.

The pyridoxine[33] requirement for laying hens has been reported as being 2 milligrams per kilogram of ration.

FIBER. Not much is known of the optimum fiber content of the ration. However, it is known that very little fiber, if any, is digested by poultry. Hence it is desirable that the amount be restricted. Also high fiber rations are lower in energy. Production does not appear to be influenced by some increase in fiber,[34] probably because of an increase in feed consumption. The weight of birds, however, might be affected. Bird and Whitson[35] reported that a level of 5.89 per cent of fiber in a laying mash exerted a detrimental effect on efficiency of feed utilization but not on egg production. High efficiency rations are favored for layers. Hill[36] places the energy requirement at 900 calories per pound.

DIETARY REQUIREMENTS

As a summary of all evidence to date, the dietary requirements or standards for layers are indicated by the Committee on Animal Nutrition of the National Research Council[37] as given

REQUIREMENTS* OF LAYING HENS

Total protein, %	15
Vitamins	
Vitamin A activity (U.S.P. units)†	2000
Vitamin D (I.C.U.)‡	225
Riboflavin, mg.	1.0
Pantothenic acid, mg.	2.1
Pyridoxine, mg.	1.3
Folacin, mg.	0.11
Minerals	
Calcium, %	2.25§
Phosphorus, %‖	0.6
Salt, %¶	0.5
Iodine, mg.	0.2
Amino acids, %	
Lysine	0.5
Methionine	0.53
or	
Methionine**	0.28
Cystine	0.25
Tryptophan	0.15

*In percentage or amount per pound of feed.

†May be fish oil vitamin A or pro-vitamin A from vegetable sources.

‡International chick units.

§This amount of calcium need not be incorporated in the mixed feed inasmuch as calcium supplements fed free choice are considered as part of the ration.

‖A portion of the phosphorus requirement must be supplied in inorganic form. All the phosphorus of nonvegetable feed ingredients is considered to be inorganic. Approximately 30 per cent of the phosphorus of vegetable products is nonphytin phosphorus and may be considered as part of the inorganic phosphorus required.

¶This figure represents added salt or sodium chloride added as such or in marine or fermentation products of high sodium chloride content.

**Cystine will replace methionine as long as the ration contains not less than 0.28 per cent methionine.

in the accompanying tabulation. The figures do not include margins of safety to compensate for possible losses of vitamins during feed processing, transportation, and storage and for variations in feed composition and environment. In earlier reports the National Research Council suggested allowances which included margins of safety of 66 per cent for vitamin A, 50 per cent for vitamin D, and 20 per cent for the water-soluble vitamins.

To meet the requirements for a laying ration, the tabulated

formula pattern is suggested for a laying mash (to be fed with grain).

AMOUNT OF FEED. Besides having a proper proportion or balance of nutrients, it is essential that the birds consume enough food. Mature fowls (not laying) eat less in proportion to live weight than younger fowls (not laying). Larger animals will

RECOMMENDED FORMULA PATTERN FOR LAYING MASH

	lb./ton
High-energy grain products (corn, wheat, wheat red dog flour, milo, oatmeal)	500 +
Medium- and low-energy grain products (oats, barley, wheat flour middlings, standard middlings, bran)	0-800
Vegetable proteins (soybean meal, corn gluten meal, peanut meal) Animal proteins; (fish meal, fish solubles, meat scraps)	400-500
Dehydrated alfalfa meal	100-150
Additional riboflavin* (if needed)	+
Additional vitamin A* (if needed)	+
Vitamin D_3 (feeding oils or D-activated animal sterols)	+
Calcium and phosphorus supplements (steamed bonemeal, dicalcium phosphate, defluorinated phosphate, limestone)	100
Salt	20
Manganese sulfate (65% feeding grade)	0.5

* Refers to the use of riboflavin supplements and vitamin A sources of guaranteed vitamin content or other vitamin-rich feedstuffs when the formula is otherwise deficient in any of these nutrients.

REQUIRED COMPOSITION

Protein, %	20
Calcium, %	2-2.5*
Phosphorus	
Total %	1.2
Available %†	0.8
Vitamin A,‡ I.U./lb.	6600
Vitamin D, I.C.U./lb.	680
Riboflavin, mg./lb.	1.3

* Free choice feeding of oyster shell or other calcium supplement recommended since this level of calcium will not meet full requirements.

† Approximately 30 per cent of the phosphorus of vegetable products is non-phytin phosphorus and may be considered as part of the inorganic phosphorus required.

‡ If corn constitutes half of scratch grain mixture, the level of vitamin A in the mash can be reduced by 1000 I.U./lb.

consume more food than smaller ones. Younger animals will consume a larger amount of food per pound of live weight. The more pounds of eggs laid, the larger the amount of food consumed. In fact, the correlation between the number of eggs laid and the amount of food consumed is very close.

Titus[38] indicates that the gross maintenance requirement of White Leghorn hens, 16 months old and weighing on an average 1632 grams (3.6 pounds), was estimated to be 64 grams (2.26 ounces) of the special feed mixture used (containing 17.5 to 18.5 per cent protein, 4.0 to 4.2 per cent ether extract, and 2.4 to 2.5 per cent fiber) per bird per day during July. The amount of this special feed mixture required, over and above the maintenance requirement, to produce an egg was estimated as being about 40 grams (1.41 ounces).

A report from Denmark[39] states that the daily ration for maintenance may be computed for practical purposes at 70 grams (2.5 ounces) of grains for laying hens of the Italian breed, weighing 1.8 kilograms (3.96 pounds); and for hens of the middleweight breeds weighing 2.7 kilograms (5.94 pounds), at 80 grams (2.86 ounces) per bird. A mixed food supplement should be given which should contain 16 per cent of digestive pure protein in order to furnish the quantity of proteins needed by the hens. For the production of 1 kilogram (2.2 pounds) of egg, 1.1 kilograms (2.42 pounds) of mixed food was necessary, containing 95 Scandinavian food units or 67 kilograms (147.4 pounds) of nutritive value in 100 kilograms (220 pounds).

From the results of various scientific and practical experiments, Axelsson[40] has calculated the general food requirement of fowls for different live weights and different intensities of production (Table 27).

TABLE 27. FOOD REQUIREMENT OF THE LAYING FOWL (POUNDS PER DAY PER 100 BIRDS)

Average Live Weight, lb.	Maintenance	Egg Production (Approx. Percentage)									
		30	35	40	44	48	52	57	61	66	70
3.85	17.5	21.7	22.1	22.8	23.3	24.0	24.5	25.2	25.6	26.3	26.8
4.40	18.6	22.8	23.3	24.0	24.5	25.2	25.6	26.3	26.8	27.5	28.0
4.95	19.8	24.0	24.5	25.2	25.6	26.3	26.8	27.5	28.0	28.7	29.1
5.50	20.7	24.9	25.4	26.1	26.6	27.3	27.7	28.4	28.9	29.6	30.1
6.05	21.7	25.9	26.3	27.1	27.5	28.2	28.7	29.4	29.8	30.5	31.0
6.60	22.6	26.8	27.3	28.0	28.4	29.1	29.6	30.3	30.8	31.5	31.9
7.15	23.3	27.5	28.0	28.7	29.1	29.8	30.3	31.0	31.5	32.2	32.6
7.70	24.0	28.2	28.7	29.1	29.8	30.5	31.0	31.7	32.2	32.9	33.3

These figures are intended to apply to birds in their first laying year. They apply to average conditions which prevail in spring and autumn. For winter conditions, they may need to be raised about 10 per cent. In very hot weather a reduction of 15 to 20 per cent may be desirable. For older birds, they may be reduced by about 5 to 15 per cent of the maintenance requirement.

Byerly[19] suggests the amounts of daily feed for 100 layers with different rates of production given in the accompanying table.

Per Cent Production	WEIGHT OF BIRD 3 lb.	4 lb.	5 lb.	6 lb.	7 lb.
0	12.8	15.5	17.9	20.2	22.3
10	14.2	16.9	19.3	21.6	23.7
20	15.6	18.3	20.7	23.0	25.1
30	17.1	19.8	22.2	24.5	26.6
40	18.5	21.2	23.6	25.9	28.0
50	19.9	22.6	25.0	27.3	29.4
60	21.3	24.0	26.4	28.7	30.8
70	22.7	25.4	27.8	30.1	32.2
80	24.2	26.9	29.3	31.6	33.7
90	25.6	28.3	30.7	33.0	35.1
100	27.0	29.7	32.1	34.4	36.5

Records at Cornell University indicate that a flock of Leghorns, averaging 4 pounds in weight and not producing, consumed $1\frac{1}{3}$ pounds of feed per hen per week. This represents about 19 pounds per day for 100 hens. The same flock, producing 50 per cent, consumed $1\frac{2}{3}$ pounds per hen per wéek, or about 23 pounds per day for 100 hens. Larger hens will require more feed, smaller ones less. Also more feed will be necessary for higher levels of production. The accompanying figures are given as suggested quantities of feed necessary for average Leghorns (weighing 4 pounds):

Per Cent Production	Pounds of Grain and Mash per Day for 100 Birds
20	21
30	22
40	23
50	24
60	25
70	26
80	27

For heavier birds, such as the American breeds, the amount should be increased 2 to 3 pounds, or approximately 2 pounds for each pound increase in body weight.

The following formulas have also been suggested for calculating the amount of food required:

(1) Total daily feed for 100 birds = 8.3 + 2.2 times the weight of the bird + 0.1 times the egg production.

(2) Feed per hen per year = 31.5 + 8 times the weight + 0.1 times the egg production.

The problem in feeding is to get the birds to consume enough feed daily. Food consumption must stay above a minimum level, which is not always easy to do. For various reasons, some of them often difficult to determine, the birds may refuse to eat what they should. At the same time they usually become inactive.

It has been the experience of many persons that food consumption can be maintained or increased by liberal grain feeding. Jones of Connecticut[41] states that the amount of grain fed 100 birds a day should not be less than 12 pounds during the fall and winter. The New Jersey Station[42] indicates that a study of egg-laying contest records shows that during November to February egg production is proportional to the amount of scratch grain consumed, up to 15 pounds daily per 100 birds; that there is no relationship during March to October; that egg production increases with the amount of mash consumed during the winter and summer-fall periods.

Decreased food consumption may be due to a decrease in the mash or the grain or both. When food consumption decreases, steps must be taken immediately to increase it. There are various means of accomplishing this, and in most cases the means need be only temporary until the birds respond.

One of the first measures resorted to for increased food consumption is the feeding of a wet mash. It usually increases mash consumption because the wet mash is more palatable and can be easily eaten. It is only a temporary measure since the birds will, after a time, adjust their intake with the dry mash.

Artificial illumination may be a means to increase food if the length of day is limited.

Another practice to increase food is to give the birds liquid milk to drink. They like it, and it acts as both food and drink.

The feeding of palatable foods, such as condensed milk, green-cut bone, fresh meat, and blood, may be justified at such times as appetizers.

Changing the grain might increase food consumption if the grain which they prefer at the time is fed.

Frequency of feeding grain or giving fresh supplies of mash may stimulate activity and increase food consumption. The feeding of pellets, as a supplementary food, has also been reported favorably in this respect.

In order to obtain sufficient food intake it is necessary to provide enough feeding space.[43] Forty-eight feet of feeding space for 100 birds is satisfactory. It has also been shown that watering equipment is important since a flock laying at a high rate of egg production will consume considerably more water than the same flock laying at a low level.

For further information concerning the amount of feed see Chap. 19, "Economics of Feeding."

METHODS OF FEEDING

Besides supplying the correct kinds and balance of nutrients, it is also necessary to make the birds consume sufficient amounts of the nutrients in order to supply the materials for the eggs as well as to maintain the body weight. To do this often involves methods and management.

It is generally agreed that it is desirable to keep the birds busy to stimulate activity. If the hens are on range and outdoors, they will get exercise; but if they are closely confined, they might be too inactive. Feeding grain in litter will help to induce activity.

A general working rule is to keep the birds a bit hungry in the early part of the day, but gradually to fill them up so that, by night, they go to roost with full crops. This usually means limiting the amount of grain fed in the morning, in order to increase mash consumption during the day, and then feeding all the grain the birds can eat at night.

METHODS OF FEEDING GRAIN. The grain may be fed by hand in a litter or it may be fed in troughs. The birds will usually eat the grain when given a choice. If the amount of grain is restricted, the fowls can be induced to consume more mash. Birds should be fed according to their condition and production. No definite rule can be given to apply to all conditions of season and production.

Grain fed in the litter should be fed scantily in the morning: about 1½ to 2 quarts to 100 hens. No grain should be left in the litter at noon, for that would indicate that too much grain had been fed in the morning. The hens should be given all the grain that they will eat in the late afternoon so that they will find it before dark and go to roost with a full crop. Usually enough is fed so that a small amount is left over for the morning. All the grain should be fed in a dry, clean, straw litter, 4 to 6 inches deep.

When grain is fed in troughs, the birds should have it available early enough in the afternoon so they can eat what they want before going to roost. About 4 P.M. is the usual time for opening the grain hoppers except during the winter months, when no artificial illumination is used at night. Then the time must be advanced. In trough feeding of grain, little or no grain is fed in the morning. Frequently a light morning feed of grain is given in the litter. Trough feeding of grain is practiced with deep-litter management.

Continuous hopper feeding of grain may be practiced. With grain available all the time, the birds usually eat large amounts of it. Thus it may be necessary to restrict the grain at times in order to regulate the proportion of grain to mash, or to use a mash that is more concentrated. If the heavier grain consumption is maintained, extra vitamin and protein carriers must be added to the ration.

Sometimes the grain is fed only at night, particularly during the more favorable seasons of the year and when the birds are on range. But sometimes grain is fed more often, as, for example, when the birds are fed grain twice during the morning in very small quantities. This is often the practice during the winter when the birds are inclined to be inactive. By feeding them a little at a time and frequently, it is sometimes possible to keep them more active than if they were fed once in the morning or fed heavily. This is particularly true of the heavier breeds, which have a tendency to be sluggish.

The amount of grain to feed depends upon the appetites of the birds. No definite rule can be given to apply to all conditions. When grain is fed both morning and night, about three-fourths of it should be given at night and the rest in the morning and at noon. The tabulated amounts are suggested as the approximate grain feedings each day for 100 laying hens, averaging 4 pounds in weight.

Month	Morning Feeding	Night Feeding	Total Grain
November—February	3	10	13
March—June	2	10	12
July	. .	11	11
August	. .	10	10
September—October	. .	9	9

The common straws for litter in the order of their desirability are wheat, oats, rye, and buckwheat. Shredded or cut corn stalks, shavings, peat moss, oat hulls, or leaves may be used if straw is not available, especially where trough feeding is practiced. The litter should be clean and free from mustiness, mold, or decay, as serious losses frequently occur when spores develop into fungus molds in the lungs or intestines of the fowls.

METHODS OF FEEDING MASH. Under most conditions it is advisable to feed the mash dry in hoppers, troughs, or boxes, having it available at all times. The open hoppers are desirable since they permit the hens to have frequent fresh supplies of mash. Open boxes, if used, should be raised from the floor. To prevent waste where a reel or wires are not used, a piece of 1-inch mesh poultry netting should be placed on top of the mash. Sufficient hopper space should be provided. A trough 20 feet long, feeding on both sides, should be furnished for 100 hens. With mechanical feeders all-mash rations are used.

Moist mashes, when fed, are usually given sometime the latter part of the day. The plan is to induce the birds to eat as much of the dry mash during the day as they will, and then to consume an additional amount in the form of the wet mash, so as to fill them up by the time they get their feeding of grain.

FEEDING GREEN FEEDS. Where fresh green foods are provided, only as much should be given as the fowls will eat the same day or before it freezes. It is best to feed it during the middle of the day. It is not advisable to feed too much succulent feeds since they might decrease grain and mash consumption. About 4 to 6 pounds a day for 100 hens is sufficient.

PROPORTIONS OF GRAIN AND MASH. It is important to follow the directions for the particular ration that is being used. Practice the recommended methods that accompany the mixtures you decide to use because the methods of feeding are devised to meet the make-up of the mixtures themselves, particularly in regard to the proportion of grain and mash to feed. The proportions of grain and mash that are recommended have a close relationship usually to the amounts of protein, minerals, and vitamins which the mash contains.

ARTIFICIAL ILLUMINATION

Although the direct effect of light is stimulation of the reproductive system, artificial illumination in the northern latitudes is also largely a nutritional consideration.[44] The birds must be given sufficient time to assimilate enough feed to produce the eggs. The naturally short days or, more important still, the naturally long nights during the fall and winter are great handicaps to the hen. First, the hen must have a sufficiently long day in which to feed and exercise. Next, the night must not be too long or the assimilated food will be drawn upon to maintain the body rather than to make eggs. Experience has shown that ordinarily the hens should not go without food for more than about 10 hours, that is, they should have a 13- to 14-hour day. In this connection, it is well to keep in mind that on September 21 and March 21 night and day are of equal length. After September 21 the nights are longer than the days. For early-laying pullets and late-laying hens, the lights should be used not later than the first of September. For the later pullets, they should be put on when the chickens are placed in winter quarters.

When artificial illumination is used in the poultry house, the grain and mash mixtures remain unchanged, but the method of feeding must be adapted to the method of illumination. Though the underlying principles are the same, the time of feeding must be arranged to fit the working hours of the birds. In order that activity may be encouraged, grain should be fed lightly at the beginning of the hen's day. If morning illumination is used, the grain may be scattered in the litter the night before. The dry mash and water should be available during the entire time that the birds are off the roost. Grain should be fed heavily at the end of the day (with either natural or artificial lighting), about one hour before the birds go to roost. Green food should be supplied in the middle of the birds' working day.

Watch the condition of the birds, since they might have a tendency to produce eggs at the expense of their bodies. Hence it is necessary to observe the birds closely, with special attention to their weight, which is one of the best measures of condition. If they begin to lose flesh, increase the amount of grain fed and supplement it with a wet mash.

MODIFICATIONS DURING THE YEAR

For the best results, it is advisable to segregate the birds according to their condition and to manage them accordingly. Better results will be obtained if the birds in the flock are nearly alike in their conditions and consequently in their requirements. Different feeds must not always be used for each group; more often the variation will come in the manner of feeding the same ration and in the management of the flock.

FEEDING PULLETS. It is particularly important that pullets have fat in the body when they commence to lay and that they be kept in good flesh. The pullets that are thin when they begin to lay are most likely to molt. If the birds are not being handled regularly, as in trapnesting, it is a good practice to band a few of them and weigh them regularly. Good food consumption is required to meet the needs of growth as well as egg production. To encourage liberal grain consumption, keep the grain in hoppers before the pullets all the time for the first month or 6 weeks of production. After that time the grain may be fed only in the morning and in the afternoon. Always let the birds eat all the grain they want at night. The urge to lay will cause pullets to produce for a considerable period of time even on a deficient ration but at the expense of their bodies. It is well to house pullets when they start to lay and thus give them proper attention before they have lost flesh laying on range. The pullets should not only maintain their weight and flesh but should actually be completing their growth during the first few months of production. To produce eggs at the expense of their body weight, or as we say "to lay themselves out," is positively detrimental.

It is better to encourage production in early hatched pullets than to retard them when they are ready to lay. Pullets at Cornell[45] fed an egg mash gave better results than pullets retarded. The forced pullets made better profit, ate less food per hen at less cost, produced more eggs of a larger size, produced more eggs during the winter, had better hatching results, made better gains in weight, showed less broodiness, had less mortality, and showed better vigor.

Pullets that, because of early hatching or rapid development, have come into production early (August or September) will show a tendency toward decreased production, owing to the shortening days late in September and October, and to cold weather. At this time a decided slump in production, followed by a molt and a period of unproductivity, often occurs. This class of birds needs careful observation. It is of prime importance to maintain the weights of the individuals. Whenever the birds are losing weight or production begins to decrease, consumption of one part of the ration or of the feed as a whole usually decreases also. Introduction of milk, pellets, wet mashes, or artificial illumination of the poultry house at the proper time will help to overcome this difficulty. The lights should usually be turned on by September 1.

For later-hatched pullets, lights need not be used until October. It is well to hopper-feed grain to these pullets all the time also for a month or more after they are placed in winter quarters.

WINTER MANAGEMENT. The winter management of layers presents problems not met with in spring and summer production. Closer confinement and unfavorable climatic conditions make it more difficult to maintain high production and the health of the individual. To prevent a slump it is again necessary to maintain the weight of the birds by proper food consumption. It is better to decrease production somewhat for a time, to build up the birds, rather than to cause a break in production. Very high production usually cannot be maintained throughout the winter without a slump or molt, unless conditions are favorable.

During the spring and summer, when the conditions are favorable, it is possible to obtain 75 to 80 per cent production without harm to the birds. With such heavy production, however, one must be sure that the birds are being favored in all respects. It means a complete ration and heavy food consumption.

CARE OF BROODY HENS. Broodiness is a natural characteristic of the birds, the natural tendency to incubate the eggs and rear the chicks. When a hen becomes broody, the ovules that are not of mature size are reabsorbed into the body. It takes about 2 to 3 weeks to develop these minute ovules to mature size. They are reabsorbed, however, in a shorter period of time. If we can take a hen right at the time she begins to get broody and stimulate production, we shall check the reabsorption of the ovules and stimulate their formation. We can make her continue to produce and show a break for only a very short period. If we get a hen right away, production will be resumed in the course of 2 or 3 days. If we allow the hen to remain broody, reabsorption of the ovules takes place and the time that it will take for that hen to come back into production again depends largely upon the time at which we arrest the reabsorption of those ovules.

In handling our flocks for egg production we are interested in breaking up broodiness and getting the hens back into production. How can we overcome this broodiness? How can we stimulate that production? First, we need to discourage inactivity of the broody hen. When the hen becomes broody, she usually stays on the nest and in so doing she starves herself, because she does not get off the nest long enough to eat what she needs for egg production. The first thing to do is to remove the bird from the nest and place her in quarters that will prevent this absolute inactivity. Put her in a broody coop, which usually has a wire or slatted bottom to discourage setting and inactivity. Then feed some stimulating feeds, feeds that will encourage production. It has been found best to give the broody hens a moist mash. Do not feed grain. Give them water or milk to drink.

Broodiness can often be induced by restricting the feed. Where the hens are not given full rations or where they are starved, we get considerably more broodiness than where they are given plentiful feed.

If we want the hen to set, we feed only for maintenance. Therefore, the ration is usually restricted to grains. The hens can be given access to the grain and grit in hoppers. Water must also be given.

LATE SUMMER AND FALL MANAGEMENT. Production during late summer and fall is accomplished under conditions that normally are not favorable. In order to hold production, the mash consumption must be increased. However, Heywang[46] concluded that it is not advantageous to reduce the proportionate amount of grain in a mash-grain diet for laying chickens during hot weather in order to increase the protein level. This usually calls for wet mashes or other supplementation during the late summer and fall. Artificial illumination of the poultry house also gives the birds a better chance. The lights should usually be turned on not later than August 15 for hens at the end of their laying year.

CARE DURING THE MOLT. The molting of a hen is a natural characteristic, but the time of the molt and the nature and length of the molt can be influenced to quite an extent by feeding and management. Molt can be brought on by restriction of the feed and by starvation. The question often arises whether it is not advisable to force the hens into a molt late in the summer with the idea that they will come back into production again during the winter and lay high-priced, winter eggs. This sounds as if it might be possible, but it has been found that, even though the hens might lay a few more winter eggs, when the production and the returns throughout the year are considered, it is not a paying proposition because some fall eggs, which are also comparatively high-priced, will be sacrificed.[47] Furthermore, to force the hens into a molt, it is necessary to restrict the feed, and by restricting the feed we are likely to get a loss in body weight. It is very difficult to force the molt of some hens successfully, except during the normal molting season. It is best to let the molt take its normal course or, if anything, to prevent the molt until late in the fall.

It is possible, however, on the other hand, to keep the birds in production for too late a period. For the central New York region, probably somewhere around the first to the middle of November is late enough for any hens to keep in production. The time to stop will depend upon our ability to get the birds far enough along with their molt so that they may have the protection of the feathers by the time cold weather sets in. If the birds are kept in production too late and shed their feathers rapidly (this is likely to happen since it is the best birds that can be kept in production and thus the best birds will drop most of their feathers at a time), they are likely to be affected by the cold weather because of not having the protection of the feathers. This will delay recovery from the molt and postpone production.

When the hen stops production in the fall and goes through the molt, she needs the various nutrients just as when she was in laying condition. She probably does not need as much of the protein, although she needs considerable to grow new feathers. She will need fattening material to make up or to replace the decreased amount of body fat which we find hens lacking at the end of the laying season, especially when they have been held in fairly high production in the late fall. Since they are likely to be thin, body fat used up, and pigment gone, we need to get all this replaced to bring the bird back into good, plump, healthy condition, and with an excess or store of fat which can be drawn upon in the next production year. That means that when the hens stop production they may be fed more heavily on the grain but that they also need mash.

Hens that have stopped laying during August and early September can be brought back into production, so as to be put under lights by October 15 to November 1, by placing them on a clover or alfalfa range and hopper-feeding grain and mash. They will then respond well for winter production.

FEEDING THE BREEDS

Are the requirements for the heavier breeds different from those of the lighter breeds? Naturally, total food requirements are greater for the larger birds. The feed records at laying contests indicate that the heavier breeds consume more of the mash in proportion to the grain than the lighter breeds. Sometimes better results seem to be obtained when heavier breeds are given a slightly narrower ration. The variation is usually not in the feeds themselves so much as in the method or system of feeding. The grain feeding of the heavier breeds is restricted in order to get the birds to consume larger amounts of the mash. The restriction of the grain also tends to keep the heavier birds more active. Their natural sluggishness is overcome to some extent in this way. For that reason it seems desirable not to change the mixture, not to put more protein in the mash and then feed heavier on grain, but to keep the same mixtures and vary the method of feeding by restricting grain, thereby reducing activity and getting the birds to eat more of the mash. Because of less activity, they probably do not need quite so much of the grain as the lighter breeds.

The results of experiments in Denmark[39] indicate different levels of protein for birds of light and medium heavy breeds. The light birds, Brown Italian, required 10.5 to 11 per cent of digestible true protein, provided by a daily ration of 65 grams of grain, with free access to a mixture containing 16 per cent of digestible true protein. The heavier breeds, Plymouth Rock, Rhode Island Red, and Sussex, required slightly more total protein and so ate more of the free access food. No advantage was gained by feeding more protein than was provided in this way, but egg yield fell in proportion as the supply fell short of this level.

It has been shown, in the case of young stock, that the requirements of different breeds may differ for some of the vitamins and minerals. It is also possible that the same may be shown to be true for the requirements of adult birds, in respect to some of the nutrients.

SLUMPS IN PRODUCTION

When birds that have been laying heavily suddenly slow down, a neck or a complete body molt is likely to accompany this slump, after which it may be weeks before the flock can be brought back into good laying again, depending upon the condition of the birds and the extent of the molt.

The actions of the birds frequently foretell slumps. General activity and singing and cackling denote that all is well. Squawking, lack of interest, huddling in the corner, and dopiness denote trouble ahead.

Slumps may be brought on by various things.

1. POOR STOCK. The birds do not have the ability to stand up under the strain of heavy production.

2. POOR ENVIRONMENT. Heavy, damp, or dirty litter and

improper ventilation will affect the condition of the birds.

3. EXTREME TEMPERATURE. Extreme cold or hot weather and sudden changes will affect the birds adversely. In cold snaps, be sure the birds eat enough. Warm the water and also the other feed if necessary. Extremely hot weather requires increased shade. Provide cool water several times a day and furnish succulent green feed.

4. POOR CONDITION OF BIRDS. (a) Loss in weight. This is usually caused by decreased food consumption. (b) Diseases, such as chicken pox and colds, will cause decided slumps.

5. TOO SHORT DAY. Food consumption can be increased by using artificial illumination. Effects can be secured usually by increasing the length of day up to 15 hours.

6. DEFICIENT RATION. Any deficiency will cause a drop in production.

7. WRONG FEEDING. (a) Lack of appetite. This is often caused by feeding too much grain in the morning. Increase palatable feeds. (b) Indigestion might affect the lay. (c) Spoiled or poor-quality feed.

CONFINEMENT

In early experiments,[48] reported by the Ohio and Pennsylvania stations, confinement of hens did not produce as good results as giving them range. However, these results were obtained before our knowledge of vitamins. Range supplements the ration with sunlight, green feed, fresh air, and contentment.

With the development of commercial poultry keeping, layers are being confined to a greater extent. It frequently has been necessary because of contaminated soil. Where weather conditions are unfavorable, the birds are benefited by being confined. Sometimes there is also decreased mash consumption, owing to the birds staying outdoors.

The key to success in keeping hens in confinement is a complete ration. Confinement also requires more exact feeding and management in order to avoid such vices as cannibalism and feather pulling. However, with proper rations and management, just as good production can be obtained from birds confined as from birds allowed to range. For example, the Ohio Station[49] reports 122 eggs from hens having a bluegrass range, as compared with 127 from hens confined but having a sun porch, and 132 from hens confined indoors but with the windows open. Reporting on the cage system for managing laying hens, the New

Mexico Station[50] shows that the average annual egg production was materially higher with White Leghorns, Rhode Island Reds, and crosses in cages, than it was with birds in floor pens. The mortality rate was also lower with the birds in cages. The feed costs were slightly higher in the cages because of higher production and a more expensive diet for cage birds.

CARE OF LAYERS IN CAGES

Because the birds are in strict confinement with restricted activity, it is necessary that conditions and management be correct in order to get the best results. Some of these provisions are adequate housing for the cages, with proper ventilation of the battery room, suitable supply of birds, and proper feeding.

The ration must be complete. Either all-mash or grain and mash rations can be used, but the former is preferred because of the difficulty of feeding grain in right amounts to each individual. Pellets have also been fed satisfactorily. A single-feed mixture is more convenient and requires less skill in use.

Fresh feed is given at least once a day and preferably twice a day. There may be times when the food intake needs to be increased. This can be accomplished by feeding supplementary wet mash or pellets.

Some rations for cage layers include oystershells and grit. If not, they can be provided separately. They can be fed either on top of the feed or in separate troughs. Enough should be supplied so that there is always a little present in the troughs.

EMERGENCY SUBSTITUTIONS FOR MASH

Sometimes an emergency might arise when the regular mash is not available. The question then arises as to what will happen to egg production and what can be done. Platt[51] reported that an absence of mash for 6 days, if grain was available on the cafeteria basis, would have no serious effect upon egg production. If, however, it was extended to a period of 12 days, a significant curtailment would be realized, and this drop in egg production could be alleviated to some extent by feeding cooked whole soybeans plus a mineral mixture, or by diluting the normal mash with an equal quantity of yellow corn meal plus a mineral mixture.

At Cornell the laying mash was taken away from a pen of layers for 10 days during January. Grain consumption increased but not enough to keep up total feed intake. There was a drop from approximately 55 per cent production to 35 per cent the week following, after which time the birds increased in production again, coming back to a normal level in about 2 weeks. In another trial the laying mash was replaced for 2 weeks during April by a mixture of 40 per cent corn meal, 20 per cent wheat middlings, 20 per cent wheat bran, and 20 per cent ground oats. Total feed consumption again decreased somewhat and there was a drop in production of about 15 per cent the week after the mash without animal protein was fed. The birds had again reached normal production in about 2 weeks after the regular laying mash was restored.

It is important to keep up feed consumption. It can be accomplished better by feeding both whole grains and ground feed. Any means can be used, such as wet mash feeding, which have been found successful for maintaining or increasing feed intake.

COMPUTING RATIONS FOR EGG PRODUCTION

The final measure of a ration is the result it actually will produce. However, it is frequently necessary, as well as interesting, to compute the various nutrients in a ration and make adjustments in their relationships.

For example, we may want to know the nutrient content and protein energy-ratio of a ration. The following mixtures may be used as a problem:

Grain, lb.	Dry mash, lb.
100 cracked corn	100 corn meal
100 wheat	100 wheat bran
	100 flour wheat middlings
(To be fed equal parts	100 ground heavy oats
by weight of grain	75 meat scrap
and mash.)	25 dried milk

In Table 3 (page 56) we see that 100 pounds of corn contain 2.0 pounds of fiber, 8.6 pounds of protein, 3.9 pounds of fat, and 69.3 pounds of nitrogen-free extract. The same table shows the amounts of fiber, protein, fat, and nitrogen-free extract in the other feeds. From this information, it is calculated that the mixtures will contain the amounts of these nutrients given in the accompanying tabulation.

As suggested in the method of feeding this ration, the hens

GRAIN MIXTURE

	Fiber	Protein	Fat	Nitrogen-Free Extract
100 lb. corn	2.0	8.6	3.9	69.3
100 lb. wheat	3.0	13.2	1.9	69.9
200 lb. grain mixture	5.0	21.8	5.8	139.2
100 lb. grain mixture	2.5	10.9	2.9	69.6

MASH MIXTURE

	Fiber	Protein	Fat	Nitrogen-Free Extract
100 lb. corn meal	2.0	8.6	3.9	69.3
100 lb. wheat bran	9.6	16.9	4.6	52.9
100 lb. flour wheat middlings	3.8	18.3	4.2	59.8
100 lb. ground oats	11.0	12.0	4.6	58.6
75 lb. meat scraps	0.9	41.9	8.2	0.4
25 lb. dried milk	. . .	8.7	0.3	12.6
500 lb. mash mixture	27.3	106.4	25.8	253.6
100 lb. mash mixture	5.5	21.3	5.2	50.7

should eat about equal parts of grain and mash. The nutrients of this ration, therefore, may be calculated as follows:

	Fiber	Protein	Fat	Nitrogen-Free Extract
100 lb. grain	2.5	10.9	2.9	69.6
100 lb. mash	5.5	21.3	5.2	50.7
200 lb. ration	8.0	32.2	8.1	120.3
100 lb. ration	4.0	16.1	4.2	60.2

This ration, then, has 4.0 pounds of fiber, 16.1 pounds of protein, 4.2 pounds of fat, and 60.2 pounds of nitrogen-free extract for every 100 pounds of feed.

It remains to compute the protein-energy ratio.

RULE FOR COMPUTING PROTEIN-ENERGY RATIO. Add the fat (4.0) multiplied by $2\frac{1}{4}$ (9.8) to the nitrogen-free extract (60.2), which gives the total energy nutrients (69.2). Total energy nutrients (69.2) divided by protein (16.1) equals protein-energy ratio (4.3). Therefore, the protein-energy ratio of this ration is 1–4.3, which means that for each pound of protein the ration contains 4.3 pounds of carbohydrates and fat.

BALANCING RATIONS. In balancing a ration, amounts of available feeds should be used as seem desirable. Then the nutrients should be calculated as above. If it is found that the protein-energy ratio is too wide (containing too large an amount of carbohydrates and fat to one part of protein), the amount of one or more feeds that contain a large proportion of carbohydrates and fat should be reduced and one or more feeds that contain a larger proportion of protein should be substituted. If it is found that the protein-energy ratio is too narrow (containing too small an amount of carbohydrates and fat to one of protein), the amount of one or more feeds that contain a large proportion of protein should be reduced and one or more feeds that contain a larger proportion of carbohydrates and fat should be substituted. After a few such trials, it should be possible to formulate a ration that will meet the requirements. One must not forget that the mixtures must be considered also from the standpoint of palatability, mechanical condition, and other factors previously discussed.

If the digestible nutrients and the nutritive ratio are desired, the same procedure is followed as above, except that the values for digestible nutrients are used instead of the crude nutrients.

RATIONS FOR EGG PRODUCTION

It is possible to formulate a large number of rations that will meet the requirements. The ingredients used will depend largely upon the availability of the feedstuffs. Some of the representative rations being recommended for layers will be found in the Appendix. (See page 554.)

REFERENCES

1. Rice, J. E. Feeding of laying hens: the principles. N. Y. (Cornell) Reading Course for Farmers. Series 4. (17) 1903.
2. Fangauf, R., and A. Haensel. The action of protein given on the laying output in examples of farm hen feeding. Archiv für Geflügelk. 11:39. 1937.
3. Halnan, E. T. Scientific principles of poultry feeding. Ministry Agr. and Fisheries (London) Bul. 7. 1930.
   Halnan, E. T. Some observations on the protein requirements of the laying fowl. Rept. Seventh World's Poultry Congress. 145. Cleveland. 1939.

4. Wilcox, J. S. The nitrogen balance of laying hens. Jour. Agr. Sci. (England) 24:636. 1934.
5. Malke, E. Über eine verhängnisvelle Folge eiweissarmer Ernährung in der Hühnerhaltung. Deutsche Tierärtzliche Wochenschrift: 623. 1930.
6. Zöllner, I., Fütterungsversuch mit verschiedenen hohen Eiweissgaben im Legehennenfutter. Deutsche Landwirtschaftliche Geflügelzeitung June 9, 1932.
Fangauf, R., and E. Kallmann. Beliebige Aufnahme von Eiweissfutter bei Legehühnern als eiweiss-sparende Fütterungstechnik. Archiv für Geflügelk 7:1. 1933.
Fangauf, R., and A. Haensel. Versuche über das Eiweissminimum bei Legehühnern. Archiv für Geflügelk 11:329. 1937.
Jaeger, J., E. Rühle, and H. Börger. Versuch zur Feststellung der MindestEiweissbedarfes zur Erreichung einer zufriedenstellenden Legeleistung. Archiv für Geflügelk 12:117. 1938.
Fangauf, R., and A. Haensel. Weitere Beobachtungen über das Eiweissminimum bei Legehühnern. Archiv für Geflügelk 13:285. 1939.
7. Graham, J. C. Individuality of pullets in balancing the ration. Poultry Sci. 13:34. 1934.
8. Fiftieth Ann. Rept. N. J. Agr. Exp. Sta. 1929:280.
9. MacDonald, A. J. The protein requirements of laying birds, Agr. Progress 15:101. 1938.
10. Heuser, G. F. The protein requirements of laying hens. Rept. Sixth World's Poultry Congress. 276. Germany. 1936.
11. Gutteridge, H. S., J. M. Pratt, and J. B. O'Neil. Level and source of protein in poultry production. II. As related to economical production of eggs. Sci. Agr. 24:240. 1944.
12. Penquite, R. Sixteen to twenty per cent protein appears best for laying hens. Okla. Rept. 1938-1940:148.
13. Heiman, V., J. S. Carver, and J. L. St. John. The protein requirements of laying hens. Wash. Tech. Paper 331. 1936.
Carver, J. S. The effects of level of protein in the laying mash on egg production. Wash. Bul. 470:69. 1945.
14. Clark, T. B., T. D. Runnels, J. H. Rietz, and C. E. Weekley, Jr. Egg production and mortality of White Leghorns fed high and low protein rations. Poultry Sci. 21:468. 1942.
15. Protein influences egg size. News Letter, Col. Agr. Moscow, Idaho. September 1936.
16. Byerly, T. C., H. W. Titus, and N. R. Ellis. Production and hatchability of eggs as affected by different kinds and quantities of proteins in the diet of laying hens. Jour. Agr. Res. 46:1. 1933.
17. Moore, E. N. Relationship of ruptured yolk to fowl paralysis. Jour. Am. Vet. Med. Assn. 96:727. 1940.
18. Bronkhorst, J. J. The influence of the protein level of the diet on the growth, egg production, egg weight and mortality of Single Comb White Leghorn pullets. Onderstepoort Jour. Vet. Sci. 10: 469. 1938.
19. Byerly, T. C. Feed and other costs of producing market eggs. Md. Tech. Bul. A1. 1941.

20. Miller, M. W., and G. E. Bearse. Feeding excess protein to laying hens. West. Wash. Bul. 18 W., N. S.:27. 1930.
21 Cravens, W. W. The effect of leucine on egg production and hatchability. Poultry Sci. 27:562. 1948.
Ingram, G. R., W. W. Cravens, C. A. Elvehjem, and J. G. Halpin. Studies on the lysine and tryptophane requirements of the laying and breeding hen. Poultry Sci. 30:426. 1951.
Ingram, G. R., W. W. Cravens, C. A. Elvehjem, and J. G. Halpin. The methionine requirement of the laying hen. Poultry Sci. 30: 431. 1951.
Leong, K. C., and J. McGinnis. An estimate of the methionine requirement for egg production. Poultry Sci. 31:692. 1952.
22. Russell, W. C., M. W. Taylor, and H. A. Walker. The absorption and retention of carotene and vitamin A by hens on normal and low fat rations. Jour. Biol. Chem. 140, No. 1:CIX. 1941.
Taylor, M. W., F. P. Jeffrey, and W. C. Russell. Fat requirements of the hen. Poultry Sci. 23:155. 1944.
23. Heywang, B. W., and H. W. Titus. Weight and quality of the yolks of eggs of chickens fed diets containing vegetable oils. Poultry Sci. 20:483. 1941.
Heywang, B. W. Hatchability in relation to the fat content of the diet. Poultry Sci. 21:521. 1942.
24. Heywang, B. W. Some results of feeding diets of varying fat content to laying pullets. Poultry Sci. 22:446. 1943.
Heywang, B. W. Hatchability in relation to the fat content of the diet. Poultry Sci. 21:521. 1942.
25. Gillis, M. B., L. C. Norris, and G. F. Heuser. Phosphorus requirements of hens. Poultry Sci. 32:977. 1953.
Heuser, G. F., M. B. Gillis, and L. C. Norris. Meeting the phosphorus needs of laying hens. Proc. Ninth World's Poultry Congress. Vol. II:52. 1951.
Kennard, D. C., and V. D. Chamberlin. The results when vitamin D and calcium fail the layers. Ohio Bimo. Bul. 232:9. 1945.
Miller, M. W., and G. E. Bearse. Phosphorus requirements of laying hens. Wash. Bul. 306. 1934.
26. Gutowska, M. S., and R. T. Parkhurst. Studies in mineral nutrition of laying hens. I. The manganese requirement. Poultry Sci. 21: 277. 1942.
Wilgus, H. S., L. C. Norris, and G. F. Heuser. The role of manganese in poultry nutrition. Proc. Seventh World's Poultry Congress. 171. 1939.
27. Almquist, H. J., and E. Mecchi. Vitamin A requirements of laying hens. Poultry Sci. 18:129. 1939.
Heywang, B. W. The level of vitamin A in the diet of laying and breeding chickens during hot weather. Poultry Sci. 31:294. 1952.
McClary, C. F., G. E. Bearse, and V. L. Miller. Vitamin A requirements of laying hens. Western Wash. Ann. Rept. 1939:45.
Russell, W. C., C. S. Platt, M. W. Taylor, and D. F. Chichester. The vitamin A requirements of the laying pullet. New Jersey Circ. 369. 1936.

Sherwood, R. M. Vitamin A requirements of poultry. Seventh World's Poultry Congress Report. 123. 1939.
Taylor, M. W., J. R. Stern, and W. C. Russell. The provitamin A requirement of hens. Poultry Sci. 26:243. 1946.
28. Carver, J. S., E. I. Robertson, D. Brazie, R. H. Johnson, and J. L. St. John. The vitamin D requirements of chickens. Wash. Bul. 299. 1934.
Couch, J. R., L. E. James, and R. M. Sherwood. The effect of different levels of manganese and different amounts of vitamin D in the diet of hens and pullets. Poultry Sci. 26:30. 1947.
Murphy, R. R., J. E. Hunter, and H. C. Knandel. The vitamin D requirement of growing chicks and laying hens. Pa. Bul. 334. 1936.
29. Norris, L. C., H. S. Wilgus, A. T. Ringrose, V. Heiman, and G. F. Heuser. The vitamin G requirement of poultry. Cornell Bul. 660. 1936.
30. Petersen, C. F., C. E. Lampman, and O. E. Stamberg. High levels of riboflavin required for hens in batteries. Idaho Agr. Exp. Sta. 54th Ann. Rept. 10. 1947.
31. Gillis, M. G., G. F. Heuser, and L. C. Norris. Pantothenic acid in the nutrition of the hen. Jour. Nutr. 35:351. 1948.
Heuser, G. F., M. B. Gillis, and L. C. Norris. The pantothenic acid requirement of poultry. Rept. 8th World's Poultry Congress 1948:114. Copenhagen.
32. Couch, J. R., and H. L. German. Pteroylglutamic acid studies with the mature fowl. Poultry Sci. 29:539. 1950.
Cravens, W. W., and J. G. Halpin. The effect of pteroylglutamic acid and an unidentified factor on egg production and hatchability. Jour. Nutr. 37:127. 1949.
Lillie, R. J., G. F. Combs, and G. M. Briggs. Folic acid in poultry nutrition I. The critical need for folic acid by laying pullets. Poultry Sci. 29:115. 1950.
Schweigert, B. S., H. L. German, P. B. Pearson, and R. M. Sherwood. Effect of the pteroylglutamic acid intake on the performance of turkeys and chickens. Jour. Nutr. 35:89. 1948.
Sunde, M. L., W. W. Cravens, H. W. Bruins, C. A. Elvehjem, and J. G. Halpin. The pteroylglutamic acid requirement of laying and breeding hens. Poultry Sci. 29:220. 1950.
Taylor, L. W. The effect of folic acid on egg production and hatchability. Poultry Sci. 26:372. 1947.
33. Cravens, W. W., E. E. Sebesta, J. G. Halpin, and E. B. Hart. Studies on the pyridoxin requirements of laying and breeding hens. Poultry Sci. 25:80. 1946.
34. Gerry, R. W. High energy rations for layers. Maine Timely Topics. Jan. 9, 1951.
35. Gerry, R. W., J. R. Smyth, and C. E. Howes. High energy-Low fiber rations. Maine Bul. 491:66. 1951.
Gerry, R. W., J. R. Smyth, and C. E. Howes. High-efficiency rations for replacement stock and laying hens. Poultry Sci. 31:917. 1952.

Bird, H. R., and D. Whitson. Effect of diet on efficiency of egg production. Poultry Sci. 25:210. 1946.

36. Hill, F. W. Energy requirements of chickens. Proc. Cornell Nutr. Conf. for Feed Mfgrs., 26. 1952.

37. Recommended nutrient allowances for domestic animals. Number 1. Recommended nutrient allowances for poultry. National Research Council. Rept. Com. Animal Nutrition. Washington. June 1944. Revised March 1950.

Nutrient requirements for domestic animals. Number 1. Nutrient requirements of poultry. Rept. Comm. Animal Nutrition National Research Council, Washington, D. C., 1954. Pub. 301.

38. Titus, H. W. Gross maintenance requirement of White Leghorns. Poultry Sci. 8:80. 1929.

39. Baelum, J. Dänische Untersuchungen über den Futter-und Proteinbedarf legender Hennen. Rept. Sixth World's Poultry Congress. 222. 1936.

Baelum, J. Forsog med forskelligt proteinindhold i foderet til aeglaeggende honer. Beretn, Kgl. Vet. Landbohojsk. landokon, Forsogslab. (Kobenhavn) 181:173. 1938.

40. Axelsson, J. The general nutritive value (energy value) of foods for poultry. Harper Adams Utility Poultry Jour. 23:43. 1937-1938.

41. Conn. Home Egg-Laying Contest Rept. for September 1928. Vol. 9 (11).

42. Clickner, F. H. Standard methods of feeding laying stock. N. J. Hints 13(9). June 1925.

43. Lee, C. E., C. L. Henry, and J. Presto. The feeding space requirements of laying birds receiving a mash, grain, and supplementary pellet ration. Poultry Sci. 31:290. 1952.

44. Bissonnette, T. H. Does increased light absorption cause increased egg production in the fowl? Poultry Sci. 12:396. 1933.

Platt, C. S. Maintaining winter egg production by the use of dim red light. Poultry Sci. 32:931. 1952.

Hall, G. O. The artificial control of egg production. Poultry Sci. 25:3. 1946.

45. Rice, J. E. Comparison of four methods of feeding early hatched pullets. N. Y. (Cornell) Bul. 249. 1907.

46. Heywang, B. W. Diet for laying chickens during hot weather. Poultry Sci. 26:38. 1947.

47. Hinds, H. B. Moulting and housing experiments. Ariz. Bul. 177. 1941.

48. Buss, W. J. Feeding experiments with laying hens. Ohio Bul. 322. 1918.

Kilpatrick, M. C., and D. E. Warner. Hens confined as compared with hens having access to open yard. Pa. Rept. 1913-1914(II): 121.

49. Kennard, D. C. Shall layers be confined? Ohio Bul. 140:156. 1929.

50. Berry, L. N. The cage system for managing laying hens. N. Mex. Bul. 276. 1941.

Berry, L. N. Feeding and management of birds in laying cages. *New Mexico Bul.* 328. 1946.

51. Platt, C. S. Emergency substitutions for laying mash in the diet of White Leghorn pullets. *Poultry Sci.* 23:126. 1944.

CHAPTER 14

FEEDING AND MANAGEMENT OF BREEDERS

There is a relationship between feeding and management of the poultry flock and hatching results. We are dealing with a reproductive process that is more exacting and apparently is influenced by more factors than only the production of eggs. It is entirely possible to secure large numbers of eggs and still not obtain eggs that will produce satisfactory hatching returns. For example, the hens in two pens at Cornell University, receiving different rations, gave satisfactory and uniform production (averaging in each case 211 eggs per bird for the year), but the hens in one pen hatched only 27.5 per cent of the fertile eggs set in February, whereas the other hens hatched 71.4 per cent. Besides numbers of eggs, especially during the hatching season, we must get eggs that not only are fertile but also are capable of producing chicks of good quality, healthy, and vigorous.

Hatchability or the ability of eggs to produce chicks is influenced by many factors,[1] some of them beyond the control of the average poultryman. For instance, some hens consistently produce eggs that are infertile or, if fertile, will not hatch.

But, in order to produce good fertile eggs that will develop vigorous chicks, it is necessary to care properly for the breeders. It is necessary to put the quality into the egg because during incubation the embryo develops within the egg independent of the hen. Thus there is inside the egg a developing individual which must be furnished suitable growth conditions.

NUTRITIONAL REQUIREMENTS FOR HATCHABILITY

Proper food or building material is a first essential which we cannot supply except through the hen. If all the necessary food nutrients are not in the egg, growth will be handicapped until the time when additional food can be furnished, which is not until after the chicks are hatched. This early, embryonic life is much more important than any other equal period and gives the chicks a start which will not easily be overcome.

In order to produce this quality in the egg, the breeding flock must be given proper attention, not only during the hatching season, but also for some time previous to it.

The nutrition of the hen is one of the most important considerations affecting hatching results. Anything that affects the condition of the birds will affect hatchability. For example, it has been reported that hatches were decreased where the hens were fed scantily. In that case, the hens probably depleted their bodies by drawing upon body reserves. Any practice that will keep up a balance of nutrients in the bird will increase or maintain hatchability. Any deficiency, be it vitamin, mineral, or protein, will decrease hatchability by affecting the health and condition of the bird.

PROTEIN. Not only is a proper amount of protein necessary, but the feeds must also furnish enough of the right amino acids.[1] An excess of protein to be eliminated will place an extra strain on the animal; a deficiency will prevent it from functioning properly.

It has been shown that rations low[2] in protein give low hatchability. This may be due in part to the fact that these rations frequently contain little or no protein concentrates. The United States Department of Agriculture[3] reports that in birds receiving a low-protein diet the trend in hatchability tended to parallel the trends in egg production and egg weight during the first year of production.

The Oklahoma Station[4] reported that, although the embryos from the high-protein hens were heavier during the greater part of the incubation period as shown by both wet weight and dry weight, the differences were shown by an analysis of variance to be insignificant. A further report indicates that in two experiments out of three the chicks produced by the hens on the high-protein levels were smaller than would be expected, whereas the chicks produced by the hens on the low levels were larger than would be expected. In hens the differences were significant, whereas in pullets they were not significant.

Some reports show no difference in hatchability between vegetable and animal protein concentrates.[5] In general, however, the use of vegetable protein concentrates has resulted in decreased hatchability. This is particularly true of cottonseed meal.[6,7]

The South Carolina Station has further shown that the addition of crude cottonseed oil to a satisfactory ration for hens markedly reduced the hatchability of the eggs, as did also refined oil produced by filtering and alkali treatment. Gossypol[8] has been shown to be a factor having an adverse effect on hatchability.

The Alabama Station[6] also reports lower hatchability from a ration containing soybean meal but comparable results with the one containing peanut meal. A number of other workers[9] have reported that soybean oil meal, as the sole protein supplement in poultry rations, fails to support good hatchability. It has been demonstrated that such rations may be deficient in manganese and riboflavin. It has also been suggested that there may be a relationship between the goitrogenicity of soybean oil meal and the poor reproduction.

The United States Department of Agriculture[10] reported that diets containing proteins from vegetable sources only increased the incidence of chondrodystrophy in embryos of hens likely to produce such embryos. Embryos in eggs from hens on such diets has a high second-week mortality.

Parkhurst[11] reported greater hatches from rations containing animal protein than from one containing no animal protein, both alone and in combination with various feeds of high vitamin content.

In comparing rations containing meat scraps with those containing milk as the source of animal protein, most experimenters report better hatchability with the milk ration.[12-18] The difference in favor of the milk has usually been about 10 to 15 per cent.

The South Carolina Station[19] indicates reduced hatchability with fish meal. Reports from Canada[20] show no influence on hatchability or viability of chicks by the addition of bone meal to the ration. Results from the Ontario Agricultural College[21] indicate that there is a difference in the protein sources as to the hatching power of the eggs produced. The best hatches came from milk and fish meal. In general, during an 11-year study with Barred Plymouth Rock pullets, the use of dried buttermilk as the protein supplement has resulted in higher hatchability than either fish meal or meat meal. During the last 6 years of this period the buttermilk showed decided superiority. The decline in meat meal may be due to the lessened amount of liver and other glandular material. It seems probable that there may be a decided variation in the value of different meat or fish meals for hatching rations, depending on the materials used in their manufacture and processing procedure.

The improved hatchability of rations containing animal proteins may be due in part to their vitamin values. This is true especially of milk, in which, no doubt, riboflavin plays an important part.

The amount of protein is the same as for layers. (See page 383.) No difference has been shown in the amino acid requirements for hatchability as compared with those for egg production only. (See page 384.)

MINERALS. Possibly some of the difference between animal and vegetable proteins may be due to the more favorable mineral content of the animal protein concentrates. The Kentucky Station[22] has shown that calcium restriction decreased hatchability. In the absence of a calcium carbonate supplement, the hatchability of fertilized eggs was diminished, finally becoming zero. When oystershells were again supplied, hatchability was increased. The Kentucky workers also found that, in the absence of a calcium carbonate supplement, the percentage of infertile eggs was increased, the chicks hatched weighed less, and the ratio of the weight of the moisture-free carcass of the chick to the original weight of the contents of the egg from which it was hatched was less.

Results reported from the National Agricultural Research Center[23] show that, in general, a high level of calcium intake adversely affected the hatchability of the eggs, and the effect was more pronounced in the hen's eggs than it was in the pullet's eggs. The hatchability of the eggs was better when calcium carbonate was used as the source of calcium than when calcium sulphate (gypsum) was used.

The level of phosphorus intake was reported[23] as having no effect on hatchability. However, the highest levels of calcium intake affected the hatchability more adversely when the level of phosphorus intake was 0.9 per cent than when it was 1.2 per cent. With a deficiency of phosphorus embryo mortality occurs mostly in the first 2 weeks. A level of 0.3 per cent of phosphorus has been shown to be sufficient.[24]

Manganese[25, 26] has also been shown necessary for good hatchability. The Kentucky Station reported a hatchability of less than 10 per cent from hens fed a low manganese ration (13 parts per million). The embryos died during the final stage of incubation and showed short legs and wings and "parrot beaks." The requirement for hens appears to be 40 to 50 parts per million of the ration.

Iodine is necessary for reproduction. Only a few investigators[27] have shown increased hatchability when feeding supplementary iodine. Most of the reports show no benefits, which indicates sufficient amounts of this mineral in ordinary rations.

Toxic grain, because of its selenium content, was reported by the South Dakota Station[28] to affect hatchability very seriously. Approximately 75 per cent of the eggs that failed to hatch contained deformed embryos.

VITAMINS. In the light of our present knowledge of nutrition, the vitamins undoubtedly constitute the most important nutritional factor affecting hatching results. Improved hatches in the spring and summer can be largely accounted for by access to green food and sunshine.

Vitamin A. It is probable that a deficiency of any vitamin that is necessary will influence hatching. Decreased hatchability reported by Kansas[29] and Oklahoma[30] in lots where white corn was fed was probably due to a vitamin A deficiency. When yellow corn or alfalfa, which are vitamin A carriers, was fed, the hatchability was improved. Fertility was good. Chicks hatched from eggs of birds fed white corn did not have a thrifty appearance. The Oklahoma Station[30] also indicates decreased hatchability from wheat. This was also likely to be caused by a vitamin A deficiency.

Reports from a number of experiment stations[31, 32] indicate that the vitamin A requirement for breeders, where a high vitamin A content of the egg is desired, is greater than for layers.

Vitamin D. It has long been noticed that hatchability improved rapidly after the birds got outdoors in the spring. The improvement was attributed to the birds getting on the ground, access to green food, increased temperature, and many other reasons. It is now generally believed that improvement was due largely to exposure to sunshine, which furnished the antirachitic factor or vitamin D.

The antirachitic factor may be furnished by means of irradiation, or exposure to the ultraviolet rays of sunshine, or artificially produced ultraviolet rays of special lamps, such as the quartz mercury-vapor or carbon-arc lamp. Wisconsin[33] was

TABLE 28. INFLUENCE OF ULTRAVIOLET LIGHT ON HATCHABILITY

Month	Irradiated *	Non-irradiated	Male Only Irradiated
February	66	35	44
March	64	20	11
April	70	0	6
			62†
May	68	0	76

* 10 minutes of ultraviolet light.
† Hens also irradiated.

one of the first stations to demonstrate that ultraviolet light greatly improved hatchability (Table 28).

The reports from other stations[34-36] also showed the influence of a ration deficient in vitamin D upon hatchability. The Kentucky Station[37] reported that pullets confined to the house and receiving sunlight only through glass windows produced eggs which progressively decreased in hatchability. Ordinary glass windows exclude most of the beneficial rays of ultraviolet light.

The antirachitic factor, or vitamin D, may be furnished by irradiation with ultraviolet light, by exposure to sunshine, or by feeding cod liver oil.[38] This is clearly shown by the following results as obtained in Kansas:

	Per Cent Hatchability
Sunshine	75.45
Ultraviolet light (Quartz lamp)	71.63
Sunshine plus ultraviolet light	67.43
Sunshine through glass	52.90
Cod liver oil (1/2 cc. per day)	74.27

If the windows of the poultry house are allowed to remain open, the birds receive considerable benefit from the sunshine that can enter. Certain glass substitutes are effective in transmitting the ultraviolet rays, but other materials are not effective. The Wisconsin Station[39] reports the following 5-year average results:

	Hatch (March) per cent
Glass closed	13
Glass closed plus irradiation from quartz mercury lamp	59
Glass open plus irradiation from quartz mercury lamp	65
Glass open	45
Glass substitute closed	45
Quartz glass closed	45
White cloth closed	23
Glass closed plus cod liver oil	49

Sunlight is very effective in furnishing the antirachitic factor and increasing hatchability. It has been pointed out by various workers that hatchability often increases more or less in proportion to the amount of sunlight available. Experiments reported from Canada[21] generally show greater hatchability during the summer months of May, June, and July, when the hours of sunshine are greater, than during the spring months of February, March, and April. With the grain ration such as used, the addition of direct sunshine or sunshine substitutes was the most important factor in producing good hatching eggs. The birds did not get the necessary amount of sunshine until there was at least 200 hours of sunshine per month.

Cod liver oil will improve hatchability by furnishing vitamin D.[40-42] When sufficient sunshine is available, cod liver oil is not necessary. Viosterol[43] has been reported not to be so effective as cod liver oil. Furthermore, an overdose of viosterol still further decreased hatchability.

Differences in hatchability are probably due to differences in egg quality. The Wisconsin Station[33] found that the developing embryo (21 days old) from eggs produced by irradiated hens contained nearly twice as much lime as the embryo from non-irradiated hens' eggs. From this, Hart and his coworkers conclude that low hatching is probably related to low power of the developing embryo to transfer lime from the shell. In this connection, Hughes and his coworkers[44] report that the antirachitic vitamin in the egg is determined by the amount of irradiation and that eggs with low antirachitic vitamin content do not have as high a hatchability as eggs having a high antirachitic vitamin content.

Experiments at the Kentucky Station[45] indicate that an absence of vitamin D decreased the percentage of eggshell and that hens receiving an adequate supply of vitamin D supplemented by pasture tend to produce chicks which grow more rapidly.

Three different yearly experiments at Cornell indicate the effect of ultraviolet irradiation and cod liver oil upon eggshell strength and hatchability (Table 29).

It is believed by some workers[46] that sunshine supplies something, besides vitamin D, that is necessary for good hatchability. The Wisconsin workers[47] also reported that the hatchability of winter eggs was much improved by adding a small amount of manganese to the mash, when soybean oil meal is the only protein supplement in the ration, but that feeding manganese has little or no beneficial effect on hatchability in spring or summer. Their records seem to indicate that the amount of direct sunlight which the hens receive affects their need for manganese, but they were unable to explain the relation of sunlight to the utilization of manganese.

Vitamin E. Vitamin E is recognized as a specific reproduc-

TABLE 29. EFFECT OF ULTRAVIOLET IRRADIATION AND COD LIVER OIL UPON EGGSHELL BREAKING STRENGTH AND HATCHABILITY

Period, 4 Weeks	Quartz Mercury Vapor Arc, lb.	Sunlight, lb.	Cod Liver Oil, lb.	Control, lb.
1	10.14	9.89	9.89	9.56
2	10.24	10.12	9.98	9.24
3	10.17	10.10	10.22	9.29
4	10.19	9.73	10.18	7.82
5	10.59	10.20	10.43	7.44
6	9.80	9.88	9.02	6.70
7	9.53	9.76	9.87	5.70
8	9.17	8.86	9.28	5.71
9	8.26	8.45	8.57	4.71
10	7.49	7.91	7.92	4.05
11	7.74	7.87	8.03	4.43
12	7.72	8.17	8.86	4.21
% hatch of fertile eggs	56.4	55.5	67.0	35.2

tive vitamin. A deficiency of it in the ration produces sterility. It is found in the germs of cereals. An ordinary mixed grain poultry ration apparently contains enough of this factor for normal reproduction. Most of the reports have shown that the addition of wheat germ oil to a mixed grain ration does not improve either fertility or hatching power. However, a few experimenters[48] have shown increasing hatchability by feeding wheat germ oil.

The necessity of this vitamin for poultry has been shown by experiments at the Illinois Station.[49] In this work the ration was treated with ferric chloride to destroy the vitamin E. It should be pointed out that, from a practical point, there is little cause for concern because all whole grains and many green feeds are good sources of this vitamin.

It has also been shown[50] that the normal diet which produced eggs of moderately high hatchability was found to be potent in vitamin E when tested with female rats. The diets which produced eggs of low hatchability, particularly marked by a high first week embryonic mortality, were found to be low or lacking in vitamin E.

Vitamin K. The Wisconsin Station[51] reports that a minimum requirement for laying hens is 1 per cent of dried cereal grass or 2 per cent of alfalfa meal in order to furnish enough vitamin

K to assure that the chicks produced will have normal blood clotting.

Thiamine. In a study of the influence of the antineuritic vitamin upon the internal organs of Single Comb White Leghorn cockerels, Souba[52] reports distinct failure of the testes to grow, with ultimate atrophy of the organs, on a ration deficient in Vitamin B_1. However, poultry rations prepared from the common grains possess an adequate supply of this vitamin.

Riboflavin is also necessary for the maintenance of health and good hatchability. The benefits of milk, already noted under the discussion of proteins, probably is due in large part to the presence of this vitamin. Also the benefits of green food and alfalfa feeding may be attributed in large part to this vitamin.[45, 53, 54]

The Ohio Experiment Station[55] shows that the inclusion in the ration of riboflavin carriers, such as alfalfa meal, dried skimmilk, dried whey, autoclaved yeast, dried liver, or wheat germ, caused an increase in the hatchability of eggs. The differences in hatching will depend upon the amount of riboflavin present. This difference may be very striking as, for example, 8.0 per cent hatchability from a ration containing none, as compared with 84.8 per cent from a ration containing 3 per cent of liver meal.

Experiments at Cornell,[56] California,[57] Wisconsin,[58] and Canada[59] show that riboflavin is required by hens in order that they may produce eggs which will hatch. The developing chick embryo dies when an insufficient amount of the vitamin is deposited in the egg. The dead embryos are smaller than normal, show curled toes, incomplete absorption of yolk, retarded growth of down, shortened legs, and a slightly edemic condition of the neck. Myelin sheath degeneration occurs in the peripheral nerves. A smaller amount of riboflavin is required for egg production than for hatchability. The riboflavin content of eggs is determined by the amount of riboflavin present in the hen's diet. Eggs of highest riboflavin content can be obtained only by feeding hens a diet rich in this vitamin. The degree of yellow coloration of the egg white is evidence of the richness of the hen's diet in riboflavin. Hens require about 230 micrograms of riboflavin per 100 grams of feed in order to produce eggs that will hatch well.

Hens may lay well on rations inadequate in riboflavin, but riboflavin supplements are needed for increased hatchability. The riboflavin requirement for good hatchability can be met by including such feeds as milk products, yeast, liver meal, alfalfa meal, and by-products of the fermentation and distillation industries.

It has also been reported that higher[60] levels of riboflavin are required for hens in batteries, owing probably to the fact that they are deprived from droppings which contain riboflavin as a result of bacterial action.

Pantothenic Acid. Experiments conducted at Cornell[61] show that pantothenic acid is necessary for hatchability. Eggs produced on a diet low in this vitamin are also low in this factor. Taylor, Thacker, and Pennington[62] reported a definite tendency for increased pantothenic acid in the egg to be associated with an increased hemoglobin concentration of the blood in the 12-day chick embryo. They also indicated that a comparatively low concentration tended to be associated with a larger than normal brain, whereas both heart and brain were depressed in relative size with higher levels of pantothenic acid. The requirement for hatchability as reported by Cornell is 750 to 1000 micrograms per 100 grams of feed.

Choline has been shown to be necessary for egg production. It has also been demonstrated to be an essential factor[63] in connection with manganese to prevent perosis. It is, therefore, highly probable that it is also necessary for hatchability. The requirements are not known, and it is undoubtedly furnished in sufficient amounts in a good ration.

Biotin has been shown by the Wisconsin workers[64] to be essential for normal embryonic development in the hen's egg. The quantitative requirements have been placed between 60 and 150 micrograms per kilogram of feed. Sufficient amounts of this vitamin are apparently supplied in a good ration.

Folic Acid.[65] The fólic acid requirement for the breeder has been determined as being 0.5 to 1.0 milligrams per kilogram of diet.

Pyridoxin.[66] The Wisconsin Station reports the pyridoxin requirements of laying and breeding hens as being 2 milligrams per kilogram of feed.

Vitamin B_{12}. Vitamin B_{12} is necessary for good hatchability.[67] The quantity reported as being required has varied considerably, but this may be accounted for by differences in the rations. With average normal rations the probable requirement is 0.5 to 1.0 micrograms per pound of ration. More is needed for hens kept on wire than for hens on litter. Heavy breeds may require a higher amount.

Other Factors. Undoubtedly other vitamins or factors not

yet identified or understood affect hatchability. Some of these have already been suggested.[68] Considerable evidence also indicates that some factor present in animal protein feeds,[69] particularly fish products, and built-up litter[70] is necessary for best hatchability and growth of the resulting progeny.[71]

Experiments at the Iowa Station[72] show that when the ration was made up of single cereals, hatchability was best with eggs from wheat-fed birds, next best for those fed oats, with eggs from those fed corn and mixed grains being approximately equal. The hens fed the wheat or oats rations produced chicks with more vigor than chicks from hens fed corn.

Experiments in Canada[73] show that hatchability is decidedly greater in eggs from hens fed a combination of cereals rather than one alone; also that improved hatchability as a result of the feeding of milk or liver meal or a combination of these protein supplements or as a result of summer sunshine and/or grass range manifests itself in a reduction in anemia, chondrodystrophy, and teratological monsters.

Landauer[1] reports that it has been claimed by Koch (1935, 1936) and Westermayer (1936) that the feeding of follicular hormone to laying hens materially increases the hatching quality of eggs. Extensive tests by Prüfer (1936), however, failed to substantiate any effect of follicular hormone on hatchability.

DIETARY STANDARD FOR BREEDERS

Considerable variation will be found in the recommendations from various sources concerning the requirements for the breeding ration. As a summary of all evidence to date, the probable dietary requirements or standards for breeders are indicated by the Committee on Animal Nutrition of the National Research Council[74] as given in the accompanying tabulation. The figures do not include margins of safety to compensate for possible losses of vitamins during feed processing, transportation, and storage and for variations in feed composition and in environment. In earlier reports the National Research Council suggested allowances which included margins of safety of 66 per cent for vitamin A, 50 per cent for vitamin D, and 20 per cent for the water-soluble vitamins.

To meet the requirements of a breeder ration the accompanying formula pattern on page 423 is suggested for a breeding mash to be fed with grain.

REQUIREMENTS* OF BREEDING HENS

Total protein, %	15
Vitamins	
Vitamin A activity (U.S.P. units)†	2000
Vitamin D (I.C.U.)‡	225
Riboflavin, mg.	1.7
Pantothenic acid, mg.	4.2
Pyridoxine, mg.	1.3
Folacin, mg.	0.16
Minerals	
Calcium, %	2.25§
Phosphorus, % ‖	0.6
Salt, %¶	0.5
Manganese, mg.	15
Iodine, mg.	0.5
Amino acids, %	
Lysine	0.5
Methionine**	0.53
or	
Methionine	0.28
Cystine	0.25
Tryptophan	0.15

*In percentage or amount per pound of feed.

†May be fish oil vitamin A or pro-vitamin A from vegetable sources.

‡International chick unit.

§This amount of calcium need not be incorporated in the mixed feed inasmuch as calcium supplements fed free choice are considered as part of the ration.

‖A portion of the phosphorus requirement must be supplied in inorganic form. All the phosphorus of nonvegetable feed ingredients is considered to be inorganic. Approximately 30 per cent of the phosphorus of vegetable products is nonphytin phosphorus and may be considered as part of the inorganic phosphorus required.

¶This figure represents added salt or sodium chloride added as such or in marine or fermentation products of high sodium chloride content.

**Cystine will replace methionine as long as the ration contains not less than 0.28 per cent methionine.

TENTATIVE REQUIREMENT

Vitamin B_{12}	0.002 mg. per lb.

RECOMMENDED FORMULA PATTERN FOR BREEDING MASH

	Lb./ton
High-energy grain products (corn, wheat, wheat red dog flour, milo, oatmeal)	500 +
Medium- and low-energy grain products (oats, barley, wheat flour middlings, standard middlings, bran)	0-800
Vegetable proteins (soybean meal, corn gluten meal, peanut meal)	300-400
Animal proteins; minimum levels (fish meal, fish solubles, meat scraps)	100-150
Other B-vitamin carriers (dried milk products, dried yeast, dried distillers' solubles, fermentation solubles)	150
Dehydrated alfalfa meal	100-150
Additional riboflavin* (if needed)	+
Additional vitamin B_{12}* (if needed)	+
Additional vitamin A* (if needed)	+
Vitamin D_3 (feeding oils or D-activated animal sterols)	+
Calcium and phosphorus supplements (steamed bonemeal, dicalcium phosphate, defluorinated phosphate, limestone)	100
Salt	20
Manganese sulfate (65% feeding grade)	0.5

* Refers to the use of riboflavin supplements, vitamin B_{12} supplements, and vitamin A sources of guaranteed vitamin content or other vitamin-rich feedstuffs when the formula is otherwise deficient in any of these nutrients.

REQUIRED COMPOSITION

Protein, %	20
Calcium, %	2-2.5*
Phosphorus	
Total %	1.2
Available %†	0.8
Vitamin A, I.U./lb.‡	6600
Vitamin D, I.C.U./lb.	680
Riboflavin, mg./lb.	2.1
Vitamin B_{12}, μg./lb.§	3-4

* Free choice feeding of oystershell or other calcium supplement recommended since this level of calcium will not meet full requirements.

† Approximately 30 per cent of the phosphorus of vegetable products is non-phytin phosphorus and may be considered as part of the inorganic phosphorus required.

‡ If corn constitutes half of scratch grain mixture, the level of vitamin A in the mash can be reduced by 1000 I.U./lb.

§ Refers to vitamin B_{12} supplied by fish products, meat scrap, and vitamin B_{12} supplements.

VALUE OF FEEDS OF HIGH VITAMIN CONTENT

Numerous experiments have been reported indicating a favorable influence upon hatchability when the ration included such feeds of high vitamin content as cod liver oil, yeast, milk, and various forms of green foods (including grass range).[11, 14, 75-77] They were effective because they made up nutritive deficiencies and thus balanced the ration.

In northern sections and where birds need to be confined, there is likely to be a deficiency of sunshine during the winter and early spring. Therefore most trials indicated benefits in hatchability when cod liver oil, cod liver meal, or liver were used.[14, 76, 78-81] The differences were usually not maintained when the birds got outdoors. The increase also was greater when the fertility was low, indicating that the birds were not in the best physical condition.

Reports from Canada[79] showed an average increase of 10.3 per cent of chicks alive at 5 weeks of age where cod liver oil was fed to the hens. Holmes[81] reported increased viability of chicks from hens fed cod liver oil.

A very definite correlation has been found between the yolk color of the egg and the intensity of the pigment in the shanks of the chick.[82] In feeding trials showing the effect of pimiento pepper, the Georgia Station[83] reported a better hatch and stronger chicks from hens receiving pimiento.

NUTRITIONAL FACTORS AFFECTING FERTILITY

In general, fertility is not influenced very much by the different nutrients even though hatchability is affected. A restriction of calcium and a lack of vitamin E decreases fertility. When rations deficient especially in vitamin A were fed, the Oklahoma Station[84] reported that the males that were on the most deficient rations produced fewer sperms, on the average, than those on more desirable rations.

RELATION OF CONDITION AND HATCHABILITY

The physical condition of the hen produced by feeding and environment has an important effect on the hatching quality of the eggs and the vigor of the chicks. To obtain the best results, breeders must be managed so that they are kept in good physical condition, not only during but also before the hatching season.

When a bird becomes sick, hatching results will become poor

and remain poor until the bird gets back into condition, as shown by the hatching records of a flock of hens at Cornell University[85] in which there was an outbreak of roup. The birds that were not affected showed constant good production and steady hatchability during March, April, and May. The hens that were sick in February showed unsatisfactory hatching until the latter part of March and continued good hatching during April and May. For the individuals that were sick in March, the hatchability early in March, before the sickness, was over 70 per cent, which rapidly fell to 50 per cent and less during and after the sickness. After the sickness, hatchability showed some improvement.

Weight can be used as an indication of health. Loss of weight in females affects hatching adversely. The effect is most noticeable at the time when the birds reach their lowest level in weight, or just after it, and when incubation conditions are unfavorable. In a study of individual hens, it was generally found that hens gaining in weight or maintaining their weight gave the best hatching results while those losing in weight had the poorest hatchability.

Shank color is another indication of condition, particularly when applied to hens just previous to and during the hatching season. Those with yellow color in the shanks might show better hatches than those with faded shanks because the presence of pigment indicates a better surplus of fat and possibly vitamins. The ability to recover pigment quickly and to retain it under heavy production is probably an indication of metabolic efficiency, resulting in a better-nourished individual.

Production, both as regards intensity at the time the eggs are saved and immediately previous to the incubation season, may have a relation to hatching results. Many references may be found in the literature. Some indicate an adverse effect; others show that there is no relation between intensity or numbers of eggs laid and hatching.[86] Where hatching results are influenced by production, it may be due to the fact that very intensive production and long periods of production previous to the hatching season make it more difficult to maintain the weight and condition of the birds.

However, production is not necessarily detrimental if the condition of the hen is not affected adversely.

Shell color[87] in brown egg laying breeds has been reported as being related to hatchability. Hatchability is in favor of the darker colored eggs. It has also been shown that darker brown egg shells are stronger and thicker than lighter brown egg shells.

MANAGEMENT OF BREEDERS

Hens that are used for breeders must be given special consideration, beginning the previous fall, particularly where early season hatching is to follow. The best producers are those that continue to lay late in the fall. Fall production can be stimulated by wet mashes, milk, and lights in order to get the benefit of high egg prices.

REST FOR THE BREEDERS. However, after a season of heavy production the breeders need a period of rest or vacation while they grow their new set of feathers, regain any lost weight and vitality, restore the color to their shanks, beaks, and skin, and store up in their bodies such reserves as vitamins, minerals, and possibly other essentials.

It is also advisable not to encourage production too late in the fall so that the birds can get well along into their molt by the time severe cold weather sets in. For Central New York conditions, production should not continue beyond November. The exact date when the birds should be thrown out of production and into the molt will depend upon the date the first chicks are wanted, the condition of the birds, and to a less extent on the season.

Artificial control[88] of egg production by restricted feeding and restricted lighting during the summer months is possible and such control may be used as a means of increasing the number of fall chicks which may be hatched from hens.

When a hen has her new feathers well grown, she is ready to go to work again. Some birds will be ready sooner than others. Two months is a safe average. If the hens finish the laying year in prime physical condition, well fleshed, and heavy, the strain of molting will not be severe. They will get their feathers back quickly. Birds that have "laid themselves out" and are thin will need more time. They must build up their weight as well as grow new feathers. For such flocks a longer rest period may be needed.

WHEN TO STOP PRODUCTION. When should the birds of a flock in average physical condition be thrown out of production? That will depend upon the time the first chicks are wanted. Let us assume that the first chicks are to be hatched on March 1. First, allow the 2 months of rest, as indicated above, at the end of which time the lights will be turned on or the length of day increased in order to bring up the production. Allow one month before saving eggs (2 weeks to get the hens started and another 2 weeks for them to get up to 50 per cent production or better).

Good hatchability is not usually obtained until production has reached a more or less steady level. Then, saving the eggs for one week plus 3 weeks for incubation makes a total of 4 months from the time the rest period starts to the time the first chicks hatch. Hence, for March 1 chicks, the prospective hen breeders should not be kept in production later than November 1. As pointed out above, in a well-conditioned flock, this time might be somewhat shortened. For instance, they might lay up to November 15 and still give a good hatch for March 1.

HOW TO STOP PRODUCTION. There are several methods of stopping production. One is to omit artificial illumination. Another is to move the birds to different quarters. A third method is to change the feeding. Eliminate wet mashes or milk if they are being fed, or omit the dry mash for a short time and feed more grain. In some flocks it may be necessary to resort to all these practices.

When the birds stop laying and molt, the amount of grain should be increased. Heavy grain feeding should be practiced during the winter since this helps to build up the body weight. As soon as laying has stopped and the molt started, keep the grain in hoppers open all the time. It is not desirable to let the breeders become overfat. However, there is little danger of this unless the birds are several years old. In that case, it may be advisable to feed the grain in clean, dry litter to induce more exercise. Keep the dry mash always available in open hoppers.

MAINTAINING HEALTH AND VIGOR OF BREEDERS

WINTER CARE OF THE MALES. There is often a real problem of feeding involved where the males are kept with the hens during the winter. On range, the cockerels have had full access to the grain mixture. For a time, the same condition exists in the breeding pen. Then the grain might be restricted to induce the hens to eat more mash. The males do not take so readily to the mash and might not get enough grain to keep them in good condition because of the shortened grain-feeding period or because they are too gallant. The result is that they become thin and inactive, with consequent poor fertility.

There are several ways to avoid this difficulty. One is to fasten boxes of grain along the wall out of reach of the hens but where the males, with their greater height, can reach them. The boxes must be narrow so that the hens cannot get a footing on them. Another plan is to divide the males into two groups and alternate these groups in the pen and in a coop, out of sight of the rest of the flock, where they can catch up on their eating.

Frozen combs and wattles often indispose the birds so that they do not eat enough. One cause of freezing is the wetting of the wattles while drinking. Fountains with narrow drinking ledges will largely overcome this trouble.

Studies at Cornell have shown that cockerels attain their greatest body weight when exposed to 9 hours, or less, of light daily. This fact is useful for poultrymen who house their breeding males in pens of pullets, exposed to 13 or 14 hours of light daily during the winter, and find it difficult to keep them in good physical condition. Males will attain greater weight and better condition if they are not exposed to supplementary illumination until the breeding season, or about 3 weeks before they are to be placed in the breeding pens, when they should be exposed to 13 hours of light daily.

GENERAL SUMMARY

Any factor which affects the condition of the bird will affect the hatching results. Therefore a deficiency in any of the nutrients can be expected to influence results.[89] A lack of the vitamins, especially, has produced lower hatchability.

Assuming that the stock has been carefully selected for vigor and vitality and breeding performance, and that environmental conditions are correct, it will be more nearly possible to "count your chicks before they are hatched" by allowing the hens a proper rest, giving them access to sunshine, and providing a complete ration by feeding a variety of cereals, animal protein feeds, green food, and other vitamin concentrates.

RATIONS FOR BREEDERS

The requirements for some nutrients are greater for breeders than for layers. Still it is possible to formulate a variety of rations for this purpose. Some representative recommendations for breeder rations will be found in the Appendix. (See page 572.)

REFERENCES

1. Landauer, W. The hatchability of chicken eggs as influenced by environment and heredity. Conn. Bul. 216. 1937. Conn. Bul. 236. 1941.
2. Albrecht. Der Einfluss verschiedener Fütterung, Eiweiss in verschiedener Menge und von verschiedener Herkunft auf Brut und Nachzucht. Deutsche Geflügel-Zeitung 1930:981.
   Heiman, V., J. S. Carver, and J. L. St. John. The protein requirements of laying hens. Wash. Bul. 331. 1936.
3. Hendricks, W. A., Trends in egg production, egg weight, and hatchability on low-protein and normal diets. Poultry Sci. 13: 290. 1934.
4. Penquite, R., and R. B. Thompson. Growth of chick embryos from hens fed different protein levels. Poultry Sci. 15:18. 1936.
   Penquite, R., and T. T. Milby. Hatching weight of chicks from hens fed different protein levels. Poultry Sci. 17:434. 1938.
5. Roemer, R. Poultry feeding in Germany. Proc. Third World's Poultry Congress. 239. Canada. 1927.
6. Ivey, J. E. Vegetable protein studies. Ala. Rept. 1927:14.
7. Ahrens, B. A. A study of the effect of cottonseed meal vs. beef scrap upon egg production, fertility and vitality of poultry. Okla. Bul. 112. 1917.
   Berry, L. N. The relative value of cottonseed meal and tankage for egg production. N. Mex. Bul. 183. 1930.
   Cottonseed meal vs. meat scraps. S. C. Rept. 1929:82.
   Morgan, C. L. Comparison of cottonseed meal and meat scraps as sources of protein for poultry. S. C. Rept. 1930:90.
   Morgan, C. L. Poultry feeding experiments. S. C. Bul. 273. 1931.
   Ringrose, R. C., C. L. Morgan, and E. J. Lease. The effect of cottonseed oil on the hatchability of eggs. Poultry Sci. 20:57. 1941.
8. Heywang, B. W., H. R. Bird, and A. M. Altschul. The effect of pure gossypol on egg hatchability and weight. Poultry Sci. 29:916. 1950.
9. Byerly, T. C., H. W. Titus, N. R. Ellis, and R. B. Nestler. Effects of light, soybean, and other diet supplements on seasonal hatchability and egg production. Poultry Sci. 16:322. 1937.
   Christiansen, J. B., J. G. Halpin, and E. B. Hart. Studies on the nature of the effective supplements for soybean oil meal in rations for the production of hatching eggs. Poultry Sci. 19:55. 1940.
   Hayward, J. W., J. G. Halpin, C. E. Holmes, G. Bohstedt, and E. B. Hart. Soybean oil meal prepared at different temperatures as feed for poultry. Poultry Sci. 16:3. 1937.
   Wilgus, H. S., Jr., and F. X. Gassner. Effect of soybean oil meal on avian reproduction. Proc. Soc. Exp. Biol. and Med. 46:290. 1941.
10. Byerly, T. C., H. W. Titus, and N. R. Ellis. Production and hatchability of eggs as affected by different kinds and quantities of proteins in the diet of laying hens. Jour. Agr. Res. 46:1. 1933.

11. Parkhurst, R. T. The value of certain feeds of high vitamin content for laying hens. Proc. Third World's Poultry Congress. 221. Canada. 1927.
12. Elford, F. C. Poultry investigations at the Dominion experimental farms. Canada Experimental Farms. Poultry Div. Rept.:1923:10.
Comparative value of water, buttermilk, and both buttermilk and water as drink in breeding pens as shown by fertility and hatchability of eggs and mortality of chicks. Lethbridge (Alta.) Exp. Sta. Rept. 1923:36.
13. Philips, A. G. The value of skimmilk and meat scraps for White Plymouth Rocks. Ind. Bul. 218. 1918.
14. Heuser, G. F. Effect of certain rations on the efficiency of breeders. Jour. Am. Assoc. Instructors and Investigators Poultry Husb. 7:15. 1920.
Heuser, G. F. Nutritional factors affecting hatchability of eggs. Proc. Third World's Poultry Congress. 207. Canada. 1927.
15. Kaupp, B. F. Operation of a four unit farm poultry plant. N. C. Bul. 251. 1927.
16. Bethke, R. M., and D. C. Kennard. The limitations of vitamin D in the production of hatchable eggs. Rept. Fourth World's Poultry Congress. 342. London. 1930.
17. Shoup, Mr. and Mrs. G. R. Western Wash. Bul. (N.S.) 10-w:28. 1928.
18. Kaupp, B. F. Influence of meat meal and milk on production and health. N. C. Rept. 1927:92.
Philips, A. G. The value of meat scrap, fish scrap, and skim milk in rations for laying pullets. Ind. Bul. 182. 1915.
19. Morgan, C. L. Fish meal vs. meat scraps for laying hens. S. C. Rept. 1930:93.
20. Elford, F. C. The effects of feeding bone meal upon fertility, hatchability, and viability. Dominion Experimental Farms. Canada Poultry Div. Rept. 1925:19.
21. Graham, W. R., J. B. Smith, and W. D. McFarlane. Results of a three-years study of certain poultry rations as they affect the hatching power of hen eggs as well as the number of eggs laid. Ont. Bul. 362. 1931.
Graham, W. R. Nutrition and hatchability. Rept. Fourth World's Poultry Congress. 207. London. 1930.
Smith, J. B. The sunshine factor in hatchability. Proc. Fifth World's Poultry Congress. 453. Rome. 1933.
Smith, J. B., and H. D. Branion. Influence of some protein supplements on hatchability. Rept. Seventh World's Poultry Congress. 195. Cleveland. 1939.
22. Buckner, G. D., J. H. Martin, and A. M. Peter. The relation of calcium restriction to the hatchability of eggs. Am. Jour. Physiol. 71:543. 1925.
Buckner, G. D., J. H. Martin, and A. M. Peter. Calcium metabolism in the laying hen. III. Calcium carbonate and hatchability. Ky. Bul. 291. 1929.
23. Titus, H. W., T. C. Byerly, N. R. Ellis, and R. B. Nestler. Effect of the calcium and phosphorus content of the diet of chickens on

egg production and hatchability. Poultry Sci. 16:118. 1937.

24. O'Rourke, W. F., H. R. Bird, P. H. Phillips, and W. W. Cravens. The hatchability effect of low phosphorus rations. Poultry Sci. 32:919. 1953.

25. Lyons, M., and W. M. Insko, Jr. Chondrodystrophy in the chick embryo produced by a mineral deficiency in the diet of the hen. Science 80:328. 1937.

Lyons, M., and W. M. Insko, Jr. Chondrodystrophy in the chick embryo produced by a mineral deficiency in the diet of the hen. Poultry Sci. 16:365. 1937.

Lyons, M., and W. M. Insko, Jr. Chondrodystrophy in the chick embryo. Ky. Bul. 371. 1937.

26. Wilgus, H. S., L. C. Norris, and G. F. Heuser. The role of manganese in poultry nutrition. Rept. Seventh World's Poultry Congress. 171. Cleveland. 1939.

Gallup, W. D., and L. C. Norris. The effect of a deficiency of manganese in the diet of the hen. Poultry Sci. 17:83. 1939.

27. Scharrer, K., and W. Schropp. Fütterungsversuche mit Jod an Hühnern. Biedermanns Zentralblatt für Tierrernährung 4:249. 1932.

Zaitschek, A. Über die Wirkung der Beifütterung Kleiner Jodmengen auf den Eierertrag von Hühnern und auf das Schlüpfergebnis. Biedermanns Zentralblatt für Tierernährung 6:102. 1934.

28. Franke, K. W., and W. C. Tully. A new toxicant occurring naturally in certain samples of plant foodstuffs. V. Low hatchability due to deformities in chicks. Poultry Sci. 14:273. 1935.

Franke, K. W., and W. C. Tully. A new toxicant occurring naturally in certain samples of plant foodstuffs. VII. Low hatchability due to deformities in chicks produced from eggs obtained from chickens of known history. Poultry Sci. 15:316. 1936.

Franke, K. W., A. L. Moxon, W. E. Poley, and W. C. Tully. Monstrosities produced by the injection of selenium salts into hen's eggs. Anatomical Record 65:15. 1936.

Moxon, A. L. Alkali disease or selenium poisoning. S. Dak. Bul. 311. 1937.

Poley, W. E., A. L. Moxon, and K. W. Franke. Further studies of the effects of selenium poisoning on hatchability. Poultry Sci. 16: 219. 1937.

Poley, W. E., and A. L. Moxon. Tolerance levels of seleniferous grains in laying rations. Poultry Sci. 17:72. 1938.

29. Effect of feeding white and yellow corn and supplementary feeds on egg production and hatchability. Kans. Rept. 1924-1926:107.

The effect of an inadequate ration on the production and hatchability of eggs. Kans. Rept. 1926-1928:103.

Payne, L. F., and J. S. Hughes. The effect of inadequate rations on the production and hatchability of eggs. Kans. Tech. Bul. 34. 1933.

30. Penquite, R., R. B. Thompson, and H. R. Naylor. The value of certain scratch grains in the poultry ration. Okla. Bul. 166. 1926.

31. Sherwood, R. M. Vitamin A requirements of poultry. Rept. Seventh World's Poultry Congress. 123. Cleveland. 1939.

32. Bearse, G. E., and M. W. Miller. The effect of varying levels of vitamin A in the hen ration on the vitamin A content of the egg yolk, hatchability and on chick livability. Poultry Sci. 16:39. 1937.
33. Hart, E. B., H. Steenbock, S. Lepkovsky, S. W. F. Kletzien, J. G. Halpin, and O. N. Johnson. The nutritional requirement of the chicken. V. The influence of ultraviolet light on the production, hatchability, and fertility of the egg. Jour. Biol. Chem. 65:579. 1925.
34. Hughes, J. S., L. F. Payne, and W. L. Latshaw. The influence of ultraviolet light on leg weakness in growing chicks and on egg production. Poultry Sci. 4:151. 1925.
35. The effect of cod liver oil and ultraviolet light on egg production and hatchability. Ohio Bul. 402:91. 1927.
36. Fiftieth Ann. Rept. N. J. Agr. Exp. Sta. 1929:9.
37. Martin, J. H., and W. M. Insko, Jr. The effect of vitamin D supplement on hatchability. Proc. Twenty-first Annual Meeting Poultry Sci. Assn. Ala. Bul. XXV. No. 1:38. 1930.
38. Hughes, J. S., L. F. Payne, and W. R. Hinshaw. Importance of ultraviolet light in the poultry industry. Proc. Third World's Poultry Congress. 214. Canada. 1927.
Payne, L. F., and J. S. Hughes. The effect of inadequate rations on production and hatchability. Kans. Tech. Bul. 34. 1933.
Charles, T. B., and B. W. Heywang. The relative effects of ultraviolet light and cod liver oil upon the eggs from foods used for breeding purposes. Pa. Bul. 213:29. 1927.
39. Halpin, J. G., C. E. Holmes, and E. B. Hart. Comparative value of different sources of vitamin D. Wis. Bul. 420. 1931:85.
40. Vitamin D studies with chickens. Ky. Rept. 1930:17.
Edson, A. W. Cod liver oil in the winter ration of pullets. Minn. Bul. 286. 1932.
41. Carver, J. S., E. I. Robertson, D. Brazie, R. H. Johnson, and J. L. St. John. The vitamin D requirement of chickens. Wash. Bul. 299. 1934.
42. Murphy, R. R., J. E. Hunter, and H. C. Knandel. The vitamin D requirement of growing chicks and laying hens. Pa. Bul. 303. 1934. Pa. Bul. 334. 1936.
43. Branion, H. D., and J. B. Smith. The influence of vitamin D on hatchability and egg production. Poultry Sci. 11:261. 1932.
44. Hughes, J. S., L. F. Payne, R. W. Titus, and J. M. Moore. Relation between the amount of ultraviolet light received by hens and the amount of antirachitic vitamin in the eggs produced. Jour. Biol. Chem. 66:595. 1925.
45. Martin, J. H., S. E. Erikson, and W. M. Insko, Jr. Effect of vitamin D supplements on laying hens. Ky. Bul. 304. 1930.
Martin, J. H., S. E. Erikson, W. M. Insko, Jr., and R. Boyden. The growth of chicks as influenced by vitamin D supplements given the mother hen. Proc. Twenty-second Annual Meeting Poultry Sci. Assn. 1930:33.
46. Titus, H. W. Nutritional factors in relation to hatchability. Rept. Seventh World's Poultry Congress. 198. Cleveland. 1939.

47. Christianson, J. G., J. G. Halpin, and E. B. Hart. Manganese and sunlight may promote hatchability of winter eggs. Wis. Bul. 446: 35. 1939.
48. Ender, F. Über die Bedeutung des E-Vitamins für die Hühnerzucht. Zeit. für Vitaminforschung 4:106. 1935.
Barbas, W. C. Over den invloed van het vruchtsbaarheids vitamine op eierleggende Kippen. Landbouwkundig Tijdschrift 48:669. 1936.
49. Card, L. E. Vitamin E requirements of poultry. Poultry Sci. 8:328. 1929.
Morris, H. P., and H. H. Mitchell. Chickens show need of vitamin E for reproduction. Ill. Rept. 1927-1928:168.
Card, L. E., H. H. Mitchell, and T. S. Hamilton. Further studies on the vitamin E requirements of poultry. II. The performance of pullets raised on a vitamin E free diet. Proc. Twenty-second Annual Meeting Poultry Sci. Assn. 1930:29.
Card, L. E., H. H. Mitchell, and T. S. Hamilton. Chickens need vitamin E to produce normal hatches. Ill. Rept. 1930:101.
Card, L. E., H. H. Mitchell, and T. S. Hamilton. Plenty of needed vitamin E in ordinary poultry feeds. Ill. Rept. 1930-1931:115.
50. Barnum, G. L. The vitamin E content of eggs as related to the diet of the hen and to hatchability. Jour. Nutr. 9:621. 1935.
51. Cravens, W. W., J. G. Halpin, S. B. Randle, and C. A. Elvehjem. Hens need vitamin K. Wis. Bul. 451:34. 1941.
52. Souba, A. J. Influence of the antineuritic vitamin upon the internal organs of S. C. W. L. cockerels. Am. Jour. Physiol. 64:181. 1923.
53. Stuart, H. O. Effect of certain green feed substitutes upon egg production and hatchability. Poultry Sci. 8:354. 1929.
54. Dutcher, R. A., and S. D. Wilkins. Vitamin Studies VII. The influence of fresh alfalfa upon the weight of testes in S. C. W. L. cockerels. Am. Jour. Physiol. 57:437. 1921.
55. Bethke, R. M., and D. C. Kennard. Nutritional factors affecting hatchability of eggs. Ohio Bul. 417:65. 1928.
Bethke, R. M., and D. C. Kennard. Nutritional factors affecting hatchability of eggs. Ohio Bul. 431:118. 1929.
Bethke, R. M., D. C. Kennard, and C. H. Kick. Nutritional factors affecting hatchability of eggs. Ohio Bul. 446:148. 1930.
Bethke, R. M., P. R. Record, and D. C. Kennard. Nutritional factors affecting hatchability of eggs. Ohio Bul. 470:186. 1931.
Bethke, R. M., P. R. Record, and D. C. Kennard. The relation of vitamin G to the hatchability of hen's eggs. Jour. Nutr. 12:297. 1936.
Hunt, C. H., A. R. Winter, and R. M. Bethke. Further studies on the riboflavin requirements of the chicken. Poultry Sci. 18:330. 1939.
56. Norris, L. C., H. S. Wilgus, Jr., A. T. Ringrose, V. Heiman, and G. F. Heuser. The vitamin G requirement of poultry. Cornell Bul. 660. 1936.
Norris, L. C., G. F. Heuser, A. T. Ringrose, H. S. Wilgus, Jr., and V. Heiman. The vitamin G requirement of poultry. Proc. Fifth World's Poultry Congress 2:512. Rome. 1934.

Davis, H. J., L. C. Norris, and G. F. Heuser. The role of vitamin G in reproduction. Poultry Sci. 17:81. 1938.

Schumacher, A. E., and G. F. Heuser. The importance of riboflavin in reproduction in poultry. Poultry Sci. 18:369. 1939.

Romanoff, A. L., and J. C. Bauernfeind. Influence of riboflavin deficiency in eggs on embryonic development (Gallus domesticus). Anatomical Record 82:11. 1942.

57. Lepkovsky, S., L. W. Taylor, T. H. Jukes. and H. J. Almquist. The effect of riboflavin and the filtrate factor on egg production and hatchability. Hilgardia 11:559. 1938.

58. Engel R. W., P. H. Phillips, and J. G. Halpin. The effect of riboflavin deficiency in the hen upon embryonic development of the chick. Poultry Sci. 19:135. 1940.

Halpin, J. G., C. E. Holmes, and E. B. Hart. Vitamin G inadequate in many rations for laying hens. Wis. Bul. 425:18. 1933.

Halpin, J. G., C. E. Holmes, and E. B. Hart. Vitamin G supplements increase egg hatchability. Wis. Bul. 428:48. 1934.

Halpin, J. G., C. E. Holmes, and W. W. Cravens. Is hatchability satisfactory on milkless egg mash? Wis. Bul. 451:33. 1941.

59. Clandinin, D. R. The significance of the level of riboflavin in the ration of breeding birds. Poultry Sci. 25:223. 1946.

60. Petersen, C. F., C. E. Lampman, and O. E. Stamberg. High levels of riboflavin required for hens in batteries. Idaho Agr. Exp. Sta. 54th Ann. Rept. 10. 1947.

61. Bauernfeind, J. C., and L. C. Norris. The antidermatosis vitamin required for reproduction in the domestic fowl. Science 89:416. 1939.

Bauernfeind, J. C., and L. C. Norris. The role of the antidermatosis vitamin and a new water-soluble growth factor in the nutrition of the mature fowl. Jour. Nutr. 18:579. 1939.

Gillis, M. B., G. F. Heuser, and L. C. Norris. The need for pantothenic acid and an unidentified factor in reproduction in the domestic fowl. Jour. Nutr. 23:153. 1942.

Gillis, M. B., G. F. Heuser, and L. C. Norris. Pantothenic acid in the nutrition of the hen. J. Nutr. 35:351. 1948.

Heuser, G. F., M. B. Gillis, and L. C. Norris. The pantothenic acid requirement of poultry. Rept. 8th World's Poultry Congress. 1948:114. Copenhagen.

62. Taylor, A., J. Thacker, and D. Pennington. The effect of increased pantothenic acid in the egg on the development of the chick embryo. Science 94:542. 1941.

63. Jukes, T. H. Prevention of perosis by choline. Jour. Biol. Chem. 134:789. 1940.

Hogan, A. L., L. R. Richardson, H. Patrick, and H. L. Kempster. Perosis due to a vitamin deficiency. Jour. Nutr. 21:237. 1941.

64. Cravens, W. W., E. E. Sebesta, J. G. Halpin, and E. B. Hart. Effect of biotin on reproduction in the domestic fowl. Proc. Soc. Biol. and Med. 50:101. 1942.

Cravens, W. W., W. McGibbon, and E. Sebesta. Lack of biotin can cause hatching difficulties. Wis. Bul. 463:37. 1944.

Cravens, W. W., W. H. McGibbon, and E. E. Sebesta. Effect of biotin

deficiency on embryonic development in the domestic fowl. Anat. Rec. 90:55. 1944.
65. Couch, J. R., and H. L. German. Pteroylglutamic acid studies with the mature fowl. Poultry Sci. 29:539. 1950.
Cravens, W. W., and J. G. Halpin. The effect of pteroylglutamic acid and an unidentified factor on egg production and hatchability. Jour. Nutr. 37:127. 1949.
Sunde, M. L., W. W. Cravens, H. W. Bruins, C. A. Elvehjem, and J. G. Halpin. The pteroylglutamic acid requirement of laying and breeding hens. Poultry Sci. 29:220. 1950.
66. Cravens, W. W., E. E. Sebesta, J. G. Halpin, and E. B. Hart. Studies on the pyridoxin requirements of laying and breeding hens. Poultry Sci. 25:80. 1946.
67. Johnson, E. L. Vitamin B_{12} requirements of hens as affected by choline and antibiotic additions to the diet. Poultry Sci. 30:919. 1951.
Milligan, J. L., and G. F. Combs. Vitamin B_{12} requirements for hatchability, viability, and growth. Poultry Sci. 29:772. 1950.
Norris, L. C., R. F. Miller, and H. Yacowitz. Studies on the vitamin B_{12} requirements of poultry. Proc. 1950 Cornell Nutr. Conf. 53. 1950.
Petersen, C. F., A. C. Wiese, G. E. Milne, and C. E. Lampman. Vitamin B_{12} requirements for hatchability and production of high quality chicks. Poultry Sci. 32:535. 1953.
Yacowitz, H., R. F. Miller, L. C. Norris, and G. F. Heuser. Vitamin B_{12} studies with the hen. Poultry Sci. 31:89. 1952.
68. Byerly, T. C., H. W. Titus, and N. R. Ellis. Effect of diet on egg composition. II. Mortality of embryos in eggs on diets containing protein supplements of different origin. Jour. Nutr. 6:225. 1933.
Nestler, R. B., T. C. Byerly, N. R. Ellis, and H. W. Titus. A new factor, not vitamin G, necessary for hatchability. Poultry Sci. 15:67. 1936.
Bauernfeind, J. C., A. E. Schumacher, A. Z. Hodson, L. C. Norris, and G. F. Heuser. A new factor required for growth in the domestic fowl. Proc. Soc. Exp. Biol. and Med. 39:108. 1938.
Bauernfeind, J. C., A. E. Schumacher, A. Z. Hodson, L. C. Norris, and G. F. Heuser. Additional evidence of a new factor required for growth and reproduction in poultry. Poultry Sci. 17:444. 1938.
Schumacher, A. E., and G. F. Heuser. Some properties of the new growth and reproduction factor with further results of its effect on chicks and hens. Poultry Sci. 18:411. 1939.
Cravens, W. W., C. E. Holmes, J. G. Halpin, and C. A. Elvehjem. The effect of alfalfa leaf meal and dried cereal grass on egg production and hatchability. Poultry Sci. 21:301. 1942.
69. Cravens, W. W., J. G. Halpin, and W. H. McGibbon. The use of various vitamin supplements in rations for laying and breeding hens. Poultry Sci. 25:99. 1946.
Cravens, W. W., W. H. McGibbon, and J. G. Halpin. Riboflavin improves some poultry breeding rations. Wisc. Bul. 469:51. 1946.
Pensack, J. M. A nutritional factor affecting hatchability. Ohio Sta. Weekly Press Bul. 32:6. 1947.

70. Kennard, D. C., R. M. Bethke, and V. D. Chamberlin. Built-up floor litter may improve the hatch. Ohio Farm and Home Res. 33:17. 1948.
71. Bethke, R. M., J. M. Pensack, and D. C. Kennard. The influence of hen's diet on growth of progeny. Poultry Sci. 26:128. 1946.
72. Call, V. D., and H. L. Wilcke. Effect of single cereal grains upon the hatchability of eggs and subsequent growth of chicks. Poultry Sci. 18:308. 1939.
73. Smith, J. B. The cereal grains and their use in poultry nutrition. I. Hatchability Studies. Sci. Agr. 16:73. 1935.
Smith, J. B., and H. D. Branion. Hatchability studies with certain feeds. Rept. Sixth World's Poultry Congress. 77. Germany. 1936.
74. Recommended nutrient allowances for domestic animals. Number 1. Recommended nutrient allowances for poultry. National Research Council. Rept. Com. on Animal Nutr. Washington. June 1944. Revised March, 1950.
Nutrient requirements for domestic animals. Number 1. Nutrient requirements of poultry. Rept. Comm. Animal Nutrition, National Research Council, Washington, D. C., 1954. Pub. 301.
75. Atwood, H. Effect of confinement and green feed on number and hatchability of eggs. W. Va. Bul. 178. 1922.
Bearse, G. E. A comparison of molasses, whey, condensed buttermilk, and condensed buttermilk containing cereal grasses as supplements to a breeding hen ration. Poultry Sci. 17:433. 1938.
76. Kennard, D. C. Hatchability and egg production as affected by the ration. Ohio Bimo. Bul. X(7):118. 1925.
Kennard, D. C., and L. B. Nettleton. Legume hays instead of green feed for chickens. Ohio Bimo. Bul. XI(4):135. 1926.
Kennard, D. C., and R. M. Bethke. Solving the green feed problem. Ohio Bimo. Bul. XII(4):120. 1927.
Hatchability of eggs as affected by feeding and management. Ohio Bul. 402:95. 1927.
Bethke, R. M., and D. C. Kennard. Producing hatchable eggs. Ohio Bimo. Bul. XIII(6):210. 1928.
77. Lewis, H. R. The influence of yeast upon fertility and hatchability of hen's eggs. Poultry Bul., issued by the Fleischmann Co., New= York. 1925.
Shoup, Mr. and Mrs. G. R. Ann. Rept. Western Washington Exp. Sta. Western Wash. Bul. N.S. 10-W:36. 1928.
Smith, R. M. The influence of certain supplements on the production, hatchability, fertility, and weight of eggs. Ark. Bul. 293. 1933.
Hart, C. P., and H. O. Stuart. The effect of certain feed supplements on the hatchability, economy, and efficiency of poultry feeding. I. Condensed buttermilk; and a mixture of cereal grasses and condensed milk. R. I. Bul. 289. 1943.
78. Taylor, E. M. Feeding breeding hens for fertility and hatchability. Canadian Poultry Review. March 1930.
79. Hopper, R. M. Cod liver oil for poultry. Its value for laying and breeding stock. Canada Exp. Farms Pamphlet 131. N.S. 1931.

80. Cod liver oil. Minn. Northwest Exp. Sta., Crookston, Rept. 1927: 55.

Holmes, A. D. Studies of the vitamin potency of cod liver oils XIX. Influence of cod liver oil on reproduction. Poultry Sci. 5:110. 1926.

Stuart, H. O., and T. B. Charles. Agricultural experiments 1929. N. H. Bul. 250:14. 1930.

81. Holmes, A. D., A. W. Doolittle, and W. B. Moore. Studies of the vitamin potency of cod liver oils. XXI. The stimulation of reproduction by fat-soluble vitamins. Am. Pharm. Assn. Jour. 16:618. 1927.

82. Work and progress of the Agricultural Experimental Station. Idaho Bul. 170:24. 1930.

83. Brown, W. L. Some effects of pimiento pepper on poultry. Ga. Bul. 160. 1930.

84. Craft, W. A., C. H. McElroy, and R. Penquite. The influence of certain feeds upon the production of spermatozoa by the domestic chicken. Poultry Sci. 5:187. 1926.

85. Van Rooyen, L. A. Some of the factors affecting the hatchability of eggs. Thesis. Cornell University. 1923.

86. Jull, M. A. Studies in hatchability. VI. Hatchability in relation to current egg production. Poultry Sci. 10:327. 1931.

Warren, D. C. The influence of some factors on the hatchability of the hen's egg. Kans. Tech. Bul. 37. 1934.

Atwood, H. A balanced and an unbalanced ration fed prior to the hatching season as affecting the hatchability of eggs and the vigor of the progeny. W. Va. Tech. Bul. 207. 1927.

87. Funk, E. M., and J. F. Forward. The relationship of egg shell color to hatchability in New Hampshires. Poultry Sci. 28:577. 1949.

Godfrey, G. F. Shell color as a measure of egg shell quality. Poultry Sci. 28:150. 1949.

Godfrey, G. F. The relationship of egg shell color to hatchability in some brown egg laying breeds. Poultry Sci. 26:381. 1947.

88. Hall, G. O. The artificial control of egg production. Poultry Sci. 25:3. 1946.

89. Payne, L. F., and J. S. Hughes. The effect of inadequate rations on the production and hatchability of eggs. Kans. Tech. Bul. 34. 1933.

CHAPTER 15

FATTENING OR FINISHING OF POULTRY

Fattening or finishing poultry for the table is one of the oldest practices of poultry husbandry. Brown[1] says:

> For a long period of time, among the dainties or finer dishes for the table, fowls of various kinds have been recognized as holding a leading place. Even as far back as the days of Solomon we find in Scripture references to "fatted fowls," though whether these words apply to ordinary poultry is a point which has led to some discussion. We may, however, leave this controversial subject on one side, for there can be no question that 4000 years ago the ancient Egyptians crammed their geese, and probably were the originators of the cramming system. A drawing, copied from one of the tablets in the Pyramid of Sakkara, represents a man engaged in the work of cramming geese by means of pators, or boluses, of food.

Wright's Book of Poultry[2] indicates that Pliny mentioned the inhabitants of Delos as the first to prepare fowls artificially for the table, by which no doubt cramming is intended, and in his time there is no doubt that the luxury-loving Romans patronized crammed poultry extensively.

Dickson[3] in his book on the general management of poultry gives information concerning early fattening practices.

Poultry has been fattened in Europe for centuries. Furthermore, the industry has been more or less localized in certain sections in the different countries. In England the counties of Surrey and Sussex have long been famous for their fatted chickens. In France the industry has been centered around La Bresse, and in Belgium around Malines.

OBJECTS OR ADVANTAGES IN FATTENING

Fattening should be looked upon as a finishing process. The carcass is improved or fitted for slaughter. In the process, an excess of nourishment is transformed into fat. The improvement is both external and internal. In the first place, the size of the bird is increased. The actual gain in weight will depend upon various factors which will be discussed later. Externally, the appearance of the bird is improved by making it more plump. The color of the flesh can also be influenced, making it paler or yellower according to the market preference.

Not only is the size increased, but usually the proportion of edible parts is enlarged. Harshaw[4] states that fattening resulted in about a 6 per cent increase in the total edible portion and that 73 per cent of the gain in weight during fattening was represented in the edible portion of the bird. The percentage of breast muscle and leg muscle decreased with fattening while the percentage of the remaining edible portion increased. The increase in fat plus water, during fattening, was from about 85 to 92 per cent of the gain in the total edible portion. In the younger birds, the increase was greater in water than in fat, but in the oldest birds the reverse was true. The increase in protein was relatively small, and its ratio to the total edible gain tended to decrease with the age of the birds.

Poley and associates[5] noted a tendency toward an inverse relationship between the fat and moisture content of edible meat. In comparing battery and range methods of finishing, an increase was found in the percentage of fat in both fryers and roasters finished in the battery. The corn- and wheat-fed fryers and roasters had significantly more total edible meat on the carcasses than the birds receiving barley. The wheat- and barley-fed fryers and roasters had a somewhat higher percentage of light meat than those receiving corn. The corn-fed fryers and roasters showed a consistent tendency to deposit more fat in the light meat, dark meat, skin and subcutaneous fat, and the abdominal fatty tissue than the other two groups. They were followed in order by the wheat- and barley-fed groups, with significantly more fat in the carcasses of the corn-fed than in those of the barley-fed group.

Fraps[6] reported that the substitution of cottonseed oil for part of the corn meal in a standard ration produced chicks with a much higher fat content. Substitution of feeds with a lower productive energy for the corn meal also produced chickens with a lower fat content. He suggests that there is probably an optimum fat content of the ration to produce chickens of good quality.

One of the important results is the internal effect or improvement in the quality of the flesh. Tiny globules of fat are distributed through the muscles. More intercellular material is formed, which softens the tissues and produces a ''marbling'' effect. This results in greater tenderness, more juiciness, and better flavor.

The increase in weight, as well as the external and internal improvement, should secure an increase in price per pound as compared with the unfinished chicken.

METHODS OF FATTENING

Various methods of fattening birds are practiced, varying from the highly intensive to the less intensive as follows: (1) stuffing or cramming; (2) crate fattening; (3) pen fattening.

STUFFING OR CRAMMING. In this method the birds are force-fed. It is practiced largely in European countries. The birds are closely confined in small and usually darkened coops. They are fed forcibly once or twice a day, which may be done in a number of ways.

1. Cramming by Hand. The food is made into a stiff paste and formed into pellets 3/4 to 1 inch long and 3/8 to 1/2 inch thick. These pellets are dipped into whey or milk, inserted into the mouth, and forced into the crop. In France, masses of food instead of pellets are sometimes used. Obviously, this method involves considerable labor. It is the method usually employed in "noodling" geese.

2. Cramming by Funnel. This method was used largely in Normandy. The food is in liquid form. A specially made funnel is inserted into the gullet and into the crop. The cream-like ration is spooned into the funnel until the crop is full.

3. Cramming by Machine. The cramming machine consists essentially of a hopper or reservoir for the feed and a force pump, controlled usually by a foot pedal. A long tube, extending from the pump, is inserted into the crop and the food forced into the crop until it is full.

Cramming puts the final finish on the birds. In Sussex (England), the birds are placed in cages out of doors and fed for a week or 10 days from troughs. Then they are placed in sheds and crammed for another period of time, usually about 10 days.

Schmidt[7] reports that cramming showed better utilization of feed than free fattening.

CRATE FATTENING. This method is used largely in the United States and Canada. Gutteridge and coworkers[8] reported the crate feeding of capons as being definitely superior to pen feeding. They also reported that crate fattening was greatly superior to ordinary range rearing methods for the production of gain, increase in fat, and grading of the dressed bird. They concluded that crate feeding was the most efficient method and was productive of very high quality stock; that caponizing for market was the next most efficient method and was very economical because of lower feed requirement during the rearing period and because of the high degree of fat even when killed off range; and that the killing of cockerels for market directly off range was the least economical procedure.

The birds are placed in small crates or coops. The crates are usually constructed of wire or slats and have wire bottoms. The feed troughs should be suspended outside.

PEN FATTENING. In pen fattening, the birds are confined to a small coop with or without yards. The birds are allowed more floor space than in crate fattening, usually about 2 square feet for old birds. For best results, the flock should be limited to 20 or 30 birds. They can be kept in pens for a longer period of time than in crates. This method is often used for broilers or young stock.

PRINCIPLES

The success of the fattening process, like success in other branches of the poultry industry, depends upon a combination of factors.

STOCK. In the first place, the birds must be healthy. Birds "off condition," of low vitality, or infested with parasites cannot be fattened profitably. Furthermore, the birds must be capable of fattening. Hens in prime laying condition will not gain by fattening.

The general-purpose and meat breeds are best for fattening purposes. However, Leghorns make good gains up to 2½ to 3 months.

QUARTERS. The pens or house in which the birds are fattened should be comfortable. They should be reasonably warm in winter and cool in summer. However, Gutteridge and O'Neil[8] reported that the temperature condition had no marked effect upon the gains made, the lowest temperature (average 36.4° F.) showing a tendency to superiority. A greater feed consumption was evident at the lower temperature. Takita,[9] comparing fowls fattened in winter (average temperature 5° C.) and in summer (average temperature 27° C.), indicated that the body fat of the former contained only about ¼ as much free fatty acid but more liquid fatty acid than of the latter. Clean quarters are necessary to insure keen appetites. The place should be quiet and free from disturbance or excitement. Subdued light will help to keep the birds quiet. The object throughout is to restrict exercise and activity since they develop tough and hard muscles.

LENGTH OF FATTENING PERIOD. The length of time depends upon keeping the birds on feed and the gains that are made. In crate fattening, gains will usually be made for 12 to 15 days. In pen fattening, the period is somewhat longer, about 2 to 3 weeks. The cost per pound of gain is lowest the first part of the fattening period, but the process may be lengthened beyond the period of cheapest cost as long as gains are being made, in order to produce the best quality of flesh. The size of the chicken also influences the most efficient length of fattening period. Jull and Maw[10] indicate a period of 10 days for large-sized birds, such as Plymouth Rocks and Rhode Island Reds (weighing 4 pounds or over), and 14 days for medium-sized birds (weighing about 3 pounds). Gutteridge and O'Neil[8] conclude that, for well-reared cockerels of roaster age, 2 weeks of fattening gave greater and more economical gains and fat increase than 1 week, but 3 weeks of fattening was not justified by the results obtained.

MANAGEMENT PRACTICES. In order that they will eat the fattening ration greedily, birds should not be fed for the first 24 hours after they are placed in the crates or the pens.

The total food intake is related to the number of feeds per day. When comparing two, three, and five feeds daily, Maw[11] reports that two feeds daily for 10 days gave definitely smaller gains than three or five feeds. The figures indicate that birds getting a larger number of feeds per day convert more of the feed consumed into gain. On the other hand, Gutteridge and O'Neil[8] report that, in crate fattening, two feedings daily were as efficient as three feedings for weight gain and fat increase.

For fattening on the farm, it has been found that feeding twice a day has given satisfactory results because the feedings can be more nearly equally spaced. There is less danger of overfeeding when feeding two times a day. The birds should be fed all they will clean up readily morning and night. Great skill is required to feed for best results in fattening, as the feed should be removed just before the bird has eaten enough.

If at any time the birds go "off feed," one feeding should be omitted. Clean pails and troughs will help to prevent this condition.

Sometimes feather picking develops. This may be overcome by feeding fresh meat or extra meat scrap. Also methods of handling the poultry before fattening should be better, and starving should not be too long.

FEEDS AND RATIONS

Fattening rations are usually restricted and need not be so complete as rations for other purposes, since the birds are not dependent upon them for a long period of time.

Whole or cracked grains are not used in fattening rations, except possibly as a light feeding in pen fattening. In a test conducted in Missouri[12] birds fed on shelled corn gained 1/5 pound in 3 weeks while birds fed on corn meal and buttermilk gained 1/2 pound in 2 weeks. The cost per pound of gain on the whole grain was 4 to 8 times as much as on the finely ground grain and buttermilk.

Grit, shell, charcoal, salt, and other accessory feeds are unnecessary and only add to the labor and expense. Green food usually is also nonessential, although sometimes it is given once or twice a week as an appetizer. Usually water is not given as such, but it must be kept in mind that less water is needed in cool than in hot weather. In very hot weather it may be necessary to give the birds water to drink. Gutteridge and O'Neil,[8] however, reported that the gain in weight of Barred Plymouth Rock roosters was increased when the birds were permitted access to drinking water between feedings.

The ground grains are mixed with the liquid until the feed runs readily in hot weather and drips freely in cool weather. Hence more liquid is used in hot weather. It usually takes about 1 pound of dry feed and 2 pounds of buttermilk to produce a sloppy mixture. In some places, particularly England, the feed is allowed to stand a number of hours to produce fermentation.

FEEDS. A variety of feeds are used in fattening rations. In the main, they are fairly concentrated and usually finely ground. In England the fattening ration is composed largely of ground oats; in Belgium buckwheat meal is used; in France the ration is made up largely of buckwheat meal and barley meal; in the United States corn meal is most often used.

Cereals and By-Products. Maw and coworkers[13, 14] show that the individual cereals, yellow corn, wheat, oats, and barley, as ground whole cereals for fattening purposes, vary in their effect on the gains made and the quantity and nature of the fats produced in the growing chicken. These grains influence the amount of fat deposited in the body in a definite order, corn being superior, with wheat, oats, and barley following in this order. The color of the fat in the carcass and the percentage of fat in the edible meat are also influenced by the cereal fed.

Results definitely show that the different cereals cause the deposition of fats in different manners. Corn meal causes a high percentage of the total body fat to be deposited in the flesh and less fat in the abdominal cavity and in the skin of the bird, whereas the cereals, barley, oats, and wheat show the reverse in varying degrees. The corn flesh showed the highest flavor and was moist, whereas the wheat flesh lacked flavor and was dry. The barley and oat flesh were intermediate.

Such factors as the age of the stock being fed and the length of the feeding period have a bearing on the results obtained. The ground whole-oat ration was found to equal ground hull-less oats in feeding broiler stock. With mature roaster stock, wheat and corn were found to be superior to oats in a 21-day feeding period, although on a 7-day period wheat and oats were of equal value, with wheat superior to corn or barley. The single cereals were equal to the best combinations of two or three cereals. No significant differences in the distribution of fat in the body were found, as between the single or combined cereals with 5-pound roaster stock. The body fats were found to differ widely in iodine value and color, according to the cereal used. Maw[14] reports the iodine value of fat from corn-fed birds to be 67.4, from wheat-fed birds to be 65.7, from oat-fed birds 63,2, and from barley-fed birds 56.5

Gutteridge and coworkers[8, 15] report that corn gave superior gain to all other feeds (wheat, oats, barley, cooked potatoes). Ground buckwheat gave as great gains as yellow corn but required considerably more feed per unit of gain and was inferior to corn in its ability to increase fat. Ground oats and ground barley were of approximately equal value. However, ground hulled oats, when coarsely ground, were superior to ground yellow corn for fattening. Jeffrey[16] states that corn proved to be superior to oats in improving the eating quality of roasters under conditions of pen fattening. The oat-fed birds, however, were superior in desirable flavor of fat. McMurray[17] indicates no significant difference in gain between Sussex ground oats and barley meal. Poley and associates[5] state that, when judged by the amount of feed required to produce a unit of gain in body weight of fryers during the growing period, wheat was most efficient, followed in order by barley and corn. In growing rations for roasters, the gain-feed ratio was practically the same for corn and wheat, but somewhat more barley was required for the same gain in body weight. In the finishing rations tested, corn, wheat, and barley ranked in this order of efficiency.

In groups of Light Sussex cockerels, fed for 12 days on a ration of 12 parts of dried skimmilk and 88 parts of Sussex ground oats, maize meal, or barley meal, Cruickshank[18] reports that the softest fat was produced by oats in mature birds and by maize in immature birds. Barley produced harder fat in both. Maize had no detrimental effect on the consistency of the fat in either mature or immature birds, when fattening was rapid and live weight gain satisfactory, but it produced a harder fat than was produced by a ration of mixed cereals with a protein supplement.

Gutteridge and O'Neil[8] report an associative complementary effect brought about by combining grains (ground oats and yellow corn). They also report that fine grinding of the grains was slightly superior to coarse grinding.

Corn oil meal is a desirable ingredient for fattening rations. It has the ability to absorb large quantities of liquids, and it has been reported to be able to hold two to seven times its weight in liquid. The fat in the corn oil meal also helps to give the bird finish.

Other feeds used are wheat middlings, low-grade flour, oat meal, oat flour, pea meal, barley meal, buckwheat middlings, buckwheat flour, graham flour, and hominy. More corn meal can be used in cool weather. The amount of middlings and ground oats are advantageously increased in hot weather, owing in part, perhaps, to the ability of these feeds to retain more water. Feeds vary widely in their nature to absorb water. Maw[19] indicates that the following feed-water ratios have been found to exist: Corn, 1:1.3; barley, 1:2; oats, 1:2.5; wheat, 1:1.75; mixtures of any two of these cereals, 1:1.5; mixtures of any three of these cereals, 1:1.65; cereal mixtures plus supplementary fats, 1:1.6. A study at the Kansas Experiment Station[20] gives information on the milk-absorbing capacity of eight single-ground grains and two-ground grain mixtures. When the grains were allowed to soak in milk at room temperature for 24 hours, the quantity of milk absorbed ranged from 21.1 gallons per 100 pounds of ground milo to 67.1 gallons per 100 pounds of ground whole oats, all others falling within a range of 30 to 45 gallons. There was no apparent relation between the moisture content of the grain and the amount of milk it would absorb.

Potatoes. Experiments reported from Germany[21] indicate that potato flakes, with an adequate protein supplement, may be used as the chief component in the ration. Potato silage and steamed potatoes may also be fed so long as the protein ratio is adjusted. It was also reported to be uneconomical to use potatoes in fattening young cockerels as compared with swine. In particular instances, however, when poultry brings a correspondingly better price than pork, feeding potatoes may be profitable. Potato flakes are more economical to use than old stored potatoes in which much of the nutriment may be lost. Gutteridge[8] reported that potatoes, either raw or cooked, and mash (equal weights) were definitely inferior to mash alone.

Sugar Beets. Sugar beet slices[21, 22] gave good results in fattening experiments in Germany. The authors concluded that, in the fattening food, up to 50 per cent of dried sugar beet slices can be used but they must be cut extremely small. Their food value is equal to that of crushed barley.

Milk. Liquid buttermilk and skimmilk have been considered an essential ingredient of all good fattening rations. They seem to whiten and soften the flesh. However, experiments at the Missouri Station[23] show the value of other forms of milk for fattening poultry. The most satisfactory gains and highest percentage of initial weight packed were obtained when 10 per cent of dried skimmilk was fed; the lowest dressing loss was obtained when 5 per cent was fed. At the feed prices used, 5 per cent of dried skimmilk and liquid buttermilk produced the cheapest gains; condensed buttermilk produced the most expensive gains. Condensed buttermilk produced the highest quality birds, with 93.6 per cent No. 1; 10 per cent dried skimmilk ranked next with 90.4 per cent No. 1 birds. Experiments in Germany[24] also showed milk as the best protein addition for fattening.

Milk is best used as a moistener for the fattening mash. Trials in Canada[25] showed that dry mash and milk fed separately ad libitum, gave much less satisfactory gains than when the two were mixed in the proportions of two parts skimmilk to one part of mash and supplied as two feeds per day. But the latter method gave optimum results only if the birds were kept in crates. Skimmilk, as a mixer[8] for a fattening mash, gave very greatly superior gains to water and was also somewhat more efficient in the production of fat. The benefit of skimmilk was not accounted for by mixing pure crystalline riboflavin with water.

Protein Concentrates. With a mixture of two or more staple grains, sour skimmilk is necessary to produce the best results. Without milk, meat scraps can be used to advantage.[8] Jull and Maw[10] conclude that 10 per cent of meat scrap is justified but 20 per cent is not justified. Where milk is used, meat scrap is unnecessary and its use not justified.

Results at North Carolina[26] indicate that animal proteins could not be replaced by vegetable proteins, and in tests lasting 1 week substantially equal gains followed the use of digester tankage, blood meal, soybean meal and dried milk, and meat scrap. Experiments in Germany[27] showed that fresh blood proved advantageous for fattening ducks and cockerels.

Fats. Fat or tallow is sometimes added to the ration. In England fat, preferably mutton fat, is included during the last 10 days of fattening. However, experiments at the South-Eastern Agricultural College[28] show no appreciable difference in the gains produced by mutton fat or palm oil. In fattening trials in Canada[8, 25] the addition of 5 per cent of mutton fat to a fattening ration increased the gain by 18 per cent, the efficiency of use of feed by 27 per cent, the increase in percentage of fat by 15 per cent, and the percentage of A grade birds by 17 per cent. A desirable fat of firm texture was produced. A level of 10 per cent of mutton fat had a tendency to impart its flavor to the fat of the bird. Corn oil, while giving very satisfactory gains and fat increase, did not maintain either gains or increase for as long a period, and a fat was produced which was decidedly soft, even to the extent of producing some fluid fat in the abdomen of some birds.

Voitellier[29] states that the nature of the fat in the feed will influence the nature of the fat in the animal and thus determine the taste, odor, and culinary quality of the flesh of the hens. Cruickshank[30] showed that the ingestion of high percentages of saturated fatty acids in the form of palm kernel oil and mutton fat definitely increased the degree of saturation of the mixed fatty acids of the depot fat, while the ingestion of unsaturated acids in the form of hempseed resulted in a marked and rapid increase in unsaturation.

Maw[14, 19] reports on the feeding of supplementary fat as follows. Hard fats (mutton fat) are difficult to feed, whereas soft fats, such as vegetable oils, are easily incorporated with the meal mixtures. Certain oils affect the flavor of the meat. Corn oil produces a very satisfactory flavor, whereas cotton oil practically causes a loss of flavor, or a very unpalatable, flat-fat flavor. Peanut oil produces a sweet flavor in the meat. The effect of feeding additional fat in the form of crude corn oil is to increase the amount of fat in the skin and the abdominal fatty tissue. Such results make for a better finish. Small stock, such as broilers, show the effect more strongly than large roasters.

Some quality loss has been reported due to bile stain in storage. Maw and Nikolaiczuk[31] report a bile depletion method, involving preslaughter fat feeding, to eliminate liver stain in stored dressed poultry. Preliminary experiments demonstrate that the inclusion of approximately 25 per cent of refined cottonseed oil, added in the final or last two feeds prior to slaughter, is effective in depleting bile volume sufficiently to overcome extensive stain damage in dressed broiler and roaster carcasses during storage.

Miscellaneous Feeds. The Hawaii Station[32] reports that fattening rations containing avocados, bananas, and sweet potatoes, mixed with wheat middlings, yellow corn meal, or with both, proved to be efficient for the production of broilers and roasters of fine quality.

Green cut bone has also been used to advantage in small amounts as an occasional appetizer.

Gutteridge and O'Neil[8] report that the addition of bone meal to the fattening mash, at a level of 5 per cent, has no beneficial effect upon gains, fat increase, or whiteness of the dressed carcass.

HORMONES. Hormones have been fed for their effect upon the carcass. The estrogenic hormones produced in the ovary cause an increased deposition of fat under the skin, in the abdominal cavity, and in the muscles. The estrogenic hormones should be of greatest use in fattening and finishing male fowls. Adult females are less likely to be improved as most of them are supplied with their own natural estrogen. The treatment should be useful for broilers of both sexes since they ordinarily grow too quickly to accumulate much fat.

Lorenz[33] reported that tissues of birds receiving subcutaneous pellet implants of the estrogen, diethylstilbestrol, had striking and consistently greater fat content. Growth was also affected by the treatment. The greatest difference was obtained at 8 weeks of age (after 5 weeks of treatment). The meat quality was improved. This was especially noticeable in older birds, which normally have tough, darkened meat. The treated bird's meat was paler and considerably more tender. Oral administration was decidedly inferior to pellet implantation, but it has certain advantages. Turkeys also showed a distinct increase in abdominal fatty tissue. The maximum effect was produced after 44 days of treatment.

In trials at Cornell, in which one pellet (15 to 20 milligrams) of diethylstilbestrol per bird was implanted under the skin of old male fowls and left for 3 to 5 weeks, the treated birds excelled in "finish" because of greater fat, especially over the back, in the skin on the breast, and in the abdomen. The eating quality was also improved by the treatment.

The Oklahoma Station[34] also reported favorable results from the use of estrogens in fattening chickens. Even on a diet high in yellow corn, the carcass was covered with a smooth layer of pale yellowish-white fat and the flesh had a bleached milk-fed appearance. Old cocks soon lost all redness, their flesh was tenderized, and they assumed the appearance of prime fowl. Cockiness is suppressed and the comb and wattles shrivel and become pale. Dianisylhexene appeared to be the most useful for fattening broilers the last 2 or 3 weeks. It is readily dissolved in feeding oils.

Many other reports[35] have shown the advantages of fattening chickens and turkeys with estrogens. There is general agreement that estrogens will improve fat deposition and market grade. Gains may or may not be effected, as is also true with improvement in eating quality.

The most common estrogen used for treating poultry is a synthetic estrogen called diethylstilbestrol (stilbestrol). Feeding these substances is prohibited at present, but they can be implanted as pellets or paste under the skin of the upper neck. The hormone is then slowly absorbed. Since some of the substance may remain under the skin at marketing time, the material must be injected high enough so that the remaining estrogen will be discarded with the head. One stilbestrol pellet, containing 12 to 15 milligrams of the estrogen and properly implanted will undergo absorption during a period of 4 to 8 weeks. In practice good results are obtained if the birds are treated 4 to 6 weeks before they are marketed.

Stilbestrol will improve the fat content and carcass grade of any meat class of males, but a popular class seems to be the "hormonized fryer" or "caponette."

Feeding thiouracil[36] depresses the formation of thyroxine. The results in general have been improved market grade and fat deposition, but weight gains are likely to be depressed. A combination of thiouracil with stilbestrol has been reported as being superior to either treatment alone.[37]

The feeding of thyroactive iodocasein[38] has also produced slightly heavier chicks and marked improvement in the amount of fat on the carcass. Early and rapid feathering was also obtained. It is useful when thyroid-blocking agents are present. It is necessary, however, to know the tolerances and to feed controlled amounts since growth is depressed and mortality increased as the levels of thyroxine are increased. Combinations[39] of thyroprotein and thiouracil or stilbestrol have also been shown to be effective.

THE RATION. Studies at the Animal Nutrition Institute, Cambridge, England,[40] indicated that the principal change in the composition of adult fowls during fattening was an increase in fat content of the body, with relatively small increases in body protein. Rations composed of dried skimmilk and Sussex ground oats in proportions of 5:95 (12.47 per cent protein) were utilized with equal efficiency by fattening fowls. Results reported from Canada[14,41] also show little effect of the amount of protein on gains in the 21-day fattening period and show that the protein and fat content of the thigh muscle are not significantly influenced by different protein levels in the fattening ration.

In young birds the finishing process involves growth as well as plumping. Hence rations containing a larger amount of protein have given better feather growth and greater gains.

In compounding the ration, feeds should be selected to give a basic reaction. Solun and Schuster[42] indicate that the maintenance of the acid-base balance in the organism is to be looked upon as one of the main factors regulating the appetite of the fowl and determining the results of fattening.

EXPERIMENTAL RESULTS AND GAINS

Increase in weight is one of the results of the fattening or finishing process. The amount which the birds will gain depends upon the age of the bird, the condition of the bird, the method of fattening, and the degree to which the various requirements are met. In growing birds, more economical gains are made during the earlier periods. The relation existing between the increase in live weight and the consumption of food is shown in the following data from Italy.[43] For each kilogram increase in the live weight of Malines Coucou, approximately 2½ kilograms of feed were required for chickens under 2 months; 3 kilograms of feed for chickens of 2 to 3 months; 3.9 kilograms for chickens of 3 to 4 months; 4.17 for chickens of 4 to 5 months; 4.80 for chickens of 5 to 6 months; 6.60 for chickens of 6 to 7 months.

Broilers show the greatest gains since they are still growing rapidly. The North Dakota Station[44] reports cockerels showing gains of 28 to 38 per cent. The Missouri Station[23] indicates broilers as gaining 24 to 30 per cent, with an average of 26.3

per cent. Results of fattening under the direction of the United States Department of Agriculture[45] show an average gain for broilers of 32.3 per cent. The gains in the case of broilers represent largely growth increases. Well-grown broilers require little or no special fattening. This is particularly true with the high-energy rations being fed at the present time.

Roasters and hens do not make as large gains as younger birds. The Missouri Station[23] indicates gains for roasters of 13 to 15 per cent, with an average of 14.3 per cent; and for hens 13 to 14 per cent, with an average of 13.5 per cent. The United States Department of Agriculture[45] indicates an average gain of 12.1 per cent for roasters and 10.4 per cent for hens.

FATTENING RATIONS

Some typical fattening rations as recommended by a number of experiment stations will be found in the Appendix. (See page 580.)

REFERENCES

1. Brown, E. Poultry fattening. London. 1895-1896.
2. Lewer, S. H. Wright's book of poultry, p. 197. The Waverly Book Co. London.
3. Dickson, W. B. Poultry. London. 1838.
4. Harshaw, H. M. Effect of diet, range, and fattening on the physical and chemical composition of cockerels. Jour. Agr. Res. 53:357. 1936.

   Harshaw, H. M. The effect of fattening at different ages on the composition of cockerels. Poultry Sci. 17:163. 1938.
5. Poley, W. E., A. L. Moxon, W. O. Wilson, and R. L. Dolocek. Effect of corn, wheat, and barley in the diet on the physical and chemical composition of fryers and roasters. Jour. Agr. Res. 61:161. 1940.
6. Fraps, G. S. Relation of the protein, fat, and energy of the ration to the composition of chickens. Poultry Sci. 22:421. 1943.
7. Schmidt, R. The production of table poultry (poulards) in Syria with special reference to the duration of the fattening process and the consumption and utilization of feeding values. Rept. Sixth World's Poultry Congress. 43. Germany. 1936.
8. Gutteridge, H. S. Experimental technique in fattening and comparative value of fattening rations. Poultry Sci. 16:358. 1937.

   Gutteridge, H. S., and J. B. O'Neil. Methods and rations for fattening poultry. III. The effects of various fats, number of feedings, and length of fattening period. Sci. Agr. 21:350. 1941.

   Gutteridge, H. S., and J. B. O'Neil. Methods and rations for fattening poultry. IV. The relative value of certain cereal grains, of bone meal, and of premixing of feeds. Sci. Agr. 21:517. 1941.

Gutteridge, H. S., and J. B. O'Neil. Methods and rations for fattening poultry. V. The comparative effect of hulled oats and yellow corn, of skimmilk and water, and of varying temperatures. Sci. Agr. 21:607. 1941.

Gutteridge, H. S., and J. B. O'Neil. Methods and rations for fattening poultry. VI. The comparative economy of range rearing, crate fattening and caponizing for production of roasters. Sci. Agr. 21:711. 1941.

Gutteridge, H. S., and J. B. O'Neil. Methods and rations for fattening poultry. VII. Comparative effect of single grains and mixtures of grains, of fine or coarse grinding, and of mixing with skimmilk or whey. Sci. Agr. 23:500. 1943.

Gutteridge, H. S., and J. B. O'Neil. Methods and rations for fattening poultry. VIII. The value of a protein supplement, of added riboflavin, and of water to drink between feedings. Sci. Agr. 23: 647. 1943.

9. Takita, T. Influence of fattening foodstuffs and temperature on the fowl's body fat. Bul. Sci. Fakult. Terkult. Kjusu. Imp. Univ. Fukuoka, Japan. Vol. 8:1. 1938.

10. Jull, M. A., and W. A. Maw. Experimental results in fattening chickens. Poultry Sci. 2:99. 1923.

11. Maw, A. J. G., and W. A. Maw. Some observations on methods of fattening chickens. U. S. Egg and Poultry Mag. 45:332. 1939.

12. Mitchell, R. V. Methods of fattening, dressing and marketing poultry. Missouri State Board of Agr. Bul. XI. (2). 1913.

13. Maw, W. A., R. Holcomb, L. H. Bemont, and A. J. G. Maw. The cereals in the fattening ration and their effect upon the edible quality of the finished carcass. Rept. Sixth World's Poultry Congress. 298. Germany. 1936.

Maw, W. A. Cereals in the fattening ration. Rept. Seventh World's Poultry Congress. 177. Cleveland. 1939.

Maw, W. A., and A. J. G. Maw. Cereals in the fattening ration. II. Their comparative values for fattening Leghorn broilers. Sci. Agr. 19:602. 1939.

Maw, W. A. The cereal grains and their use in poultry nutrition. II. Influence on live weight gains and distribution of fat in fattening stock. Sci. Agric. 16:77. 1935.

14. Maw, W. A. How breeding and feeding control poultry character and meat quality. U. S. Egg and Poultry Mag. 45:608. 1939.

15. Gutteridge, H. S. Feeding practices and nutritional problems affecting grade. Conference Associate Com. Market Poultry. Ottawa. p. 55. March 2, 1936.

16. Jeffrey, F. P. Meat production in chickens. N. J. Bul. 656. 1938.

17. McMurray, M. Table poultry experiments. Rept. XIX Ann. Poultry Conf. Harper Adams Agr. Col. p. 495. 1935.

18. Cruickshank, E. M. A note on the effect of different cereals in the fattening ration on the composition of the body fat of the fowl. Jour. Agr. Sci. 27:309. 1937.

19. Maw, W. A. Feeding station problems. U. S. Egg and Poultry Mag. 43:142. 1937.

Maw, W. A., and I. E. Puddington. Supplementary fats in the fattening ration. Poultry Sci. 16:366. 1937.

20. Payne, L., and F. Santo. A factor in the milk fattening ration: the milk absorbing efficiency of certain grains and rations used for crate fattening poultry. Am. Creamery and Poultry Review 81: 806. 1936.

21. Stahl, W., and F. Haring. Beitrage zur Junghähnchenmast mit Kartoffel. Archiv für Geflügelk 7:97. 1933.

Stahl, W. Junghähnchenmast mit Kartoffeln. Archiv für Geflügelk 12:276. 1938.

22 Ferber, K. E., and M. Chodziesner. Junghähnchenmast mit einfachen Magermilchschrotgemischen unter besonderer Berücksichtigung des getrockneten Zuckerrübenschrotes. Biedermanns Zentralblatt 5:639. 1933.

23. Kempster, H. L., and E. E. Schnetzler. Experiment Station Research. Mo. Bul. 285:98. 1930.

Funk, E. M., H. L. Kempster, and C. G. Bryan. The value of dried skimmilk for fattening poultry. Mo. Bul. 309. 1932.

24. Fangauf, R., and R. Deditius. Über die Verwendung und Verwertung von Milch und Milchabfällen in der Geglügelmast. Zentralblatt für Tierernährung 5:469. 1933.

25. Gutteridge, H. S. Methods and rations for fattening poultry. II. Experimental technique and comparative value of fattening rations. Sci. Agr. 18:198. 1937.

26. Studies in feeding problems. N. C. Rept. 1921:43.

27. Richter, K., and H. Brüggemann. Frisches Schlachtblut als Eiweissfutter bei der Mast van Schweinen, Enten und Hähnchen. Züchtungskunde 113. 1936.

28. Fermor, C. E. Experiments in fattening with palm oil in lieu of mutton fat. Bul. Imp. Inst. London:390. 1933.

29. Voitellier, C. Influence of fat on the quality of the flesh and eggs of hens. La revue avicole 45:9. 1934.

30. Cruickshank, E. M. Studies in fat metabolism in the fowl. I. The composition of the egg fat and depot fat of the fowl as affected by the ingestion of large amounts of different fats. Biochem. Jour. 28:965. 1934.

Cruickshank, E. M. Feeding of different fats to poultry. Agric. Progress 11:147. 1934.

31. Maw, W. A., and N. Nikolaiczuk. A bile depletion method to eliminate liver stain in stored dressed poultry. U. S. Egg and Poultry Mag. 48:275. 1942.

32. Bice, C. M. Poultry feed supplements. Hawaii Circ. 4. 1932.

33. Lorenz, F. W. Fattening cockerels by stilbestrol administration. Poultry Sci. 22:190. 1943.

Lorenz, F. W. The influence of diethylstilbestrol on fat deposition in turkeys. Poultry Sci. 23:458. 1944.

Lorenz, F. W. The fattening action of orally administered synthetic estrogens as compared with diethylstilbestrol pellet implants. Poultry Sci. 24:91. 1945.

Lorenz, F. W. The influence of diethylstilbestrol on fat deposition and meat quality in chickens. Poultry Sci. 24:128. 1945.

34. Thayer, R. H., R. G. Jaap, and R. Penquite. Fattening chickens by feeding estrogens. Poultry Sci. 23:555. 1944.

Jaap, R. G., and R. B. Thompson. Fattening poultry by feeding "female" hormones. U. S. Egg and Poultry Mag. 51:108. 1945.

35. Almquist, H. J. Effects of male sex hormone on gains and feed conversions of hen turkeys. Poultry Sci. 31:747. 1952.

Almquist, H. J., and J. B. Merritt. Effects of diethylstilbestrol on gains and feed conversions of turkeys. Poultry Sci. 31:748. 1952.

Black, J. G., and R. G. Booth. Capon production by the use of synthetic oestrogen (stilbestrol). Vet. Jour. 102:41. 1946.

Davidson, J. A., L. F. Wolterink, and E. P. Reineke. Some effects of high dosages of synthetic estrogens in young turkeys. Poultry Sci. 25:400. 1946.

Davis, G. T., and R. Thayer. Finishing market turkeys with estrogens. Poultry Sci. 27:79. 1948.

Gassner, F. X., and H. S. Wilgus. Observation on the estrogen fattening of chickens. Poultry Sci. 27:663. 1948.

Hixson, F. M., and R. B. Thompson. The use of estrogens for improving the market finish of turkeys in hot weather. Poultry Sci. 30:393. 1951.

Jaap, R. G. Activity of synthetic estrogens on oral administration in the domestic fowl and turkey. Endocrinology 37:369. 1945.

Jaap, R. G. The duration of subcutaneously administered estrogens in cockerels. Poultry Sci. 25:403. 1946.

Stadelman, W. J., C. M. McCartan, E. L. Baum, and B. A. McLaren. Growth and processing shrinkage of diethylstilbestrol treated fryers. Poultry Sci. 30:512. 1951.

Sturkie, P. D. The effect of estrogens upon the meat quality of old cocks and hens. Poultry Sci. 25:365. 1946.

Sturkie, P. D. Of what value are female sex hormones (estrogens) in fattening chickens. N. Jersey Hints to Poultrymen 33 (2). March, 1950.

Sykes, J. F., J. A. Davidson and F. N. Barrett. The effect of feeding diethylstilbestrol to cockerels. Poultry Sci. 24:542. 1945.

Taylor, M. W. Tests with female sex hormones for fattening birds. Modern Poultry Keeping. LV: 230. 1946.

Thayer, R. H., and G. T. Davis. Use of estrogens in turkey broiler production. Poultry Sci. 27:176. 1948.

Thayer, R. H., R. G. Jaap, and R. Penquite. Fattening chickens by feeding estrogens. Poultry Sci. 24:483. 1945.

Westermarck, H., and A. Aaltonen. Omkapunering av tuppar med stilbestrol. Nordisk Veterinarmed. 2:405. 1950.

36. Andrews, F. N., and E. E. Schnetzler. Influence of thiouracil on growth and fattening in broilers. Poultry Sci. 25:124. 1946.

Blakely, R. M., and R. W. Anderson. The influence of thiouracil on growth, fattening, feed consumption, and thyroid weight of turkey broilers. Poultry Sci. 28:185. 1949.

Mixner, J. P., B. A. Tower, and C. W. Upp. The effect of feeding thiouracil on the body weight of New Hampshire cockerels. Poultry Sci. 25:536. 1946.

Reineke, E. P., J. A. Davidson, L. F. Wolterink, and F. N. Barrett. The effect of thiouracil on fattening turkeys. Poultry Sci. 25:410. 1946.

37. Andrews, F. N., and B. B. Bohren. Influence of thiouracil and stilbestrol on growth, fattening, and feed efficiency in broilers. Poultry Sci. 26:447. 1947.

Baum, E. L., H. G. Walkup, W. J. Stadelman, and J. E. Faris. Some economic implications of thiouracil and diethylstilbestrol treatment of turkeys. Poultry Sci. 31:723. 1952.

Detwiler, R. W., F. N. Andrews, and B. B. Bohren. The influence of thiouracil and stilbestrol on broiler quality. Poultry Sci. 29:513. 1950.

Stadelman, W. J. The use of thiouracil and diethylstilbestrol in finishing turkey roasters. Washington Sta. Circ. 141. 1951.

Stadelman, W. J. The use of thiouracil and diethylstilbestrol in finishing turkeys for market. Poultry Sci. 31:310. 1952.

Robblee, A. R., A. B. Morrison, and D. R. Clandinin. The use of thiouracil and diethylstilbestrol for finishing turkeys. Poultry Sci. 30:772. 1951.

38. Graham, W. R. Jr. The use of thyroxine-like products in animal feeding. Texas Nutr. Conf. Abstracts 3. 1950.

Olsson, N. Försök med thyreoaktivt jodkasein. Nordisk Fääderfättidskrift. No. 1. 1949.

Wheeler, R. S., E. Hoffman, and C. L. Graham. The value of thyroprotein in starting, growing, and laying rations. I. Growth, feathering, and feed consumption of Rhode Island Red broilers. Poultry Sci. 27:103. 1948.

Wheeler, R. S., and E. Hoffman. The value of thyroprotein in starting, growing and laying rations. Poultry Sci. 27:509. 1948.

Irwin, M. R., E. P. Reineke, and C. W. Turner. Effect of feeding thyroactive iodocasein on growth, feathering, and weights of glands of young chicks. Poultry Sci. 22:374. 1943.

Turner, C. W., E. P. Reineke, and A. B. Schultze. The use of thiourea in the fattening of meat animals. Jour. Animal Sci. 3:448. 1944.

Kempster, H. L., and C. W. Turner. The effect of feeding thiouracil on the fleshing of New Hampshire broilers. Poultry Sci. 24:94. 1945.

39. Glazener, E. W., and M. A. Jull. Effects of thiouracil, desiccated thyroid, and stilbestrol derivatives on various glands, body weight, and dressing appearance in the chicken. Poultry Sci. 25:236. 1946.

Henderson, W., J. S. Carver, and E. L. Stephenson. Finishing turkeys using thiouracil, iodinated casein, and diethelstilbestrol. Poultry Sci. 27:667. 1948.

Moreng, R. E., and C. S. Shaffner. A thiouracil-thyroprotein treatment for fattening poultry. Poultry Sci. 28:504. 1949.

Quisenberry, J. H., and W. F. Krueger. Effects of feeding various

combinations of protamone, oestrogens, and thiouracil on growth and fattening of broilers and fryers. Poultry Sci. 27:681. 1948.
40. Halnan, E. T. On the influence of protein on the fattening of fowls. Jour. Agr. Sci. (Eng.) 28:341. 1938.
41. Maw, W. A., A. J. G. Maw, R. Holcomb, and L. H. Bemont. Protein levels in the fattening ration as influencing the composition of the thigh muscle with varying ages of poultry meat stock. Sci. Agr. 17:453. 1937.
42. Solun, A. S., and M. Schuster. Zur Frage des Saure-Basen Gleichgewichtes während der Geflügelmastung. Die Tierernährung 6: 515. 1934.
43. Giuliani, R., and C. Ruiz. The economic fattening of Rhode Island Red cockerels. Proc. Third World's Poultry Congress. 250. Canada. 1927.
44. Barton, O. A. Feeding. N. Dak. Bul. 217:93. 1928.
45. Lee, A. R. The commercial fattening of poultry. U.S.D.A. Bul. 21. 1914.

CHAPTER 16

FEEDING TURKEYS

The feeding of turkeys, especially the young stock, has undergone considerable change. It is only natural that it should follow in the wake of the advances made in chick feeding. As was also true of chicks, the older methods of feeding were usually complicated and laborious. The following statement taken from the bulletin "Raising Turkeys in Wisconsin"[1] describes the old order.

> For a long time a turkey ration was used that changed in amount, composition, and time of feeding each day. The principal ingredients were cracker crumbs, stale bread, boiled eggs, dandelion greens, lettuce, and milk; and no one ever had any plausible reason for using a ration of that sort. It was just accepted.

At the present time turkey rations are being developed along the same lines as chicken rations. The information gained in the feeding of chickens is being applied to the feeding of turkeys. In fact, many persons have used the usual poultry rations with fairly good success, especially where the turkeys have good range. The chicken rations are not the best, however, since in many respects the requirements of turkeys differ from those of chickens. Turkeys show greater relative gains than chickens, especially early in life. These greater gains are reflected in larger demands for some of the nutrients. This is particularly true for energy, protein, and unidentified vitamins.[2]

REQUIREMENTS OF THE TURKEY RATION

PROTEIN. Most experiment stations now recommend high-protein rations for young turkeys. This no doubt is necessary because of the greater rate of growth. The California Station[3] showed that turkey poults require more protein than chicks. Funk[4] pointed out that turkeys make greater relative gains than chickens and that there is a relation between early and later growth.

In 1932 the Pennsylvania Station[5] indicated the protein requirement of poults, based on the amount of milk consumed by them, to be 26 per cent for the first two weeks, 21.7 per cent for the third week, and 19.5 to 21.3 per cent for the fourth to eighteenth weeks.

Similarly, results from other sources[2, 4-6] show the advantages and necessity of high-protein rations for starting turkeys.

In turkey feeding trials at the Washington Station,[7] in which the birds had free access to both grain and mash, they consumed 19 per cent scratch grain and 81 per cent mash from the twelfth to the sixteenth week, as compared with 72 per cent scratch and 28 per cent mash during the last four weeks of the trial. The protein content of the feed consumed averaged 13 per cent at the end of the twenty-eighth week.

In experiments reported by the U. S. Department of Agriculture,[8] in which mash and scratch were fed ad libitum, with the protein content of the mashes ranging from 18 to 30 per cent, it was found that the ratio of mash to grain consumed varied inversely with the protein content of the mash. During the first 16 weeks, the average live weight of the several lots was, in general, in the same order as the quantity of protein consumed. However, after 16 weeks the gains per 4-week period were not so closely associated with the quantity of protein consumed. The birds fed the mash that contained about 28 per cent of protein weighed the most at all ages after 12 weeks, and those fed the mash that contained about 18 per cent of protein weighed the least at all ages. Between 21 and 28 weeks of age, the turkeys consumed mash and grain in such proportions as to provide a ration averaging about 16 per cent protein. The quantity of protein consumed had no consistent effect on mortality or malformation of leg or breast bones.

The results to date would indicate that for the most rapid and economical gains the protein level of a turkey starting ration should be 28 per cent. After 8 weeks a growing ration containing 20 per cent protein is sufficient. In the later growing period (after 4 months) the protein can be reduced to 16 per cent. The breeding ration should furnish 15 per cent protein.

AMINO ACIDS. Some information has also been obtained concerning the amino acid requirements of turkeys. The arginine[9] requirement has been placed at 1.35 per cent for the starting ration. Approximately 0.8 per cent of the sulfur amino acids[10] were required for optimum growth in a ration containing 24 per cent crude protein. This amount includes a minimum of 0.5 per cent methionine. Methionine may completely replace cystine, but cystine is not changed to methionine.

Lysine[11] is necessary for growth and the prevention of the occurrence of white feathers in Bronze turkeys. The requirement has been placed at 1.3 per cent, although this requirement may be increased under certain conditions.

Methionine and lysine appear to be the limiting amino acids on low-protein turkey poult diets. Supplementing a 20 per cent corn-soybean diet with lysine and methionine has produced growth equivalent to a 28 per cent protein ration.[12]

Approximately 0.9 per cent of total glycine[13] has been reported as the smallest amount which is necessary for optimum growth. Glycine may be concerned with "hock trouble" which occurs in turkeys.

The tryptophan[14] requirement of the poults has been reported as being 0.19 to 0.28 per cent.

MINERALS. A proper amount and a balance of minerals are necessary. For the growing poult, calcium and phosphorus must be furnished in largest amounts. The quantities to furnish will depend somewhat on the amount of vitamin D present.[15] Mussehl and Ackerson[16] report that growing poults are able to adjust themselves to a considerable variation of the calcium-phosphorus ratio. When the vitamin D was withheld, the poults receiving the higher levels of calcium, provided by calcium carbonate, appeared to adjust themselves best to the vitamin limitation.

The calcium and phosphorus requirements[15, 17] vary somewhat depending upon other factors. The rate of growth might have some influence. A smaller amount appears more satisfactory for growth than for good bone calcification. The calcium requirement has been indicated as being 1.6 per cent to 2.0 per cent. A diet containing 0.6 per cent of available phosphorus has given excellent calcification.

The total phosphorus of the ration should not be too high since it might aggravate the occurrence of perosis and decrease growth. However, the ration must have sufficient manganese and choline[18] and niacin to secure proper bone development and prevent perosis.

Usually one-half to 1 per cent of salt is added to turkey rations. Turkeys have been reported to tolerate salt up to 4 per cent of the ration.[19] The other minerals are ordinarily present in sufficient amounts in the average practical ration.

VITAMINS. The same vitamins are necessary for turkeys as for chickens and are supplied in the same feeds. However, special consideration must be given to species reactions or requirements. Turkeys require larger amounts of vitamins than do chickens.[20]

Vitamin A. The vitamin A requirement of poults is higher than for chicks. Sherwood[21] reported that turkeys require twice the amount of vitamin A as do chickens. Poley and Tulley[22] report more rapid gains from birds receiving yellow corn than those receiving white corn. They attribute the difference to a possible vitamin A deficiency due to drought conditions, which did not permit the growth of vegetation.

Hinshaw[23] observed in turkeys receiving various levels of dehydrated alfalfa meal as the source of vitamin A that the percentage of mortality associated with A-avitaminosis varied inversely as the amount of alfalfa in the ration. No mortality due to A-avitaminosis occurred in turkeys receiving either 8 per cent of dehydrated alfalfa meal or freshly cut alfalfa.

The vitamin A requirement[24] of turkey poults has been reported as ranging from 500 to 700 International units per 100 grams of feed.

Vitamin D. In applying the feeding of cod liver oil to turkeys to prevent rickets, it was soon noticed that the turkey's requirement of this vitamin was greater than the chicken's. This was shown by the Kansas workers[25] when they reported that turkeys developed rickets earlier than chicks. Baird and Greene[26] state that chickens weighing 1000 grams or better at 12 weeks required a minimum of approximately 18 U.S.P. units of vitamin D per 100 grams of feed, whereas turkeys weighing 1900 grams or better in 12 weeks required a minimum of 60 to 70 U.S.P. units of vitamin D per 100 grams of feed. Other workers[27] have also concluded that 70 to 100 A.O.A.C. (52.5 to 75 International chick) units of vitamin D per 100 grams of ration seemed to be ample for satisfactory calcification in the poult.

Murphy[28] reported that the requirement for poults appears to be 175 A.O.A.C. (131.25 International chick) units of vitamin D per 100 grams of feed. Jukes and Sanford,[29] using a fish-oil blend as the source of vitamin D, concluded, in 1939, that while the vitamin D requirement of turkeys cannot be precisely stated in terms of A.O.A.C. chick units, the value of 200 chick units per 100 grams of diet was approximately the amount required to support normal development of turkeys to 4 weeks of age. Later they found this to be true for one source of vitamin D but not for two other sources of the vitamin.

The above difference can be explained by later experiments,[30] which show that the source of phosphorus influences the efficiency of vitamin D, that the response of turkey poults to vitamin D from different sources is not the same, and that the poult utilizes certain forms of vitamin D with degrees of efficacy that differ from the chick, and hence vitamin D potency expressed in chick units is not necessarily a true measure of the value of a vitamin D supplement for turkeys.

Robertson, Rhian, and Wilhelm[31] showed that the growth of poults to 4 weeks of age on a ration devoid of vitamin D was in direct proportion to the level of vitamin D in the breeding hens' ration. The effect of the level of vitamin D in the hens' ration upon the response of poults is greater the first two weeks, and thereafter the influence of vitamin D in the poults' ration is greater. Wilhelm, Robertson, and Rhian[32] reported no benefits in egg production or hatchability from the addition of cod liver oil beyond 100 units of vitamin D per 100 grams of ration.

Vitamin E. Vitamin E has also been reported as benefitting the hatchability of turkey eggs.[33]

Riboflavin. Riboflavin deficiency in turkeys is characterized by retarded growth, dermatitis, perosis, and poor feathering.[34] Most turkey rations containing a large amount of milk have given good growth, owing in part to the fact that the milk furnished enough riboflavin. Experiments at Cornell indicated that turkey rations for the first 4 weeks should contain a minimum of 320 micrograms of riboflavin per 100 grams of feed. During the second 4-week period the riboflavin requirement dropped to 200 micrograms. After the turkeys were 8 weeks old, the riboflavin requirement was not greater than 140 micrograms. The quantitative requirements for riboflavin for the first two periods of 4 weeks each were in proportion to the relative growth rate. The riboflavin requirement of turkeys was approximately 25 per cent greater than for chicks at the same age, which represented roughly the difference in the rate of growth of these two species. Jukes,[35] however, did not find such difference but reports that the riboflavin requirement for poults is about the same as for chickens.

The Nebraska Station[36] reported that turkeys have a relatively high vitamin B requirement. Since this conclusion was based on the feeding of yeast, it is probable that the response was due to the riboflavin of the yeast.

Other reports[37] have indicated the riboflavin requirement for normal growth and hatchability to be between 270 and 350 micrograms per 100 grams of ration.

Pyridoxine. The California Station[38] reported pyridoxine deficiency in turkeys similar to that in chicks, being characterized by loss of appetite, poor growth, apathy, hyperexcitability when disturbed, convulsions, and death. The requirement was indicated as 300 micrograms per 100 grams of ration.

Choline. Choline[39] has been shown to be necessary to prevent perosis. The requirement for poults has been indicated as being 800 to 1100 milligrams per pound. The requirement for turkey breeders is lower, 370 milligrams per pound being reported as sufficient for hatchability.

Folic Acid. A deficiency of folic acid[40] will result in slow growth, cervical paralysis, anemia, and high mortality. Several of the reports indicate the requirement for poults as being 80 micrograms per 100 grams of feed. Approximately half that amount seems to be sufficient for hens.

Niacin. A deficiency of niacin[41] will result in retarded growth, perosis, diarrhea, poor feathering, mouth inflammation, and high mortality. The deficiency symptoms were prevented by including 3 to 5 milligrams of niacin per 100 grams of ration. Higher levels may be needed for optimum growth, at least 5 milligrams probably being necessary. Niacin also helps in preventing the enlarged hock condition.

Pantothenic Acid. A ration deficient in pantothenic acid[42] will result in slow growth and dermatitis of the mouth. Approximately 10.5 milligrams per kilogram of diet are required for optimum growth.

Biotin. The Pennsylvania Station[43] concluded that biotin protected turkey poults from dermatitis.

Vitamin B_{12}. The vitamin B_{12} requirement for starting turkey poults has been reported as 5 to 10 micrograms per kilogram of ration.[44]

Other vitamins as yet unrecognized are also essential. This is true for at least one factor involved in the production of the enlarged hock disorder in turkeys.[45]

FIBER.[46] Turkeys can tolerate more fiber than can chickens. Good gains and good quality have been reported for growing turkeys with diets containing up to 20 per cent. However, feed efficiency was best with lower levels. Quality of plumage was improved and feather pulling retarded with the higher fiber rations. The level of fiber in the mash did not affect weight since the per cent of whole grain selected was related to mash fiber levels.

SUMMARY. As a summary of the information available to date, the nutrient requirements for turkeys are indicated by the Committee on Animal Nutrition of the National Research Council[47] (Table 30). The figures do not include margins of safety

TABLE 30. NUTRIENT REQUIREMENTS* OF TURKEYS

	Starting Poults, 0–8 weeks	Growing Turkeys 8–16 weeks	Breeding Turkeys
Total protein, %†	28	20	15
Vitamins			
Vitamin A activity (U.S.P. units)‡	2400	2400	2400
Vitamin D (I.C.U.)§	400	400	400
Riboflavin, mg.	1.7	?	1.5
Pantothenic acid, mg.	5.0	?	?
Choline, mg.	750	?	?
Folacin, mg.	0.4	?	?
Minerals			
Calcium, %‖	2.0	2.0	2.25
Phosphorus, %¶	1.0	1.0	0.75
Manganese, mg.	25.0	?	15.0
Salt, %**	0.5	0.5	0.5
Amino acids, %			
Arginine	1.6	—	—
Lysine	1.5	—	—
Methionine††	0.87	—	—
or			
Methionine	0.52	—	—
Cystine	0.35	—	—
Tryptophan	0.26	—	—
Glycine‡‡	1.0	—	—
Isoleucine	0.84	—	—

* In percentage or amount per pound of feed.

† The protein content of rations for growing turkeys from 16 weeks to market weight may be reduced to 16 per cent.

‡ May be vitamin A or pro-vitamin A.

§ International chick units.

‖ This amount of calcium need not be incorporated in the mixed feed inasmuch as calcium supplements fed free choice are considered as part of the ration.

¶ At least 0.50 per cent of the total feed of starting poults should be inorganic phosphorus. All the phosphorus of nonvegetable feed ingredients is considered to be inorganic. Approximately 30 per cent of the phosphorus of vegetable products is nonphytin phosphorus and may be considered as part of the inorganic phosphorus required. Presumably a portion of the requirement of growing and breeding turkeys must also be furnished in inorganic form.

** This figure represents added salt or sodium chloride added as such or in marine or fermentation products of high sodium chloride content.

†† Cystine will replace methionine as long as the ration contains not less than 0.52 per cent methionine.

‡‡ Glycine can be synthesized, but the synthesis does not proceed at a rate sufficient for maximum growth.

to compensate for possible losses of vitamins during processing, transportation and storage, and for variations in feed composition and in environment. In earlier reports the National Research Council suggested allowances which included margins of safety of 66 per cent for vitamin A, 50 per cent for vitamin D, and 20 per sent for the water-soluble vitamins.

MAKING UP A TURKEY RATION

Most of the common cereals have been used in turkey rations.[48-53] No appreciable differences in the rate of growth have been reported for corn, wheat, oats, barley, rye, milo or kafir, sorghums, and proso millet. However, oats showed a lower feed efficiency.

The Wyoming Station[54] reported on the influence of various feeds upon the quality of meat in turkeys. None of the grains had any significant effect on the dressing shrinkage, but the corn- and wheat-fed birds averaged a higher market grade. Oats and corn produced softer fats than barley or wheat, with rye intermediate. Oats produced a more intense and desirable aroma in the roasted bird. Corn, oats, and rye produced a texture of breast meat superior to the texture produced by wheat and barley. The corn-fed birds were slightly more tender when roasted and had the greatest amount of juice. Corn gluten meal produced a decidedly yellow-colored dressed turkey. Dry skimmilk produced a less intense aroma in the breast meat. Soybean oil meal and cottonseed meal produced a coarser texture in the breast meal after roasting. The least desirable flavor was found in birds fed cottonseed meal. Corn gluten meal produced a better quality of juice than any of the other concentrates.

The Utah Station[55] reported that alfalfa meal could be fed in large quantities to growing turkeys and could be used up to 35 per cent of the mash when a good grade of alfalfa meal could be purchased at a lower cost per pound than ground wheat, barley, or millrun bran and shorts.

The California Station[56] indicated that raisins may be used as a cereal substitute in rations for growing turkeys, replacing 30 per cent of the grain portion or 16 per cent of the entire ration.

The various vegetable protein concentrates[57] have been fed successfully to furnish protein in turkey rations, when such deficiencies as calcium, phosphorus, and lysine have been corrected. Soybean oil meal, corn gluten meal, and cottonseed meal have all been fed. Corn gluten meal has been reported as producing a superior fleshing condition.

Wilgus[58] reported that hatchability of turkey eggs was markedly improved by adding 2.5 to 5 per cent of dried whey to an ordinary poultry ration, thus showing that the requirements of turkeys for riboflavin are fairly high.

In experiments conducted in Michigan[59] in which mash, whole corn, gravel, and drink were before the birds at all times, and chopped fresh alfalfa was fed daily, the poults receiving liquid skimmilk consumed less mash per pound of gain, but ate more corn, than poults receiving water to drink. The Ontario Station[60] concluded that rations for starting poults were improved by including some buttermilk powder.

Grasshoppers[61] have also been fed to turkeys. Milby and Penquite reported that, when grasshoppers are abundant, they may prove to be a valuable protein feed for turkeys if properly prepared for feeding and adequately supplemented with other feedstuffs. McHargue concluded that the value of insects as a food for poultry was probably due to their high protein and lysine content. Wickware reported a potential danger in feeding grasshoppers to turkeys. Turkeys died in Canada after eating two species found in Ontario. The loss was reported as "poisoning" but was found to consist of enteritis due to injury caused by the legs of the insects which even punctured the intestines. This loss, however, could be avoided by feeding a liberal quantity of mash in the morning before the birds ate the grasshoppers.

THE RATION

A large number of satisfactory turkey rations have been recommended. The successful ones have shown certain common characteristics. The general pattern is suggested in Table 31.

The mash mixtures should not be sticky when moistened, because stickiness affects the proper eating of it. The mash should not be too bulky because the ration must have a high available energy content. Neither should it be ground too coarsely or too finely, except that the oats for young turkeys should be finely pulverized.[62]

Penicillin added to a turkey breeder mash has been reported as decreasing hatchability, egg production, egg weight, and food consumption.[63]

GROWTH RATE AND FEED CONSUMPTION

The rate at which turkeys grow will depend upon many factors, such as breed and strain, the ration, rearing conditions, environment, and management. As a guide[64] for turkey growers the

TABLE 31. FORMULA PATTERN FOR TURKEY MASHES

	Starting Mash 0–4 wks. (all-mash) lb./ton	Growing Mashes 4–8 wks. (all-mash) lb./ton	Growing Mashes After 8 wks. (with grain) lb./ton	Breeding Mash (with grain) lb./ton
Corn meal, yellow Milo, ground Wheat, ground or crushed Oat groats Wheat flour middlings	800–1000	700–900	600–800	400–600
Wheat standard middlings Wheat bran	0	0	300–400	200–400
Oats, pulverized Barley, ground	100–200	100–200	100–200	100–200
Soybean meal* Corn gluten meal Peanut meal	400–600	300–500	150–200	150–200
Fish meal† Fish solubles Meatscrap (50–55% protein)	200–300	200–300	200–300	200–300
Dried whey product‡ Buttermilk, dried Yeast, dried brewers'§ Distillers' dried solubles Skimmilk, dried	100–200	100–200	100–200	100–300
Alfalfa meal	40–60	100	100–200	100–200
Steamed bone meal Dicalcium phosphate Defluorinated phosphate Ground limestone	30–40	40–50	50–60	70–90
Salt	5–10	5–10	10–20	10–20
Manganese sulfate (feeding grade)	0.5	0.5	0.5	0.75
Vitamin A and D supplements	+	+	+	+
Riboflavin supplement (if needed)	+	+	+	+
Choline (if needed)	+	+	+	+
Antibiotic feed supplement	+	+	+	—
Niacin and vitamin E	+	+	+	+
Required Nutrient Content:				
Protein, %	28	24	20	24
Calcium, %	1.5	1.5	1.5‖	‖
Phosphorus, %	0.9	0.9	1	1.5
Riboflavin, mg/lb	2	2	¶	5.8
Choline, mg/lb	900	900	¶	¶
Vitamin A, U.S.P./lb	4000	4000	8000	12,000
Vitamin D, I.C.U./lb	600	600	1200	1800

* Soybean meal to represent at least 3/4 of total in this class.

† Fish meal to represent at least 2/3 of total in this class for starting and breeding mashes.

‡ Preferably dried whey product containing 50% or less lactose; wheys with higher lactose levels less effective.

§ Dried brewers' yeast to represent at least 1/2 of total in this class.

‖ Extra feeding of oyster shell or other calcium supplement recommended; no definite calcium content required for breeding mash.

¶ Requirement unknown.

weights and feed consumption for Broad Breasted Bronze turkeys reared under conditions of confinement or dry lot rearing are given in Table 32. Similar information for Beltsville Small White turkeys is given in Table 32A.

For further information concerning growth and feed consumption see Chap. 19, "Economics of Feeding."

FEEDING METHODS AND MANAGEMENT

Experiments conducted at the Washington Station[10] resulted in no significant difference, at 28 weeks, in the body weights of either the hens or the toms fed mash, mash and pellets, or pellets supplemented with scratch grain and green feed. The three lots ate practically the same amounts of feed. However, the pelleted feed was more attractive and palatable than mash to the young turkey poults 2 to 10 days old. In another experiment, no difference in weight after 20 weeks was found in lots receiving no scratch grain, hand-fed scratch grain, or hopper-fed scratch grain. The Kansas Station[65] concluded that at least during the early stages of growth mash feeding is preferred over pellet feeding. The Ontario Station[66] reported greater weights for the groups receiving pellets than those receiving mash. The advantage of pellets was greater for the groups containing the higher amounts of dehydrated alfalfa and dehydrated cereal grass.

The Washington Station[67] reported greater weight at maturity and higher efficiency in converting feed in turkeys fed a high-protein concentrate and a choice of four whole grains than in similar turkeys fed developing mash and a mixture of whole grains. When the turkeys were changed to the concentrate at 4 weeks of age, they adjusted the protein content of the ration quite readily. On the other hand, the Missouri Station[68] concluded that the use of concentrates containing high percentages of protein could not be recommended. The difference is probably due to climate. Turkeys grown in warmer climates will not shift to grains sufficiently to balance their ration.

Turkeys can utilize pasture to advantage and so effect a saving in feed. Reports on the amount of feed saved vary, but frequently savings in feed of 10 to 20 per cent are reported. Under certain conditions, even greater savings have been found. Westermarck[69] controlled the consumption of food by turkeys from the day of hatching up to the time they were killed and used the following three groups: (I) in pens; (II) on cultivated land;

TABLE 32. GROWTH RATE AND FEED CONSUMPTION OF BROAD BREASTED BRONZE TURKEYS
(Cornell University)

Age in Months	Age in Weeks	Average Weight of Toms and Hens Combined, lb.	Gain in Weight for Period, lb.	Feed Consumed Each week (Mash and Grain), lb.	Total Cumulative Feed Required, lb.	Successive Weekly Feed Required per Pound of Gain, lb.	Feed Required per Pound of Gain to Date, lb.
		0.12					
	1	0.28	0.16	0.19	0.19	1.2	1.2
	2	0.55	0.27	0.37	0.56	1.3	1.3
	3	0.90	0.35	0.61	1.17	1.7	1.5
	4	1.40	0.50	0.88	2.05	1.8	1.6
1	Total	1.40	1.28	2.05	2.05	1.5	1.6
	5	2.0	0.6	1.15	3.2	1.9	1.7
	6	2.7	0.7	1.4	4.6	2.0	1.8
	7	3.5	0.8	1.8	6.4	2.2	1.9
	8	4.3	0.8	2.4	8.8	3.0	2.1
2	Total	4.3	2.9	6.75	8.8	2.3	2.1
	9	5.2	0.9	2.9	11.7	3.2	2.3
	10	6.2	1.0	3.3	15.0	3.3	2.5
	11	7.2	1.0	3.4	18.4	3.4	2.6
	12	8.2	1.0	3.4	21.8	3.4	2.7
3	Total	8.2	3.9	13.0	21.8	3.3	2.6
	13	9.2	1.0	3.6	25.4	3.6	2.8
	14	10.2	1.0	3.8	29.2	3.8	2.9
	15	11.2	1.0	4.0	33.2	4.0	3.2
	16	12.2	1.0	4.3	37.5	4.3	3.1
4	Total	12.2	4.0	15.7	37.5	3.9	3.1
	17	13.1	0.9	4.0	41.5	4.4	3.2
	18	14.0	0.9	4.3	45.8	4.7	3.3
	19	14.9	0.9	4.5	50.3	5.0	3.4
	20	15.8	0.9	4.6	54.9	5.1	3.5
5	Total	15.8	3.6	17.4	54.9	4.8	3.5
	21	16.7	0.9	4.8	59.7	5.3	3.6
	22	17.6	0.9	5.0	64.7	5.5	3.7
	23	18.4	0.8	4.8	69.5	6.0	3.8
	24	19.2	0.8	4.9	74.4	6.1	3.9
6	Total	19.2	3.4	19.5	74.4	5.7	3.9
	25	20.0	0.8	5.1	79.5	6.3	4.0
	26	20.8	0.8	5.3	84.8	6.6	4.1
	27	21.5	0.7	7.1	91.9	10.0	4.3
	28	22.2	0.7	7.5	99.4	10.7	4.5
7	Total	22.2	3.0	25.0	99.4	8.4	4.5
	29	22.8	0.6	7.6	107.0	12.6	4.7
	30	23.4	0.6	7.7	114.7	12.8	4.9
	31	24.0	0.6	7.7	122.4	12.8	5.1
	32	24.5	0.5	7.7	130.1	15.4	5.3
8	Total	24.5	2.3	29.7	130.1	13.3	5.3

TABLE 32A. GROWTH RATE AND FEED CONSUMPTION OF BELTSVILLE SMALL WHITE TURKEYS

Age in Months	Age in Weeks	Average Weight of Toms and Hens Combined lb.	Gain in Weight for Period, lb.	Feed Consumed Each Week (Mash and Grain), lb.	Total Cumulative Feed Required lb.	Successive Weekly Feed Required per Pound of Gain, lb.	Feed Required per Pound of Gain to Date, lb.
		0.11					
	1	0.22	0.11	0.17		1.5	1.5
	2	0.40	0.18	0.33	0.5	1.8	1.7
	3	0.60	0.2	0.5	1.0	2.5	2.0
	4	.90	0.3	0.8	1.8	2.7	2.3
1	Total	0.90	.79	1.8	1.8	2.3	2.3
	5	1.2	0.3	0.8	2.6	2.8	2.4
	6	1.6	0.4	1.1	3.7	2.8	2.5
	7	2.1	0.5	1.4	5.1	2.8	2.6
	8	2.6	0.5	1.4	6.5	2.8	2.6
2	Total	2.6	1.7	4.7	6.5	2.8	2.6
	9	3.2	0.6	1.6	8.1	2.8	2.6
	10	3.8	0.6	1.7	9.8	2.9	2.7
	11	4.5	0.7	2.1	11.9	3.0	2.7
	12	5.2	0.7	2.1	14.0	3.0	2.8
3	Total	5.2	2.6	7.5	14.0	2.9	2.8
	13	5.9	0.7	2.2	16.2	3.1	2.8
	14	6.6	0.7	2.4	18.6	3.4	2.9
	15	7.2	0.6	2.5	21.1	4.1	3.0
	16	7.8	0.6	2.7	23.8	4.5	3.1
4	Total	7.8	2.6	9.8	23.8	3.8	3.1
	17	8.4	0.6	3.0	26.3	5.0	3.2
	18	8.9	0.5	3.4	29.7	6.8	3.4
	19	9.3	0.4	3.8	33.5	9.5	3.7
	20	9.6	0.3	4.4	37.9	14.5	4.0
5	Total	9.6	1.8	14.6	37.9	8.1	4.0

(III) on woodland. The two free-running groups were later put on wheat stubble. The saving in food in both grassland and stubble was 40 per cent. The difference between the cultivated and woodland groups was of no importance.

The Michigan Station[51] reports that the inclusion of green feed, as alfalfa, lawn grass, or green oats in the ration, had little apparent influence on the rate of growth, feathering, or other features of development, but did result in a slight saving in the total feed cost in some instances. The Pennsylvania Station[70] obtained better weight and better market quality more rapidly with turkeys fed grass clippings artificially dried and soaked in water overnight than those allowed only dry forage.

The Kansas Station[71] found that restricting the diet to grain and young grass range a few weeks before marketing reduced the size somewhat but materially lowered the cost of production.

Turkeys have been reared successfully in confinement. The Michigan Station[72] reported that rearing in confinement to maturity was slightly more efficient than rearing in yards. Control of mortality from diseases and predators gave satisfactory results in cobblestone yards over a 7-year period. The Oklahoma Station[73] reported no difference between birds grown in complete confinement and those grown on Bermuda grass range. Feed consumption in the confined groups is usually greater than in the range groups. Feather picking might occur in confined groups, which might reduce the market quality of some of the turkeys. The North Dakota Station[74] reported somewhat better growth for the turkeys on range than for those kept in cages.

FEEDING AND MANAGING THE BREEDERS. A good hatching egg is a fertile egg that contains in the correct amounts all the protein, carbohydrates, fat, minerals, and vitamins; in fact, all the ingredients (except oxygen) that are necessary for life and growth of the embryo during the 28-day incubation period.

Breeders in confinement cannot lay eggs that contain all the food ingredients required by the embryo, unless these ingredients are supplied in the breeder ration. Breeders that have been confined and wintered on grain alone cannot be expected to produce good hatchable eggs until after a more complete ration has been supplied or until the spring grass, sunshine, bugs, and the like have enabled them to balance the ration for themselves.

The ration for growing poults may be continued through the winter and until about 30 to 60 days prior to the mating season, at which time a breeder ration should be substituted.

The Kansas Station[75] reported on restricting food intake during the nonlaying period, with free access to feed thereafter. Neither the number of eggs laid nor their hatchability was influenced by reducing the intake to 78 per cent of that of the free-choice group. Reducing the intake to 61 per cent, however, significantly reduced hatching power.

Although the date at which the breeders start laying depends largely on the influence of artificial lights and housing conditions, feed also hastens or retards this laying period, besides influencing the production and hatchability of the eggs and the livability of the poults.

A 12- to 14-hour day should be provided for the breeders by

the use of morning, afternoon, or morning and afternoon lights, depending upon the convenience of the operator. The lights should be started about 30 days prior to the desired production date.

When the breeders have been kept on a growing ration the breeder ration should be started about 30 days prior to the start of lay. When they have been roughed through the winter on grain alone, the breeder ration should be started 30 days earlier.

All feed should be hopper fed, and the hoppers and fountains should be kept on the wire-covered platforms. The feed should be in open hoppers before the birds at all times. Should the breeders tend to consume more grain than mash, the grain hoppers may be kept closed part of the time and opened at regular periods.

FEEDING AND MANAGING THE POULTS. Feed and water should be put in small feeders and fountains and placed before the poults when they are 36 to 48 hours old, or as soon as they are placed in the brooder house. Early feeding lessens the danger of the poults' eating litter and eliminates the trouble of teaching the poults to eat, provided the brooder house is maintained at a comfortable temperature and is free from drafts around the feeders and fountains. Hammond[76] reported that poults starved for 3 or 4 days had to be taught individually to eat after feed was available and that poults may fail to learn to eat or drink in the presence of other poults that are eating and drinking. He concluded that lack of water is the primary cause of loose, slimy gizzard linings that accompany early nonspecific mortality in turkey poults. Chilson and Patrick[77] concluded that turkey poults should be supplied with feed and water as soon after hatching as possible since withholding feed and water for 24, 48, and 72 hours after hatching resulted in 4.8, 11.5, and 29.3 per cent mortality respectively up to 12 weeks of age.

FEEDERS AND FOUNTAINS. Many different types of good commercial feeders and fountains, also homemade ones, are in use on turkey farms. The amount of feeder and fountain space, rather than the kind of feeder, is the important factor to consider. Fifteen feet of feeder space to 150 poults will permit 30 to 50 per cent of them to eat at one time during the first 4-week period. Not more than 150 poults should be brooded in a 10- by 12-foot compartment or under one hover. However, lack of feeder and fountain space is as serious a brooding fault as crowded brooder houses.

FINISHING TURKEYS. The poults that have been properly

grown on a full and well-balanced ration will usually need little or no extra fattening to get them ready for the market. Turkeys that have been merely maintained during the growing season and then fattened rapidly just prior to the time of marketing lack the tenderness, juiciness, and excellent flavor of a rapidly grown bird. Turkeys that will not fatten or finish properly until practically full grown are the slow-maturing kind that should be eliminated from the flock by the proper selection of breeders.

The North Dakota Station[78] reported that broad-breasted turkeys marketed at 28 weeks of age after an 8-week finishing period were in satisfactory market condition. Use of a moist mash twice daily made considerable extra work not warranted by returns. Feeding of the grower mash with the whole grains fed separately produced the heavier males and females after 8 weeks of finishing and at the lowest feed cost per pound of gain.

Fish products affect the flavor. Bryant and Stevenson[79] reported that fishy flavor was detected in the roasted carcasses of turkeys receiving 10 per cent or more of fish meal. Fishy flavor was eliminated within 7 weeks after the 10 per cent level of fish meal feeding was discontinued and within 8 weeks after the 20 per cent level was discontinued. The drippings had a more pronounced fishy flavor than did the meat, and male birds exhibited a slightly stronger fishy flavor than females. The Pennsylvania Station[80] also reported fishy flavor and odor in the roasted carcasses of turkeys 28 weeks old, fed either 1 per cent of cod liver oil or 10 per cent of fish meal. The removal of both cod liver oil and fish meal from the diet 8 weeks prior to slaughtering time practically eliminated the occurrence of both fishy flavor and odor. The California Station[81] reported that high-grade fish meal, at a level of 25 per cent of the entire ration, did not apparently produce an off flavor when the birds were properly handled. When the birds were not starved before killing and were kept in a warm room overnight, the flavor was adversely affected, and, when so treated, birds fed inferior fish meals had a poorer flavor than birds fed a high-grade fish meal. Birds fed 2 to 5 per cent of fish oil showed an off flavor and odor when cooked. Marsden and coworkers[82] found that fishy off-flavors persisted 4 to 13 weeks after turkeys were removed from starting diets. They recommend that the feeding of fish meals and oils in turkey starting diets be restricted in quantities and that fish products be excluded from growing diets.

TURKEY RATIONS

It is possible to formulate many rations which will be satisfactory. Some of the representative turkey rations being recommended will be found in the Appendix. (See page 586.)

REFERENCES

1. Hayes. J. B., and G. E. Annin. Raising turkeys in Wisconsin. Wis. Circ. 231. 1929
2. Scott, M. L. Poult, chick rations differ. Yearbook 1950-51. Poultry Improvement Board of New York. 72.
   Scott, M. L. G. F. Heuser, and L. C. Norris. Energy, protein, and unidentified vitamins in poult nutrition. Poultry Sci. 27:773. 1948.
3. Rept. Agr. Exp. Sta. Univ. Calif. 1929-1930:91.
4. Funk, E. M. Rate of growth in Bronze and White Holland turkeys. Poultry Sci. 9:343. 1930.
5. Funk, E. M., and P. H. Margolf. Feed consumption and costs in raising turkeys. Pa. Bul. 250. 1932.
6. Learmouth, R. Milk in the feeding of poults. Jour. Am. Vet. Med. Assn. 79:206. 1931.
   Moore, J. M. Feeding different amounts of protein to growing turkeys. Mich. Quart. Bul. 14:148. 1932.
   Smith, E. Y., and L. E. Weaver. Turkeys. Cornell Ext. Bul. 359. 1936.
   Mussehl, F. E., and C. W. Ackerson. Protein requirements for finishing turkeys. Neb. Bul. 298. 1936.
   Macdonald, A. J. Turkey rearing experiment, 1937. Harper Adams Utility Poultry Jour. 23(7):207. 1938.
   Headley, F. B., and E. W. Knight. Turkey feeding experiments. Nev. Bul. 148. 1938.
   Roberts, R. E. Levels of protein in rations for young turkeys. I. Starting rations—first twelve weeks. II. Growing rations—after twelve weeks. Ind. Bul. 448. 1940.
   Mussehl, F. E., C. W. Ackerson, and R. H. Thayer. Protein utilization by the growing poult. Poultry Sci. 20:469. 1941.
   Fritz, J. C., J. L. Halpin, and J. H. Hooper. Studies on the nutritional requirements of poults. Poultry Sci. 26:78. 1947.
   Roberts, R. E. Effect of high- and low-protein starting rations on subsequent growth of turkeys. Purdue Univ. Agr. Exp. Sta. 60th Ann. Rept. 1947: 48.
   Almquist, H. J. Protein requirements of growing turkeys. Feedstuffs 24:44. 1952.
   Ackerson, C. W., and F. E. Mussehl. The utilization of food elements by growing poults. 2. A comparison of diets containing 25 and 30 per cent protein. Poultry Sci. 32:958. 1953.

7. Carver, J. S., E. I. Robertson, and J. W. Cook. Effects of methods of feeding on growth and finishing of Bronze turkeys. Wash. Bul. 368:69. 1938.

Carver, J. S., L. A. Wilhelm, and J. W. Cook. Methods of feeding turkeys. Wash. Bul. 356. 1938.

Draper, C. I., R. J. Evans, M. Rhian, and A. W. Brant. Protein requirements of Broad Breasted Bronze turkeys. Wash. V. Circ. 14. 1943.

8. Hammond, J. C., and S. J. Marsden. The effect of the level of the protein intake on the growth and feed utilization of turkeys. Poultry Sci. 18:11. 1939.

9. Kratzer, F. H., F. H. Bird, V. S. Asmundson, and S. Lepkovsky. The arginine requirement of young turkey poults. Jour. Nutr. 34: 167. 1947.

10. Kratzer, F. H., D. E. Williams, and Blanche Marshall. The sulfur amino acid requirements of turkey poults. Jour. Nutr. 37:377. 1949.

11. Fritz, J. C., J. H. Hooper, J. L. Halpin, and H. P. Moore. Failure of feather pigmentation in bronze poults due to lysine deficiency. Jour. Nutr. 31:387. 1946.

Grau, C. R., F. H. Kratzer, and V. S. Asmundson. The lysine requirements of poults and chicks. Poultry Sci. 25:529. 1946.

Kratzer, F. H., D. E. Williams, and Blanche Marshall. The relation of lysine and protein level in the ration to the development of feather pigment in turkey poults. Poultry Sci. 29:285. 1950.

Slinger, S. J., K. M. Gartley, W. F. Pepper, and D. C. Hill. The influence of animal protein factor supplements and antibiotics on the incidence and severity of white feathers in turkeys. Jour. Nutr. 43:345. 1951.

12. Baldini, J. T., H. R. Rosenberg, and J. Waddell. Low-protein diets for the turkey poult. Poultry Sci. 32:888. 1953.

13. Kratzer, F. H., and D. Williams. The glycine requirement of young poults. Jour. Nutr. 35:315. 1948.

14. Bird, F. H. The tryptophane requirement of turkey poults. Poultry Sci. 29:737. 1950.

Kratzer, F. H., D. E. Williams, and Blanche Marshall. The tryptophane requirement of young turkey poults. Jour. Nutr. 43:223. 1951.

15. Hammond, J. C., H. E. McClure, and W. L. Kellogg. The minimum phosphorus requirements of growing turkeys. Poultry Sci. 23:239. 1944.

Fritz, J. C., J. H. Hooper, and H. P. Moore. Calcification in the poult. Poultry Sci. 24:324. 1945.

16. Mussehl, F. E., and C. W. Ackerson. Calcium and phosphorus requirements of growing turkeys. Poultry Sci. 14:147. 1935.

17. Motzok, I., and S. J. Slinger. Studies on the calcium and phosphorus requirements of Broad Breasted Bronze turkeys. Poultry Sci. 27:486. 1948.

Singsen, E. P., L. D. Matterson, and H. M. Scott. Phosphorus in poultry nutrition. III. The relationship between the source of the vitamin D and the utilization of cereal phosphorus by the poult. Jour. Nutr. 33:13. 1947.

Wilcox, R. A., C. W. Carlson, W. Kohlmeyer, and G. F. Gastler. Calcium and phosphorus requirements of poults fed purified diets. Poultry Sci. 32:1030. 1953.

18. Evans, R. J., E. I. Robertson, M. Rhian, and L. A. Wilhelm. Development of perosis in turkey poults and its prevention. Poultry Sci. 21:422. 1942.

Kozeff, Anna, E. P. Singsen, and L. D. Matterson. The relative effect of manganese, choline, and nicotinic acid deficiencies on growth rate and perosis in the turkey poult. Poultry Sci. 28:771. 1949.

19. Foss, J. O. Salt tolerance of turkey poults. N. Dak. Bimo. Bul. 4:7. 1941.

20. Kratzer, F. H. Vitamins for turkeys: nutritive requirements for adequate rations under continuing study. California Agric. 3(2): 15. 1949.

21. Sherwood, R. M. Vitamin A requirements of poultry. Seventh World's Poultry Congress Rept. 1939:123.

22. Poley, W. E., and W. C. Tully. The values of white corn and milk in growing turkeys. Poultry Sci. 14:311. 1935.

23. Hinshaw, W. R. A-avitaminosis of turkeys. Poultry Sci. 13:300. 1934.

24. Van Reen, R., M. W. Taylor, and W. C. Russell. The vitamin A requirement of the turkey poult fed a purified diet. Jour. Nutr. 43: 235. 1951.

Wharton, F. D., L. D. Matterson, H. M. Scott, and C. I. Bliss. The vitamin A requirement of growing turkeys. Jour. Nutr. 39:543. 1949.

25. Scott, H. M., J. S. Hughes, and H. W. Loy. Rickets in young turkeys. Poultry Sci. 11:177. 1932.

26. Baird, F. D., and D. J. Greene. The comparative vitamin D requirements of growing chicks, turkeys and pheasants. Poultry Sci. 14: 70. 1935.

27. Hammond, J. C. The vitamin D requirement of turkey poults. Poultry Sci. 20:204. 1941.

Carver, J. S., and M. Rhian. The vitamin D requirements of turkey poults. Poultry Sci. 21:260. 1942.

Fritz, J. C., J. H. Hooper, and H. P. Moore. Calcification in the poult. Poultry Sci. 24:324. 1945.

Olsson, N. Investigations on the vitamin D requirements of chicks, poults, ducklings, and goslings. Annals of the Royal Agr. Coll. of Sweden 16. 1949.

28. Murphy, R. R. Vitamin D requirements of turkeys are measured. In "Science for the farmer." Pa. Bul. 429:28. 1942.

29. Jukes, T. H., and T. D. Sanford. The vitamin D requirement of young turkeys. Jour. Nutr. 18:71. 1939.

Sanford, T. D., and T. H. Jukes. Further observations on the vitamin D requirement of turkey poults. Poultry Sci. 23:221. 1944.

30. Bird, H. R. Comparison of response of turkey poults and of chicks to different forms of vitamin D. Jour. Nutr. 27:377. 1944.

Boucher, R. V. Efficacy of vitamin D from different sources for turkeys. *Jour. Nutr.* 27:403. 1944.

Matterson, L. D., H. M. Scott, and E. P. Singsen. The influence of sources of phosphorus on the relative efficiency of vitamin D_3 and cod liver oil in promoting calcification in poults. *Jour. Nutr.* 31: 599.

McGinnis, J., and R. J. Evans. Response of turkey poults to vitamin D from different sources. *Poultry Sci.* 25:521. 1946.

31. Robertson, E. I., M. Rhian, and L. A. Wilhelm. Growth and calcification of Bronze turkey poults from hens fed different levels of vitamin D. *Poultry Sci.* 20:357. 1941.

32. Wilhelm, L. A., E. I. Robertson, and M. Rhian. The effect of the level of vitamin D on egg production and hatchability of Bronze turkey hens. *Poultry Sci.* 20:565. 1941.

33. Jensen, L. S., G. F. Heuser, M. L. Scott, and L. C. Norris. The effect of vitamin E and niacin in the nutrition of turkey breeder hens. *Poultry Sci.* 32:907. 1953.

34. Heuser, G. F. A preliminary report on the vitamin G requirement of turkeys. *Poultry Sci.* 14:376. 1935.

McGinnis, J., and J. S. Carver. The effect of riboflavin and biotin in the prevention of dermatitis and perosis in turkey poults. *Poultry Sci.* 26:364. 1947.

35. Jukes, T. H. The vitamin G requirements of young poults. *Poultry Sci.* 17:227. 1938.

36. Mussehl, F. E. Turkey production. *Neb. Rept.* 1928:34.

37. Boucher, R. V., H. Patrick, and H. C. Knandel. The riboflavin requirement of turkeys for hatchability and growth. *Poultry Sci.* 21: 466. 1942.

Patrick, H., M. I. Darrow, and C. L. Morgan. The role of riboflavin in turkey poult nutrition. *Poultry Sci.* 23:146. 1944.

Bird, F. H., V. S. Asmundson, F. H. Kratzer, and S. Lepkovsky. The comparative requirements of chicks and turkey poults for riboflavin. *Poultry Sci.* 25:47. 1946.

Jukes, T. H., E. L. R. Stokstad, and M. Belt. Deficiencies of certain vitamins as studied with turkey poults on a purified diet. *Jour. Nutr.* 33:1. 1947.

MacGregor, H. I., J. McGinnis, and J. S. Carver. The effect of different intakes of riboflavin on growth of Broad Breasted turkeys after 8 weeks of age. *Poultry Sci.* 27:675. 1948.

38. Bird, F. H., F. H. Kratzer, V. S. Asmundson, and S. Lepkovsky. Pyridoxine deficiency in turkeys. *Proc. Soc. Exp. Biol. and Med.* 52:44. 1943.

Kratzer, F. H., F. H. Bird, V. S. Asmundson, and S. Lepkovsky. The comparative pyridoxine requirements of chicks and turkey poults. *Poultry Sci.* 26:453. 1947.

39. Jukes, T. H. Prevention of perosis by choline. *Jour. Biol. Chem.* 134:789. 1940.

Jukes, T. H. Effect of choline and other supplements on perosis. *Jour. Nutr.* 20:445. 1940.

Jukes, T. H. Studies of perosis in turkeys. I. Experiments related to choline. *Poultry Sci.* 20:251. 1941.

Evans, R. J., M. Rhian, and C. I. Draper. Perosis in turkey poults and the choline content of their diets. Poultry Sci. 22:88. 1943.
Evans, R. J. Choline requirements of turkey poults. Poultry Sci. 22:266. 1943.
Singsen, E. P., L. D. Matterson, Anna Kozeff, and Lois Decker. The choline requirements of turkey breeders. Poultry Sci. 29: 780. 1950.
Gartley, K. M., S. J. Slinger, A. M. Morphet, and C. R. Cameron. The choline requirements of broadbreasted bronze turkeys in the presence of APF concentrates. Poultry Sci. 30:913. 1951.
40. Scott, M. L., G. F. Heuser, and L. C. Norris. Studies in turkey nutrition using a purified diet. Poultry Sci. 27:770. 1948.
Jukes, T. H., E. L. R. Stokstad, and M. Belt. Deficiencies of certain vitamins as studied with turkey poults on a purified diet. Jour. Nutr. 33:1. 1947.
Richardson, L. R., A. G. Hogan, and H. L. Kempster. The requirement of the turkey poult for vitamin B_c. Jour. Nutr. 30:151. 1945.
Russell, W. C., M. W. Taylor, and J. V. Derby, Jr. The folic acid requirement of turkey poults on a purified diet. Jour. Nutr. 34: 621. 1947.
Schweigert, B. S., H. L. German, P. B. Pearson, and R. M. Sherwood. Effect of the pteroylglutamic acid intake on the performance of turkeys and chickens. Jour. Nutr. 35:89. 1948.
41. Briggs, G. M. Nicotinic acid deficiency in turkey poults and the occurrence of perosis. Jour. Nutr. 31:79. 1946.
Jukes, T. H., E. L. R. Stokstad, and M. Belt. Deficiencies of certain vitamins as studied with turkey poults on a purified diet. Jour. Nutr. 33:1. 1947.
Koseff, Anna, E. P. Singsen, and L. D. Matterson. The relative effect of manganese, choline, and nicotinic acid deficiencies on growth rate and perosis in the turkey poult. Poultry Sci. 28:771. 1949.
Lance, B. G., and A. G. Hogan. Vitamin B_c, inositol and nicotinic acid in the nutrition of the turkey. Jour. Nutr. 36:369. 1948.
Slinger, S. J., W. F. Pepper, A. M. Morphet, and E. V. Evans. Effect of penicillin on the niacin requirement of turkeys and a carry-over effect of penicillin from dams to progeny. Poultry Sci. 32:754. 1953.
42. Kratzer, F. H., and D. Williams. The pantothenic acid requirement of poults for early growth. Poultry Sci. 27:518. 1948.
43. Patrick, H., R. V. Boucher, R. A. Dutcher, and H. C. Knandel. Biotin and prevention of dermatitis in turkey poults. Proc. Soc. Expt. Biol. and Med. 48:456. 1941.
44. Sherwood, D. H. Studies with corn-soy type rations for starting turkey poults. Dissertation (Publ. 4351) Univ. of Minn. 1952.
45. Scott, M. L. Studies on the enlarged hock disorder in turkeys. Evidence of the detrimental effect of fish liver oil and the beneficial effect of dried brewers' yeast and other materials. Poultry Sci. 30:846. 1951.
Scott, M. L. Effect of dried distillers' solubles, whey, and lactose upon the enlarged hock disorder. Poultry Sci. 31:175. 1952.

46. Almquist, H. J., and J. B. Merritt. Effect of fiber level in mash on gain and economy of Beltsville White turkeys. Poultry Sci. 32:548. 1953.

Dymsza, H., R. V. Boucher, and M. G. McCartney. Response of growing turkeys to variations in the fiber and energy content of mash and pelleted diets. Poultry Sci. 32:898. 1953.

Goff, O. E. Observations of turkey poults receiving rations varying in fiber content. Okla. Rept. 1932-1934:138.

Goff, O. E. Observations of Bronze turkey poults receiving rations varying in fiber content. Poultry Sci. 13:295. 1934.

47. Recommended nutrient allowances for domestic animals. No. 1. Recommended nutrient allowances for poultry. Rept. Com. on Animal Nutr. National Research Council. Washington. 1944. Revised Mar., 1950.

Nutrient requirements for domestic animals. Number 1. Nutrient requirements of poultry. Rept. Comm. Animal Nutrition, National Research Council., Washington, D. C., 1954. Pub. 301.

48. Poley, W. E., and W. O. Wilson. Cereal grains in turkey rations. S. Dak. Bul. 330. 1939.

Carlson, C. W., and W. Kohlmeyer. Oats for growing turkeys. S. Dakota Farm & Home Research III(2):42. 1952.

49. Goodearl, G. P., and F. E. Moore. Turkey feeding. I. Proso millet—a substitute for yellow corn in the ration for growing turkeys. N. Dak. Bul. 303. 1941.

Goodearl, G. P. Millet feeding for turkeys. N. Dak. Bimo. Bul. 1(5):3. 1939.

50. Wilson, W. O., and W. E. Poley. Turkeying-off sorghums and proso. S. Dak. Circ. 38. 1942.

51. Barrett, F. N., C. G. Card, and A. Berridge. Feeding and confinement rearing experiment with turkeys during 1938. Mich. Quart. Bul. 22(2):79. 1939.

Barrett, F. N., C. G. Card, and A. Berridge. Feeding and confinement rearing experiment with turkeys during 1939. Mich. Quart. Bul. 23(2):85. 1940.

Barrett, F. N., C. G. Card, and A. Berridge. Feeding and confinement rearing experiment with turkeys during 1943. Mich. Quart. Bul. 27:169. 1944.

52. Robertson, E. I., J. S. Carver, and J. W. Cook. Finishing rations for turkeys. Wash. Bul. 372. 1939.

53. Gish, C. L. Feeding cereal grains to growing turkeys. National Collegiate Poultry Club News Letter, Kansas State Edition. Jan., 1948.

Payne, L. F., and A. B. Erhart. A study of animal versus plant protein, restricted diets after 18 and 20 weeks of age and finished condition of Bronze and Beltsville White turkeys at 28 and 24 weeks of age as related to economic production. Kansas Agr. Exp. Sta. C-Form 33, Oct., 1951.

54. North, M. O. Influence of cereal grains upon quality of meat in turkeys. Wyo. Bul. 248. 1941.

North, M. O. The influence of protein concentrates upon the quality of meat in turkeys. Wyo. Bul. 264. 1943.

55. Alder, B. Economical turkey production in Utah. Utah Agr. Exp. Sta. Mimeo Service No. 323. 1946.
56. Kratzer, F. H., and D. E. Williams. Raisins for turkeys fed at will with no harmful effects on growth and quality. California Agric. 5:13. Apr., 1951.
57. Hunter, J. E., D. R. Marble, and H. C. Knandel. Vegetable protein in turkey rations. Pa. Bul. 321. 1935.
Headley, F. B., and E. W. Knight. Turkey feeding experiments. Nev. Bul. 148. 1938.
Funk, E. M., and H. L. Kempster. The use of vegetable protein concentrates for raising turkeys. Mo. Bul. 414. 1940.
Headley, F. B. The effect of substituting vegetable protein for meat protein in a ration for growing turkeys. Nev. Bul. 168. 1944.
Brant, A. W., C. I. Draper, and R. J. Evans. Growing turkeys on rations low in animal protein. Wash. Bul. 441. 1944.
Hammond, J. C., S. K. Haynes, S. J. Marsden, and H. W. Titus. Vegetable protein diets for turkeys. Poultry Sci. 23:105. 1944.
58. Wilgus, H. S., Jr. Common laying rations without supplement may not be sufficient for breeder turkeys. Colo. Farm Bul. 1939:16.
59. Barrett, F. N., C. G. Card, and A. Berridge. Summary of feeding and confinement rearing experiment with turkeys during 1935. Mich. Sta. Quart. Bul. 19:24. 1936.
60. Slinger, S. J., J. J. Macilraith, and E. V. Evans. The use of crystalline riboflavin and of supplementary choline in starting and growing rations for turkeys. Poultry Sci. 25:628. 1946.
61. Milby, T. T., and R. Penquite. Feeding grasshoppers to turkeys. Poultry Sci. 18:407. 1939.
Milby, T. T., and R. Penquite. Feeding grasshoppers to turkeys. Poultry Sci. 19:332. 1940.
McHargue, J. S. A study of the proteins of certain insects with reference to their value as food for poultry. Jour. Agr. Res. 10: 633. 1917.
Wickware, A. B. Grasshoppers. A potential danger to turkeys. Canadian Jour. Comp. Med. and Vet. Sci. 9:80. 1945.
62. Couch, J. R., H. L. German, L. E. James, and R. M. Sherwood. Coarsely ground oats versus finely pulverized oats for young turkeys. Poultry Sci. 26:176. 1946.
63. Slinger, S. J., A. M. Morphet, E. C. Hunt, and W. F. Pepper. Effect of penicillin on the reproductive performance of turkeys. Poultry Sci. 32:660. 1953.
64. Scott, M. L., Growth rate and feed consumption of Broad Breasted Bronze and Beltsville Small White turkeys. Cornell Ext. Stencil 200. Revised Dec. 1953.
65. Payne, L. F., T. B. Avery, and D. C. Warren. Mash versus pellets for feeding growing turkeys. Kansas Agr. Exp. Sta. 13th Biennial Rept. 53. 1946.
66. Slinger, S. J., K. M. Gartley, and E. V. Evans. Pelleted and unpelleted diets high in dehydrated green feeds for turkeys grown in confinement. Poultry Sci. 28:556. 1949.
67. Robertson, E. I., and L. A. Wilhelm. Concentrate feeding of broad breasted Bronze turkeys. U. S. Egg and Poultry Mag. 46:597. 1940.

Robertson, E. I., and J. S. Carver. Concentrate feeding of turkeys. Wash. Bul. 402. 1941.
68. Funk, E. M. Protein content of concentrates for turkeys. Mo. Bul. 471. 1943.
69. Westermarck, N. Ueber des Weidefüttern der Puten. Maatalousr. Aikakauskirja 8:183. 1936. (Reference in Züchtungskunde 1937.)
70. Margolf, P. H. Turkeys fed grass clippings gain weight more rapidly and are marketable sooner. Pa. Sta. Bul. 463, Supp. 3:2. 1945.
71. Payne, L. F., and A. B. Erhart. A study of animal versus plant protein, restricted diets after 18 and 20 weeks of age, and finished condition of Bronze and Beltsville White turkeys at 28 and 24 weeks of age as related to economic production. Kansas Agr. Exp. Sta. C-Form 33. Oct., 1951.
72. Barrett, F. N., C. G. Card, and A. Berridge. Feeding and confinement rearing experiment with turkeys during 1942. Mich. Quart. Bul. 26(2):134. 1943.
73. Milby, T. T., and R. B. Thompson. Limited range for growing turkeys. Poultry Sci. 21:243. 1942.
74. Goodearl, G. F. Selection of feeds by growing turkeys. North Dak. Bul. 335:19. 1945.
75. Scott, H. M., and L. F. Payne. The influence of restricted food intake on the reproductive performance of breeding turkeys. Poultry Sci. 20:395. 1941.
76. Hammond, J. C. Lack of water a cause of loose, slimy gizzard linings accompanying early mortality in poults. Poultry Sci. 23: 477. 1944.
77. Chilson, W. T., and H. Patrick. Effect of withholding feed and water on early poult mortality and growth. Poultry Sci. 25:86. 1946.
78. Goodearl, G. P. Feeding turkeys for market finish. N. Dak. Bul. 328. 1943.
79. Bryant, R. L., and G. T. Stevenson. Fishy flavor in turkey meat caused by feeding menhaden fish meal. Va. Bul. 321. 1939.
80. Marble, D. R., J. E. Hunter, H. C. Knandel, and R. A. Dutcher. Fishy flavor and odor in turkey meat. Poultry Sci. 17:49. 1938.
81. Asmundson, V. S., T. H. Jukes, H. M. Fyler, and M. L. Maxwell. The effect of certain fish meals and fish oils in the ration on the flavor of the turkey. Poultry Sci. 17:147. 1938.
82. Marsden, S. J., L. M. Alexander, G. E. Schopmeyer, and J. C. Lamb. Starting diet as a factor in edible quality of turkey. Poultry Sci. 31:451. 1952.

CHAPTER 17

FEEDING WATERFOWL

FEEDING DUCKS

The rations for ducks are similar to rations for hens. This similarity applies particularly to the feeds that are used. However, ducks can make use of a larger amount of green feeds than hens, and fresh-cut greens can be fed if the flock does not get an abundance of green feed on range. It is not necessary to furnish water for swimming, but the ducks make better use of their feed and are more contented if water is available at feeding and until the feed is eaten up.

METHODS OF FEEDING. Duck mashes have usually been fed moist. In this case, sufficient water should be added to cause the materials to stick together, but the feed should never be so wet as to be sloppy. Since ducks seem to prefer a sticky mash, low-grade flour or similar feeds are frequently added to make the mixture more sticky.

In comparing methods of feeding ducks, the Indiana Station[1] produced satisfactory gains when an all-mash chick starting ration was fed ad libitum to ducklings as a dry mash. The same ration fed as a moist mash four times daily gave only a slight increase over the dry mash. When the ration was fed as a moist mash ad libitum, it apparently produced a significant increase in the rate of growth as compared to the other two methods of feeding.

Of five methods of feeding ducklings in the Philippines[2] it was observed that the best method was giving them uncooked mash and allowing them free access to all the green feed they would eat. Cooking the mash increased the amount of feed consumed. The addition of green food reduced the amount of feed consumed.

In recent years, the use of pellets has increased for duck feeding. This method simplifies the feeding very considerably since the pellets are fed in pans, troughs, or hoppers, and the birds are allowed to eat what they care to. The pellets are usually made available at all times, and fresh water is supplied continuously. The pellets are usually the same composition as the regular mash mixture. The results are practically the same as with wet-mash feeding. In comparing pellets versus wet mash for table duck production, experiments conducted in England[3] showed in one case that slightly greater final weights were obtained from the mash-fed ducklings whereas in another trial the ducklings reared on pellets were heavier than those reared on mash.

At Cornell[4] feeding pellets to ducklings resulted in the highest average weight. Following the pellet-fed ducks in order were the ducklings getting dry mash ad libitum supplemented with 3 wet mash feedings daily, dry mash ad libitum, wet mash ad libitum, and wet mash fed four times daily.

FEEDS. The feeds commonly given to chickens are also given to ducks.

Animal feeds seem to be particularly adapted to the feeding of ducks. It has been reported[5] that even such forms of animal food as scales of fish, which are digested only with great difficulty by other animals, are digested by ducks in a very short space of time.

Horton[6] reported that a ration containing milk produced a market duckling of better quality than a ration without milk. In experiments reported from Germany[7] a combination of fish meal and soybean oil meal gave better results than sour skim-milk curd. Roberts[8] concluded that an all-mash ration containing 10 per cent of meat and bone scraps and 5 per cent of dried milk fed ad libitum as a dry mash proved satisfactory for growing ducks during the first 10 weeks. This combination was superior to 10 per cent of meat scraps with no milk. There seemed to be little to be gained by using more than 10 per cent of meat scraps in combination with 5 per cent of dried milk in this type of ration.

In rations for egg production, it was shown in experiments conducted in the Philippines[9] that 30 per cent of fish meal in the ration gave a better egg yield than either 20 per cent or 50 per cent. Mortality was excessive at the higher levels of fish meal, but the 20 per cent level was considered most economical. For growing ducklings 30 per cent of fish meal as the only protein supplement in the ration was found to be optimal. Weight increase, mortality, and feather development were adversely affected when higher or lower percentages were used. Experiments reported from England[10] showed no significant difference in the egg production of ducks receiving fish meal or meat and bone meal, but because the latter was lower in price it was more economical.

Weight for weight, fish meal was reported as being greatly superior to shrimp meal as a protein supplement for laying ducks.[11] The rations containing 40 per cent shrimp meal proved slightly superior to those containing 30 per cent fish meal only as to percentage of egg production, but such rations were too expensive owing to the higher price of the shrimp meal.

Substitution of copra meal[12] for fish meal in standard rations for laying ducks proved detrimental to egg production. The health of the birds did not suffer, but there was a decreased food consumption when the copra meal was fed. Soybean meal has been shown to be a satisfactory source of protein for ducks.[13]

Egg production was maintained at a fairly high level in groups of ducks receiving a ration in which 50 per cent of the dry matter was provided by town food waste, or by equivalent parts of town food waste and steamed potatoes.[14] Difficulty was experienced with higher levels of substitution because of the very bulky nature of the rations.

At Cornell[15] potato meal was substituted for corn meal and wheat standard middlings or a combination of these feeds. Thirty per cent of potato meal was the maximum amount that could be fed.

GROWTH AND FOOD CONSUMPTION. Ducklings make very rapid gains early in life. Green ducks or fancy ducklings can be fed so that they will weigh about 6 pounds in 8 to 9 weeks.

The growth rates and feed consumption for White Pekin ducklings given in Table 33 were obtained by Heuser and associates.[15]

The average rate of growth and weekly consumption of feed

TABLE 33. GROWTH RATE AND FEED CONSUMPTION OF WHITE PEKIN DUCKLINGS

Week	Average Weight Per Duckling, lbs.	Cumulative Feed Consumption Per Duckling, lbs.	Amount of Feed to Produce 1 Pound of Duck, lbs.
When hatched	.133	——	——
1	.334	.28	.84
2	1.01	1.17	1.16
3	1.64	3.17	1.93
4	2.53	5.72	2.26
5	3.32	8.54	2.57
6	4.42	11.75	2.66
7	5.31	14.96	2.82
8	6.08	18.69	3.07
9	6.62	23.06	3.48

per duckling of different breeds of ducks up to 12 weeks of age have been reported by Elford[16] as follows:

Breed	Average Weight, lb.	Feed Consumed, lb.
Pekins	7.09	28.03
Rouens	5.98	28.00
White Muscovies	5.09	24.97
Colored Muscovies	5.73	21.91
Indian Runners	4.07	29.40
Khaki Campbells	4.13	23.46

FEEDING DUCKLINGS

REQUIREMENTS. Relatively few experimental results are available dealing with the nutritive requirements of ducks.

Protein. Horton[17] reported that a well-balanced 19 per cent protein chick mash to which approximately 10 per cent of flour was added was satisfactory for growing White Pekin ducklings. He further stated that they could be grown successfully on a low-protein mash but that the total feed consumption was greater and the cost of feed was higher. Hamlyn, Branion, and Cavers[18] reported that a total protein level of about 25 per cent is approaching an excess of this nutrient in a ration for growing ducks and the optimum protein level would seem to be about 18 per cent or less. In comparing a 17 per cent ration with one containing 14 per cent of protein, Miller[13] showed slight differences in weight during the growing period between the high- and low-protein groups. Scott and Heuser[19] produced satisfactory gains in ducklings to 8 weeks of age on a ration containing approximately 15 per cent of protein. However, there was some indication of a slight advantage in early growth for rations containing 17 per cent or more of protein.

Demers and Bernard[20] concluded that in the presence of 0.4 per cent cystine, approximately 0.5 per cent methionine is required for normal growth.

Vitamins. Reporting on the vitamin D requirements of ducklings, Fritz, Archer, and Barker[21] concluded that the vitamin D requirements of White Pekin ducklings are approximately the same as those of chicks and that 30 A.O.A.C. (22.5 International) chick units of vitamin D per 100 grams of feed will produce optimum calcification. Motzok and associates[22] conclude that the vitamin D requirement of ducklings appears to be between 30 and 40 A.O.A.C. (22.5 and 30 International) chick units per 100 grams of ration. Olsson[23] places the requirement at 80 A.O.A.C. (60 International) chick units per 100 grams of feed.

Hegsted[24] reported the symptoms of niacin deficiency as lack of growth, diarrhea, and general weakness, indicating a requirement of 2.5 milligrams of niacin per 100 grams of ration. Results at Cornell[25] showed that a bowed leg disorder in ducklings was entirely prevented by supplementing the diet with 5 to 7.5 per cent of dried brewers' yeast or by adding 10 milligrams of synthetic niacin per pound of ration. Satisfactory growth was obtained with the addition of 3.8 per cent of dried brewers' yeast or 5 milligrams of synthetic niacin per pound of ration.

Other water soluble[26] vitamins are also necessary. The riboflavin requirement of ducklings has been reported as being 300 to 400 micrograms per 100 grams of diet, the pantothenic acid requirement as 1100 micrograms per 100 grams of diet, and the pyridoxine requirement as 250 micrograms per 100 grams of ration. Neither riboflavin nor pantothenic acid deficiencies produce characteristic symptoms. Pyridoxine deficiency is characterized by growth failure and anemia in young ducklings and also convulsions and paralysis in older ducklings. Biotin is required by the duck, but the only effect of a deficiency is very poor growth.

Scott and Heuser[19] concluded that dried skimmilk and dried brewers' yeast contain some unidentified factor or factors of importance in the nutrition of ducklings.

Minerals. Bernard and Demers[27] concluded that 15 parts per million of manganese in the ration was sufficient to prevent perosis in ducklings but that it required 60 parts per million to bring the alkaline phosphatase activity of blood serum near normal values. Van Reen and Pearson[28] indicate the magnesium requirement as being 50 milligrams per 100 grams of diet.

Fiber. Serfontein[29] reported that for ducklings a ration which was low in fiber produced the highest average weight at 10 weeks. Although growth after the age of 4 weeks was apparently not much affected by the high percentage of fiber, it appeared to be best to feed a ration low in fiber throughout the growing period.

As a summary of available information the Committee on Animal Nutrition of the National Research Council[28a] recommends the tabulated nutrient requirements for ducks on the next page.

Feeding Management. Ducklings are usually fed within 36 hours after the hatch is completed or as soon as they are placed in the brooder house.

If crumbly wet mash is fed, it is given four or five times a

NUTRIENT REQUIREMENTS* OF DUCKS

	Starting and Growing Ducks
Total protein, %	17
Vitamins	
Vitamin D (I.C.U.)†	100
Riboflavin, mg.	1.8
Pantothenic acid, mg.	5.0
Niacin, mg.	25.0
Pyridoxine hydrochloride, mg.	1.2

*In percentage or amount per pound of feed.
†International chick unit.

day during the first week or two. Later the number of feedings is reduced to three or four.

Fresh drinking water should be provided at each feeding period. The fountains should be arranged so that the ducklings can submerge their bills in the water but cannot get into it to wet their bodies. This permits them to drink and also allows them to clean their nostrils by squirting water through them. Any wet mash left over after the ducklings have had their fill should be removed. Sand or grit should be kept before them at all times.

If pellets are fed they are kept before the ducklings all the time, with a plentiful water supply available.

Chopped fresh green feed or cooked vegetables are often used in the ration for ducklings, as well as for older ducks. No grain is fed to ducks grown for market. In developing ducks for egg production, grain is sometimes fed at night after they are 4 months old.

Enough feeding space should be provided for the ducks to eat without crowding. Ducks should be fed only what they will clean up in 20 minutes, when the wet mash system of feeding is used.

FATTENING. When fattening or finishing of the ducklings is carried on it is usually done 2 to 3 weeks before marketing. A heavy daily feed consumption is necessary during the fattening period. During this period it is best to give a light noon feeding and then a heavy feeding at night. Fattening ducks require less range than growing ducks, and it is advisable to have the source of drinking water near the feed trays for heavy ducks.

FEEDING AND MANAGEMENT OF YOUNG BREEDERS. From the time ducklings are selected as breeders, at about 8 weeks of age, until the breeding season begins, every effort should be made to develop and condition them for egg production. Both drakes and ducks should be fed pellets or given a good growing mash, mixed grain, and green foods. It is highly desirable to run them on pasture if it is available. About equal parts of mash and grain may be fed. They should complete their growth after they molt and reach the laying stage in good-bodied flesh. About a month or 6 weeks before eggs for hatching are desired, a breeding ration should be substituted for the growing ration. The same method should be followed with the laying type of ducks, such as the Indian Runner.

FEEDING THE MATURE DUCKS. The rations for laying ducks are similar to rations for hens. The breeders should have a breeder ration. If pellets are not fed, the mash part of the ration is moistened and the ducks are given all the wet mash they will eat morning and night. This wet mash should be neither too crumbly nor too wet but of such a consistency that it will hold together when squeezed with the hand or, if dropped, will fall apart in lumps. A mixture of grain is usually fed in addition to wet mash. In England it is customary to feed laying ducks a hard grain in the water trough. About two parts of mash are fed to one part of grain. Oystershell or high-grade limestone grit should be supplied to provide calcium for eggshell formation. In addition, granite grit or gravel should be available in each pen.

Feed is usually given twice a day, with a light feeding in the morning (10 minutes) and a heavy feeding at night (20 minutes). The drinking water should be near the troughs. The average daily feed consumption for about 200 ducks is 100 pounds of feed, of which 40 pounds should be fed in the morning and 60 pounds at night.

Considerable attention has been given to the breeding and management of ducks in England. At the Harper Adams College laying trials an average egg production of about 250 eggs per duck has been obtained. The feeding method employed was as follows.[30] The first feed is given when the ducks are being released from the trapnest. It consists of 1 ounce of grain per duck, given in the water trough. The second feed, given at 11 A.M., is wet mash, the quantity allowed being rather less than one-half of the total daily mash ration. The third feed, given in the afternoon, is the rest of the mash and also 1 ounce of grain placed in the water trough as in the morning. Each duck therefore receives about 2 ounces of grain and 4 ounces of mash daily.

RATIONS FOR DUCKS. Some rations that have been recommended for ducks will be found in the Appendix. (See page 609.)

FEEDING GEESE

Geese are generally reared where they have a good grass range or pasture as they are good grazers and, except during the winter months, usually pick up most of their living. They are not adapted to intensive conditions.

FEEDING THE ADULT GEESE. The pasture may be supplemented with light feedings of home-grown grains or wet mash daily, the necessity and quantity of this feed depending on the condition of the pasture.

During the winter, when pasture is not available, geese should have both grain and roughage, but great care should be taken not to overfeed the breeders so that they will become fat. Oats make a desirable grain feed for breeding geese, but a limited portion of corn, wheat, or barley may be added for variety. The greater part of the feed should be made up of roughage such as vegetables, clover or alfalfa hay, chopped corn stover, or silage.

As the breeding season approaches, it is necessary to increase the quantity of feed and add to it a mash which is usually given in the morning. A good duck breeder or hen breeder mash can be fed. A simple mixture which has given satisfactory results is made up of 3 parts of wheat by-products, 1 part of corn meal, and 1 part of meat scrap. Buttermilk may be used in place of the meat scrap.

Grit and oystershells should be kept before the geese when they are laying and may be provided all the time to advantage. Drinking water, which should be available at all times, is best supplied in drinking fountains or vessels so constructed that the stock cannot get their feet into the water.

FEEDING THE GOSLINGS. Goslings do not need feed until they are 36 to 48 hours old, when they can be fed a chick or duckling ration. This can be fed as pellets or in the form of wet mash, or they can be fed stale bread soaked in milk or water, scalded cracked corn, or a mash made of 4 parts corn meal and 1 part middlings. Green grass should make up most of their feed, and only a very limited amount of grain should be used. Plenty of fresh clean drinking water should be supplied. After 2 or 3 weeks, if the goslings have plenty of grass, they will usually not need much other feed until fattening time.

If the goslings are confined the ration should include vitamin

D. Olsson[23, 31] indicates the requirement for goslings as 30 to 35 chick units per 100 grams of feed. Choline, folic acid, and nicotinic acid have been shown necessary for goslings fed purified diets.[32] Folic acid deficient geese showed cervical paralysis.

Experiments reported from England[33] showed that little advantage was gained by feeding concentrates to goslings throughout the growing period, provided they have free access to good grazing. The final weights of birds at 34 weeks of age that had received mash throughout the experimental period were only slightly greater than the average weights of those birds that had no supplementary feeding from the age of 5 weeks to 26 weeks and from 5 weeks to 30 weeks. All the birds were in good marketable condition at the end of the experiment. It was concluded that a satisfactory carcass could be produced without the use of concentrates from the age of 5 weeks until a month before marketing. On the other hand, it was reported[34] that confining the goslings and providing cut grass as a sole food was insufficient to promote a normal growth rate.

Geese can consume relatively larger quantities of potatoes than hens. It has been reported[35] that goslings, 2 to 3 months old, could eat 300 to 400 grams of potatoes per day. Potatoes can also be fed to adult geese, but care must be taken that they do not become too fat during the laying period.

PREPARING FOR MARKET. In the final fattening or finishing period grain is usually fed. Corn is commonly fed to geese for fattening. Sometimes corn on the cob is fed. The geese may be fattened on range or in pens.

One recommended method for pen fattening is to feed 3 times daily, 1 feed of a moist but not sloppy mash made up of 1/3 shorts and 2/3 corn meal and 2 feeds of corn with some oats or barley. Some roughage or vegetables should be provided.

Such feeds as dried sugar beets, molasses, and skimmilk have been used satisfactorily in fattening geese in Germany.[36]

Noodling Geese. The following method for noodling geese is described by Lee.[36] This method, which produces a much better-fattened goose than ordinary procedures but involves considerably more work, is to stuff large geese with noodles for 3 or 4 weeks. The feeders stuff the birds with noodles, usually beginning by feeding 3 to 5 noodles three times daily and gradually increasing to 6 or 7 noodles five times daily at 4-hour intervals. The noodles are made of scalded corn meal, ground oats, ground barley, and ground wheat or wheat flour, about equal parts of each being used. Add salt as for bread, thoroughly mix the feed, and put it through a sausage stuffer, cutting the product into pieces $2\frac{1}{2}$ or 3 inches long. Boil them 10 to 15 minutes, or until they float, in a wash boiler containing a wire rack which stands $1\frac{1}{2}$ inches above the bottom of the boiler. Dip the noodles in cold water and roll in flour to keep them from sticking together. Pour hot water over the noodles, just before they are fed, to make them slippery and keep them warm. The number of noodles fed depends on the size and condition of the bird and the judgment of the feeder. The noodles are put into the mouth, one at a time, and worked down by using the hands on the outside of the neck. At the next feeding time, if any feed can be felt in the crop, no noodles are given; otherwise the bird will go off its feed. Keep plenty of drinking water before the geese. This method of feeding involves a large amount of work and long hours but will produce a gain of 6 to 10 pounds. One effect of noodling is the production of enormous livers that in Europe have been used for making pate de foie gras.

REFERENCES

1. Roberts, R. E. Methods of feeding ducks. Poultry Sci. 13:338. 1934.
2. Ancheta, L. M. Observations on the influence of various methods of feeding ducklings. Philippine Agriculturist 29:262. 1940.
3. McMurray, M. Table poultry experiment, 1935. Table ducklings. Harper Adams Utility Poultry Jour. 20:495. 1934-1935.
   Tallent, V. K. Pellets vs. mash for table duck production. Harper Adams Utility Poultry Jour. 17:539. 1931-1932.
4. Heuser, G. F., and M. L. Scott. Studies in duck nutrition. I. Methods of feeding. Poultry Sci. 30:161. 1951.
5. Morstadt, E. Wie schnell verdauen Enten tierische Nahrungsmittel? Deutsche Landwirtschaftliche Geflügelzeitung 39. 1936.
6. Horton, D. H. The value of dried skimmilk in feeding ducklings. Poultry Item 36(8):5. 1934.
7. Bünger, H., A. Werner, and Brandenburg. Mastversuche mit Jungenten. Biedermanns Zentralblatt 5:140. 1933.
   Bünger, H., A. Werner, J. Schultz, H. Krüger, and J. Keseling. Mastversuche mit Jungenten. Biedermanns Zentralblatt 5:507. 1933.
8. Roberts, R. E. Levels of meat scraps and dried milk in rations for ducks. Poultry Sci. 15:136. 1936.
9. Castillo, J. V. Determination of the optimum amount of fish meal in rations for growing ducklings. Philippine Agriculturist 27:18. 1938.
   Fronda, F. M. Fish meal for growing ducklings. Philippine Agriculturist 27:18. 1938.

Fronda, F. M., and L. L. Mencias. The use of fish meal in duck rations for egg production. Philippine Agriculturist 26:290. 1937.
10. Tallent, V. K. A comparison of fish meal with meat and bone meal for laying ducks. Harper Adams Utility Poultry Jour. 18:350. 1932-1933.
11. Fronda, F. M., L. L. Mencias, and E. Basio. Effects of rations containing different amounts of shrimp meal on the egg production of ducks. Philippine Agriculturist 27:278. 1938.
12. Fronda, F. M., and E. Basio. Use of copra meal in duck rations for egg production. Philippine Agriculturist 27:173. 1938.
13. Miller, M. S. Progress report on the National Institute of Poultry Husbandry duck feeding experiment. Harper Adams Utility Poultry Jour. 18:600. 1933.
14. Wright, M. M., and F. J. Dudley. Feeding of town food waste and steamed potatoes to laying ducks. Harper Adams Utility Poultry Jour. 28:63. 1943.
15. Heuser, G. F., M. L. Scott, R. K. Eskew, and P. W. Edwards. Studies in duck nutrition. 3. The feeding of potatoes to ducks. Poultry Sci. 30:672. 1951.
16. Elford, F. C. Duck feeding experiments. Rept. Dominion Poultry Husbandman. (Ottawa, Canada.) 1925:49. 1926.
Elford, F. C. Duck feeding experiments. Rept. Dominion Poultry Husbandman. (Ottawa, Canada.) 1927:38. 1928.
17. Horton, D. H. A comparison of feeding a twelve per cent and a nineteen per cent protein ration to White Pekin ducklings. Poultry Sci. 11:106. 1932.
18. Hamlyn, W. L., H. D. Branion, and J. R. Cavers. The influence of protein on the growth of ducks. Poultry Sci. 13:333. 1934.
19. Scott, M. L., and G. F. Heuser. Studies in duck nutrition. II. Studies of protein and unidentified vitamin requirements. Poultry Sci. 30:164. 1951.
20. Demers, J. M., and R. Bernard. Further work on the nutrition of ducklings. A. Lipotropic factors. B. Sulphur amino acid requirements. Canadian Jour. Res. Sect. E. Med. Sci. 28:202. 1950.
21. Fritz, J. C., W. Archer, and D. Barker. Vitamin D requirements of ducklings. Poultry Sci. 20:151. 1941.
22. Motzok, I., and H. D. Branion. The vitamin D requirements of growing ducks. Poultry Sci. 27:482. 1948.
Motzok, I., W. D. Graham, H. D. Branion, and F. N. Slinger. The vitamin D requirement of ducklings. Poultry Sci. 25:298. 1946.
23. Olsson, N. Investigations on the vitamin D requirements of chicks, poults, ducklings, and goslings. Annals of the Royal Agr. Coll. of Sweden 16. 1949.
24. Hegsted, D. M. Nutritional studies with the duck. III. Niacin deficiency. Jour. Nutr. 32:467. 1946.
25. Heuser, G. F., and M. L. Scott. Studies in duck nutrition. 5. Bowed legs in ducks, a nutritional disorder. Poultry Sci. 32:137. 1953.
Scott, M. L., and G. F. Heuser. Studies in duck nutrition. 4. Bowed legs in ducks caused by niacin deficiency. Poultry Sci. 31:752. 1952.

26. Fritz, J. C., W. Archer, and D. Barker. Riboflavin requirements of ducklings. Poultry Sci. 18:449. 1939.

Hegsted, D. M., and R. L. Perry. Nutritional studies with the duck. V. Riboflavin and pantothenic acid requirements. Jour. Nutr. 35: 411. 1948.

Hegsted, D. M., and M. N. Rao. Nutritional studies with the duck. II. Pyridoxine deficiency. Jour. Nutr. 30:367. 1945.

Hegsted, D. M., and F. J. Stare. Nutritional studies with the duck. I. Purified rations for the duck. Jour. Nutr. 30:37. 1945.

27. Bernard, R., and J. M. Demers. Le manganese dans la nutrition du caneton (Pekin Blanc). Revue Canadienne de Biologie 11:147. 1952.

28. Van Reen, R., and P. B. Pearson. Magnesium deficiency in the duck. Jour. Nutr. 51:191. 1953.

28a. Nutrient requirements for domestic animals. Number 1. Nutrient requirements of poultry. Rept. Comm. Animal Nutrition, National Research Council, Washington, D. C., 1954. Pub. 301.

29. Serfontein, P. J. Feeding experiments with ducks. Farming in South Africa. Nov. 1943.

30. Hedges, T. The feeding and management of the laying duck. Harper Adams Utility Poultry Jour. 18:597. 1933.

31. Olsson, N. Undersökningar över gasungarnas behov av D-vitamin samt utprovning av en praktisk metod för uppfödning av gäss. Lantbr. Hogsk. Husdjurforsokanst. Meddel. 21:32. 1946.

32. Briggs, G. M., E. G. Hill, and T. H. Canfield. The need for choline, folic acid, and nicotinic acid by goslings fed purified diets. Poultry Sci. 32:678. 1953.

33. Wright, M. M., and F. J. Dudley. Rearing geese on grass alone and with supplementary feeding. Harper Adams Utility Poultry Jour. 27:135. 1942.

Wright, M. M., and F. J. Dudley. Rearing geese for the Christmas market on grass alone and with supplementary feeding. Harper Adams Utility Poultry Jour. 26:81. 1941.

34. Wright, M. M. An observation on the feeding of cut grass to goslings. Harper Adams Utility Poultry Jour. 27:117. 1941-1942.

35. Rabinovich, A. B. Potatoes in the food ration of goslings. Problemy Zhivotnovodstva 4-5:200. 1935.

Fangauf, R., and E. Kallman. Weidemast bei Enten, Gänsen, und Puten. Archiv für Geflügelk. 7:109. 1933.

Ferber, K. E., and M. Chodziesner. Junggänsemast mit Zuckerschnitzeln, Mellassemischfütter und Magermilch. Archiv für Geflügelk. 7:177. 1933.

36. Lee, A. R. Goose raising. U.S.D.A. Farmers' Bul. 767. 1931.

CHAPTER 18

FEEDING OTHER SPECIES OF BIRDS

GAME BIRDS

In general, game birds grow more rapidly than chickens. For that reason their requirements for many of the nutrients are higher. They have, therefore, made better growth response to rations containing higher amounts of protein, riboflavin, and vitamin D.

Formerly a large variety of rations, most of which were very complex, were fed game birds. In most cases, the rations also included special feeds or ingredients. Many game breeders considered it impossible to grow a bird except by using worms and other natural feeds, such as artificially produced larvae.

In recent years rations similar to those developed for the feeding of chickens and turkeys have also been fed game birds. There have also been made available by commercial feed companies feed mixtures designed particularly for certain species of game birds such as pheasants and quail.

In comparing the value of grains[1] for winter game feeding, it has been found that pheasants, quail, and partridge like yellow corn better than any other feed. Next in the order of consumption preference are wheat, scratch feed, and buckwheat, followed by white corn, popcorn, barley, sweet corn, and sudan grass seed. The smallest amounts consumed were sorghum seed, soybeans, oats, and rye.

PHEASANTS

It has been shown that it is possible to rear pheasants without resorting to complex rations or complicated systems of feeding. In fact, rations and methods similar to those for the rearing of chickens and turkeys have proved satisfactory. The pheasant chick resembles the chick in its response to energy and the animal protein factor.[2] It is necessary, of course, to adapt the ration to meet the particular nutritive requirements of the pheasant.

Requirements. The pheasant is a rapidly growing animal. It has been known to increase from a hatching weight of approximately 19 grams to an average weight of about 450 grams at 8 weeks of age, and nearly 700 grams at 12 weeks of age. Callenbach, Murphy, and Hiller[3] showed that better growth was obtained on a high-protein ration than on a lower-protein ration suitable for chicks of the domestic fowl. Later Callenbach and Hiller[4] reported best growth and feathering on a 28 per cent protein ration. Norris, Elmore, and Bump[5] obtainted maximum growth in ring-necked pheasant chicks during the first eight weeks of life by feeding a ration containing 30 per cent protein. Excellent growth, however, was also obtained on rations containing 21 per cent, 24 per cent, and 27 per cent protein. They concluded that, in practice, satisfactory growth without undue forcing will be obtained by feeding a ration containing 24 per cent protein. Skoglund[6] reported improved results for starting ring-necked pheasants by substituting soybean oil meal for part of the meat scrap and fish meal. Besides slower growth on low-protein rations, cannibalism and feather pulling have also been reported to be more prevalent in low-protein lots.

The pheasants also have a relatively high riboflavin requirement. Norris[7] concluded that the riboflavin requirement of pheasants during early growth was satisfied when approximately 4 per cent of dried pork liver was included in the ration, approximately twice the amount necessary for chicks. In a practical pheasant-rearing ration, approximately 20 per cent of dried skimmilk, or its equivalent in other riboflavin carriers, will be required to meet the requirements of pheasant chicks for this vitamin.

Baird and Greene[8] concluded that pheasants require a minimum of approximately 50 to 60 U.S.P. units of vitamin D per 100 grams of feed. This is approximately three times the quantity necessary to prevent the development of rickets in chicks.

The calcium requirement has been reported to be 1.5 per cent and the phosphorus requirement 0.75 per cent.[6] When meat scrap and fish meal are fed to supply the necessary high level of protein, perosis is frequently encountered because of the high calcium and phosphorus content of these ingredients. However, with a ration containing 35 parts per million of manganese no particular difficulty was experienced when the calcium was kept under 2.84 per cent and the phosphorus under 1.08 per cent.

Growth and Feed. Callenbach and Hiller[4] reported that it required 3.44 pounds of feed per bird up to 8 weeks of age and 6.77 pounds up to 12 weeks of age. Skoglund[6] indicates a requirement of 3.55 pounds per pheasant to 8 weeks of age.

Methods of Feeding. For the feeding of young pheasants, the all-mash method has proved satisfactory. The mash is kept constantly available in hoppers. Some feeders prefer to give moist mash to young pheasants. In some cases, commercial chick grain is also introduced after the birds are 3 to 4 weeks old. Callenbach and Hiller[4] reported that the free-choice or cafeteria system of feeding did not give satisfactory results. Pellets have also been fed.

Grit can be fed on top of the feed for the first few weeks, after which time it can be made available in hoppers. Fresh drinking water should also be given each day.

Mature birds are fed rations similar to those fed breeding hens, which usually consists of a grain mixture and a mash mixture. The mash might be fed as a dry mash or a wet mash in the morning. The grain is fed in the afternoon. Usually all the grain that the birds will clean up before dark is fed. Mash feeding is begun at least 3 weeks before the birds are likely to lay in order to get the body in condition for production. Mash feeding can be discontinued when eggs are no longer needed for hatching. The birds should also have access to medium-sized grit and oystershell and fresh water.

Rations. Some ready-mixed rations are available for pheasants which are compounded to meet the specific nutritive requirements of this species. Satisfactory results have also been reported in growing pheasants by using turkey-growing rations or by feeding chick starters supplemented with milk.

The following rations have also been reported as giving satisfactory growth.

Cornell.[2]

	Pounds
Yellow corn meal	21
Wheat standard middlings	14
Pulverized oats	10
Soybean oil meal	30
Fish meal	5
Meat scrap	5
Dried skimmilk	5
Dried brewers' yeast	4
Dried whey	2
Dicalcium phosphate	1
Ground limestone	1.5
Fish liver oil (2000 A, 400 D)	1.0
Salt	0.5
Manganese sulfate	0.025

Pennsylvania. (The Pennsylvania State College Department of Poultry Husbandry, State College, Pennsylvania, Stencil G 134, 1951.)

STARTING MASH FORMULAS FOR RING-NECKED PHEASANTS

	No. 1	No. 2
Ground yellow corn	100	170
Wheat flour middlings	100	100
Wheat bran	100	100
Ground oats	100	100
Alfalfa meal, low fiber	50	50
Dried whey	50	50
Brewers' dried yeast (1)	30	30
Meat scrap (not less than 50% protein)	30	120
Fish meal (not less than 55% protein)	20	30
Soybean oil meal	400	250
Steamed bonemeal	10	——
Ground limestone	10	——
Salt	5	5
Fish liver oil (400 A.O.A.C. units of D per gram) (2)	2.5	2.5
Anhydrous manganese sulfate (3)	.125	.125
	1007.625	1007.625

1. If necessary, a riboflavin concentrate composed of natural ingredients may be substituted for the brewers' yeast. A pound for pound substitution may be made if the riboflavin concentrate contains 35 micrograms of riboflavin per gram of concentrate. Adjustments can be made for concentrates of greater potency. If, for example, a product containing 70 micrograms per gram is used, 15 pounds in place of 30 pounds should be added and the ground yellow corn increased 15 pounds in the mash mixtures.

2. If desired, 0.5 pound of D-activated animal sterol, containing 2000 A.O.A.C. chick units of vitamin D per gram may be substituted for the fish liver oil provided good quality alfalfa meal is used.

If oil is used, it should be premixed with 50 pounds of the bran before adding to the other ingredients.

If D-activated animal sterol is used, it should be premixed with 50 pounds of the soybean oil meal before adding to the other ingredients.

3. The anhydrous manganese sulfate should be premixed with the ground limestone or salt before adding to the other ingredients.

GRAIN MIXTURE

200 lb.	coarse cracked yellow corn
100 lb.	whole wheat
50 lb.	whole oats
350 lb.	

Barley or buckwheat may be substituted for one-half the corn with satisfactory results.

FEEDING DIRECTIONS

Pheasant chicks should be placed in brooding quarters and fed as soon as they complete their "after-hatching" sleep. Such quarters should be amply provided with filled chick-size mash hoppers and water receptacles. For 1 or 2 days some mash should also be sprinkled on egg flats, small pieces of newspaper, or cardboard. Each feeding of mash should be lightly covered with a small amount of insoluble grit until such time as the chicks are able to feed from a regular grit and shell hopper. The grit is shiny and seems to attract the attention of the tiny chicks. This helps teach them to eat, as does a small amount of finely chopped green feed sprinkled on top of the mash. When the chicks eat mash readily, the green feed may be discontinued.

After the chicks are 6 to 8 weeks of age, oystershells (or a high calcium limestone grit) and insoluble grit should be constantly available in hoppers. At this time, scratch grain may also be fed although this practice may be delayed until the chicks are twelve weeks of age. The simplest way to feed the grain is to keep it constantly before the birds in hoppers. A lower protein mash, similar to the Pennsylvania State chick mash, may be used after the twelfth week.

Until 5 weeks of age, Ring-necked pheasants may be kept very closely confined with excellent results. Thereafter, if the chicks are confined too closely much difficulty will be experienced from feather picking and mortality from cannibalism may be near. A good grass pasture, such as provided by clover and timothy, alfalfa, or some other vegetation that furnishes shade and cover, will be most helpful in supplying food and shelter after the birds are 5 weeks of age.

QUAIL

In recent years quail have also been successfully reared by methods similar to those applied to chicks. Feed ingredients are similar, but the amounts are adjusted to meet the nutritive requirements of the species. The information available concerning the nutritive requirements of the quail is somewhat limited.

Requirements. Norris[9] showed that the bobwhite required 27 per cent of protein in a diet for rapid growth. However, the difference between the results at the 24 per cent and the 27 per cent level was not great. Baldini, Roberts, and Kirkpatrick[10] reported a ration containing 28 per cent protein supplied by soybean oil meal as being adequate. Later they reported the lysine requirement as being higher for the quail than for the chick and concluded that 20 per cent protein was sufficient if the lysine of the ration was increased. Bass[11] concluded that 40 to 100 parts per million of manganese in a diet for bobwhites will prevent perosis.

Nestler and Llewellyn[12] reported an abnormal juvenile feather growth in which primary and secondary wing feathers were curved, twisted, stunted, and, in many cases, frizzled, among pen-reared bobwhites. It was most prevalent on the diet containing no dried milk products. The incidence diminished as the percentage of milk products in the diet was increased but appeared in a few birds, even on the diet containing 15 per cent of dried buttermilk and 3 per cent of dried whey. They concluded that a deficiency of riboflavin apparently was the major but not the sole cause of the abnormality.

In experiments dealing with pen-reared bobwhites, Nestler and Llewellyn[12] balanced the ration so as to contain approximately 28 per cent crude protein, 1.1 per cent calcium, 0.7 per cent phosphorus, 2400 International units of vitamin A, 530 International units of thiamin, and 540 International units of vitamin D.

Feeding Management. Nestler and Bailey[13] suggest the following feeding and management for the propagation of bobwhites. All-mash diets are fed exclusively, and they are kept constantly before the birds. A supply of clean fresh water should always be available. The birds should also have access to insoluble grit. Green leaves are good sources of certain of the dietary factors but are not essential from the nutritive standpoint when the vitamins are furnished in sufficient amounts in the feed. However, fresh-cut greens can be fed to add relish to the diet.

For the mature birds the breeding diet is made available 1 month before the breeding season and continued as long as eggs are to be used for hatching purposes.

The growing diet is kept constantly before the birds for the first 12 weeks of their lives. After 6 weeks of age, the maintenance ration is also fed in separate hoppers and the birds allowed to eat what they wish of either of these diets.

The maintenance diet is fed alone, after the bird is 12 weeks of age, and continued until it is changed to the breeding diet.

Rations.

Breeding Diet (26% protein)

Ground yellow corn	25
Wheat standard middlings	10
Dehydrated alfalfa meal	10
Soybean oil meal	36
Dried buttermilk	12
Bonemeal	3
Limestone	2 1/2
Salt mixture	1
Feeding oil (400A, 3000D)	1/2

Growing Ration (28% protein)

Ground yellow corn	24
Ground millet	10
Dehydrated alfalfa meal	5
Soybean oil meal	42
Dried buttermilk	16
Bonemeal	0.9
Salt mixture	1
Vitamin A-D oil	0.3

Maintenance Diet (12% protein)

Ground yellow corn	85.6
Dehydrated alfalfa meal	5
Soybean oil meal	7
Bonemeal	1.2
Salt mixture	1
Vitamin A-D oil	0.2

The salt mixture used in the above rations is made up as follows:

Common salt	50.000
Anhydrous manganous sulfate	0.850
Anhydrous ferrous sulfate	0.550
Anhydrous copper sulfate	0.020

If iodine is needed, the following is also added:

Potassium iodide	0.035
Anhydrous sodium thiosulfate	0.032
Calcium carbonate	0.035

It will require about 2½ pounds of feed to rear the quail to 10 weeks of age.

Coburn and Nestler[14] reported that of 9 cereals used as the sole grain millet gave the best results. Any of the cereals could replace half the corn; millet, wheat, and rye were the leading three.

The Pennsylvania[15] station obtained the best results with the following mash mixture in experiments evaluating 15 mash mixtures.

	Pounds
Ground yellow corn	9.5
Wheat bran	10.0
Wheat flour middlings	10.0
Ground oats	10.0
Alfalfa leaf meal	5.0
Dried whey	5.0
Soybean oil meal	40.0
Fish meal	2.0
Meat scraps	3.0
Dried brewers' yeast	3.0
Ground limestone	1.0
Steamed bonemeal	1.0

PIGEONS

Pigeons are primarily grain eaters. The feeding of pigeons, therefore, differs from the feeding of other poultry in that they are not fed any mash or green feed but are given a ration of whole grains, a mineral mixture, and water. Usually some high-protein grains such as cow peas, field peas, or peanuts are included in order to increase the protein content in the ration since the ordinary scratch mixture used for chickens is usually low in protein.

Grains. The most important part of the pigeon diet is a mixture of dry, hard grains that are clean, of good quality, and free from mold and decay. Levi[16] gives the basic feeds as being corn, wheat, kafir, and peas in the proportion of one part of peas to four parts of the other grains.

Corn is one of the best feeds for pigeons. Yellow corn is a good source of vitamin A. Soft corn should not be fed, and whole corn is better than cracked corn. Kafir and milo are also good feeds. Corn and kafir together usually constitute the major part of the pigeon ration.

Field or Canada peas are most commonly used as the high-protein feed. However, other feeds such as cow peas, peanuts, soybeans, or vetch are also fed.

Wheat is also included in fairly large quantities in most pigeon rations. The hard red wheat is preferred to the softer varieties.

Other grains may also be fed, but they are usually included only in small quantities. Such grains are oats, hempseed, millet, buckwheat, rice, rape, and rye.

Hemp is very palatable and is sometimes fed to stimulate feed intake. Sunflowerseeds are not palatable and must be restricted.

Mineral Mixtures. A suitable mineral mixture is necessary for the pigeons since the grains and seeds are usually low in minerals. The mineral mixture usually supplies a grit for grinding and material which will furnish calcium, phosphorus, iron, and salt. Platt[17] reported that a combination of 85 per cent oystershell, 10 per cent charcoal, and 5 per cent salt appeared to meet the needs for squab production.

Water. A plentiful supply of clean, fresh drinking water should be provided. Some arrangement, however, should be made to prevent the pigeons from bathing in the water supply.

Green Feed. Green feed is not necessary, especially when

the birds get outdoors. Some feeders like to supply some green feed as a relish to pigeons when they are confined.

METHODS OF FEEDING. The usual method is to feed the grain by hand, two or three times daily. A common practice is to feed the grain in the morning and afternoon, giving as much as will be cleaned up in 1½ to 2 hours. The grain is fed either on the floor or in open troughs. Feeding in troughs is preferred since it is more sanitary.

The grain may also be fed to the pigeons by making it available at all times in self-feeding hoppers. If the pigeons show a preference for certain of the grains, it might be advisable to put only about 1 day's supply of grain in the hopper at one time.

The quantity of feed that a given number of pigeons will eat depends on the weather, on their appetite, the breed, and on the number of squabs in the nest. One hundred pairs of Kings, or breeds of that size, will eat an average of about 27 pounds of grain each day.

Platt and Dare[18] reported very unsatisfactory results when attempting to feed an all-mash ration consisting of regular grain mixtures ground in mash form. However, the feeding of pellets has been done satisfactorily.

REQUIREMENTS OF THE RATION. Lee and Haynes[19] state that a good pigeon feed usually contains 13 to 15 per cent protein, 60 to 70 per cent carbohydrates, 2 to 5 per cent fat, and not more than 5 per cent fiber.

Supplementation of the ration with riboflavin and vitamin B_{12} has been reported as increasing the squab number owing to increased hatchability.[20] Livability was also increased with added riboflavin.

RATIONS. The following rations have been used with good results.

Cornell.[21]

	Per Cent
Cracked corn	30
Red wheat	20
Kafir corn	20
Canada peas	25
Rice, barley, or oats	5

U. S. Department of Agriculture.[19]

	Per Cent
Whole yellow corn	35
Kafir or milo	20
Cow peas	20
Hard red wheat	15
Oat groats	5
Hempseed	5

New Jersey.[22]

700 pounds whole yellow corn
400 pounds wheat
500 pounds milo
400 pounds green peas

Feed grain twice daily, giving the birds all they will eat. In addition, see that a regular pigeon grit and drinking water are available at all times.

New Jersey State Pigeon Breeding Test at Mellville.[23] From January to September, the birds were fed the following mixture:

	Pounds
Whole yellow corn	270
Cracked yellow corn	270
Wheat	260
Green peas	200

After October first, the mixture was changed to the following:

	Pounds
Whole yellow corn	300
Cracked yellow corn	150
Kafir corn	150
Wheat	200
Green peas	200

Many breeders of homing pigeons believe that a special feed is of value to induce the birds to enter the lofts promptly upon returning home after a flight. A mixture of this type, as well as a simpler combination, are recommended by Platt and Dare,[24] on the next page.

Some pigeon feeders change the ration during the summer. The chief change is to decrease the amount of corn. For example Levi[25] suggests the following:

Grains	Winter	Summer
Corn	35–56	20–40
Wheat	10–30	15–30
Kafir	9–18	15–35
Peas	18–20	20–25
Other	0–5	0–5

NEW JERSEY RATION FOR HOMING PIGEONS[24]

	Mixture 1	Mixture 2
Whole yellow corn (domestic)	30	. .
Red wheat	20	15
Alaskan green peas	20	. .
Kafir corn	15	25
Cracked yellow corn (domestic)	15	. .
Argentine corn	. .	30
Canada field peas	. .	17
Maple peas	. .	10
Hemp	. .	2
Millet	. .	2
Rice	. .	2
Buckwheat	. .	2
Hulled oats	. .	3
Vetch	. .	2
	100	100

FEEDING THE SQUABS. Squabs are reared and fed by both the parent birds on a thick, creamy mixture called pigeon milk, produced in the crop of the pigeons. The pigeons usually feed their squabs shortly after they themselves are fed and should not be disturbed at that time. If the parent birds become sick or die, the young birds may be fed by hand after they are a week old by dropping some of the smaller grain into the squab's mouth. They should be fed two or three times a day on grain that has been soaked for about 8 hours.

Squabs are usually ready for the market at about 28 days of age. Shortly after that time the squabs will leave the nest and feed for themselves, and then they will no longer have the quality of meat desired in the squab market. Squabs being saved for breeders can be removed from their parents at about the sixth week.

ECONOMICS OF FEEDING. Squabs will reach the weight of 14 ounces in about 25 days or about 1 pound in 4 weeks. There is some variation among the various breeds of pigeons in regard to the annual production of squabs, size of squabs, and feed consumption. The following averages were reported for ten different breeds at the New Jersey State Pigeon Breeding Test for a 5-year period:[18]

Squabs per pair annually	11.4
Grain per pair annually (lb.)	101.0
Grit per pair annually (lb.)	5.9
Grain to produce 1 lb. of squab dressed weight (lb.)	8.6
Weight per squab dressed (oz.)	16.3

CANARIES

The food requirements of canaries are very simple if the birds are not to be bred and young canaries reared. The chief requisite is a supply of canary seed to which may be added a small quantity of rape seed and a little hemp. Cuttle bone and water should always be available to the canary. In addition to the grain, occasionally such supplements as lettuce, chick weed, or a bit of apple may be fed. Bread that has been moistened in scalded milk or other soft foods may also be fed occasionally.

During the breeding season, the canary seed should be supplemented with egg food. It should be given daily from the first day the birds are placed in the breeding cage. Commercial nestling foods are also available which may be used in place of the home-mixed egg food.

The egg food can be made as follows: Mashed or riced hard-boiled eggs are mixed with fine crumbs, made from plain crackers or rebaked bread. Approximately 2 tablespoons of crumbs are used for each egg. A teaspoon of cod liver oil is used for every two eggs.

Both the male and female help to feed the little ones. The parent birds predigest and regurgitate their food in the form of pap which is fed to the baby directly. The babies will usually be out of the nest and feeding when less than 3 weeks old. By the time they are a month old, they are usually cracking their own seed but should have egg food for some time.

The young birds should be removed from the feeding cage just as soon as they commence shelling seed. The egg food is continued in decreasing quantities until they are 6 to 7 weeks old.

The Wisconsin Station[26] reported that canaries will do exceptionally well on good chick rations. Over a period of 2 years, they grew well and, upon reaching maturity, produced eggs with a high degree of hatchability. Especially noticeable was the bright yellow color of the birds, no doubt owing to the abundant carotene in the chick mash since this factor is one of the yellow pigments in feathers. On the other hand, a mixture of canary and rape seed, such as commonly used for pet birds, produced either poor growth or actual loss in weight in every case when it made up the only food of experimental animals. Neither did canaries thrive on such a ration. This was probably due to the fact that a diet of seeds is deficient in vitamins and minerals.

OSTRICHES

Very little information is available concerning the feeding of ostriches. The Arizona Station[27] reports having fed daily an average of 3 pounds of alfalfa hay, 1 pound of dried beet pulp, and 1 pound of grain per bird. The grain consisted chiefly of whole wheat, but milo and barley have also been fed. The Texas Station gives the following amounts as a breeding ration per pair of birds:

	Pounds
Alfalfa meal	8
Whole corn	1
Wheat bran	1
Bonemeal	1/2

REFERENCES

1. Hawkins, A. S., E. B. Moore, and A. Leopold. Compare value of grains for winter game feeding. Wis. Bul. 439:49. 1937.
2. Scott, M. L., and R. E. Reynolds. Studies on the nutrition of pheasant chicks. Poultry Sci. 28:392. 1949.
3. Callenbach, E. W., R. R. Murphy, and C. A. Hiller. The artificial propagation of ring-necked pheasants. Poultry Sci. 11:150. 1932.
4. Callenbach, E. W., and C. A. Hiller. The artificial propagation of ring-necked pheasants. Pa. Bul. 299. 1933.
5. Norris, L. C., L. J. Elmore, and G. Bump. The protein requirement of ring-necked pheasant chicks. Poultry Sci. 15:454. 1936.
6. Skoglund, W. C. An improved ration for starting ring-necked pheasants. Pa. Bul. 389. 1940.
7. Norris, L. C. Some studies of the nutritive requirements of pheasants. Trans. Twentieth Am. Game Conf. 304. January 1934.
8. Baird, F. D., and D. J. Greene. The comparative vitamin D requirements of growing chicks, turkeys, and pheasants. Poultry Sci. 14:70. 1935.
9. Norris, L. C. Protein requirements of bobwhite chicks. New York State Conservation Dept. Reports 1933-1936.
10. Baldini, J. T., R. E. Roberts, and C. M. Kirkpatrick. A study of the protein requirements of bobwhite quail reared in confinement in battery brooders to eight weeks of age. Poultry Sci. 29:161. 1950.
    Baldini, J. T., R. E. Roberts, and C. M. Kirkpatrick. Protein studies with the bobwhite quail. Poultry Sci. 30:906. 1951.
    Baldini, J. T., R. E. Roberts, and C. M. Kirkpatrick. Low protein rations for the bobwhite quail. Poultry Sci. 32:945. 1953.
11. Bass, C. C. Occurrence of slip tendon in quail in close confinement. Game Breeder and Sportsman 42(8):128. 1938.

12. Nestler, R. B., and L. M. Llewellyn. Abnormal feathering of pen-reared bobwhites. Poultry Sci. 23:73. 1944.
13. Nestler, R. B., and W. W. Bailey. Bobwhite quail propagation. U. S. Department of the Interior Fish and Wildlife Service. Conservation Bul. 10. 1941.
14. Coburn, D. R., and R. B. Nestler. Food particle size and quality in relation to disease in artificially propagated quail chicks. Jour. Am. Vet. Med. Assn. 110 (838):30. 1947.
15. Stadelman, W. J., E. W. Callenbach, R. R. Murphy, and R. V. Boucher. Rations for bobwhite quail. Pennsylvania Agr. Exp. Sta. Paper No. 1266, journal series, 1945.
16. Levi, W. M. Making pigeons pay. Orange Judd Co. New York. 1946.
17. Platt, C. S., A study of the composition of mineral mixtures for pigeons. Poultry Sci. 30:196. 1951.
18. Platt, C. S., and R. S. Dare. Squab production. N. J. Bul. 634. 1937.
19. Lee, A. R., and S. K. Haynes. Squab raising. U.S.D.A. Farmers' Bul. 684. 1942.
20. Schultz, F. T., C. R. Grau, and P. A. Zweigart. Vitamin supplements and squab production. Poultry Sci. 32:762. 1953.
21. Botsford, H. E. A 4-H pigeon loft. Cornell 4-H Club Bul. 74. 1946.
22. Platt, C. S. Records of squab production in New Jersey. 1931-1949. New Jersey Bul. 761. 1951.
23. Platt, C. S. A monthly standard for squab production. N. J. Hints 28(3). 1941.
24. Platt, C. S., and R. S. Dare. The care of homing pigeons. N. J. Hints 31(3). 1944.
25. Levi, W. M. The Pigeon. Sumter, S. C. 1941.
26. Kline, B. E., and C. A. Elvehjem. Canary birds thrive on chick rations. Wis. Bul. 439:10. 1937.
27. Williams, R. H., and W. S. Cunningham. Ostrich investigations. Ariz. Rept. 1916:290.

CHAPTER 19

ECONOMICS OF FEEDING

The amount of feed which birds consume is a major item in the cost of production. For example, the cost of feed for mature birds represents at least 50 to 60 per cent of the cost of producing eggs. The net return to the producer, however, is influenced also by production and the value of the product as well as the price of the feed.

AMOUNT OF FEED

The amounts of feed which the birds are likely to consume will vary, depending upon conditions. There are a number of factors that influence food consumption.

SIZE OF BIRD. Larger animals (other things being equal) will consume a larger amount of food. Sometimes it is stated that the breed will influence the feed consumed, but it is not so much the breed as it is the actual size of the individual. A 3-pound bird will not consume as much feed as the 4-pound bird, and the 4-pound bird, in turn, not as much as the 5-pound bird under the same conditions of production. That is true because we have an extra amount of body tissue to maintain and, as indicated previously, the maintenance requirements take up by far the greatest proportion of feed consumed. Consequently, such breeds as Plymouth Rocks, Wyandottes, and Rhode Island Reds will consume more feed in a year than Leghorns or Anconas.

INFLUENCE OF PRODUCTION. The heavier the production, either as regards numbers or pounds of eggs laid, the greater the amount of food consumed. The variation in feed consumption throughout the year is due largely to variation in production as shown in the accompanying tabulation of 6-year averages of high versus low pens at the New York State Laying Trials.[1]

The maintenance requirements remain fairly constant for a bird of given size. Additional feed is required for production in direct relation to the number of eggs laid. However, the proportion of feed needed for the production of the eggs is small,

Month	High Pens		Low Pens	
	Feed, lb.	Eggs	Feed, lb.	Eggs
October	8.4	23.0	6.7	12.6
November	8.7	24.5	7.3	15.4
December	9.3	25.3	8.0	17.3
January	9.8	25.2	8.6	17.9
February	9.0	21.9	8.0	14.4
March	9.4	23.9	8.6	14.8
April	9.4	23.5	8.2	14.7
May	9.1	24.3	8.2	14.6
June	8.7	23.2	7.7	12.6
July	8.6	22.8	7.3	10.9
August	8.3	21.4	7.1	9.6
September	5.2	13.7	4.6	5.5
Total	104.5	273.2	91.7	160.8

relative to that required for maintenance. Hence the pounds of feed consumed per dozen eggs produced decreases very rapidly with increased production, as shown in the accompanying estimates for White Leghorn pullets.

RELATION OF FOOD CONSUMPTION TO EGG PRODUCTION IN WHITE LEGHORN PULLETS

Yearly Egg Production	Pounds of Feed			
	For Maintenance	For Eggs	Total	Per Dozen Eggs
80	64.00	7.14	71.14	10.67
120	64.00	10.69	74.69	7.47
160	64.00	14.24	78.24	5.87
200	64.00	17.81	81.81	4.91

This is also shown in the accompanying estimates of feed per bird per year, with various rates of production, as given by Byerly.[2]

Eggs per Year	Weight of Bird		
	4 lb.	5 lb.	6 lb.
0	56.5	65.3	73.6
100	70.5	79.5	87.8
150	77.8	86.6	94.9
200	84.9	93.7	102.0

Similar relations between feed consumption and egg production have been shown by a number of experiment stations.[3–7]

The above relationship occurs because feed consumption is made up of the maintenance needs plus a certain amount of food to produce each egg.

The National Research Council[8] presented a practical guide for the poultryman and feed man (Table 34).

TABLE 34. FEED REQUIRED BY CHICKENS OF DIFFERENT LIVE WEIGHTS FOR MAINTENANCE AND FOR THE PRODUCTION OF 0, 100, 200, AND 300 EGGS, RESPECTIVELY, PER YEAR

	Average Total Feed Required per Bird per Year for Maintenance and the Production of the Indicated Number of Eggs			
Average Live Weight, lb.	0 Eggs per Year, lb.	100 Eggs per Year, lb.	200 Eggs per Year, lb.	300 Eggs per Year, lb.
3.0	47	61	75	89
3.5	52	67	81	95
4.0	57	71	85	99
4.5	61	75	89	104
5.0	65	80	94	108
5.5	70	84	98	112
6.0	74	88	102	116
6.5	78	92	106	120
7.0	81	96	110	124

INFLUENCE OF AGE. Mature fowls (not laying) eat less in proportion to live weight than younger fowls (not laying). Age influences feed consumption probably from two standpoints. First, birds in their second and later years of production are mature and are no longer growing as during the first or pullet year. We find that the birds usually continue to increase in weight nearly to the end of the first laying season. Pullets in the fall mature sexually but they are not mature physiologically. Thus we need to furnish feed for both production of eggs and production of body tissues. Second, the natural performance of the bird is to produce fewer eggs the second year than it did the first and fewer the third than the second so that we have production again as a factor influencing it.

Lamon and Lee[6] show that hens are more efficient in egg production during the first year than in succeeding years, as shown by the pounds of feed required to produce a dozen eggs (Table 35). The difference in actual feed consumption in pounds is not so marked, but, because of the lowered production, the efficiency is decreased.

SEASON AS A FACTOR. Birds will consume larger amounts of feed in colder weather in order to supply the extra heat necessary to overcome the greater difference in temperature between the air and body. Gutteridge, MacGregor, and Pratt[9] reported that the maximum saving in feed accomplished through the

TABLE 35. POUNDS OF FEED REQUIRED TO PRODUCE ONE DOZEN EGGS

Pen	First Year	Second Year	Third Year
1	6.2	9.2	14.1
2	4.9	9.2	16.0
3	7.0	10.3	13.1
4	4.7	5.6	6.0
5	7.3	8.6	11.0
6	8.1	10.6	12.9
Average	6.4	8.9	12.2

decreased requirement of feed for the maintenance of body temperature under heated conditions was 4.7 pounds per bird annually, with a mean saving of 2.85 pounds. The mean inside pen temperature range in the tests was from 32° F. to 58.9° F.

INFLUENCE OF RANGE. Birds on good range have access to a supply of natural food in the grass. Its consumption will decrease the amounts of grain and mash the birds will consume. The difference in food consumption may be as much as 20 per cent.

Similarly birds in cages usually consume less feed than birds kept in pens on the floor.[10]

SUGGESTED AMOUNTS OF FEED

Records at Cornell University indicate that a flock of Leghorns, averaging 4 pounds in weight and not in production, consumed 1⅓ pounds of feed per hen per week. This represents about 19 pounds per day for 100 hens. This same flock, producing 50 per cent, consumed 1⅔ pounds per hen per week or about 23 pounds per day for 100 hens. Larger hens will require more feed, smaller ones less. Also more feed will be required for higher levels of production.

The following are given as suggested quantities of feed necessary for average Leghorns (weighing 4 pounds):

Per Cent Production	Pounds of Grain and Mash per Day for 100 Birds
20	21
30	22
40	23
50	24
60	25
70	26
80	27

For heavier birds, such as the American breeds, the amount should be increased by 2 to 3 pounds, or approximately 2 pounds for each pound increase in weight.

The accompanying estimates for feed required per 100 layers a day are given by Byerly.[2]

Per Cent Production	Weight of Birds 4 lb.	5 lb.	6 lb.
0	15.5	17.9	20.2
10	16.9	19.3	21.6
20	18.3	20.7	23.0
30	19.8	22.2	24.5
40	21.2	23.6	25.9
50	22.6	25.0	27.3
60	24.0	26.4	28.7
70	25.4	27.8	30.1
80	26.9	29.3	31.6
90	28.3	30.7	33.0
100	29.7	32.1	34.4

The following formulas have been suggested for calculating the amount of food required.

(1) Total daily feed for 100 birds =

(a) 8.3 + 2.2 × the average weight of the bird + 0.1 × the egg production.

(b) [2] Leghorns

4.11 × the weight + change in body weight + number of eggs divided by 8.

Heavies

3.56 × the weight + change in body weight + number of eggs divided by 8.

(2) Feed per hen per year =

(a) 31.5 + 8 × the weight of the bird + 0.1 times the egg production.

(b) [2] Leghorns

15 × the weight + change in body weight + number of eggs divided by 8.

Heavies

13 × the weight + change in body weight + number of eggs divided by 8.

SOME REPRESENTATIVE RECORDS

YEARLY FEED CONSUMPTION OF MATURE BIRDS. Some variation is found in actual food consumption records, depending upon the various factors already discussed. In general, however, there is considerable agreement. As an average of seven contests, the Utah Station[11] reported a grain consumption of 44.1 pounds and a mash consumption of 30 pounds per bird, with an average first-year production of 204 eggs. The Maryland Station[12] reported a feed consumption per year of 80.5 pounds for Leghorns, 88.7 pounds for Plymouth Rocks, and 92.2 pounds for Rhode Island Reds. In a 6-year experiment, Cornell[13] gave an average feed consumption of 80.4 pounds for Leghorns, with an average production of 183 eggs.

The accompanying records give average figures for the 5-year period, 1913-1918, of the Connecticut[14] contest.

RELATION BETWEEN FOOD CONSUMPTION AND EGG PRODUCTION
(Connecticut Contest)

	Plymouth Rocks	Wyandottes	Rhode Island Reds	Leghorns
Egg production	153	163	151	162
Lb. grain per bird	45.5	44.3	45.1	43.6
Lb. mash per bird	51.6	45.4	50.1	39.6
Lb. total feed	97.1	89.7	95.2	83.2

Results reported from British Columbia[15] are tabulated.

RELATION BETWEEN FOOD CONSUMPTION AND EGG PRODUCTION
(British Columbia)

	White Leghorns	White Wyandottes	Plymouth Rocks	Rhode Island Reds
Egg production	204	194	182	170
Average wt. (lb.)	4.2	6.4	6.5	5.8
Lb. grain	41.8	43.4	43.4	43.5
Lb. mash	45.5	53.7	56.7	50.5
Lb. total feed	87.3	97.1	97.1	94.0
Lb. oystershell	4.51	3.92	3.57	3.00
Lb. grit	0.25	0.35	0.36	0.31

The 5-year average of the New York Egg-Laying Tests is given in the accompanying table.

FIVE YEAR AVERAGE OF NEW YORK EGG-LAYING TESTS

	White Leghorn	Rhode Island Red	White Plymouth Rock	Barred Plymouth Rock
Production (eggs)	219.1	215.0	182.4	213.6
Weight beginning (lb.)	3.8	5.1	5.1	5.2
Weight end (lb.)	4.7	6.4	6.4	6.6
Feed (lb.)	97.4	108.1	91.2	101.4

The food consumption record of 350 two-year-old hens, producing 152 eggs each, in the Advanced Registry at Cornell[16] (1920-21) was:

	Pounds
Grain	39.5
Mash	43.1
Oyster shells	3.1
Grit	0.6
Cabbage	10.9
Sprouted wheat	3.0
Semi-solid buttermilk	1.9

From a survey of feed records[17] on 120 poultry farms in New York State, Darrah reported a feed consumption of 95 pounds for the light breeds and 107.8 pounds for the heavy breeds in 1940-1941. This represented, respectively, 6.9 and 7.9 pounds of feed to produce a dozen eggs. Feed records from 143 farms in 1946-47 indicate an average feed consumption of 108.6 pounds for the light breeds and 116.8 pounds for the heavy breeds. This represents, respectively, 7.2 and 7.5 pounds of feed to produce a dozen of eggs.

MONTHLY FEED CONSUMPTION OF MATURE BIRDS. There is some variation in monthly feed consumption. The difference is due chiefly to the fluctuation in egg production. Table 36 shows monthly food consumption for a vlock at Cornell.[13]

POUNDS OF FEED TO PRODUCE ONE DOZEN EGGS. The economy of producing eggs can be measured by the pounds of feed necessary to produce one dozen eggs. The lighter breeds, in general, are more efficient in this respect. The efficiency is also closely associated with egg production. The efficiency of production goes up with increased egg production. The Maryland Station[12] reports the highest efficiency for a flock of Leghorns which required 3.75 pounds of feed to produce a dozen eggs.

In the New York Laying Trials, flocks producing 217 eggs required 4.56 pounds of feed to produce a dozen eggs whereas the flocks producing 154 eggs required 6.96 pounds. For twelve flocks over a period of 6 years, Cornell[13] shows an average of 6.21 pounds of feed needed to produce a dozen eggs, with a range of 5.35 pounds to 7.92 pounds for the year. The New Jersey Station[3] indicated 6.76 pounds for the average of thirty-two commercial farms. The Oklahoma Station[18] showed that the average feed required to produce one dozen eggs per year for the 5-year egg-laying contests was 2.4 pounds of grain and 2.1 pounds of mash, with a production of approximately 200 eggs.

TABLE 36. FEED CONSUMPTION AND EGG PRODUCTION PER 100 HENS

Month	Grain, lb.	Dry Mash, lb.	Dry Mash in Moist Mash, lb.	Total Feed, lb.	Feed per Day, lb.	Production, %
October	205	129	9	343	21.5	8.4
November	400	292	18	710	23.7	51.8
December	441	219	55	715	23.1	50.0
January	390	247	61	698	22.5	35.7
February	361	281	57	699	24.1	40.3
March	396	321	74	791	25.5	54.1
April	400	374	19	793	26.4	69.1
May	387	399	. . .	786	25.3	70.6
June	346	366	. . .	712	23.7	68.7
July	327	280	32	639	20.6	52.9
August	278	238	123	639	20.6	45.3
September	267	204	121	592	19.7	31.4
October	52	46	24	122	13.5	19.8
Total or average	4250	3396	593	8239	22.3	46.0

There is some difference between the various breeds in this respect (Table 37). Size of bird and production are important factors.

TABLE 37. POUNDS OF FEED REQUIRED TO PRODUCE ONE DOZEN EGGS

	Plymouth Rocks	Wyandottes	Rhode Island Reds	White Leghorns	New Hampshires
Connecticut[14]	7.6	6.6	7.6	6.2	. . .
Maryland[12]	5.7	. . .	6.1	4.8	. . .
Jull[19]	6.1	8.8	5.6	5.2	6.4

It has already been pointed out that the efficiency of production increases with an increase in egg production. This is shown by the accompanying estimates of Byerly,[2] which give the feed required to produce one dozen eggs.

Percentage Egg Production	Weight of Bird 4 lb.	5 lb.	6 lb.
20	11.0	12.4	13.8
40	6.4	7.1	7.8
60	4.8	5.3	5.7
80	4.0	4.4	4.7

For average conditions on commercial farms Misner and Lee[20] concluded that it required 7 pounds of feed to produce one dozen eggs.

The variations on the monthly basis are much greater than on the yearly basis, owing probably to the greater differences in egg production for the different months. For instance, records at Cornell[13] show monthly variations from 3.95 pounds to 28.60 pounds. The accompanying table is representative of the quantity of feed necessary to produce one dozen eggs for each month throughout the laying year. It will be noted that the amounts are closely associated with the percentage of production.

Month	Pounds of Feed Required to Produce One Dozen Eggs	Per Cent Production
October	28.6	8.4
November	5.5	51.8
December	5.5	50.0
January	7.6	35.7
February	7.2	40.3
March	5.7	54.1
April	4.6	69.1
May	4.3	70.6
June	4.1	68.7
July	4.7	52.9
August	5.5	45.3
September	7.6	31.4
October	12.2	19.8
Average	7.9	46.0

FEED REQUIRED FOR YOUNG STOCK. Food consumption is rather closely related to growth. For example, for the first 26 weeks[21] American-breed pullets consumed 5 pounds more feed than was consumed by Leghorn pullets. However, they also weighed more. When put on the basis of pounds of feed per pound of body weight, the consumption amounts to 6.86 pounds for the Leghorns and 6.48 pounds for the heavy breeds. The American cockerels to 30 weeks of age consumed 4.3 pounds more food than was consumed by the Leghorn cockerels. However, they are considerably heavier so that their food consumption per pound of weight amounts to 6.15 pounds, as compared with 7.51 pounds for the Leghorns. In both instances, the food consumption was relatively greater for the Leghorns, probably because they reached maturity at an earlier age.

These amounts of feed agree closely with those reported by Card and Kirkpatrick,[22] who give a food consumption of approximately 24 pounds for White Leghorns and 27 pounds for Rhode Island Reds, to 24 weeks of age.

The Arizona Station[23] reported that it took 25 pounds of feed to rear a Single Comb White Leghorn pullet to 26 weeks of age, with an average weight of 3 pounds, and that it took 21 pounds of feed to rear a Rhode Island Red pullet, with an average weight of 3 pounds and 6 ounces. The North Carolina Station[24] indicated that it took approximately 23 pounds of feed to put Rhode Island Red pullets into lay.

In a survey of 80 farms in New York[17] in 1940-41 it was found that 23.1 pounds of feed were required to rear a pullet of the light breeds to maturity and 31.4 pounds for a heavy breed pullet. This represented 5.6 pounds and 4.7 pounds of feed to produce 1 pound of pullet for the light and heavy breeds, respectively. In 1947[25] it took an average of 33.5 pounds of feed per pullet on 137 farms.

In Tables 19 and 20 (Chap. 12) are presented the feed consumption for chicks under a normal rearing program. Both large and small strains are represented in the case of Leghorns and in the case of the heavy breeds, New Hampshires, Rhode Island Reds, Barred Cross and Indian River Cross are represented.

The rate of growth, as well as the actual gains, decreases as the chicks grow older. On the other hand, the amount of food consumed gradually increases with the increase in the size of the bird. Therefore the number of pounds of feed required to produce a pound of gain is relatively low at the start and increases as the chicks grow older.[21]

There exists fair agreement on the amount of feed to produce a pound of gain for the different kinds of poultry. It takes approximately 3.0 pounds of feed to produce a pound of gain up to 3 months of age for chickens, ducks, turkeys, and geese and 5.0 to 6.0 pounds of feed to produce a pound of gain up to 24 to 28 weeks of age for chickens, ducks, and turkeys.

Feed efficiency, as expressed by pounds of feed to produce a pound of gain, varies considerably depending upon many factors. Some of these are the kind of ration fed, rate of growth, age, and sex. Feed conversion also varies between breeds and strains of the same breed. The Maryland Station[26] has presented data that strongly indicate that the efficiency of feed utilization is inherited.

FEED REQUIRED FOR BROILERS. In the production of broilers considerable improvement has been made in feed efficiency. Earlier reports[27] indicate weights of 2¼ to 3½ pounds per bird in 11 to 14 weeks on 3.5 to 4.8 pounds of feed to produce 1 pound of bird. At the present time 3 to 4 pounds of meat are being produced in 9 to 12 weeks with a feed efficiency of 3 pounds or less of feed to produce a pound of meat.[28] Singsen reports an average weight of 2.6 pounds for 8-week-old male chicks in one experiment with a feed efficiency of 2.03 pounds of feed per pound of gain.

Figures reported for large-scale broiler production show the commercial possibilities (Table 38).

Some further reported broiler results are given in Tables 39 and 40.

TABLE 38. GROWTH AND FEED FOR 10–11 WEEK BROILERS

	Average Weight, lb.	Pounds of Feed to Produce a Pound of Meat
Lot 1	3.12	2.69
2	3.41	2.72
3	3.49	2.72
4	3.69	2.47
5	3.53	2.77
6	3.50	2.80
7	3.56	2.87
8	3.40	2.85
9	3.14	2.66
10	3.20	2.73
11	3.41	2.67
12	3.02	2.59
13	3.75	2.97
14	3.70	2.87

TABLE 39. RELATION BETWEEN AGE AND FEED CONSUMPTION AND GROWTH OF BROILERS*

	Body Weight per Bird		Total Pounds of Feed (to date)			
Age	Cockerels and Pullets		Leghorns		Heavies	
(weeks)	Leghorns	Heavies	Per Bird	Per lb.	Per Bird	Per lb.
At start	.09	.08				
4	.72	.96	1.37	1.90	1.70	1.77
6	1.37	1.81	3.30	2.41	3.80	2.11
8	2.01	2.74	5.19	2.58	6.63	2.42
10	2.54	3.42	7.90	3.10	8.93	2.61

* Published with the permission of the Beacon Milling Company from _Profitable Broiler Battery and Laying Gage Management_, 6th Edition, 1951. C. E. Lee. Copyrighted by The Beacon Milling Company, Inc., Cayuga, New York.

TABLE 40. RELATION OF BREED AND AGE TO GROWTH AND FEED EFFICIENCY OF BROILERS

Breed	Age	Average Weight	Feed per Pound of Bird
New Hampshires	12 wks.	4.03	3.05
New Hampshires	12 wks.	3.60	3.16
New Hampshires	10 wks., 6 days	3.30	3.75
New Hampshires (cockerels)	9 wks.	3.02	2.57
		3.03	2.64
		3.15	2.58
		3.09	2.69
White Rocks	12 wks.	4.36	2.88
		4.32	2.72
Heavies	12 wks.	4.50	3+
Crosses mixed	10 wks., 3 days	3.75	3.60
Crosses cockerels	13 wks.	5.25	4.60
Crosses cockerels	11 wks.	3.63	2.92

See also Table 26 (Chap. 12) for the amounts of feed required by heavy breed broilers at various ages.

In a study of Leghorn cockerels as broilers, the Oregon Station[29] showed that the feed required per pound of gain was somewhat less than 3 pounds for battery-reared birds and slightly less than 4 pounds for floor-reared birds. The battery-reared birds were about 1 week ahead of the floor-reared birds in growth.

FEED REQUIRED BY TURKEYS. About 50 pounds of mash and 20 pounds of grain are required to produce a 19-pound turkey at 24 weeks of age under the complete confinement method of rearing. More pounds of feed are required to produce a pound of gain as the poults grow older. This is shown in the accompanying table giving the amount of grain and mash fed per pound of gain in weight.[30] (See also Table 32, Chap. 16.)

Age in Weeks	Average Weight, lb.	Pounds of Feed per Pound of Gain: Period	Pounds of Feed per Pound of Gain: Total
1–4	1.4	1.7	1.7
5–8	4.1	2.4	2.2
9–12	7.6	3.1	2.6
13–16	11.8	3.7	3.0
17–20	15.5	4.7	3.4
21–24	19.1	5.6	3.8
25–28	22.1	8.3	4.5
29–32	24.5	12.2	5.2

Feed consumption and growth data, as reported for Broad Breasted Bronze and Beltsville Small White turkeys by Almquist,[31] are given in Tables 41 and 42.

TABLE 41. GROWTH AND FEED CONSUMPTION FOR BROAD BREASTED BRONZE TURKEYS
(average data for mixed sexes)

Age in Weeks	Weight, lb.	Mash to Date, lb.	Grain to Date, lb.	Total Feed, lb.	Feed Efficiency
2	0.49	0.7	0.0	0.7	1.42
4	1.15	2.5	0.0	2.5	2.18
6	2.15	4.7	0.3	5.0	2.33
8	3.70	8.1	1.1	9.2	2.49
10	5.45	11.8	2.3	14.1	2.58
12	7.40	16.3	3.8	20.1	2.71
14	9.40	21.6	5.3	26.9	2.86
16	11.42	27.2	7.7	34.9	3.06
18	13.38	33.6	10.2	43.8	3.27
20	15.35	40.7	13.2	53.9	3.51
22	17.30	48.0	16.2	64.2	3.71
24	19.20	55.4	22.0	77.4	4.03
26	21.00	62.5	29.0	91.5	4.36

TABLE 42. GROWTH AND FEED CONSUMPTION FOR BELTSVILLE SMALL WHITE TURKEYS
(Average data for mixed sexes)

Age in Weeks	Weight lb.	Mash to Date, lb.	Grain to Date, lb.	Total Feed, lb.	Feed Efficiency
2	0.40	0.6	0.0	0.6	1.50
4	0.85	1.8	0.1	1.9	2.24
6	1.58	3.3	0.5	3.8	2.40
8	2.60	5.3	1.1	6.4	2.46
10	3.82	7.9	1.9	9.8	2.56
12	5.13	10.9	2.9	13.8	2.69
14	6.50	14.3	4.3	18.6	2.86
16	7.72	18.7	5.7	24.4	3.16
18	8.80	23.4	7.7	31.1	3.53
20	9.66	27.6	9.9	37.5	3.88

The average feed consumption and weight of White Holland and Bronze turkeys are reported from Massachusetts[32] in Table 43.

The accompanying growth and feed consumption data are reported from Nevada[33] for Broad Breasted Bronze turkeys.

When turkeys are confined, they will consume somewhat more total feed and also require more pounds of feed to produce a pound of gain than when they are allowed to range.[34, 35]

Age	Average Weight, lb.	Total Feed Required, lb.	Cumulative Pounds of Feed per Pound of Gain
First month	1.3	1.4	1.1
Second month	3.9	6.9	1.8
Third month	7.4	15.4	2.1
Fourth month	11.2	26.9	2.4
Fifth month	14.8	41.0	2.8
Sixth month	18.0	57.1	3.2
Seventh month	21.3	78.3	3.7
Eighth month	24.4	103.8	4.2

TABLE 43. CUMULATIVE QUANTITY OF FEED CONSUMED (100 BIRDS) AND WEIGHT OF TURKEYS
(Massachusetts)

	Feed, lb.		Weight, lb.			
			Bronze		White Holland	
Age, weeks	Bronze	White Holland	Male	Female	Male	Female
1	28.26	28.26				
2	58.59	58.59	0.31	0.29	0.34	0.32
3	101.95	101.95				
4	162.51	162.51	0.72	0.63	0.78	0.69
5	234.44	234.44				
6	316.54	316.54	1.38	1.15	1.42	1.23
7	423.24	420.28				
8	559.05	544.17	2.41	1.97	2.33	1.97
9	717.28	705.28				
10	886.81	887.31	3.82	3.24	3.78	3.09
11	1136.42	1116.31				
12	1394.95	1351.34	5.80	4.76	5.38	4.31
13	1690.39	1651.75				
14	2039.79	1992.84	8.14	6.48	7.51	5.78
15	2405.26	2352.83				
16	2794.93	2756.32	10.06	7.69	9.39	6.95
17	3218.73	3201.40				
18	3705.63	3630.22				
19	4160.78	4041.57				
20	4742.65	4575.42	15.02	10.64	13.15	8.88
21	5313.32	5147.56				
22	5797.60	5624.61				
23	6347.91	6122.01				
24	6941.61	6604.32	19.01	12.46	16.46	10.78

Most of the experimental results show fair agreement in the utilization of feed by growing turkeys. The pounds of feed required to produce a pound of gain as reported by a number of stations is as follows:

Station	Pounds of Feed Required to Produce a Pound of Gain
Pennsylvania[36]	
Bronze	4.49
White Holland	4.73
U.S.D.A.[37]	4.12
Oklahoma[34]	
Bronze	3.82
	4.12
	4.45
South Carolina[35]	
Broad Breasted Bronze	4.00
	4.37
Small type Broad Breasted White	4.39
	4.53
Massachusetts[32]	
Bronze	4.41
White Holland	4.85
Cornell[38]	
White Holland	4.19
	4.37
	3.91

Marsden[39] reports that feed consumption of young Bronze breeding hens, fed ad libitum, averaged 3.23 pounds per week per hen for the 8-week winter period; 2.73 pounds per week for the 16-week spring period; and 3.50 pounds per week for the 4-week fall fattening period, after having been held on limited maintenance rations of 1.40 pounds of scratch grain per hen per week during the summer period of 20 weeks. For the 48-week year, the total feed consumed was 111.52 pounds. By adding 4 weeks to the summer maintenance period, the total was 117.12 pounds for the full year of 52 weeks. The males ate nearly twice as much feed per average bird as the females, the requirement for the 48-week year being 226.88 pounds and for the 52-week year 240.88 pounds.

In an economic study of Washington's[40] turkey breeding flocks, it was found that the total amount of feed, excluding shell, fed by growers in different parts of the state did not vary much. For 61 farms it averaged 31.2 pounds of mash, 1.2 pounds of hay, and 40.3 pounds of grain, or a total of 72.7 pounds.

Jull[41] gives the following feed consumption per month during the breeding season:

Broad Breasted Bronze	17–19 pounds
Standard Bronze	16–18 pounds
White Holland	14–16 pounds
Beltsville	11–13 pounds

Parker and Barton[42] report that during a 5 month's period turkey breeding hens and toms consumed 90.5 pounds of feed per bird of which 52 pounds was mash and 38.5 pounds whole grain.

COST OF FEEDING

If the amounts of feed are known for the various purposes, it is easy to figure the cost of production. Costs will be influenced by the actual cost per 100 pounds of the different feeds used to make up the ration. These feed costs vary considerably, depending upon a large number of factors.

Under normal conditions, there are seasonal variations in feed prices which often can be used to advantage.[43] For example, we ordinarily find that grains are at their lowest price soon after harvest. This is true because, as grain is held, the costs of shrinkage, interest, insurance, and destruction must be added. Corn is usually lowest in November to February and highest in July to August; wheat reaches the low point about September to November; oats are lowest during late summer and early fall and highest during May and June. The wheat by-products are usually lowest during the summer and highest during the winter. There is usually a falling off in the demand for meat scraps during the summer months, with a somewhat lower trend in price during July to September.

Any advantage that can be obtained in the price of feeds may mean considerable in the total cost of producing eggs or meat since feed cost represents the largest single item in the cost of production. It usually does not fall much below 50 per cent of the total cost, and in some cases may represent as much as 75 per cent of the cost.

The feed costs on a number of poultry farms for 2 years, as reported from England,[44] represented 60 and 54 per cent of the total cost. On 172 New York farms[45] the feed cost per layer represented 60.0 per cent of the total cost in 1946-47. The feed cost for rearing on commercial poultry farms in New York[46] represented 46 per cent of the total cost in 1940-41. In an economic study of the broiler industry in Western Indiana[47] feed cost was 54.3 per cent of the total cost of producing broilers.

Under normal conditions, feed will represent approximately 60 per cent of the cost of producing eggs and about 50 per cent of the cost of rearing chickens.

REFERENCES

1. Ogle, R. C. Six years of Central and Western New York official egg-laying tests. Cornell Bul. 394. 1938.
2. Byerly, T. C. Feed and other costs of producing market eggs. Md. Tech. Bul. A1. 1941.
3. Aubry, V. G. Lessons to be learned by keeping records. N. J. Hints 7(5). 1919.

   Allen, W. H. Egg production, monthly costs, and receipts on New Jersey poultry farms. N. J. Hints 12(4). 1924.
4. Wing, H. H. Cooperative experiments on the cost of egg production. Cornell Bul. 204. 1902.

   Wing, H. H. The yearly record of three flocks. Cornell Bul. 211. 1903.

   Rice, J. E. Comparison of four methods of feeding early hatched pullets. Cornell Bul. 249. 1907.
5. Kazmeier, F. W. Report of the first Texas National Egg-laying Contest. Texas Bul. 246. 1919.
6. Lamon, H. M., and A. R. Lee. Feed cost of egg production. U.S.D.A. Farmers' Bul. 561:5. 1917.
7. Philips, A. G. Feeding laying hens. Ind. Circ. 101. 1929.
8. Nutrient requirements for domestic animals. Number 1. Nutrient requirements for poultry. Nat. Res. Council Rept. Com. on Animal Nutr. Washington. 1954. Pub. 301.
9. Gutteridge, H. S., H. I. MacGregor, and J. M. Pratt. The effect of heat, insulation and artificial light on egg production and feed consumption of pullets. Sci. Agr. 25:1. 1944.
10. Bird, S., and J. W. Sinclair. Economic aspects of poultry keeping in Canada, with special reference to egg production. Sci. Agr. 19:551. 1939.
11. Alder, B. Results of seven years of egg-laying contests. Utah Bul. 248. 1934.
12. Waite, R. H. Feed consumption studies based on six Maryland egg laying contests. Md. Bul. 359. 1934.
13. Huttar, J. C., F. L. Fairbanks, and H. E. Botsford. Ventilation of poultry houses for laying and breeding hens. Cornell Bul. 558. 1933.
14. Card, L. E., and W. F. Kirkpatrick. Egg Laying Contest. Conn. (Storrs) Bul. 100. 1919.
15. Lloyd, E. A., and V. S. Asmundson. Feeding for egg production. Dept. Agr. (B. C.) Bul. 93. 1928.
16. Heuser, G. F. Advanced registry poultry breeding project at Cornell University. Poultry Sci. 1:83. 1921.
17. Darrah, L. B. Costs and returns from the laying flock on commercial poultry farms, 1940-1941. Cornell Bul. 802. 1943.

    Kearl, C. D. Commercial poultry management in New York State, 1946-47. Cornell Bul. 864. 1950.

    Kearl, C. D. Seasonal costs and returns in producing eggs, New York, 1946-47. Cornell Bul. 865. 1950.
18. Willham, O. S. The feed required to produce a dozen eggs. Okla. (Panhandle) Bul. 35:3. 1932.

19. Jull, M. A. Produce more eggs with less feed. World's Poultry Sci. Jour. 5:94. 1949.
20. Misner, E. G., and A. T. M. Lee. Economic studies of poultry farming in N. Y. I. Commercial poultry farms, 1926, 1929, 1930, 1931, 1932, 1933. Cornell Bul. 684:38. 1937.
21. Heuser, G. F., and F. E. Andrews. Weight changes in chickens. Cornell Ext. Bul. 240. 1932.
22. Card, L. E., and W. F. Kirkpatrick. Rearing chickens. Part I. Normal rate of growth in White Leghorns and Rhode Island Reds. Conn. (Storrs) Bul. 96. 1918.
23. Embleton, H. Poultry feeding experiments. Ariz. Bul. 143:89. 1933.
24. Cost of putting pullets into lay. N. C. Rept. 1929:105.
25. Pickler, M. J. Costs of raising pullets on New York farms, 1947. Cornell Bul. 859. 1950.
26. Hess, C. W., T. C. Byerly, and M. A. Jull. The efficiency of feed utilization by Barred Plymouth Rock and Crossbred broilers. Poultry Sci. 20:210. 1941.
27. Young, E. C. An economic study of the broiler industry in Western Indiana. Ind. Bul. 441. 1939.
Tomhave, A. E. Broiler feeding experiments. Del. Bul. 210. 1938.
Poffenberger, P. R. Merchandising Directory. Hatchery Tribune. 1942. Mt. Morris, Ill.
Platt, C. S. Feed consumption and growth of White Leghorn chicks in batteries. N. J. Circ. 316. 1934.
28. Combs, G. F. Are you getting good feed efficiency? Worlds Poultry Sci. Jour. 9:26. 1953.
Singsen, E. P. The effect of high efficiency diets on the nutrient intake of chickens. Sixth Calif. Animal Ind. Conf. Proc. 17. 1953.
29. Cooney, W. T., and F. E. Price. Surplus Leghorn cockerels as broilers. Ore. Bul. 386. 1940.
30. Scott, M. L. Growth rate and feed consumption of Broad Breasted Bronze and Beltsville Small White turkeys. Cornell Dept. of Poultry Husbandry, Ext. Stencil 200. 1950. Revised Dec. 1952.
31. Almquist, H. J. Comparative mash consumption, grain consumption, and feed efficiency of Broad Breasted Bronze and Beltsville Small White turkeys. World's Poultry Sci. Jour. 7:103. 1951.
32. Massachusetts Poultry Year Book. 1939:61.
33. Cline, L. E. How fast do turkeys grow? Turkey World January 1943:36.
34. Thompson, R. B., E. E. Schnetzler, and W. P. Albright. Growing turkeys in confinement. Okla. Bul. 202. 1932.
35. Darrow, M. I., and C. L. Morgan. Large vs. small type turkeys. S. C. Bul. 350. 1944.
36. Funk, E. M., and P. H. Margolf. Feed consumption and costs in raising turkeys. Pa. Bul. 250. 1930.
37. Marsden, L. J. Progress report of turkey investigations at the United States Range Livestock Experiment Station, Miles City, Nevada. Mimeographed Rept. U.S.D.A. 1931.
38. Smith, E. Y. Growing turkeys. Cornell Bul. 717. 1947.

39. Marsden, S. J. Feed consumption and cost of feeding of Bronze turkey breeding stock. Poultry Sci. 15:400. 1936.
40. Berryman, C. N., and M. T. Buchanan. An economic study of Washington's turkey industry in 1942. Part I: Breeding flocks. Wash. Bul. 440. 1944.
41. Jull, M. A. Managing turkey breeders in winter. Southern Planter 108(Dec.): 27. 1947.
42. Parker, J. E., and O. A. Barton. Observations with Broad Breasted Bronze turkey breeding stock. North Dakota Bimo. Bul. 8:3. 1945.
43. Richards, P., F. L. Thomsen, and J. W. Burch. Seasonal variation in feed prices. Mo. Circ. 226. 1929.
Haag, H. M., and N. St. John. Seasonal variation and economy of basic feeds, 1924-1940. Mo. Bul. 422. 1941.
44. General notes on the results of the poultry survey for 1938-39. Harper Adams Utility Poultry Jour. 25:151. 1940.
45. Kearl, C. D., Commercial poultry farm management in New York State, 1946-47. Cornell Bul. 864. 1950.
46. Darrah, L. B. Cost of incubation and rearing on commercial poultry farms. 1940-1941. Cornell Bul. 797. 1943.
47. Young, E. C. An economic study of the broiler industry in Western Indiana. Ind. Bul. 441. 1939.

APPENDIX

In the main chapters we discussed the requirements that need to be met in order to make the various rations complete and effective. In the application of these requirements to actual rations it is possible to formulate a large number of mixtures for any specific purpose. These mixtures will vary in different localities depending to a large extent upon the feed ingredients that are available.

In the appendix are given representative rations for definite purposes. Selections have been made of typical rations as recommended in different sections of the United States and Canada. The kinds of rations given are as follows:

(Rations for geese will be found in Chap. 17; for pigeons and other species, in Chap. 18.)

SECTION I. RATIONS FOR YOUNG CHICKENS

CORNELL. (Department of Poultry Husbandry, New York State College of Agriculture, *Stencil* 205, January, 1953, Recommendations for formulating poultry rations; *Stencil* 210, February, 1954, Broiler rations.)

Chick Starter Mashes. To be fed as an all-mash ration to chicks until 6 weeks of age. Limited amounts of grain, not to exceed 20 per cent of the daily feed intake, may be fed with it in the following 2 weeks.

Confinement Grower Mashes. To be fed to growing chicks from 8 weeks to maturity in confinement or on poor pasture. Designed for free-choice feeding along with grain.

Pasture Grower Mashes. To be used with free-choice grain feeding only on good pasture supplying abundant succulent forage.

Broiler Starter Mashes. To be fed at least the first 8 weeks of the growth period. They may be used until broilers reach market age. When they have reached that age, a limited amount of grain, not to exceed 20 per cent, can be fed after 8 weeks.

Broiler Grower Mashes To be fed after 8 weeks of age. The all-mash grower ration is fed without grain. The mash to be fed with grain can be fed after 8 weeks with free access to a grain mixture. The grain intake should not exceed 40 per cent of daily feed consumption.

Mixing Mashes. Mash concentrates to be used with local grain (see Section VII).

CORNELL CHICK STARTER MASHES

	lb./ton	lb./ton	lb./ton	lb./ton
Yellow corn meal	900	895	940	855
Ground wheat	250	200	. . .	. . .
Wheat flour middlings	. . .	. . .	. . .	200
Wheat standard middlings	. . .	. . .	200	. . .
Ground barley	. . .	. . .	. . .	200
Ground oats	100	200	100	. . .
Soybean meal	450	425	350	350
Corn gluten meal	. . .	. . .	100	. . .
Peanut meal	. . .	. . .	. . .	100
Fish meal	50	100	. . .	. . .
Fish solubles	. . .	. . .	50	. . .
Meat scrap	50	. . .	50	100
Corn distillers' dried solubles	50	. . .	100	. . .
Dried whey	50	50	. . .	100
Molasses distillers' dried solubles	. . .	25	. . .	. . .
Dehydrated alfalfa meal	50	50	50	50
Riboflavin supplement to supply (mg. riboflavin)	500 mg.	500 mg.	700 mg.	. . .
Vitamin B_{12} supplement to supply (mg. B_{12})	1 mg.	. . .	. . .	2.5 mg.
D-activated animal sterols (1500 I.C.U./gm.)	0.8	0.8	0.8	0.8
or				
Vitamin feeding oil (300 D, 1500 A)	4	4	4	4
Steamed bonemeal	15	20	25	10
Limestone	30	30	30	30
Salt (iodized)	5	5	5	5
Manganese sulfate (65% feeding grade)	0.4	0.4	0.4	0.4
Antibiotic feed supplement	+	+	+	+
Protein, %	20.5	20.3	20.6	20.5
Calcium, %	1.3	1.2	1.3	1.3
Phosphorus, total, %	0.7	0.7	0.7	0.7
available, %	0.4	0.4	0.4	0.4
Vitamin A,* I.U./lb.	3400	3400	4200	3400
Vitamin D., I.C.U./lb.	270	270	270	270
Riboflavin, mg./lb.	1.6	1.6	1.7	1.7
Vitamin B_{12},† μg./lb.	2	2	2	2

*Assuming use of alfalfa meal containing 100,000 International Units vitamin A activity per pound, and no feeding oil.

† From animal proteins and vitamin B_{12} supplement.

CORNELL CONFINEMENT GROWER MASHES

	lb./ton	lb./ton	lb./ton	lb./ton
Yellow corn meal	710	575	640	605
Ground wheat	300	200	...	...
Wheat flour middlings	...	...	...	300
Wheat standard middlings	...	300	200	...
Ground barley	...	...	100	300
Ground oats	200	200	200	...
Soybean meal	400	350	350	310
Corn gluten meal	...	...	100	...
Peanut meal	...	...	...	100
Fish meal	50	100	...	...
Fish solubles	...	...	50	...
Meat scrap	50	...	50	100
Corn distillers' dried solubles	100	...	50	...
Dried whey	...	50	50	100
Molasses distillers' dried solubles	...	25	...	...
Dehydrated alfalfa meal	100	100	100	100
Riboflavin supplement to supply (mg. riboflavin)	...	...	...	...
Vitamin B_{12} supplement to supply (mg. B_{12})	1 mg.	...	...	2 mg.
D-activated animal sterols (1500 I.C.U./gm.)	0.8	0.8	0.8	0.8
or				
Vitamin feeding oil (300 D, 1500 A)	4	4	4	4
Steamed bonemeal	60	60	70	55
Limestone	20	30	30	20
Salt (iodized)	10	10	10	10
Manganese sulfate (65% feeding grade)	0.5	0.5	0.5	0.5
Antibiotic feed supplement	±	±	±	±
Protein, %	20.6	20.4	20.4	20
Calcium, %	1.8	1.8	1.9	1.8
Total phosphorus, %	1.0	1.0	1.0	0.9
available, %	0.7	0.7	0.7	0.7
Vitamin A,* I.U./lb.	5700	5600	5600	5600
Vitamin D, I.C.U./lb.	270	270	270	270
Riboflavin, mg./lb.	1.3	1.5	1.7	1.8
Vitamin B_{12},† μg./lb.	1.9	2.0	2.1	1.8

*Assuming use of alfalfa meal containing 100,000 International Units vitamin A activity and no vitamin feeding oil.

† From animal proteins and vitamin B_{12} supplement.

CORNELL PASTURE GROWER MASHES

	lb./ton	lb./ton	lb./ton	lb./ton
Yellow corn meal	665	715	665	905
Ground wheat	300	. . .	200	. . .
Wheat flour middlings	. . .	200	. . .	. . .
Wheat standard middlings	. . .	200	200	200
Pulverized oats	300	100	. . .	100
Ground barley	. . .	100	200	100
Soybean meal	600	400	450	450
Corn gluten meal	. . .	100	. . .	. . .
Peanut meal	. . .	. . .	100	. . .
Fish meal	. . .	. . .	. . .	50
Meat scrap	. . .	. . .	. . .	50
Corn distillers' dried solubles	. . .	50	. . .	. . .
Dried whey	. . .	. . .	50	. . .
Molasses distillers' dried solubles	. . .	. . .	. . .	25
Steamed bonemeal	85	85	85	60
Limestone	30	30	30	40
Salt (iodized)	20	20	20	20
Manganese sulfate (65% feeding grade)	0.5	0.5	0.5	0.5
Antibiotic feed supplement	±	±	±	±
Protein, %	20.7	20.4	20.5	20.5
Calcium, %	1.9	1.8	1.9	2.0
Total phosphorus, %	1.0	1.0	1.0	1.0
available, %	0.7	0.7	0.7	0.7

CORNELL BROILER STARTER MASHES

Ingredients	lb./ton	lb./ton	lb./ton
Ground yellow corn	975	970	780
Crushed (or coarse ground) wheat	300	...	400
Wheat flour middlings	...	200	...
Pulverized oats	...	100	...
Soybean meal (solvent)	400	330	420
Corn gluten meal	...	100	100
Fish meal	50	100	...
Fish solubles	...	...	50
Meat scraps	100	...	50
Corn distillers' dried solubles	50	50	75
Dried whey	50	50	...
Molasses fermentation solubles	...	...	25
Alfalfa meal (minimum 17% protein)	50	50	50
Ground limestone	20	30	30
Dicalcium phosphate	...	20	20
Salt	5	5	5
Manganese sulfate (feed grade)	0.5	0.5	0.5
D-activated animal sterols (1500 D)	0.5	0.5	0.5
or			
Vitamin feeding oil (300 D, 1500 A)	2	2	2
Riboflavin supplement to supply (gm. riboflavin)	1 gm.	1.5 gm.	1 gm.
Vitamin B_{12} supplement to supply (mg. B_{12})	4 mg.	4 mg.	4 mg.
Antibiotic feed supplement	+	+	+
Calculated composition:			
Protein, %	20.9	20.9	21.1
Calcium, %	1.2	1.2	1.3
Phosphorus, total, %	0.67	0.77	0.72
available, %	0.42	0.50	0.45
Vitamin A,* USP units/lb.	4500	3500	4200
Vitamin D, I.C.U./lb.	170	170	170
Riboflavin, mg./lb.	1.9	1.9	1.9
Vitamin B_{12}, μg./lb.	4	4	4
Niacin, mg./lb.	16	17	21
Pantothenic acid, mg./lb.	4.7	4.5	5.0
Productive energy, cal./lb.	925	885	895

* Calculated assuming alfalfa meal contains 100,000 USP units per pound, and without use of vitamin feeding oil in formula.

CORNELL BROILER GROWER MASHES

Ingredients	All-Mash Grower lb./ton	Mash-Grain Grower lb./ton
Ground yellow corn	1125	845
Crushed (or coarse ground) wheat	300	300
Soybean meal (solvent)	250	350
Corn gluten meal	75	100
Fish meal	50	50
Meat scrap	50	100
Corn distillers' solubles	50	50
Dried whey	. . .	50
Alfalfa meal	50	75
Dicalcium phosphate	15	30
Limestone	30	40
Salt	5	10
Manganese sulfate (feed grade)	0.5	1
D-activated animal sterol (1500 D)	0.5	1
or		
Vitamin feeding oil (300 D, 1500 A)	2	4
Riboflavin supplement to supply (gm. riboflavin)	2 gm.	2.5 gm.
Vitamin B_{12} supplement to supply (mg B_{12})	2 mg.	4.5 mg.
Antibiotic feed supplement	+	+
Calculated composition:		
Protein, %	18.1	21.5
Calcium, %	1.3	2.0
Phosphorus, total, %	0.69	0.97
available, %	0.45	0.72
Vitamin A, USP units/lb.	4300	5600
Vitamin D, I.C.U./lb.	170	340
Riboflavin, mg./lb.	2	2.7
Vitamin B_{12}, μg./lb.	2.4	4
Niacin, mg./lb.	16	16
Pantothenic acid, mg./lb.	4	4.7
Productive energy, cal./lb.	960	870

BRITISH COLUMBIA. (University of British Columbia and Department of Agriculture, U. B. C. Feed Formulas for Poultry, Poultry Circular 37, 1954.)

Chick Starting Mash. Designed to be fed to chicks for the first 4 to 8 weeks. Depending upon the rate of growth of the chicks, scratch grain may be fed in gradually increasing amounts, beginning with the fifth week. In case of cannibalism, ground or crushed oats should be self-fed.

Chick Growing Mash. To be fed with scratch grain in approximately equal amounts.

Broiler Mash. All-mash ration to be fed up to 8 weeks of age. Small amounts of scratch grain may be fed from the ninth week until marketing. If white skin, flesh, and fat are preferred, wheat may be used as the only grain. If yellow pigmentation is preferred, then equal amounts of wheat and corn should be fed. In case of cannibalism, whole oats should be fed in small quantities several times a day.

BRITISH COLUMBIA MASHES FOR YOUNG CHICKENS

Ingredients	Chick Starting Mash (per ton) lb.	Chick Growing Mash (per ton) lb.	Broiler Mash (per ton) lb.
Coarse ground wheat	805	770	700
Ground yellow corn	300	200	400
Pulverized oats	100	200	. . .
Ground barley	100	100	. . .
Wheat bran	. . .	100	. . .
Wheat middlings	100	100	200
Fish meal (65-70% protein)	100	50	100
Meat and bone scrap (50% protein)	100	100	100
Dried milk by-products	50	. . .	50
Soybean oil meal (44% protein)	200	150	300
Dehydrated green feed	50	100	40
Distillers' dried solubles or fermentation solubles	50 lb.	50 lb.	60 lb.
Ground limestone	30	40	25
Steamed bonemeal	. . .	20	10
Iodized salt	10	15	10
Manganese sulfate	4 oz.	8 oz.	5 oz.
Feeding oil (2250 I.U., A; 300 I.C.U., D per gram)	5 lb.	5 lb.	5 lb.
Choline chloride	1-2 lb.	. . .	1-2 lb.
Riboflavin	3 gm.	3 gm.	3 gm.
Vitamin B_{12}	1-2 mg.	1-2 mg.	4 mg.
Antibiotic	2-10 gm.	2-10 gm.	4-10 gm.
Recommended protein level	20%	18%	22%

CALIFORNIA. (California Official Random Sample Chicken Meat Production Test, Modesto, 1954.)

MASH FORMULA

Ingredient	Lb./ton
Alfalfa meal, dehydrated	80
Barley, ground	100
Bonemeal, special steamed	15
Corn, yellow ground	600
Fish meal, 65% protein minimum	200
Milo, ground	400
Ground limestone	40
Soybean oil meal, 44% protein minimum	250
Wheat, ground	200
Salt, fine	10
Vitamin A and D oil (2250, 400 D)	2
Butyl fermentation product (3630 mg. riboflavin per lb.)	1/2
Manganese sulfate, feeding grade	1/2
Antibiotic supplement	4

FLORIDA. (University of Florida, 1954.)

FLORIDA MASHES FOR YOUNG CHICKENS

Ingredients	Chick Starting and Growing* Ration, lb.	Broiler Ration, lb.
Wheat bran	3	...
Wheat middlings	7	...
Yellow corn meal	36	50
Ground oats	5	...
Distillers' solubles	3	...
Alfalfa leaf meal	6	3
Soybean meal	30	35
Meat scraps	3	...
Fish meal	...	3
Dried whey	3	3
Steamed bonemeal	2	1.5
Oystershell flour	1	1.5
Salt	1	0.5
Manganese sulfate	5.7 gm.	5.7 gm.
Delsterol	9.0 gm.	9.0 gm.
Vitamin A	...	14 gm.
Calcium pantothenate	...	1 gm.
Riboflavin	...	0.15 gm.
Nicotinic acid	...	1.5 gm.
Choline chloride		12.7 gm.
Aurofac 2A	...	57 gm.

*Grain to be added after 6 to 8 weeks.

IOWA. (Iowa State College Poultry Department, 1954.)

IOWA RATIONS FOR YOUNG CHICKENS

Ingredient and Protein Content	Starting 20%	Growing 20%	Broiler No. 1	Broiler No. 2
Ground yellow corn	1000	580	1135	1001
Ground whole oats	100	200	. . .	100
Wheat bran	100	200	. . .	. . .
Wheat middlings	100	200	100	100
Dehydrated alfalfa meal (17%)	100	200	50	50
Soybean oil meal (44%)	360	400	450	500
Meat and bone scrap (50%)	100	100	100	50
Fish meal (65%)	50	. . .	50	50
Dried whey or buttermilk	30	. . .	50	50
Steamed bonemeal (or equivalent)	20	50	20	40
Ground oystershell or limestone	20	30	10	20
Iodized salt	9	18	9	9
Manganese sulfate	1	1	1	1
Vitamin D concentrate (1500 I.C.U. per gm.)	1	2	1	1
Vitamin A concentrate (2250 I.U. per gm.)	5	5	. . .	. . .
Vitamin A-D concentrate (2250 A, 300 D)	. . .	. . .	4	4
Riboflavin concentrate (500 mcg./gm.)	. . .	. . .	20	20
Riboflavin concentrate (227 mg./lb.)	10	10	. . .	. . .
Niacin (grams)	20	20	20	20
Choline chloride (25%)	4	4	4	4
Pantothenic acid (grams)	. . .	. . .	10	10
Vitamin B_{12} (milligrams)	8	4	5	5
Total pounds	2000	2000	2000	2000

Note: The starting mash is to be fed as "all-mash." Grain is to be fed with the other mashes. Vitamins are usually provided in the form of concentrates. Adjustments must be made to compensate for differences in potency. Antibiotic supplements should be fed as supplements to the starting ration. The manufacturers' recommendations will be a satisfactory guide for the level to include with the specific antibiotic concentrate.

Antibiotics should be added to either of the above broiler rations. Penicillin at 2–4 grams per ton or aureomycin, terramycin, or bacitracin at 6–10 grams per ton are the commonly recommended levels. Methionine may be added at the rate of 0.5–1.0 pound per ton.

NEBRASKA. (University of Nebraska, Leaflet 109, 1953.)

NEBRASKA MASHES FOR YOUNG CHICKENS

Ingredients	Chick Starter 53-C, lb.	Broiler Ration 53 Br, lb.
Ground yellow corn	390	580
Wheat shorts or pulverized oats	200	50
Soybean meal	150	150
Alfalfa meal (17% protein plus)	50	50
Meat scraps (50% protein plus)	100	100
Fish meal	20	30
Dried whey	30	. . .
Fish solubles blend	20	. . .
Nebraska Vitamin Concentrate No. 4* or equivalent	10	10
Mineral Mixture No. 57†	30	30

*Each pound of Vitamin Concentrate No. 4 to carry the following minimum values:

Riboflavin		0.2 gm.
Calcium pantothenate		0.4 gm.
Niacin		0.6 gm.
Choline chloride		2.0 gm.
D_3		135,000 I.C.U.
B_{12}		0.3 mg.
Antibiotic	(procaine penicillin)	200 mg.
	(aureomycin)	1 gm.
	(terramycin)	1 gm.
	(bacitracin)	1 gm.

†Mineral Mixture No. 57	Parts by weight
Steamed bonemeal (or equivalent)	403
Limestone	403
Salt	161
Trace Mixture No. 1‡	33
	1000

‡Trace Mixture No. 1 carries enough manganese, iodine, iron, cobalt, copper, zinc, and other minor mineral elements when included at a level of 33 parts per 1000, and the complete mineral supplement is used at a level of either 2 or 3 per cent to supplement ingredients as called for in these formulas.

NEW ENGLAND COLLEGE CONFERENCE. (High efficiency poultry feed formulas, revised, June, 1954.)

RATIONS FOR YOUNG CHICKENS

Ingredients		All-Mash Chick Starting and Broiler, lb.	All-Mash Grower, lb.	Mash and Grain (14), Grower, lb.
Ground yellow corn (1)		1100	1050	950
Ground barley or pulverized oats (2)		. . .	200	100
Standard wheat middlings		100	250	200
Soybean oil meal (44%)		500	200	350
Fish meal (60%) (13)		100	50	50
Meat and bone scrap (50%)		. . .	50	75
Alfalfa meal (17%) (100,000 A per lb.)		60	75	100
Distillers dried solubles (3) (4)		50	50	75
Butyl fermentation product (3)(4)		20	20	20
Dicalcium phosphate or equivalent (5)		24	24	36
Ground limestone (feeding grade)		30	25	50
Iodized salt		10	10	15
Dry vitamin D (1500 D per gram) (6)		0.5	0.5	0.7
Manganese sulfate or equivalent (7)		0.25	0.25	0.4
Antibiotic supplement		* (8)	. . .	. . .
Vitamin B_{12} supplement		* (9)	* (9)	* (9)
Niacin		18 gm.	18 gm.	30 gm.
Choline chloride (dry, 25%)		2.5	. . .	. . .
DPPD (Diphenyl-p-phenylene-diamine)		0.25	* (10)	* (10)
Coccidiostat		* (11)	* (11)	* (11)
Totals (12)		1997.50	2004.75	2022.10
Calculated Analysis				
Energy	cal./lb.	898	891	903.0
Protein	%	21.1	16.2	16.2
Fat	%	3.2	3.7	3.6
Fiber	%	3.7	4.2	4.4
Calcium	%	1.36	1.34	1.43
Total phosphorus	%	0.77	0.82	0.77
Readily available phosphorus	%	0.50	0.53	0.50
Manganese	mg./lb	24.0	27.0	27.0
Vitamin A	I.U./lb	4308.0	5007.0	4463.0
Vitamin D	I.U./lb	170.0	170.0	157.0
Riboflavin	mg./lb	2.4	2.3	1.9
Pantothenic acid	mg./lb	5.3	5.2	4.9
Choline	mg./lb	684.0	431.0	424.0
Niacin	mg./lb	23.0	29.0	26.0

(1) Two to four hundred pounds of coarsely ground wheat may be used to replace an equal amount of corn. Add 0.4 pound of vitamin A and D oil for each 100 pounds of corn removed.

(2) On a nutrient content basis, barley is preferred to oats. Both barley and oats may be replaced by corn if a higher energy level is desired.

(3) 20 pounds of a butyl fermentation product containing at least 250 micrograms of riboflavin per gram (or 113.5 milligrams per pound) and 50 pounds of dried distillers solubles, or 40 pounds yeast or 40 pounds of dried whey plus a riboflavin supplement to furnish not less than 2.0 milligrams per pound in the final ration. To determine the amount of riboflavin supplement to use above, divide the number of milligrams desired by the manufacturer's guaranteed potency. Example: needed to furnish 454 milligrams, using a product having a guaranteed potency of 113.5 milligrams per pound. Solution: 454 divided by 113.5 equals 4 pounds needed in addition to either the yeast or the solubles. This is an example only, not an actual case.

(4) A vitamin concentrate containing not less than 2 grams of riboflavin and 4 grams of pantothenic acid and possibly other vitamins may be used to replace part or all of the fermentation products, and the total weight made up by adding corn meal.

(5) Steamed bonemeal or defluorinated rock phosphate may replace the dicalcium phosphate on a phosphorus basis. Raw rock phosphate containing not more than 3.5 per cent fluorine may replace one-half of the phosphorus in the dicalcium phosphate in the grower.

(6) Vitamin A and D feeding oil may be substituted on a unit basis.

(7) Manganese sulfate (70 per cent feeding grade) or equivalent amount of manganese from other sources.

(8) Use one to five pounds per ton depending upon the product used. Suggested levels are aureomycin, bacitracin, or terramycin, 9 gm.; or procaine penicillin, 2 to 4 grams per ton of finished ration, or equivalent.

(9) Use a vitamin B_{12} concentrate contributing not less than 6 milligrams of vitamin B_{12} per ton of ration.

(10) DPPD (diphenyl-p-phenylenediamine) is an antioxidant used in the chick starting and broiler ration at the 0.0125 per cent level to prevent the appearance of encephalomalacia (crazy chick disease). If desired it may also be added at the 0.0125 per cent level (one-quarter pound per ton) to the other rations to help prevent the destruction of the fat soluble vitamins.

(11) A coccidiosis controlling drug may be used in these rations at the level recommended by the manufacturer.

(12) If an even 2000 pounds is desired, adjust by removing or adding middlings.

(13) If a high salt fish meal is used, omit the added salt.

(14) Feeding ratio equals two parts of mash to one part of grain. Grain mixture contains fifty parts of corn, twenty-five parts of wheat and twenty-five parts of oats.

NORTH CAROLINA. (North Carolina State College of Agriculture and Engineering, University of North Carolina, 1954.)

NORTH CAROLINA RATIONS FOR YOUNG CHICKENS

Ingredients	No. 43 Broiler or Starter 20% lb.	No. 44 Finisher 17% lb.	No. 45 Grower All-Mash 16% lb.	No. 48 Grower Grain-Mash 20% lb.
Ground yellow corn	1143	1275	975	910
Pulverized oats	. . .	100	250	100
Wheat middlings	100	. . .	300	200
Corn gluten meal	50	50	. . .	. . .
Alfalfa meal (17% protein) 100,000 A per lb.	75	75	75	100
Fish meal (60% protein)	100	75	50	50
Soybean oil meal (44% protein)	400	300	225	425
Whey, dried	30	30	20	20
Butyl fermentation solubles (250 mg.) riboflavin per gm.)	40	40	20	20
Steamed bonemeal or equivalent	50	50	30	60
Salt	9	9	10	20
Feeding oil (300 D, 1500 A per gm.)	0.5	0.5	0.5	2.50
D-activated animal sterol (1500 D per gm.)	1	1	0.75	1
Meat and bone scrap (50% protein)	. . .	. . .	25	75
Antibiotic supplement	grams ++ *	grams ++ *	. . .	. . .
Vitamin B_{12} supplement	6–10 mg.	6–10 mg.	6 mg.	10–12 mg.
Choline chloride (dry 25%)	2	2	. . .	. . .
Niacin	20 gr.	20 gr.	18 gr.	20 gr.
Manganese sulfate	0.5	0.5	0.25	0.50
Pulverized oystershells or equivalent	. . .	. . .	20	20
Total	2001+	2008+	2002+	2004+

*Aureomycin, bacitracin, penicillins, and terramycin are added to broiler mashes for the purpose of stimulating growth in young chickens. Two arsonic compounds are also being used commercially in broiler feeds to stimulate growth in young chickens. The quantity of antibiotic as well as arsonic compound added to a broiler mash should be governed by the recommendation of the manufacturer.

Suggestions on feeding:

1. Self-feed the chicks broiler or starter mash without grain for 7 weeks. Replace the broiler mash with the finisher at 8 weeks, and feed it until the broilers are marketed. Some broiler growers, instead of using a finishing mash, prefer to feed the broiler mash throughout the growing period and finish the birds by feeding all the cracked yellow corn the broilers will clean up in 20 to 30 minutes in the late afternoon. The feeding of corn is started at 8 weeks of age.
2. Self-feed the replacement stock starter or broiler mash without grain for 7 weeks. Change the replacement stock from starter to grower at 8 weeks of age.
3. Do not feed a scratch mixture or separate grains with the all-mash 16 per cent protein mashes.
4. Feed a scratch mixture or separate grains with the 20 per cent protein mashes.
5. Keep crushed oystershells or limestone before the birds that are fed the 20 per cent protein grower. It is not necessary to feed crushed oystershells or limestone to the chickens receiving the all-mash 16 per cent protein mashes.
6. The growing chickens fed a scratch mixture or separate grains should have access to insoluble hard grit or gravel. Crushed granite, quartz, and feldspar are examples of hard grit.

ONTARIO AGRICULTURAL COLLEGE. (S. J. Slinger, W. F. Pepper, and J. R. Cavers. O.A.C. Chicken Starting, Growing, and Fattening Feed Formulas, O.A.C. Circular 142, revised, January, 1954; O.A.C. Broiler Feed Formulas, O.A.C. Circular 143, revised, June, 1953.)

Starter Mash. The feeding of chick grain as the sole feed, at the start, is often helpful in preventing pasting-up. It is recommended that chick grain not be fed for longer than 24 hours. This mash contains about 20 per cent protein (N × 6.25). It is designed to be fed for the first 8 weeks of life. It should be used as an all-mash ration for the first 7 weeks. For the period from 7 to 8 weeks of age a small amount of whole oats may be fed in conjunction with the mash. The feeding of insoluble grit is particularly important when grain feeding begins.

Chick Starter Concentrate. This concentrate when mixed in the proportion of 100 parts of concentrate to 225 parts of ground grains will make a chick starter mash containing about 20 per cent protein (N × 6.25). To have the chick starter mash similar in composition to the mash shown it is suggested that the ground grains be used in the proportions of 4 parts wheat, 1 part corn, 1 part barley, and 1 part oats by weight. The resultant starter mash should be used as already indicated for the chick starter mash.

Chick Confinement Grower Mash. This mash contains about 19 per cent protein (N × 6.25). It is designed to be fed to confined birds in conjunction with whole grain from 8 weeks of age until the birds begin to lay. The mash should be fed free choice, and grain should be hand fed in accordance with mash consumption, gradually increasing the level of grain feeding as the birds grow. As a guide, it is suggested that by 12 weeks of age the birds should be eating 75 parts of mash and 25 parts of grain; by 14 weeks of age, 60 of mash and 40 of grain; and at 16 weeks of age, 50 of mash and 50 of grain. For confinement-reared pullets it is not desirable at any time to have the grain consumption greater than that of mash.

Chick Confinement Grower Concentrate. This concentrate when mixed in the proportions of 100 of concentrate to 225 of ground grains will result in a confinement grower mash containing about 19 per cent protein. To make a grower mash similar in composition to the confinement mash presented, the ground grains should be used in the proportions of 6 parts wheat, 3 parts barley, 3 parts oats, and 2 parts corn by weight. The confinement grower mash made in this way should be used in the manner indicated previously.

Chick Range Grower Mash. This mash contains about 17.7 protein (N × 6.25). It is designed to be fed to birds on range from about 8 weeks of age until egg production begins. Mash should be freely accessible and grain limited until the birds are 12 weeks of age. After this time mash and grain may be made freely available in separate hoppers. If the range is succulent and short, the birds will gradually tend to consume more grain in proportion to mash as they grow. As a guide they should be consuming about 50 parts of mash to 50 parts of grain at 12 weeks of age, 40 parts of mash to 60 parts of grain by 16 weeks, and 30 parts of mash to 70 parts of grain by 20 weeks of age. It may be necessary to adjust these proportions somewhat during the latter part of the growing period, depending upon the rate of maturity. For birds reared out of doors but with little or no pasture available, the mash designed for confinement-reared birds should be used in preference to the range grower mash.

Chick Range Grower Concentrate. This concentrate when mixed in the proportions of 100 parts of concentrate to 300 parts of ground grains will make a range grower mash containing about 17.7 per cent protein (N × 6.25). To have a mash similar in composition to the range grower mash shown, the ground grains should be used in the proportions of 7 parts wheat, 3 parts barley, 3 parts oats, and 2 parts of corn by weight. The range mash made in this way should be used as suggested above for the range grower mash.

Broiler Feed. Regardless of the program used (Number 1, 2, or 3) the birds should be fed the starter mash for the first 6 weeks of age. At this time they should be changed to the formulas listed under 7 to 10 weeks. The change should be made gradually over a period of about 3 days. They should be fed this diet until they are 10 to 11 weeks old if they are to be marketed as broilers. The diets listed under "11 to 15 weeks" were devised for light roasters.

The feeding of chick grain as the sole feed for 24 hours is often helpful in preventing pasting-up. After this time no grain or additional minerals should be fed in conjunction with these mashes. Mash should be available for from 12 to 14 hours a day.

Insoluble grit such as granite should be sprinkled on the feed twice weekly or made freely accessible to the birds in separate hoppers. Chick-size grit is advisable for the first 6 weeks, after which grower-size grit is preferable.

Clean, fresh water should be easily accessible at all times. Placing waterers close to all feed hoppers is a distinct advantage.

O.A.C. CHICKEN STARTING AND GROWER MASHES

Ingredients	Chick Starter Mash, lb.	Chick Starter Concentrate, lb.	Chick Confinement Grower Mash, lb.	Chick Confinement Grower Concentrate, lb.	Chick Range Grower Mash, lb.	Chick Range Grower Concentrate, lb.
Ground wheat	760	...	600	...	700	...
Ground yellow corn	200	...	200	...	200	...
Ground barley	200	...	300	...	300	...
Pulverized oats	200	...	300	...	300	...
Dehydrated alfalfa meal (100,000 I.U. vitamin A activity/lb.) or cereal grass	63	200	93	300	50	207
Meat meal (50% protein)	20	60	70	240	60	240
Fish meal (65% protein)	50	160	25	80	20	80
Dried buttermilk or skimmilk	40	120	40	130	40	160
Soybean oil meal (44% protein)	400	1275	300	1000	250	1000
Ground limestone	15	60	20	90	25	100
Steamed bone meal or equivalent	40	90	40	120	45	165
Iodized salt	10	30	10	34	10	40
Vitamin A oil (10,000 I.U./gm.)	0.75	2	0.75	2	0.75	2
Dry vitamin D_3 (1650 I.C.U./gm.)	1	3	1	3	1	3
Manganese sulfate (feed grade)	0.25	0.75	0.4	1.25	0.4	1.5
	gm.	gm.	gm.	gm.	gm.	gm.
Riboflavin	2	7	3	10	2	8
Antibiotic*	2–10	6–30	3–15	10–50	2–10	8–40
Arsonic acid†	45–90	135–270	45–90	135–270	45–90	135–270
	mg.	mg.	mg.	mg.	mg.	mg.
Vitamin B_{12}	3	10	3	10	3	12
Calculated analysis:	%	%	%	%	%	%
Min. crude protein	20.4	38.6	19.0	35.5	17.7	35.2
Min. crude fat	2.3	1.6	2.6	2.1	2.6	2.1
Max. crude fiber	5.4	6.9	6.1	7.6	5.6	6.3
Calcium	1.2	3.3	1.4	5.0	1.5	5.7
Total phosphorus	0.8	1.4	0.8	1.8	0.8	2.1
Inorganic phosphorus	0.48	1.08	0.56	1.56	0.56	1.85

*If penicillin is used, the lower level is satisfactory. If aureomycin, terramycin, or bacitracin are used, the higher levels should be employed.

† Either 3-nitro, 4-hydroxyphenylarsonic acid at the lower levels indicated or arsanilic acid or sodium arsanilate at the higher levels may be used.

Substitutions. An equal mixture of wheat shorts and bran may be used to replace ground wheat or barley. For the starting diet an equal-parts mixture of wheat middlings and wheat shorts is more desirable.

Dried whey may replace dried buttermilk or dried skimmilk. For every 40 pounds of dried milk replaced, increase the amount of soybean oil meal by 30 pounds and reduce the ground wheat by 30 pounds.

Vitamin A feeding oil and dry vitamin D_3 may be replaced by fish oil on an equal unitage basis. The vitamin A oil may be replaced by dry vitamin A products or by vitamin A oils of other potency on an equal unitage basis.

Steamed bonemeal may be replaced by defluorinated rock phosphate. Other calcium and phosphorus carriers may also be used. Replacement should be based on the calcium and phosphorus content.

Manganese sulfate may be replaced by other manganese carriers to supply equal levels of manganese.

Ground limestone may be replaced by calcium carbonate.

O.A.C. BROILER FEED FORMULAS

Ingredients	Program No. 1 Age in Weeks 0-6	7-10	11-15	Program No. 2 Age in Weeks 0-6	7-10	11-15	Program No. 3 Age in Weeks 0-6	7-10	11-15
	lb.	lb.	lb.	lb.	lb.	lb.	lb.	lb.	lb.
Ground wheat	1000	900	900	1200	1100	1100	280	300	300
Ground yellow corn	200	550	600	100	400	450	900	1055	1100
Pulverized oats	–	–	100	–	–	100	–	–	100
Soybean oil meal (44% protein)	570	350	230	–	–	–	590	450	330
Soybean oil meal (50% protein)	–	–	–	470	300	180	–	–	–
Soybean oil	20	20	–	20	20	–	20	20	–
Dehydrated alfalfa meal or cereal grass	40	40	40	40	40	40	40	40	40
Meat meal (50% protein)	20	20	20	20	20	20	20	20	20
Fish meal (65% protein)	60	40	40	60	40	40	60	40	40
Dried buttermilk or skimmilk	40	30	30	40	30	30	40	30	30
Ground limestone	10	15	15	10	15	15	10	10	10
Steamed bonemeal	35	25	20	35	25	20	35	30	25
Iodized salt	5	5	5	5	5	5	5	5	5
Vitamin A oil (10,000 I.U./gm.)	0.75	0.75	0.75	0.75	0.75	0.75	0.75	0.75	0.75
Dry vitamin D_3 (1500 I.C.U./gm.)	1	1	1	1	1	1	1	1	1
DL Methionine (feed grade)	0.5	0.5	–	0.5	0.5	–	0.5	0.5	–
Manganese sulfate (feed grade)	0.3	0.3	0.3	0.3	0.3	0.3	0.35	0.35	0.35
	gm.	gm.	gm.	gm.	gm.	gm.	gm.	gm.	gm.
Riboflavin	3	2	2	3	2	2	3	2	2
Niacin	–	10	10	–	5	5	15	15	15
Antibiotic*	2–10	2–10	2–10	2–10	2–10	2–10	2–10	2–10	2–10
Arsonic acid†	45–90	45–90	45–90	45–90	45–90	45–90	45–90	45–90	45–90
	mg.	mg.	mg.	mg.	mg.	mg.	mg.	mg.	mg.
Vitamin B_{12}	5	3	3	5	3	3	5	3	3
Calculated analysis	%	%	%	%	%	%	%	%	%
Min. crude protein	23.4	18.4	16.6	23.4	18.9	16.7	21.9	18.8	16.8
Min. crude fat	3.9	4.1	3.3	4.1	4.2	3.4	4.0	4.0	3.2
Max. crude fiber	4.4	3.8	4.1	3.1	3.2	3.7	4.2	3.9	4.1
Calcium	1.0	0.9	0.8	1.0	0.9	0.8	1.0	0.9	0.8
Total phosphorus	0.8	0.6	0.6	0.8	0.6	0.6	0.8	0.6	0.6
Inorganic phosphorus	0.47	0.36	0.33	0.47	0.37	0.33	0.47	0.39	0.35

*Penicillin, 2 grams; aureomycin, terramycin or bacitracin, 10 grams.

†3 nitro-4 hydroxyphenylarsonic acid, 45 grams; arsanilic acid or sodium arsanilate, 90 grams.

Substitutions. Soybean oil may be replaced by corn or wheat when the feed is fed as pellets or crumbles.

Dried buttermilk or skimmilk may be replaced by dried whey provided proper adjustment is made for protein.

Steamed bonemeal may be replaced by other calcium and phosphorus carriers on the basis of their calcium and phosphorus content.

Vitamin A feeding oil and dry vitamin D_3 may be replaced by fish oil on an equal unitage basis.

Manganese sulfate may be replaced by other manganese carriers to supply equivalent amounts of manganese.

OHIO. (Ohio State University Extension Bulletin 343, 1954)

OHIO RATIONS FOR YOUNG CHICKENS

Ingredients	Chick Starting Mash 20% protein lb.	Broiler Mash, 22% protein lb.
Corn, yellow	400	488
Middling, standard or ground wheat	150	50
Wheat bran	70	. . .
Soybean oil meal (44% protein)	225	300
Meat scrap (50% protein)	50	50
Alfalfa, 17% protein dehydrated	50	30
Fish meal (58% protein) or fish solubles*	30	30
Rock phosphate, defluorinated or steamed bone meal (15% phos.)	10	12
Limestone (95% or more calcium carbonate)	10	10
Iodized salt	5	5
Manganese sulfate	0.25	0.25
Stabilized animal fat* or ground corn	0	25
	1,000	1,000
Additives per 1,000 lb. of mash:		
Vitamin A, I.U.	1,000,000	1,500,000
Vitamin D_3, I.U.	225,000	300,000
Riboflavin, gm.	1.6	2.0
Calcium pantothenate, gm.	1.0	2.0
Choline chloride, gm.	125	180
Vitamin B_{12}, mg.	0	6
Antibiotic	†	†
Niacin, gm.	6	10
Methionine (optional)	†	†
Sodium arsanilate or arsanilic acid, gm. (optional)	0	†

*Preferred.

†Should be used at manufacturers' recommended level.

TEXAS. (Agricultural and Mechanical College of Texas, 1954)

TEXAS RATIONS FOR YOUNG CHICKENS

Ingredients	Chick Starter and Broiler All-Mash %	Chicken Grower All-Mash %	Broiler Finisher All-Mash %
Ground milo	27*	39*	25*
Ground yellow corn	27 1/2*	25*	44*
Soybean oil meal (44% protein)†	30	22	18
Fish meal (60% protein)	2 1/2	2	2 1/2
Fish solubles	2 1/2	. . .	. . .
Dried whey	2 1/2	3	2 1/2
Dehydrated alfalfa leaf meal	4	5	4
Steamed bonemeal or equivalent phosphorus supplement	2	2	2
Ground limestone or oystershell	1 1/2	1 1/2	1 1/2
Salt	1/2	1/2	1/2
Supplements‡			

*Milo and corn can be used interchangeably depending upon price and availability.

†Soybean oil meal may be replaced by cottonseed meal meeting the following quality specifications: (1) containing no more than 0.1 per cent free gossypol; (2) having a nitrogen solubility of at least 70 per cent in 0.02 N sodium hydroxide. Ten per cent in the starter and broiler all-mash; 8 per cent in the chicken grower, all-mash; 6 per cent in the all-mash broiler finisher.

‡To be added per ton of feed:

1. Manganese sulfate: 1/2 pound.
2. Antibiotics: Use either 10 grams of aureomycin, 10 grams of bacitracin, 10 grams of terramycin or 4 grams of penicillin. A combination of two, three or four of the antibiotics may be used. In making up the combination, use a proportionate part of the above given levels on a per ton basis.
3. Vitamin A: 2,270,000 International units. Any source of vitamin A available may be used just so the total number of units added per ton is that given above.
4. Vitamin D_3: 1,200,000 International chick units.
5. B vitamins: 4 gm. riboflavin; 10 gm. calcium pantothenate (Dextrorotatory); 25 gm. niacin; 100 gm. choline chloride. It will probably be necessary to obtain choline chloride in the dry form as a 25 per cent supplement.
6. Vitamin B_{12}: 6 milligrams.
7. Methionine: 1 pound.
8. Arsonic acids: Add level according to manufacturers' recommendations (add to broiler, broiler finishing, and starting rations only).

WASHINGTON. (Washington Poultry Feed Formulas, Poultry Science Department, State College of Washington, Ext. Mimeo. 1057, 1065, and 1582, 1954.)

CHICKEN FRYER AND STARTER MASHES

Ingredients	1 %	2 %	3 %	4 %	5 %	6 %
Ground yellow corn or milo*	64.7	63.7	59.8	65.8	66.5	68.8
Dehydrated alfalfa or grass (carotene, 12mg./100gm.)	2.5	2.5	2.5	2.5	2.5	2.5
Fish meal (70% protein)	5.0	3.5	2.0	3.5	3.5	10.0
Soybean oil meal (44% protein)	24.0	26.5	28.8	20.7	18.2	15.3
Meat and bonemeal (50% protein)	...	...	...	5.0	7.5	...
Whey, dried	...	...	3.0	...	...	...
Limestone or shell flour	1.6	1.5	1.6	1.6	1.5	1.6
Steamed bonemeal or defluorinated phosphate	1.9	2.0	2.0	0.6	...	1.5
Salt (iodized, fine)	0.3	0.3	0.3	0.3	0.3	0.3
Add the following to each ton of feed						
Riboflavin (grams)	1.0	1.0	0.22	1.0	1.0	1.0
Vitamin D_3, millions of I.C.U.	0.27	0.27	0.27	0.27	0.27	0.27
Methionine (97-100% pure)	0.5	0.5	0.5	0.5	0.5	0.5
Manganese sulfate, lb. (100% pure)	0.25	0.25	0.25	0.25	0.25	0.25
Antibiotic†						

Suggested analysis: protein, 20 per cent; calcium, 1.4 per cent; phosphorus, 0.7 per cent; vitamin A, 1200 International units per pound; vitamin D_3, 135 International chick units per pound; and riboflavin 1.6 milligrams per pound.

The suggested method of feeding fryers is as follows: During the first 2 weeks keep mash or crumbles only before the chicks. From 2 weeks to market age feed mash, crumbles or pellets. An amount of scratch that will be cleaned up in 20 minutes may be fed once a day after 6 weeks of age.

The suggested method of feeding replacement stock is as follows: During the 8-week starting period keep mash, crumbles or pellets (after second week) always before the chicks. Start grain feeding the fourth week. Keep grain in hoppers continuously or feed all they will eat three times daily in the litter or yard. Feed granite or silica grit of the proper size 1 day each week.

*Up to 20.0 per cent of ground wheat, ground barley, or finely ground oats may be used to replace an equivalent amount of corn or milo; however, substitutions of oats and barley will noticeably decrease feed efficiency.

†If using diamine or procaine penicillin use at rate of 3 grams per ton. If using aureomycin, bacitracin or terramycin use at rate of 10 grams per ton.

WASHINGTON CHICKEN DEVELOPER MASHES
(8 weeks to maturity)

Ingredients	1 %	2 %	3 %	4 %	5 %	6 %
Ground corn or ground milo	...	...	...	...	...	66.1
Ground grains*	48.8	49.6	51.9	46.7	48.9	...
Wheat mixed feed (mill-run)*	20.0	20.0	20.0	20.0	20.0	...
Fish meal (70% protein)	2.5	...	2.5	...	2.5	2.5
Meat and bonemeal (50% protein)	...	5.0	5.0	...	...	...
Soybean oil meal (44% protein)	12.7	10.7	6.3	17.1	7.6	20.0
Cottonseed meal (43% protein; maximum free gossypol, 0.003%)	...	...	...	...	5.0	...
Dehydrated alfalfa or grass (carotene, 12 mg./100 gm.)†	10.0	10.0	10.0	10.0	10.0	5.0
Limestone or shell flour	2.0	1.5	1.5	2.0	2.3	1.6
Steamed bonemeal or defluorinated phosphate	3.2	2.4	2.0	3.4	2.9	4.0
Salt (iodized, fine)	0.8	0.8	0.8	0.8	0.8	0.8
Add the following to each ton of feed						
Vitamin A, millions I.U.	...	...	...	...	...	6.9
Vitamin D_3, millions I.C.U.	0.27	0.27	0.27	0.27	0.27	0.27
Riboflavin (grams)	1.6	1.6	1.6	1.6	1.6	2.5
Vitamin B_{12} (milligrams)	...	...	...	4.8	...	...
Manganese sulfate lb. (100% pure)	0.4	0.4	0.4	0.4	0.4	0.4

Suggested analysis: protein, 17.5 per cent; calcium, 2.0 per cent; phosphorus, 1.0 per cent; vitamin A, 8000 International units per pound; vitamin D_3, 540 International chick units per pound; riboflavin, 2.0 milligrams per pound.

These mashes are formulated to be fed free choice with whole grains. Adequate vitamins are provided to meet requirements when pullets consume up to 75 per cent whole grain. Granite or silica grit should be fed one day each week.

*Ground corn, milo, wheat, barley or oats may be used singly or in any combination with 0 to 20 per cent millrun as long as the combined amounts of barley, oats, and millrun to not exceed 55 per cent of the mash.

†Dehydrated alfalfa or grass may be reduced 5 per cent in rations 1 through 5; and the ground grain may be increased by 5 per cent if vitamin A is added at the rate of 6.9 million International units per ton of mash. Less vitamin A supplement will be required if a higher carotene dehydrated alfalfa or grass is used.

WASHINGTON ALL INCLUSIVE DEVELOPER MASHES

Ingredients	No. 1 %	No. 2 %
Ground grains and millrun*	74.6	75.6
Fish meal (70% protein)	2.0	2.0
Meat and bonemeal	. . .	5.0
Soybean oil meal (44% protein)	15.0	10.0
Dehydrated alfalfa or grass (carotene 12mg./100g.)	5.0	5.0
Limestone or shell flour	1.7	1.3
Steamed bonemeal or defluorinated phosphate	1.7	0.6
Salt (iodized, fine)	0.5	0.5
Add the following to each ton of feed		
Vitamin D_3, millions of I.C.U.	0.27	0.27
Manganese sulfate, lb. (100% pure)	0.3	0.3

Suggested analysis: protein, 16 per cent; riboflavin, 0.9 per cent, milligrams per pound; vitamin A, 2000 International units per pound; vitamin D_3, 135 International chick units per pound; phosphorus, 0.7 per cent; calcium, 1.4 per cent.

These diets are designed to be used as the only feed fed to the birds.

*Ground corn, milo, wheat, barley, or oats may be used singly or in any combination with 0-10 per cent millrun as long as the combined amounts of barley, oats, and millrun do not exceed 35 per cent of the diet.

WISCONSIN. (University of Wisconsin, 1954.)

WISCONSIN RATIONS FOR YOUNG CHICKENS

Ingredients	20% Chick Starter and Broiler Mash	Chick Grower with Good Pasture
Ground yellow corn	515	350
Wheat bran	50	100
Wheat middlings	50	150
Pulverized oats	. . .	150
Dehydrated alfalfa meal	50	. . .
Meat scrap	50	50
Fish meal	. . .	. . .
Soybean oil meal	250	150
Steamed bonemeal or defluorinated rock phosphate or equivalent	10	20
Chick size oystershell or hi-calcium limestone	20	20
Iodized salt	5	10
Riboflavin*	Yes	No
Vitamin B_{12} supplement†‡	Yes	No
Antibiotic feed supplement†	Yes	No
400 D Fish oil or powder§	1 1/2	. . .
Manganese sulfate (feeding grade)	1/4	. . .

Grains to be fed free choice with all above rations, except 20 per cent chick starter and broiler mash.

Oystershell and granite grit fed free choice in all rations.

* Riboflavin: 1.0 milligrams per pound of feed from any source.

† Use according to manufacturers' directions.

‡ Some commercial supplements do not meet the minimum standards for this product but may be good sources.

§ Based on A.O.A.C. units. If new International chick unit is used, 75 per cent of the above will be sufficient.

WISCONSIN RATIONS FOR BROILERS

Ingredients	I	Ia	II	III	IV	V	VI	VII
Ground yellow corn	43	43	43	38	43	43	44	43
Wheat bran	5	5	5	5	5	5	5	5
Wheat middlings	5	5	5	5	5	5	5	5
Soybean oil meal	22	32	32	32	30	20	26	27
Meat scrap	...	...	...	...	...	...	5	...
Fish meal	...	...	...	...	2	2	...	...
Fish solubles	3	3	...	...	...	...	...	...
Dried yeast	...	...	...	...	...	...	...	5
Dried whey (fortified)	...	...	...	5	...	...	...	...
Dehydrated alfalfa meal	5	5	5	5	5	5	5	5
Steamed bonemeal	2	2	2	2	2	2	1	2
Chick size oystershell	2	2	2	2	2	2	2	2
Granite grit	2	2	2	2	2	2	2	2
Iodized salt	0.5	0.5	0.5	0.5	0.5	0.5	0.5	0.5
Corn gluten meal	10	...	...	...	...	10	...	...
Feeding oil (300 D)*	0.2	0.2	0.2	0.2	0.2	0.2	0.2	0.2
Riboflavin supplement†	+	+	+	...	+	+	+	+
$MnSO_4$ oz./100 lb. (feeding grade)	0.25	0.25	0.25	0.25	0.25	0.25	0.25	0.25
Vitamin B_{12} supplement‡	...	...	+	+	+	+	+	+
Antibiotic feed supplement‡	+	+	+	+	+	+	+	+

*New International chick unit (I.C.U.)

† To supply 1 milligram riboflavin per pound of feed from any source.

‡ Use according to manufacturer's directions. Certain supplements not of antibiotic origin may give equivalent growth.

SECTION II. RATIONS FOR LAYERS

CORNELL. (Department of Poultry Husbandry, New York State College of Agriculture, Stencil 205, January, 1953.)

Cornell Layer Mashes. To be fed with approximately equal grain intake according to any good mash-grain feeding program.

Mixing Mashes. Mash concentrates to be used with local grain (see Section VII).

CORNELL LAYER MASHES

	Lb./ton	Lb./ton	Lb./ton	Lb./ton
Yellow corn meal	795	580	750	630
Ground wheat	300	300	...	...
Wheat flour middlings	...	...	300	200
Wheat standard middlings	...	300	...	200
Pulverized oats	100	...	200	...
Ground barley	...	...	...	200
Soybean meal	475	425	370	380
Corn gluten meal	...	...	...	50
Peanut meal	...	100	...	...
Fish meal	...	...	50	50
Meat scrap	100	...	50	...
Corn distillers' dried solubles	...	...	50	...
Dried whey	...	...	...	50
Molasses distillers' dried solubles	...	25	...	...
Dehydrated alfalfa meal	100	100	100	100
Riboflavin supplement to supply (mg. riboflavin)	400 mg.	200 mg.	200 mg.	...
D-activated animal sterols (1500 I.C.U./gm.)	2	2	2	2
or				
Vitamin feeding oil (300 D, 1500 A)	10	10	10	10
Steamed bonemeal	90	120	90	100
Limestone	20	20	20	20
Salt (iodized)	20	20	20	20
Manganese sulfate (65% feeding grade)	0.5	0.5	0.5	0.5
Protein, %	20.6	20.7	20.5	20.6
Calcium, %	2.3	2.3	2.2	2.1
Total phosphorus, %	1.2	1.2	1.2	1.2
Available, %	0.9	0.9	0.9	0.9
Vitamin A,* I.U./lb.	5800	5600	5800	5600
Vitamin D, I.C.U./lb.	680	680	680	680
Riboflavin, mg/lb.	1.3	1.3	1.3	1.6

* Assuming use of alfalfa meal containing 100,000 units of vitamin A activity per pound and no vitamin feeding oil.

CORNELL. (All-mash ration for hens, F. W. Hill, *Cornell Feed Service*, November, 1952.)

	lb.
Yellow corn meal	945
Ground wheat	500
Alfalfa meal (17%)	40
Soybean meal (44%)	250
Fish meal	50
Meat scraps (50%)	50
Distillers' dried solubles	50
Dried whey	50
Dicalcium phosphate	25
Ground limestone	30
Salt	10
Manganese sulfate	0.5
Vitamin A oil (4500/gm.)	1
Dry D (1500/gm.)	1
	2002.5

Calculated composition:

Protein, %	16.1
Calcium, %	1.4*
Phosphorus, %	0.78
Available phosphorus, %	0.56
Vitamin A, I.U./lb.	4400.
Vitamin D, I.C.U./lb.	340.
Riboflavin, mg./lb.	1.3

*Calcium level insufficient to meet requirements for high egg production. Free-choice feeding of oystershell or other calcium supplement necessary.

BRITISH COLUMBIA. (University of British Columbia and Department of Agriculture U.B.C. Feed Formulas for Poultry, 1954, Poultry Circular 37.)

Pullet Laying Mash. To be fed with scratch grain: approximately 60 parts of mash to 40 parts of grain. Clean oystershell should be freely accessible.

All-Mash Laying Ration. This is an all-mash ration which need not be supplemented with oystershell. It may be fed either to birds in laying cages or birds ordinarily housed.

BRITISH COLUMBIA LAYING MASHES

Ingredients	Pullet Laying Mash (per ton), lb.	All-Mash Laying Ration (pelleted) (per ton), lb.
Coarse ground wheat	800	1035
Ground yellow corn	100	300
Pulverized oats	200	100
Ground barley	100	100
Wheat bran	100	...
Wheat middlings	100	...
Fish meal (65-70% protein)	100	50
Meat and bone scrap (50% protein)	200	...
Soybean oil meal (44% protein)	100	150
Dehydrated green feed	100	80
Distillers' dried solubles or fermentation solubles	...	50
Ground limestone	50	70
Steamed bonemeal	20	50
Iodized salt	20	10
Manganese sulfate	8 oz.	4 oz.
Feeding oil (2250 I.U., A; 300 I.C.U., D per gram)	10	5
Choline chloride	...	1-2
Riboflavin	2 gm.	1 gm.
Recommended protein level	20%	16%

CALIFORNIA. (California Egg Laying Test, Modesto, 1954.)

LAYING MASH FORMULA

Ingredients	Lb./ton
Alfalfa meal, dehydrated	150
Barley, ground	200
Corn, yellow ground	400
Fish meal, 70% protein minimum	158
Meat and bone scraps, 50% protein minimum	50
Milo, ground	200
Ground limestone	40
Wheat, ground	200
Soybean oil meal, 44% protein	250
Wheat bran	300
Whey, dried	50
Salt, fine	10
Vitamin D source (1500)	2
Manganese sulfate, 85% pure	1/4
Riboflavin (or concentrate to provide this amount)	1 gm.

Free choice barley, granite grit, oystershell

CONNECTICUT. (A high-efficiency ration for laying and breeding hens, E. P. Singsen, L. D. Matterson, and Anna Kozeff, Conn. Bul. 286, 1952.)

	Pounds
Ground yellow corn	1223
Standard wheat middlings	250
Soybean oil meal	200
Meat scrap (50%)	100
Fish meal (60%)	40
Alfalfa meal (100,000 A/lb.)	50
Butyl fermentation product (250 riboflavin/lb.)	20
Steamed bonemeal	40
Ground limestone	60
Salt	10
Vitamin A and D feeding oil (2000 A-400 D/gm.)	5
Vitamin B_{12} concentrate (3 mg./lb.)	2
Manganese sulfate	0.25
Nicotinic acid	20 gm.
	2000.25

This ration to be fed as an all-mash ration or as all-mash and pellets. The pellets are made from the same mash.

FLORIDA. (University of Florida, 1954.)

Ingredients	Laying and Breeding Ration lb.	National Egg Laying Test lb.	Low-Energy All-Mash lb.	Cage-Layer High-Efficiency All-Mash lb.
	Mash			
Yellow corn meal	200	100	287	52
Shorts	100	100	287	10
Wheat bran	100	100	100	. . .
Ground oats	100	100	287	10
Soybean meal	150	70	70	10
Meat scrap	100	20	20	5
Fish meal	. . .	15	15	2.5
Dried whey	80	10	10	
Alfalfa leaf meal	100	25	25	5
Steam bonemeal	30	10	10	3
Shell	20	7	7*	2
Salt	10	3	3	0.25
Delsterol (vitamin D)	450 gm.	. . .	†	
Vitamin A	454 gm.	. . .	‡	
Vitamin supplement	. . .	. . .	. . .	§
	Grain			
Whole yellow corn	100	100		
Wheat	100	200		
Oats	100	100		

* Keep oystershell in hopper.

† 200 units per pound.

‡ 2000 units per pound.

§ Must supply the following amounts of each vitamin per pound of mash:

Vitamin A	4000 units.
Vitamin D_3	600 units.
Riboflavin	2 mg.
Pantothenic acid	3 mg.
Niacin	9 mg.
Vitamin B_{12}	1.5 μg.

IOWA. (Iowa State College, Poultry Department, 1954.)

IOWA RATIONS FOR LAYING AND BREEDING HENS

Ingredient and Protein Content	15%	20%	26%
Ground yellow corn	1120	573	134
Ground whole oats	200	200	200
Wheat bran	100	200	200
Wheat middlings	100	200	200
Dehydrated alfalfa meal (17%)	100	200	300
Soybean oil meal (44%)	200	400	600
Meat and bone scrap (50%)	100	100	150
Steamed bonemeal (or equivalent)	40	60	100
Ground oystershell or limestone	20	30	55
Iodized salt	9	18.5	28
Manganese sulfate	1	1.5	2
Vitamin D concentrate (1500 I.C.U. per gr.)	1 lb.	2 lb.	3 lb.
Riboflavin concentrate (227 mg./lb.)	6 lb.	10 lb.	20 lb.
Niacin (grams)	5 gm.	10 gm.	20 gm.
Vitamin B_{12} (milligrams)*	2 mg.	3 mg.	4 mg.
Vitamin A concentrate (2250 I.U. per gr.)	3 lb.	5 lb.	8 lb.
Total pounds	2000	2000	2000

Note: The 15 per cent laying mash is to be fed as "all-mash." Grain is to be fed with the other mashes. Vitamins are usually provided in the form of concentrates. Adjustments must be made to compensate for differences in potency. If the laying mashes are to be used as breeder rations, 40-100 pounds of fish solubles should be added per ton.

* Vitamin B_{12} to be added to laying rations if they are to be used as breeder rations.

NEW ENGLAND COLLEGE CONFERENCE, JUNE, 1954.

RATIONS FOR LAYERS

	Mash and Grain	All-Mash
Feeding ratio; mash to scratch	2/1	. . .
Mash ingredient	lb.	lb.
Ground yellow corn (1)	950	1125
Ground barley or pulverized oats (2)	100	100
Standard wheat middlings	200	200
Soybean oil meal (44%)	350	250
Fish meal (60%) (3)	40	25
Meat and bone scrap (50%)	75	50
Alfalfa meal (17%; 100,000 A/lb.)	100	75
Distillers' dried solubles (4) (5)	75	50
Dicalcium phosphate or equivalent (6)	40	32
Ground limestone (feeding grade)	65	75
Iodized salt	15	10
Dry vitamin D (1500 D/gm.) (7)	1.5	1
Manganese sulfate or equivalent (8)	0.4	0.25
Vitamin B_{12} supplement	(9)	(10)
Niacin	30 gm.	18 gm.
DPPD (diphenyl-p-phenylenediamine)	(11)	(11)
Totals (12)	2011.9	1993.25

(1) Two to four hundred pounds of coarsely ground wheat may be used to replace an equal amount of corn. Add 0.4 pounds of vitamin A and D oil for each 100 pounds of corn removed.

(2) On a nutrient content basis, barley is preferred to oats. Both barley and oats may be replaced by corn if a higher energy level is desired.

(3) If a high salt fish meal is used, omit the added salt.

(4) Twenty pounds of a butyl fermentation product containing at least 250 micrograms of riboflavin per gram (or 113.5 milligrams per pound) and 50 pounds of dried distillers' solubles; or 40 pounds yeast or 40 pounds of dried whey plus a riboflavin supplement to furnish not less than 2.0 milligrams per pound in the final ration. To determine the amount of riboflavin supplement to use above, divide the number of milligrams desired by the manufacturer's guaranteed potency. Example: Needed to furnish 454 milligrams using a product having a guaranteed potency of 113.5 milligrams per pound. Solution: 454 divided by 113.5 equals 4 pounds needed in addition to either the yeast or the solubles. This is an example only, not an actual case.

(5) A vitamin concentrate containing not less than 2 grams of riboflavin and 4 grams of pantothenic acid and possibly other vitamins may be used to replace part or all of the fermentation products, and the total weight may be made up by adding corn meal.

(6) Steamed bonemeal or defluorinated rock phosphate may replace the dicalcium phosphate on a phosphorus basis. Raw rock phosphate

containing not more than 3.5 per cent fluorine may replace one-quarter of the phosphorus in the dicalcium phosphate in the layer rations.

(7) Vitamin A and D feeding oil may be substituted on a unit basis.

(8) Manganese sulfate (70 per cent feeding grade) or equivalent amount of manganese from other sources.

(9) Use 9 milligrams of vitamin B_{12} per ton of ration.

(10) Use a vitamin B_{12} concentrate contributing not less than 6 mg. of vitamin B_{12} per ton of ration.

(11) DPPD (diphenyl-p-phenylenediamine) is an antioxidant and may be added at the 0.0125 per cent level (one-quarter pound per ton) to help prevent the destruction of the fat soluble vitamins.

(12) If an even 2000 pounds is desired, adjust by removing or adding middlings.

NEW YORK EGG-LAYING TESTS, 1952-1953. This is an all-mash formula. No supplements need to be fed, though water may be sprinkled on the mash as a feeding stimulus.

	Lb.
Yellow corn meal	945
Ground wheat	500
Alfalfa meal (17%)	40
Soybean meal (44%)	250
Fish meal	50
Meat scraps (50%)	50
Distillers' dried solubles	50
Dried whey	50
Dicalcium phosphate	25
Ground limestone	30
Salt	10
Manganese sulfate	0.5
Vitamin A oil (4500/gm.)	1
Dry D (1500/gm.)	1
	2002.5

OHIO. (Ohio Poultry Rations, Ohio Ext. Bul. 343, 1954.)

Laying and Breeding Mash, 20 per cent protein. This mash is adequate in the vitamins essential to good hatchability, therefore it can be fed to breeding flocks as well as market-egg flocks.

Keep the mash before the layers at all times. Feed whole grains (corn, wheat, or oats) at the rate of 40 pounds of grain to each 60 pounds of mash consumed. Another system is keep the mash before the birds all the time and limit the grain to from 2 to 6 quarts per 100 birds per day. Feed the smaller amount of grain when egg production is low.

Breeding Mash Concentrate, 26 per cent protein. Feed free choice as a laying and breeding mash for chickens and turkeys. Grains such as corn, wheat, and oats also can be fed free choice.

High-Energy Ration. This ration should be fed without the addition of any other feedstuff except a good source of calcium.

OHIO LAYING AND BREEDING RATIONS

Ingredients	Laying and Breeding Mash, 20% Protein lb.	Breeding Mash Concentrate, 26% Protein lb.	High-Energy Laying, Breeding, All-Mash lb.
Corn, yellow	400	292	600
Middling, standard or ground wheat	140	100	100
Wheat bran	70	...	...
Soybean oil meal (44% protein)	200	320	160
Meat scrap (50% protein)	50	50	25
Alfalfa, 17% protein dehydrated	50	75	40
Fish meal (58% protein) or fish solubles*	25	50	25
Rock phosphate, deflurinated or steamed bonemeal (15% phos.)	30	48	20
Iodized salt	10	15	5
Manganese sulfate	0.25	0.75	0.2
Dried whey (low lactose) or dried buttermilk*	25	50	25
	1,000	1,000	1,000
Additives per 1,000 lb. of mash			
Vitamin A, I.U.	2,000,000	3,000,000	500,000
Vitamin D_3, I.U.	1,000,000	1,350,000	500,000
Riboflavin, gm.	2.0	3.0	1.5
Calcium pantothenate, gm.	2.0	2.0	1.0
Vitamin B_{12}, mg.	6	12	6

* Preferred.

NORTH CAROLINA. (North Carolina State College of Agriculture and Engineering of the University of North Carolina, 1954.)

NORTH CAROLINA RATIONS FOR LAYERS

Ingredients	No. 46 All-Mash 16% lb.	No. 49 Grain-Mash 20% lb.
Ground yellow corn	925	870
Standard wheat middlings	300	50
Pulverized oats	250	100
Meat and bone scrap (50% protein)	50	75
Fish meal (60% protein)	25	50
Soybean oil meal (44% protein)	225	475
Alfalfa meal (17% protein) 100,000 A/lb.	75	100
Butyl fermentation solubles (250 micrograms riboflavin per gm.)	20	20
Steamed bonemeal or equivalent	50	120
Pulverized oystershells or equivalent	70	20
Salt	10	20
Feeding oil (300 D, 1500 A per gm.)	2	2
D-activated animal sterol (1500 D per gm.)	1	2.25
Manganese sulfate	0.25	0.50
	gm.	gm.
Niacin	18	20
	mg.	mg.
Vitamin B_{12} supplement	3-6	6-12
Total	2003+	2004+

Suggestions on Feeding:

1. Do not feed a scratch mixture or separate grains with the all-mash, 16 per cent protein mash.
2. Feed a scratch mixture or separate grains with the 20 per cent protein mash.
3. Keep crushed oystershells or limestone before the birds that are fed the 20 per cent protein layer mash. It is not necessary to feed crushed oystershells or limestone tò the chickens receiving the all-mash, 16 per cent protein mash.
4. The laying chicken fed a scratch mixture or separate grains should have access to insoluble hard grit or gravel. Crushed granite, quartz, and feldspar are examples of hard grit.

ONTARIO AGRICULTURAL COLLEGE. (S. J. Slinger, W. F. Pepper, and J. R. Cavers. O.A.C. Chicken Laying and Hatching Feed Formulas, O.A.C. Circular 142A, revised, January, 1954.)

Laying Mash No. 1. This is a conventional type laying mash containing about 20 per cent protein (N × 6.25). Laying mashes containing this level of protein have an advantage over those with 18 per cent protein or less in that they permit the use of more home-grown grain in relation to mash.

Laying Mash No. 2. This is a high-energy laying mash containing about 21 per cent protein (N × 6.25). The feed efficiency for egg production has been shown to be greater with high-energy diets such as this, than with conventional type laying mashes. There has recently been a growing interest in the use of high-energy diets for laying stock. A prime consideration in the use of such diets should be the relative cost and availability of the high-energy grains such as wheat and corn as compared with oats, barley, and mill feeds.

Laying Mash No. 3. This is an all-mash, high-energy ration containing about 16.5 per cent protein (N × 6.25). This mash should be freely accessible to the birds at all times, and no grain should be given. A free-choice supply of oystershell or other suitable calcium source should be available in separate hoppers at all times. The all-mash system of feeding is simpler than the mash-grain method since no error can be made in the proportions of mash and grain to be fed. The all-mash method also fills a need where automatic feeders are used.

Laying Concentrate. This concentrate may be mixed with ground grains to make laying mashes similar to numbers 1, 2, or 3. To make a conventional type laying mash such as No. 1, mix 100 parts of concentrate with 200 parts of ground grains. The ground grains in this case could be a mixture of 6 parts wheat, 3 of corn, 2 of barley, and 2 of oats by weight. This mixture will give a conventional-type laying mash containing about 20 per cent of protein. Mixing 100 parts of concentrate with 200 parts of ground wheat and corn will make a high-energy laying mash such as No. 2. If the proportions of wheat and corn are 9 to 4, the diet will contain about 20 per cent protein. If it is desired to make an all-mash, high-energy laying diet similar to No. 3, mix 100 parts of concentrate with 300 parts of ground wheat and 100 of ground corn.

Hatching Mash. If eggs are not wanted for hatching purposes immediately after the birds are housed, the birds may be maintained on laying mash until 6 weeks before eggs are desired for setting. At this time they should be changed gradually to hatching mash and grain.

Hatching Concentrate. This concentrate when mixed with ground grains in the proportions of 100 parts of concentrate to 200 parts of ground grains will make a hatching mash containing about 20 per cent protein. Using ground grains in the ratio of 7 parts wheat, 3 of corn, 1 of barley, and 2 parts oats, by weight, will give a mash similar in composition to the hatching mash shown.

O.A.C. CHICKEN LAYING AND HATCHING FEED FORMULAS

Ingredients	Laying Mash No. 1 lb.	Laying Mash No. 2 lb.	Laying Mash No. 3 lb.	Laying Concentrate lb.	Hatching Mash lb.	Hatching Concentrate lb.
Ground wheat	600	840	1100	...	685	...
Ground yellow corn	300	400	455	...	300	...
Ground barley	180	...	...	...	100	...
Pulverized oats	200	...	...	...	200	...
Dehydrated alfalfa meal or cereal grass	80	80	50	225	100	270
Meat meal (50% protein)	50	75	50	180	70	200
Fish meal (65% protein)	50	50	30	140	70	200
Dried buttermilk or skimmilk	50	50	30	140	60	160
Soybean oil meal (44% protein)	375	400	200	1000	310	870
Ground limestone	40	40	40	120	40	110
Steamed bonemeal or equivalent	55	45	35	140	45	130
Iodized salt	15	15	10	40	15	40
Vitamin A oil (10,000 I.U./gm.)	2	2	1	6	2.5	7
Dry vitamin D_3 (1,650 I.C.U./gm.)	2	2	1	6	2.5	7
Manganese sulfate (feed grade)	0.5	0.5	0.25	1.5	0.5	1.5
	gm.	gm.	gm.	gm.	gm.	gm.
Riboflavin	2	2	1	6	4	10
Antibiotic*	4-20	4-20	2-10	12-40	4-20	12-40
	mg.	mg.	mg.	mg.	mg.	mg.
Vitamin B_{12}	3	3	3	9	5	15
Calculated Analysis:	%	%	%	%	%	%
Minimum crude protein	20.1	20.9	16.6	35.5	20.2	35.8
Minimum crude fat	2.5	2.4	2.5	2.2	2.7	2.5
Maximum crude fiber	5.4	4.2	3.6	6.5	5.3	6.8
Calcium	2.0	2.0	1.7	5.6	2.0	5.5
Total phosphorus	0.9	0.9	0.7	1.9	0.9	2.0
Inorganic phosphorus	0.64	0.64	0.48	1.63	0.66	1.71

*If penicillin is the antibiotic being employed use the lower level; if aureomycin, terramycin, or bacitracin are used, the higher level should be added.

Substitutions. An equal-parts mixture of wheat shorts and bran may be used to replace ground wheat in laying mash No. 1 or in the hatching mash.

Dried whey may replace dried buttermilk or skimmilk. For every 40 pounds of dried milk replaced by dried whey, increase the amount of soybean oil meal by 30 pounds and reduce the ground wheat by 30 pounds.

Vitamin A feeding oil and dry vitamin D_3 may be replaced by fish oil on an equal unitage basis. The vitamin A oil may be replaced by dry vitamin A or by vitamin A oils of other potency on an equal unitage basis.

Steamed bonemeal may be replaced by defluorinated rock phosphate. Other calcium and phosphorus carriers may also be used. Replacement should be based on the calcium and phosphorus content.

Manganese sulfate may be replaced by other manganese carriers to supply equal levels of manganese.

Ground limestone may be replaced by calcium carbonate.

WASHINGTON. (Washington Poultry Feed Formulas, Poultry Science Department, State College of Washington, Ext. Mimeo. 1107 and 1582, 1954.)

CHICKEN LAYER MASHES

Ingredients	1 %	2 %	3 %	4 %	5 %
Ground grains*	60.7	43.7	45.2	41.0	45.8
Wheat mixed feed (millrun)*	...	20.0	20.0	20.0	20.0
Fishmeal (70% protein)	4.0	...	5.0	1.5	...
Meat and bonemeal (50% protein)	...	5.0	5.0	...	10.0
Soybean oil meal (44% protein)	23.0	20.0	13.0	25.0	15.0
Dehydrated alfalfa or grass (carotene, 12 mg./100 gm.)	5.0	5.0	5.0	5.0	5.0
Limestone or shell flour	3.0	3.0	3.0	3.2	2.7
Steamed bonemeal or defluorinated phosphate	3.8	2.8	3.3	3.8	1.0
Salt (iodized, fine)	0.5	0.5	0.5	0.5	0.5
Add the following to each ton of feed					
Vitamin A, millions I.U.	2.0	2.0	2.0	2.0	2.0
Vitamin D_3, millions I.C.U.	1.2	1.2	1.2	1.2	1.2
Manganese sulfate, lb. (100% pure)	0.5	0.5	0.5	0.5	0.5

Suggested analysis: protein, 19.0 per cent; calcium, 2.5 per cent; phosphorus, 1.1 per cent; vitamin A, 5500 International units per pound; vitamin D_3, 560 International chick units per pound; riboflavin, 1.2 milligrams per pound.

The feeding of cracked or whole grains on the basis of the birds eating 60 per cent mash and 40 per cent grain is suggested. It is recommended that one third of the grain be fed in the morning and two thirds in the afternoon. All the grain may be fed at one time if more convenient, preferably in late afternoon. Shell or limestone grit should be available to the birds at all times. Granite or silica grit should be fed 1 day each week.

*Ground corn, milo, wheat, barley, or oats may be used singly or in any combination with 0 to 20 per cent millrun as long as the combined amounts of barley, oats, and millrun do not exceed 45 per cent in any mash. Barley may be used as the only cereal grain and in place of millrun if the feed is pelleted.

WASHINGTON ALL INCLUSIVE LAYER AND BREEDER MASHES

Ingredients	1 %	2 %	3 %	4 %
Ground grains and millrun*	78.0	79.5	76.1	77.6
Fish meal (70% protein)	2.5	2.5	2.5	2.5
Meat and bonemeal	. . .	5.0	. . .	5.0
Soybean oil meal (44% protein)	12.0	7.0	12.0	7.0
Dehydrated alfalfa or grass (carotene, 12 mg./100 gm.)	3.0	3.0	3.0	3.0
Limestone or shell flour	1.7	1.3	3.6	3.2
Steamed bonemeal or defluorinated phosphate	2.3	1.2	2.3	1.2
Salt (iodized, fine)	0.5	0.5	0.5	0.5
Add the following to each ton of feed				
Vitamin A, millions I.U.	1.0	1.0	1.0	1.0
Vitamin D_3, millions I.C.U.	0.68	0.68	0.68	0.68
Riboflavin, gm.	1.5	1.5	1.5	1.5
Manganese sulfate, lb. (100% pure)	0.3	0.3	0.3	0.3

Suggested analysis: protein, 15 per cent; riboflavin, 1.7 milligrams per pound; vitamin A, 3300 I.U./lb.; vitamin D_3, 340 I.C.U./lb.; phosphorus, 0.8 per cent; calcium, mashes 1 and 2, 1.6 per cent; mashes 3 and 4, 2.25 per cent.

These diets are designed to be used as the only feed fed to the birds with the exception that a supplementary supply of calcium carbonate must be provided for laying or breeding hens fed layer and breeder mashes 1 and 2. This may be supplied in the form of hen-size oystershell or limestone. Layer and breeder mashes 3 and 4 contain all the calcium necessary for shell formation.

These layer and breeder diets may be fed with 1 or 2% whole grain, which is fed in the litter as an aid to keeping the litter stirred up.

*Ground corn, milo, wheat, barley, or oats may be used singly or in any combination with 0-10 per cent millrun as long as the combined amounts of barley, oats, and millrun do not exceed 25 per cent of the diet.

WISCONSIN. (University of Wisconsin, 1954.)

WISCONSIN LAYING MASHES

Ingredients	Laying Mash, lb.	26% Laying Supplement, lb.
Ground yellow corn	250	. . .
Wheat bran	100	100
Wheat middlings	100	200
Pulverized oats	150	. . .
Dehydrated alfalfa meal	100	200
Meat scrap	75	150
Soybean oil meal	175	250
Steamed bonemeal or defluorinated rock phosphate or equivalent	30	60
Iodized salt	10	20
400 D fish oil or powder*	6	12
Manganese sulfate (feeding grade)	1/4	1/2

Grains to be fed free choice with above rations.
Oystershell and granite grit fed free choice in all rations.

* Based on A.O.A.C. units. If new International chick unit is used, 75 per cent of the above will be sufficient.

WISCONSIN ALL-MASH FEEDS FOR LAYING HENS PRODUCING MARKET EGGS

	%	%	%	%	%
Ground yellow corn	56.2	55.9	52.2	62.7	58.2
Ground oats or wheat	10.0	10.0	. . .	10.0	. . .
Wheat middlings	. . .	. . .	15.0	. . .	15.0
Alfalfa meal	5.0	5.0	5.0	5.0	5.0
Soybean oil meal	22.0	22.0	21.0	10.0	10.0
Meat meal	. . .	. . .	. . .	8.0	7.5
Steamed bonemeal or defluorinated superphosphate	3.0	. . .	3.0	1.0	0.5
Dicalcium phosphate	. . .	2.5	. . .	. . .	. . .
Pulverized limestone or oystershell	3.0	3.8	3.0	2.5	3.0
Salt	0.5	0.5	0.5	0.5	0.5
Vitamin A and D feeding oil (300 I.C.U. vitamin D, 1500 I.U. vitamin A per gm.)	0.3	0.3	0.3	0.3	0.3
Riboflavin (grams/100 lb.)	0.02	0.02	0.02	0.02	0.02
Manganese sulfate (grams/100 lb.)	5.0	5.0	5.0	5.0	5.0

The level of riboflavin supplement is indicated in grams of the pure vitamin per 100 pounds of feed because of the wide range of potencies of riboflavin supplements. Unfortified dried whey, a widely-used "natural" supplement, contains 0.013 gram of riboflavin per pound, and so would be used at 1.6 per cent of the mash to provide the level indicated in the table.

One to two per cent of stabilized animal fat could be used in any of these formulas in place of an equal quantity of corn and would have a beneficial effect on the texture of the feed.

Limestone or oystershell grit should be supplied to birds receiving these mashes.

SECTION III. RATIONS FOR BREEDERS

See also Appendix, Section II, since some rations are designated as laying and breeding rations.

CORNELL. (Department of Poultry Husbandry, New York State College of Agriculture, Stencil 205, January, 1953.)

Cornell Breeder Mashes. To be fed with approximately equal grain intake according to any good mash-and-grain program. Breeding ration should be fed for at least 4 weeks before eggs are taken for hatching.

Mixing Mashes. Mash concentrates to be used with local grain (see Section VII).

CORNELL BREEDER MASHES

	lb./ton	lb./ton	lb./ton	lb./ton
Yellow corn meal	750	570	620	640
Ground wheat	300	200	. . .	. . .
Wheat flour middlings	. . .	. . .	300	200
Wheat standard middlings	. . .	200	. . .	150
Pulverized oats	100	200	200	. . .
Ground barley	. . .	. . .	. . .	200
Soybean meal	375	325	350	250
Corn gluten meal	. . .	50	. . .	. . .
Peanut meal	. . .	. . .	. . .	50
Fish meal	75	100	. . .	. . .
Fish solubles	. . .	. . .	75	. . .
Meat scrap	75	. . .	75	150
Corn distillers' dried solubles	50	. . .	100	75
Dried whey	50	100	50	75
Molasses distillers' solubles	. . .	25	. . .	. . .
Dehydrated alfalfa meal	100	100	100	100
Riboflavin supplement to supply (mg. riboflavin)	2300 mg.	1500 mg.	1000 mg.	1500 mg.
Vitamin B_{12} supplement to supply (mg. B_{12})	4 mg.	4 mg.	. . .	5 mg.
D-activated animal sterols (1500 I.C.U./gm.)	2	2	2	2
or				
Vitamin feeding oil (300 D, 1500 A)	10	10	10	10
Steamed bonemeal	75	90	90	70
Limestone	30	20	20	20
Salt (iodized)	20	20	20	20
Manganese sulfate (65% feeding grade)	0.5	0.5	0.5	0.5
Protein, %	20.7	20.5	20.6	20.5
Calcium, %	2.4	2.1	2.2	2.3
Total Phosphorus, %	1.2	1.2	1.2	1.2
Available, %	0.9	0.9	0.9	0.9
Vitamin A,* I.U./lb.	5800	5600	5600	5600
Vitamin D, I.C.U./lb.	680	680	680	680
Riboflavin, mg./lb.	2.7	2.6	2.5	2.6
Vitamin B_{12},† μg./lb.	4	4	3.2	3.6

* Assuming use of alfalfa meal containing 100,000 International units vitamin A activity and no vitamin feeding oil.

† From animal proteins and vitamin B_{12} supplement.

BRITISH COLUMBIA. (University of British Columbia and Department of Agriculture U.B.C. Feed Formulas for Poultry, 1954, Poultry Circ. 37.)

Hen Breeding Mash. To be fed with scratch grain in similar proportions as in the case of laying mash. To insure high hatchability, a distillers' feed product and/or liver meal should be included 30 days previous to collecting hatching eggs.

BRITISH COLUMBIA HEN-BREEDING MASH

Ingredients	lb. per ton
Coarse ground wheat	720
Ground yellow corn	100
Pulverized oats	100
Ground barley	100
Wheat bran	100
Wheat middlings	100
Fish meal (65-70% protein)	100
Meat and bone scrap (50% protein)	100
Dried milk by-products	70
Soybean oil meal (44% protein)	200
Dehydrated green feed	100
Distillers' dried solubles or fermentation solubles	100
Ground limestone	50
Steamed bonemeal	30
Iodized salt	20
Manganese sulfate	8 oz.
Feeding oil (2250 I.U., A; 300 I C.U., D per gram)	10
Riboflavin	4 gms.
Vitamin B_{12}	3 mg.
Recommended protein level	20%

NEW ENGLAND COLLEGE CONFERENCE, JUNE, 1954.

RATIONS FOR BREEDERS

	Mash and Grain	All-Mash
Feeding ratio; mash to scratch	2/1	. . .
Mash ingredient	lb.	lb.
Ground yellow corn (1)	975	1125
Ground barley or pulverized oats (2)	100	100
Standard wheat middlings	200	200
Soybean oil meal (44%)	250	175
Fish meal (60%) (3)	100	75
Meat and bone scrap (50%)	75	50
Alfalfa meal (17%; 100,000 A/lb.)	100	75
Distillers' dried solubles (4) (5)	75	50
Butyl fermentation products (4) (5)	25	25
Dicalcium phosphate or equivalent (6)	24	32
Ground limestone (feeding grade)	65	75
Iodized salt	15	10
Dry vitamin D (1500 D/gm.) (7)	1.5	1.0
Manganese sulfate or equivalent (8)	0.4	0.25
Vitamin B_{12} supplement	(9)	(10)
Niacin	30 gm.	18 gm.
DPPD (Diphenyl-p-phenylenediamine)	(11)	(11)
Totals (12)	2005.9	1993.25

(1) Two to four hundred pounds of coarsely ground wheat may be used to replace an equal amount of corn. Add 0.4 pound of vitamin A and D oil for each 100 pounds of corn removed.

(2) On a nutrient content basis, barley is preferred to oats. Both barley and oats may be replaced by corn if a higher energy level is desired.

(3) If a high salt fish meal is used, omit the added salt.

(4) Twenty pounds of a butyl fermentation product containing at least 250 micrograms of riboflavin per gram (or 113.5 milligrams per pound) and 50 pounds of dried distillers' solubles, or 40 pounds yeast or 40 pounds of dried whey plus a riboflavin supplement to furnish not less than 2.0 milligrams per pound in the final ration. To determine the amount of riboflavin supplement to use above, divide the number of milligrams desired by the manufacturer's guaranteed potency. Example: Needed to furnish 454 milligrams using a product having a guaranteed potency of 113.5 milligrams per pound. Solution: 454 divided by 113.5 equals 4 pounds needed in addition to either the yeast or the solubles. This is an example only, not an actual case.

(5) A vitamin concentrate containing not less than 2 grams of riboflavin and 4 grams of pantothenic acid and possibly other vitamins may be used to replace part or all of the fermentation products, and the total weight may be made up by adding corn meal.

(6) Steamed bonemeal or defluorinated rock phosphate may replace

the dicalcium phosphate on a phosphorus basis. Raw rock phosphate containing not more than 3.5 per cent fluorine may replace one-quarter of the phosphorus in the dicalcium phosphate in the rations.

(7) Vitamin A and D feeding oil may be substituted on a unit basis.

(8) Manganese sulfate (70% feeding grade) or equivalent amount of manganese from other sources.

(9) Use 9 milligrams of vitamin B_{12} per ton of ration.

(10) Use a vitamin B_{12} concentrate contributing not less than 6 milligrams of vitamin B_{12} per ton of ration.

(11) DPPD (diphenyl-p-phenylenediamine) is an antioxidant and may be added at the 0.0125 per cent level (one-quarter pound per ton) to help prevent the destruction of the fat soluble vitamins.

(12) If an even 2000 pounds is desired, adjust by removing or adding middlings.

NORTH CAROLINA. (North Carolina State College of Agriculture and Engineering of the University of North Carolina, 1954.)

NORTH CAROLINA RATIONS FOR BREEDERS

Ingredients	No. 47 All-Mash 16%* lb.	No. 50 Grain-Mash 20%† lb.
Ground yellow corn	945	850
Standard wheat middlings	250	200
Pulverized oats	250	100
Meat and bone scrap (50% protein)	25	75
Fish meal (60% protein)	75	100
Soybean oil meal (44% protein)	200	375
Alfalfa meal (17% protein) 100,000 A/lb.	75	100
Whey, dried	20	20
Butyl fermentation solubles (250 micrograms riboflavin per gram)	30	40
Steamed bonemeal or equivalent	50	100
Pulverized oystershells or equivalent	70	20
Salt	10	20
Feeding oil (300 D, 1500 A per gram)	2	2
D-activated animal sterol (1500 D per gram)	1	2.25
Manganese sulfate	0.25	0.50
	grams	grams
Niacin	20	20
	milligrams	milligrams
Vitamin B_{12} supplement	6	12
Total	2003+	2004+

* Do not feed a scratch mixture or separate grains with the all-mash, 16 per cent protein mash.

† Feed a scratch mixture or separate grains with the 20 per cent protein mash. Keep crushed oystershells or limestone before the birds that are fed the 20 per cent breeder mash.

TEXAS. (Agricultural and Mechanical College of Texas, 1954.)

TEXAS ALL-MASH BREEDER-LAYER RATION

Ingredients	lb./ton
Soybean oil meal (44% protein)	350
Fish meal	80
Dried whey	50
Dehydrated alfalfa leaf meal	80
Ground yellow corn	650*
Ground milo	650*
Bonemeal or defluorinated phosphate	40
Oystershell flour or calcium carbonate	40
Salt	10
Vitamin and mineral mixture†	50
Total	2000

*Milo and corn may be used interchangeably, depending on price and availability.

† Vitamin and mineral mixture in soybean oil meal:

Riboflavin	4 gm.
Calcium pantothenate	10 gm.
Niacin	25 gm.
B_{12}	6 mg.
Antibiotic	‡
Vitamin A (stable, dry A)	2,270,000 I.U.
Vitamin D_3 (stable, dry D)	1,200,000 I.C.U.
Manganese sulfate	227 gm.
Soybean oil meal	Enough to make total equal to 50 lb.

‡ Use 10 grams aureomycin, 10 grams bacitracin, 10 grams of terramycin or 4 grams penicillin. A combination of two, three, or four of the antibiotics may be used. If a combination is used, take a proportionate part of the above levels on a per ton basis.

WASHINGTON. (Washington Poultry Feed Formulas, Poultry Science Department, State College of Washington, Ext. Mimeo. 1183, 1954.)

CHICKEN BREEDER MASHES

Ingredients	1 %	2 %	3 %	4 %	5 %	6 %
Ground corn or ground milo	...	...	...	...	...	62.9
Ground grains*	45.2	42.9	46.9	38.8	40.8	...
Wheat mixed feed (millrun)*	20.0	20.0	20.0	20.0	20.0	...
Fishmeal (70% protein)	5.0	2.0	3.5	...	...	5.0
Meat and bonemeal (50% protein)	...	...	5.0	5.0	...	...
Soybean oil meal (44% protein)	13.0	18.0	9.2	13.0	21.8	20.0
Dehydrated alfalfa or grass (carotene, 12mg./100 gm.)†	10.0	10.0	10.0	10.0	10.0	5.0
Dried whey	...	...	...	2.5	...	...
Distillers' dried solubles	...	...	...	5.0	...	...
Limestone or shell flour	2.7	2.6	2.3	2.6	2.8	2.2
Steamed bonemeal or defluorinated phosphate	3.6	4.0	2.6	2.6	4.1	4.4
Salt (iodized, fine)	0.5	0.5	0.5	0.5	0.5	0.5
Add the following to each ton of feed						
Vitamin A, millions I.U.	...	...	...	...	...	1.9
Vitamin D_3, millions I.C.U.	1.2	1.2	1.2	1.2	1.2	1.2
Riboflavin (gm.)	2.1	2.2	2.0	1.1	2.2	2.8
Vitamin B_{12} (mg.)	...	6.0	...	8.0	11.0	...
Manganese sulfate, lb. (100% pure)	0.5	0.5	0.5	0.5	0.5	0.5

Suggested analysis: Protein, 19 per cent; calcium, 2.5 per cent; phosphorus, 1.1 per cent; vitamin A, 5500 International units per pound; vitamin D_3, 600 International chick units per pound; riboflavin, 2.8 milligrams per pound.

These mashes are formulated for hand feeding of grain on the basis of the birds eating 60 per cent mash, pellets, or crumbles and 40 per cent cracked or whole grains. It is recommended that one third of the grain be fed in the morning and two thirds in the afternoon. All the grain may be fed at one time if more convenient, preferably in late afternoon. Supplemental calcium in the form of limestone grit or shell should always be available in separate hoppers. Granite or silica grit should be fed one day each week.

*Ground corn, milo, wheat, barley, or oats may be used singly or in any combination with 0 to 20 per cent millrun as long as the combined amounts of barley, oats, and millrun do not exceed 45 per cent of the mash.

†Dehydrated alfalfa or grass may be reduced to 5 per cent and the ground grain increased by 5 per cent if 1,916,000 International units of vitamin A are added per ton of mash. Vitamin A supplement will not be required if a dehydrated alfalfa or grass assaying 15 milligrams per 100 grams or more of carotene is used.

WISCONSIN. (University of Wisconsin, 1954.)

WISCONSIN BREEDER MASHES

Ingredients	No. 1	No. 2
Ground yellow corn	300	325
Wheat bran	100	100
Wheat middlings	100	100
Pulverized oats	100	100
Dehydrated alfalfa meal	100	100
Meat scrap	50	40
Fish meal	. . .	40
Soybean oil meal	200	160
Steamed bonemeal or defluorinated rock phosphate or equivalent	30	20
Iodized salt	10	10
Riboflavin*	Yes	Yes
Vitamin B_{12} supplement†,‡	Yes	No
400 D fish oil or powder§	6	6
Manganese sulfate (feeding grade)	1/4	1/4

Grains to be fed free choice with above rations.

Oystershell and granite grit fed free choice in all rations.

* Riboflavin, 1.0 milligram per pound of feed from any source.

† Use according to manufacturer's directions.

‡ Some commercial supplements do not meet the minimum standards for this product, but they may be good sources.

§ Based on A.O.A.C. units. If new International chick unit is used, 75 per cent of the above will be sufficient.

SECTION IV. FATTENING RATIONS

CORNELL. (G. F. Heuser, Poultry rations, Cornell Bul. 45, revised, 1941.)

CORNELL FATTENING RATIONS

	To Be Fed with Liquid Milk*	To Be Fed without Liquid Milk†
Corn meal	50	50
Wheat flour middlings	20	20
Ground heavy oats	10	10
Dried buttermilk or skimmilk		10
Meat scrap		10

*Mixed to a batter, fresh at each feeding, with buttermilk or skimmilk. Will require approximately 2 pounds (1 quart) of milk to 1 pound (1 quart) of mash.

†Mixed to a batter, fresh at each feeding, with water. Will require approximately 3 pounds (1 1/2 quarts) of water to 2 pounds (2 quarts) of mash.

BRITISH COLUMBIA. (University of British Columbia and Department of Agriculture U.B.C. Feed Formulas for Poultry, 1954. Poultry Circ. 37.)

Fattening Mash. All-mash ration to be fed moistened with water or liquid skimmilk. The feeding oil should be discontinued 1 to 2 weeks before marketing the birds. If yellow corn is expensive, it may be replaced with other grains. When available and not too expensive, 3 to 5 per cent of corn oil or soybean oil may be fed to advantage during the last 10 days of fattening.

BRITISH COLUMBIA FATTENING MASH

Ingredients	lb. per ton
Coarse ground wheat	650
Ground yellow corn	600
Pulverized oats	200
Ground barley	100
Wheat middlings	100
Meat and bone scrap (50% protein)	50
Dried milk by-products	50
Soybean oil meal (44% protein)	150
Dehydrated green feed	50
Ground limestone	25
Steamed bonemeal	10
Iodized salt	10
Manganese sulfate	4 oz.
Feeding oil (2250 I.U., A; 300 I.C.U., D per gram)	5
Riboflavin	2 gm.
Recommended protein level	14%

CALIFORNIA. (H. J. Almquist, T. H. Jukes, and W. E. Newlon, Feeding chickens, Calif. Circ. 108, revised, 1940.)

	Pounds
Ground yellow corn	100
Ground whole barley	100
Ground oat groats or oatmeal	50
Dried skimmilk	50
Water to mix to the consistency of a thick soup	

KANSAS. (Poultry rations, Kans. Agr. Exp. Sta., Dept. Poultry, C Form 1, Oct., 1943.)

Crate Feeding

	Pounds
Corn meal	60
Oatmeal or shorts	40
Buttermilk	200

When liquid milk is not available, add 40 pounds of condensed milk to 100 pounds of grain and enough water to give the consistency of thick cream.

Pen or Lot Feeding

	Pounds
Shelled corn, kafir or milo	85
Semi-solid or condensed buttermilk	15

This ration should be fed in hoppers 4 to 6 weeks. The milk paste is added to the grain once daily at the rate of 3 to 3½ pounds for 100 chickens and 5 to 6 pounds daily per 100 turkeys.

MACDONALD COLLEGE, CANADA. (Macdonald College fattening rations. Canadian Poultry Review, Sept., 1940.)

MACDONALD COLLEGE FATTENING RATIONS

Feed	1 lb.	2 lb.	3 lb.	4 lb.	5 lb.	6 lb.	7 lb.
Ground yellow corn	22.75	22.50	30.00	23.25	31.00	16.00	...
Ground wheat	22.75	22.50	...	23.25	...	...	...
Ground oats	22.75	22.50	30.00	23.25	31.00	30.00	31.00
Ground barley	22.75	22.50	30.00	23.25	...	30.00	31.00
Ground buckwheat	...	...	...	...	30.00	...	31.00
Rice feed*	...	...	...	...	...	16.00	...
Beef meal	3.50	3.50	3.50	3.50	3.50	3.50	3.50
Powdered milk	2.50	2.50	2.50	2.50	2.50	2.50	2.50
Crude corn oil	2.00	2.00	2.00	...	...	...	...
Bone char or charcoal	...	1.00	1.00	...	1.00	1.00	...
Salt	1.00	1.00	1.00	1.00	1.00	1.00	1.00
	100.00	100.00	100.00	100.00	100.00	100.00	100.00

*Ground broken rice and polishings.

The following suggestions are offered concerning the purpose for which each of the foregoing rations is intended:

1. For commercial feeding on short periods—4 to 8 days—any class of stock.
2. For commercial feeding where white skin and fat finish are desired. Add 1 per cent bone char or English nut charcoal to the ration.
3. For pen feeding or range finishing of broilers. Dry mash fed ad libitum in hoppers and two wet-mash feedings per day, giving as much as will be cleaned up readily.
4. For farm fattening (confinement in crates or pen feeding) 14-day feeding period.
5. Recommended for heavy roasters and fowl where yellow fat and skin are not objectionable.
6. Where rice feed is available, this ration should give excellent results with any class of stock.
7. For heavy stock, such as roasters and fowl especially. Will produce a white finish.

ONTARIO AGRICULTURAL COLLEGE. (S. J. Slinger, W. F. Pepper, and J. R. Cavers. O.A.C. Chicken Starting, Growing, and Fattening Formulas, *O.A.C. Circular* 142, revised, Jan., 1954.)

Roaster Fattening Mash. This mash contains about 14 per cent protein (N × 6.25). It is designed to aid in the fattening of mature or relatively mature stock and is not recommended for fattening broilers. It is fed without grain in the form of a thin gruel or "pour batter" made by mixing with water or liquid skimmilk or buttermilk. For fattening roasters or fowl, it is recommended that the birds be given the amount they will just clean up in 15 minutes, three times daily, for a period of 10 to 12 days. Water should be available at all times to birds being fattened.

O.A.C. FATTENING MASH

Ingredient	lb.
Ground wheat	750
Ground yellow corn	600
Ground barley	100
Pulverized oats	278
Dehydrated alfalfa meal (100,000 I.U. vitamin A activity/lb. or cereal grass)	20
Meat meal (50% protein)	50
Dried buttermilk or skimmilk	50
Soybean oil meal (44% protein)	100
Ground limestone	20
Steamed bonemeal or equivalent	20
Iodized salt	10
Vitamin A oil (10,000 I.U./gm.)	0.75
Dry vitamin D_3 (1,650 I.C.U./gm.)	1
Manganese sulfate (feed grade)	0.25
	gm.
Riboflavin	1
Antibiotic*	2-10
	mg.
Vitamin B_{12}	3
Calculated analysis:	%
Minimum crude protein	14.1
Minimum crude fat	3.0
Minimum crude fiber	4.5
Calcium	1.0
Total phosphorus	0.6
Inorganic phosphorus	0.35

*If penicillin is the antibiotic, use the lower level. If aureomycin, terramycin, or bacitracin are used, the higher level should be employed.

Substitution. Wheat middlings can replace ground wheat.

SECTION V. RATIONS FOR TURKEYS

CORNELL. (Turkey rations, New York State College of Agr. Dept. of Poultry Husbandry, Stencil 208, revised, July, 1953.)

Starting Mash. The starting mash is kept available at all times as an all-mash ration to 4 or 8 weeks of age.

Growing Mashes. The growing mash to be fed during the 4- to 8-week period should be fed as an all-mash ration. After 8 weeks of age both grain and mash are fed. Scratch grains may be fed free choice after 12 weeks. It also would be advisable to feed extra oystershell or some other source of calcium. When turkeys are to be marketed as turkey broilers, the fish meal should be replaced by high quality meat scrap in order to prevent "fishy flavor" in the broilers. If the turkeys are to be reared in confinement or if the available range is not in good condition, care must be taken to supply adequate amounts of vitamin A.

Breeding Mash. The breeding mash recommendations are designed for a grain-and-mash feeding system. The grain intake should constitute at least half but should not exceed 2/3 the total daily feed consumption. Free-choice oystershell or other calcium supplement should be provided.

CORNELL TURKEY STARTING RATION
Feed as all-mash ration to 4 or 8 weeks of age

Ingredients	lb./ton	
Corn, ground yellow	588	
Wheat flour middling	300	
Oats, pulverized	100	
Soybean meal, solvent, 44% protein	580	
Fish meal	100	
Meat and bone scrap	150	
Dried skimmilk, or dried whey product*	60	
Dried brewers' yeast	40	
Alfalfa meal, 17% protein	40	
Ground limestone	30	
Salt, iodized	10	
Manganese sulfate, feed grade, 70% $MnSO_4$	0.5	
Choline chloride, 70% solution, to supply	1.5	
Niacin supplement, to supply	40	gm./ton
Mixed-tocopheryl acetate supplement, to supply	5	gm./ton
Vitamin A supplement to supply	3000	units/lb.
D-activated animal sterol supplement to supply	600	units/lb.
Riboflavin supplement, to supply	0.5	mg./lb.
Antibiotic feed supplement, to supply	10	gm./ton

Approximate analyses:

Protein, %	28
Fat, %	3.6†
Fiber, %	4.3
Calcium, %	1.9
Phosphorus, %	0.9
Riboflavin, mg./lb.	2.3
Niacin, mg./lb.	42
Choline, mg./lb.	1028
Pantothenic acid, mg./lb.	5.7
Vitamin A, units/lb.	5690
Vitamin D, units/lb.	600

* Dried whey product containing approximately 50 per cent or less lactose; dried whey containing more lactose is less effective, probably because it is not well tolerated.

† Fat value depends upon fat content of animal protein supplements. If these supplements have been solvent-extracted, the fat value will be somewhat lower.

CORNELL TURKEY GROWING MASHES

Ingredient	Growing Mash 4-8 Weeks (All Mash) lb./ton		Growing Mash after 8 Weeks (with Grain)* lb./ton	
Corn meal, yellow	628.5		669.5	
Wheat middlings	300	(flour)	400	(standard)
Oats, pulverized	200		200	
Soybean meal, solvent, 44% protein	400		200	
Fish meal	100*		. . .	
Meat and bone scrap	100		200	
Dried brewers' yeast	40		40	
Dried whey product or dried skim-milk	60		60	
Alfalfa meal, 17% protein	100†		140†	
Ground limestone	30		30	
Steamed bonemeal or dicalcium phosphate	30		40	
Salt, iodized	10		20	
Manganese sulfate, feed grade, 70% $MnSO_4$	0.5		0.5	
Choline chloride, 70% solution to supply	1		. . .	
Riboflavin supplement to supply	0.5	mg./lb.	2.0	mg./lb.
Niacin supplement to supply	40	gm./ton	40	gm./ton
Mixed-tocopheryl acetate supplement	5	gm./ton	5	gm./ton
Vitamin A supplement to supply	5000	units/lb.	1000	units/lb.
D-activated animal sterol supplement	600	units/lb.	1200	units/lb.
Antibiotic feed supplement to supply	10	gm./ton	10	gm./ton

Approximate analyses

Protein, %	24.6	20.0
Fat, %	3.7	4.2
Fiber, %	5.1	5.7
Calcium, %	1.9	2.3
Phosphorus, %	1.0	1.1
Riboflavin, mg./lb.	2.3	3.8
Choline, mg./lb.	822	740
Pantothenic acid, mg./lb.	6	7
Vitamin A, units/lb.	5750	8740
Vitamin D, units/lb.	600	1200

* Fish meal should be replaced by meat scrap if turkeys are to be marketed early as broilers so as to prevent "fishy flavor."

† Formula calculations based on alfalfa containing 100,000 units of vitamin A activity per pound. If lower-potency alfalfa is used, the required vitamin A level should be maintained by additional high-potency vitamin A supplement.

CORNELL TURKEY BREEDING MASH

Ingredients	Breeding Mash (Fed with Grain) lb. per Ton
Corn meal, yellow	404.5
Wheat standard middlings	400
Oats, pulverized	200
Soybean meal, solvent, 44% protein	240
Fish meal	100
Meat and bone scrap	200
Dried skimmilk or dried whey product	100
Distillers' dried solubles	100
Alfalfa meal, 17% protein	150*
Dicalcium phosphate or steamed bonemeal	60
Ground limestone	25
Salt, iodized	20
Manganese sulfate, feed grade, 70% $MnSO_4$	0.5
Riboflavin supplement, to supply	3.5 mg./lb.
Mixed-tocopheryl acetate supplement to supply	5 gm./ton
Vitamin A supplement to supply	5000 units/lb.
D-activated animal sterol supplement to supply	1800 units/lb.

Approximate analyses

Protein, %	24
Fat, %	4.6
Fiber, %	5.8
Calcium	2.8
Phosphorus	1.4
Riboflavin, mg./lb.	6.1
Choline, mg./lb.	686
Pantothenic acid, mg./lb.	6.3
Vitamin A, units/lb.	12,950
Vitamin D, units/lb.	1,800

* Formula calculations based on alfalfa containing 100,000 units of vitamin A activity per pound. If lower potency alfalfa is used, the required vitamin A level should be maintained by additional high-potency vitamin A supplement.

CALIFORNIA. (V. S. Asmundson and F. H. Kratzer, Turkey Production in California, *Calif. Circ.* 110, 1951.)

Poult Starting Mashes. Poults should be started on an all-mash ration. Slightly more rapid early growth may be produced by feeding the high-energy mash. The poults may be fed this ration for the first 2 to 4 weeks and then changed to the regular starter.

Poultry Growing and Developing Rations. After poults are 6 weeks old they are fed some grain. The grain should be started very gradually, because sudden changes in the ration will slow up growth. A little grain may be scattered on top of the mash in the afternoon at first. A suitable growing ration for poults that are running outside may consist of any starting mash with the fish oil omitted or of the growing, or high-protein, mashes with whole grains added.

Developing and Finishing Rations. The developing and finishing ration may consist of the growing mash fed with whole grains or of a high-protein mash fed with large amounts of scratch grains.

Feeding Breeder Hens. During the cloudy months, some vitamin D should be included in the mash. The mash should be fed with equal parts of scratch grain. Fresh greens may be fed when available; and, if they are abundant, the alfalfa meal may be reduced to 200 pounds and the ground grains increased to 1000 pounds. Additional calcium may be furnished by placing cracked oystershell or limestone before the birds.

CALIFORNIA POULT STARTER MASHES

Feedstuff	Regular 1 lb.	2 lb.	3 lb.	4 lb.	High-Energy lb.
Fish meal	200	140	150	100	293
Meat scrap	. . .	140	50	100	100
Soybean oil meal	500	450	500	525	500
Liver meal	. . .	. . .	. . .	. . .	40
Molasses	. . .	. . .	. . .	. . .	50
Alfalfa meal*	100	100	100	100	100
Wheat bran	200	200	200	200	. . .
Ground wheat	200	200	200	200	200
Ground barley	265	270	270	255	. . .
Ground corn	400	400	400	400	600
Bonemeal, special steamed†	25	0	30	20	10
Ground limestone	50	40	40	40	30
Salt, iodized	10	10	10	10	10
Manganese sulfate	1/2	1/2	1/2	1/2	1/2
Dried whey	40	40	40	40	50
Fish oil (2250 A, 300 D)‡	3	3	3	3	3
Vitamin D carrier (1500 D/gm.)	1 1/2	1 1/2	1 1/2	1 1/2	1 1/2
Riboflavin supplement§	5	5	5	5	7
Choline chloride	1	1	1	1	. . .
Antibiotic supplement	+	+	+	+	+

* Should contain carotene equivalent to at least 67,000 International units of vitamin A per pound.

† Other products of equivalent calcium and phosphorus content may be used.

‡ Proportionate amounts of products of other potency may be used.

§ Containing 225 milligrams of riboflavin per pound. A proportionate amount of a product of different potency may be used.

CALIFORNIA TURKEY GROWING MASHES (20 per cent protein)

Feedstuff	1 lb.	2 lb.	3 lb.	4 lb.	5 lb.
Fish meal	100	. . .	50	100	. . .
Meat scrap	. . .	100	. . .	. . .	100
Soybean oil meal*	400	400	450	400	400
Alfalfa meal†	200	200	200	300	300
Wheat bran	300	300	300	300	300
Ground grains	897	907	849	779	789
Molasses	. . .	. . .	. . .	20	20
Bonemeal, special steamed‡	40	30	40	40	30
Ground limestone	40	40	40	40	40
Salt, iodized	20	20	20	20	20
Manganese sulfate	1/2	1/2	1/2	1/2	1/2
Dried whey	. . .	. . .	50	. . .	. . .
Vitamin D carrier (1,500 D/gm.)	1	1	1	1	1
Riboflavin§	2	2	. . .	. . .	. . .

* Soybean oil meal may be partly replaced by cottonseed meal, 10 per cent (200 pounds); or sesame seed oil meal, 5 per cent (100 pounds).

† Should contain carotene equivalent to at least 67,000 International units of vitamin A per pound.

‡ Other products of equivalent calcium and phosphorus content may be used.

§ Containing 225 milligrams of riboflavin per pound. A proportionate amount of a product of different potency may be used.

CALIFORNIA CONCENTRATE TURKEY GROWING MASHES
(30 per cent protein)

Feedstuff	1 lb.	2 lb.	3 lb.
Fish meal	200	100	200
Meat scrap	. . .	100	. . .
Soybean oil meal*	800	800	800
Alfalfa meal†	400	500	500
Wheat bran	300	250	250
Ground grains	94	68	. . .
Molasses	. . .	. . .	50
Bonemeal, special steamed‡	80	60	80
Ground limestone	80	80	80
Salt, iodized	40	40	40
Manganese sulfate	3/4	3/4	3/4
Vitamin D carrier (1,500 D/gm.)§	2	2	2
Riboflavin supplement‖	4	. . .	. . .

* Soybean oil meal may be partly replaced by cottonseed meal, 20 per cent (400 pounds); or sesame seed oil meal, 10 per cent (200 pounds).

† Should contain carotene equivalent to at least 67,000 International units of vitamin A per pound.

‡ Other products of equivalent calcium and phosphorus content may be used.

§ Proportionate amounts of products of different potency may be used.

‖ Containing 225 milligrams per pound. A proportionate amount of a product of different potency may be used.

CALIFORNIA TURKEY BREEDER MASHES

Feedstuff	1 lb.	2 lb.	3 lb.	4 lb.
Fish meal	100	200	50	100
Meat scrap	100	. . .	150	. . .
Soybean oil meal	200	200	250	350
Alfalfa meal*	300	300	300	300
Wheat bran or millrun	300	300	300	300
Ground grains	805	843	813	773
Bonemeal, special steamed†	20	30	10	50
Ground limestone	40	40	40	40
Salt, iodized	20	20	20	20
Manganese sulfate	1/2	1/2	1/2	1/2
Dried whey	100	50	50	50
Vitamin A and D feeding oil (2,250 A, 300 D/gm.)‡	6	6	6	6
Vitamin D source (1,500 D/gm.)‡	3	3	3	3
Riboflavin source§	6	8	8	8

* Should contain carotene equivalent to at least 67,000 International units of vitamin A per pound.

† Other products of equivalent calcium and phosphorus content may be used.

‡ Proportionate amounts of products of other potency may be used.

§ Containing 225 milligrams of riboflavin per pound. A proportionate amount of a product of different potency may be used.

IOWA. (Iowa State College Poultry Department, 1954.)

IOWA STARTING RATIONS FOR TURKEY POULTS

Ingredients	1	2	3	4
Ground yellow corn	544	648	465	529
Ground oats	100	100	100	100
Wheat bran	200	100	100	100
Wheat midds	200	200	200	100
Dehydrated alfalfa meal	100	100	100	100
Soybean oil meal (44%)	450	400	600	600
Meat and bone scrap (50%)	100	150	150	200
Fish meal (65%)	100	50	100	50
Fish solubles	...	50	...	50
Dried buttermilk	100	100	100	100
Steamed bonemeal (or equivalent)	25	30	20	...
Ground limestone or oystershell	40	30	25	30
Iodized salt	9.5	9.5	9.5	9.5
Manganese sulfate	0.5	0.5	0.5	0.5
Riboflavin concentrate (227 mg./lb.)	15.0	15.0	15.0	15.0
2250 A, 300 D concentrate	7	7	7	7
1500 D concentrate	2	2	2	2
Choline chloride (25%)	7	7	6	6
Niacin (100%)	20 gr.	20 gr.	20 gr.	20 gr.
Pantothenic acid	10 gr.	10 gr.	10 gr.	10 gr.
Methionine	...	1.0	...	1.0
Antibiotic*	+	+	+	+
Total pounds	2000	2000	2000	2000
Calculated analysis:				
Protein (minimum), %	24.0	24.0	28.0	28.0
Fat, %	3.9	4.1	3.8	3.9
Fiber, %	5.4	5.0	5.3	5.1
Calcium, %	2.1	2.1	2.0	2.0
Phosphorus, %	1.0	1.0	1.1	1.0

* Antibiotics may be used according to the manufacturer's recommendations with any of these rations. Vitamins are usually added as concentrates, and adjustments must be made to compensate for the variation in potency of these concentrates.

Methionine may be added at 1/2 to 1 pound per ton to any of these rations.

IOWA RATIONS FOR GROWING TURKEYS

Ingredients	1*	2	3	5	6*	7
Ground yellow corn	547	397	496	332	378	238
Ground whole oats	100	100	120	. . .	. . .	. . .
Wheat bran	100	100	100	100	100	100
Wheat middlings	100	100	100	100	100	100
Bonemeal or defluorinated phosphate	150	220	150	160	160	200
Ground limestone or oystershell	50	20	25	20	20	20
Iodized salt	18	18	18	18	18	18
Manganese sulfate	2	2	2	2	2	2
Dehydrated alfalfa meal (17% protein)	100	100	100	100	100	100
Fish meal (65% protein)	100	. . .	. . .	. . .	100	. . .
Condensed fish solubles (33% protein)	. . .	100	. . .	. . .	. . .	100
Meat and bone scrap (50% protein)	150	100	200	225	175	125
Soybean meal (41-44% protein)	540	700	550	800	800	950
2250 A, 300 D concentrate (oil or dry)†	14	14	14	15	15	15
Vitamin D concentrate (1500 I.C.U. per gm.)†	5	5	5	6	6	6
Riboflavin concentrate (227 mg. per lb.)†	20	20	16	18	22	22
Dried milk	. . .	. . .	100	100	. . .	. . .
Choline chloride (25% or equivalent)†	4	4	4	4	4	4
Niacin	20 gr.	20 gr.	20 gr.	20 gr.	20 gr.	20 gr.
Pantothenic acid	6 gr.	6 gr.	6 gr.	6 gr.	6 gr.	6 gr.
Total pounds	2000	2000	2000	2000	2000	2000
Calculated analysis:						
Protein, %	24.1	24.0	23.7	28.1	28.6	28.3
Fat, %	2.4	2.2	2.6	2.2	2.1	1.7
Fiber, %	6.1	6.2	6.3	6.3	6.3	6.6
Calcium, %	4.3	4.2	3.9	4.2	4.0	4.1
Phosphorus, %	1.9	2.3	2.0	2.1	2.1	2.2

* Rations 1 and 6 preferred.

† Concentrates of these nutrients with different potencies may be used if adjustments are made to compensate for variation in potency. Antibiotics may be used according to manufacturers' recommendations as supplements to these rations. Mash and grain are to be available to the turkeys at all times.

IOWA RATIONS FOR TURKEY BREEDING HENS

Ingredients	1	2	3	4	5	6	7	8	9
Ground yellow corn	448	444	496	446	222	...	...	...	...
Wheat bran	200	200	200	200	200	300	150	150	100
Ground whole oats	200	200	250	200	...	...	...	...	...
Wheat middlings	200	200	200	200	200	300	250	250	100
Bone meal or defluorinated phosphate	100	100	100	100	120	100	180	150	130
Ground limestone or oystershell	...	...	...	...	...	50	...	...	...
Iodized salt	19	19	19	19	18	18	18	18	20
Manganese sulfate	1	1	1	1	2	2	2	2	2
Dehydrated alfalfa meal (17% protein)	200	200	200	200	300	300	300	300	300
Fish meal (65% protein)	...	...	100	...	...	150	...	...	...
Condensed fish solubles (33% protein)	...	100	...	50	...	...	100	...	...
Meat and bone scrap (50% protein)	200	150	150	100	100	300	250	300	400
Soybean meal (44% protein)	300	350	200	400	750	400	700	600	720
2250 A, 300 D concentrate (oil or dry)*	12	12	12	12	15	16	16	16	18
Vitamin D concentrate (1500 I.C.U. per gm.)*	4	4	4	4	5	6	6	6	7
Riboflavin concentrate (227 mg. per lb.)*	16	20	18	18	18	18	20	16	18
Vitamin B_{12} (mg.)*	...	...	...	...	5 mg.	...	...	...	...
Dried milk	100	...	50	50	50	50	...	200	200
Total pounds	2000	2000	2000	2000	2000	2010	1992	2008	2015
Calculated analysis:									
Protein, %	20.6	20.5	20.2	20.2	26.2	28.5	28.0	28.6	32.0
Fat, %	3.1	3.0	3.3	2.8	1.8	2.9	2.1	2.6	2.4
Fiber, %	7.5	7.6	7.5	7.7	8.8	8.8	8.7	8.5	7.9
Calcium, %	2.8	2.5	2.7	2.3	2.6	4.7	4.3	4.3	4.5
Phosphorus, %	1.6	1.5	1.6	1.4	1.6	2.1	2.2	2.2	2.3

* Concentrates of different potencies may be used to supply these nutrients if adjustments are made to compensate for potency variation. The first four rations are to be used in a limited-grain feeding program so that approximately equal parts of mash and grain will be consumed. All other rations are to be fed with grain at all times. A source of calcium such as oystershell must be available for the hens at all times.

NEBRASKA. (*University of Nebraska Leaflet* 109, 1953.)

NEBRASKA TURKEY RATIONS

Ingredient	Turkey Starter 53-T lb.	Turkey Grower 53-TG lb.
Ground yellow corn	340	247
Wheat shorts or pulverized oats	150	200
Whole oats	...	200
Soybean meal	250	150
Alfalfa meal (17% protein plus)	50	50
Meat scraps (50% protein plus)	100	100
Fish meal	20	20
Fish solubles blend	20	...
Dried whey	30	...
Nebraska Vitamin Concentrate No. 4 (or equivalent)*	10	3
Mineral Mix No. 57†	30	30
Total	1000	1000
Calculated protein level (per cent)	24.2	22.2

* Each pound of Vitamin Concentrate No. 4 to carry the following minimum values:

Riboflavin	0.2 gm.
Calcium pantothenate	0.4 gm.
Niacin	0.6 gm.
Choline chloride	2.0 gm.
D_3	135,000 I.C.U.
B_{12}	0.3 mg.
Antibiotic (procaine penicillin)	200 mg.
(aureomycin)	1 gm.
(terramycin)	1 gm.
(bacitracin)	1 gm.

† Mineral Premix Formula No. 57

	Parts by Weight
Limestone	403
Steamed bonemeal (or equivalent)	403
Salt	161
Trace Mix No. 1‡	33

‡ Trace Mix No. 1 to carry enough manganese, iodine, iron, cobalt, copper, zinc, and other minor mineral elements when included at a level of 33 parts per 1000 and the complete mineral supplement is used at a level of either 2 or 3 per cent to supplement ingredients as called for in these formulas.

NEW ENGLAND COLLEGE CONFERENCE, JUNE, 1954.

TURKEY RATIONS

Mash ingredient	Starter (1), (2)	Grower (1)	Grower (3), (4)	Breeder (1)
Ground yellow corn	800	950	800	1000
Standard wheat middlings	100	200	200	300
Ground oats	...	...	...	150
Fish meal (60%)	200	50	50	100
Meat scrap (50%)	100	...	50	50
Soybean oil meal (44%)	650	580	680	200
Alfalfa meal (17%) (100,000 A/lb.)	60	60	60	60
Butyl fermentation product (5)	40	40	50	40
Dicalcium phosphate or equivalent (6)	8	52	40	32
Ground limestone (feeding grade)	30	40	55	55
Iodized salt (7)	5	10	10	10
Antibiotic supplement	(8)	...	...	...
Vitamin B_{12} supplement	...	...	...	(9)
Niacin	45 gm.	45 gm.	45 gm.	45 gm.
Choline chloride (dry, 25%)	4.0	2.0	2.0	2.0
Dry vitamin D (1500 D/gm.)	1.0	1.0	1.0	1.0
Dry vitamin A (5000 A/gm.)	1.8	1.8	1.8	1.8
Manganese sulfate or equivalent (10)	...	...	...	0.25
Vitamin E concentrate (20,000 I.U./lb.)	0.4	0.2	0.2	0.4
Totals (11)	2000.2	1987.0	2000.0	2002.45

(1) To be fed as all-mash rations. Feed starting ration until birds are 10 weeks old.

(2) A coccidiosis-controlling drug may be used at the level recommended by the manufacturer.

(3) To be fed with grain after the birds are at least 12 weeks old. (60 to 80 per cent mash and 20 to 40 per cent grain).

(4) May be converted to a finishing ration by reducing soybean oil meal by 200 pounds and adding a like amount of ground yellow corn. May be fed after birds are 20 weeks old.

(5) Based on a product containing 250 gamma of riboflavin per gram. Three per cent of corn distillers' dried solubles may be used; and the ration, fortified to contain not less than 2 milligrams of riboflavin and 6 milligrams of pantothenic acid per pound of ration.

(6) Steamed bonemeal or defluorinated rock phosphate may replace the dicalcium phosphate on a phosphorus basis. Raw rock phosphate containing not more than 3.5 per cent fluorine may replace one-half of the phosphorus in the dicalcium phosphate in the grower and one-fourth in the breeder rations.

(7) If a high salt fish meal is used, omit the added salt.

(8) Use 1 to 5 pounds per ton depending upon the product used. Suggested levels are: 9 grams of aureomycin, bacitracin, or terramycin; or 2 to 4 grams of procaine penicillin per ton of finished ration, or equivalent.

(9) Use a vitamin B_{12} concentrate contributing not less than 6 milligrams of vitamin B_{12} per ton of ration.

(10) Manganese sulfate (70 per cent feeding grade) or equivalent amount of manganese from other sources.

(11) If an even 2000 pounds is desired, adjust by removing or adding middlings.

NORTH CAROLINA. (North Carolina State College of Agriculture and Engineering of the University of North Carolina, 1954.)

NORTH CAROLINA TURKEY MASHES

	No. 51 Starter 28% lb.	No. 52 Grower 28% lb.	No. 53 Breeder 20% lb.
Ground yellow corn	600	425	863
Wheat middlings	100	100	200
Pulverized oats	100	. . .	100
Meat and bone scraps (50% protein)	100	300	100
Fish meal (60% protein)	125	. . .	100
Soybean oil meal (44% protein)	750	700	300
Alfalfa meal (17% protein) 100,000 A per lb.	75	200	125
Whey, dried	50	75	75
Butyl fermentation solubles (500 micrograms riboflavin per gram)	30	30	30
Steamed bonemeal or equivalent	30	150	75
Pulverized oystershells or equivalent	40	. . .	. . .
Salt	10	25	20
Feeding oil (300 D, 1500 A per gram)	2.5	5	5
D-activated animal sterol (1500 D per gram)	1.75	5	3.5
Choline chloride (dry 25%)	3.0	2	2
Manganese sulfate	0.5	0.7	0.5
	grams	grams	grams
Niacin	60	60	55
Antibiotic supplement*	+	. . .	. . .
			milligrams
Vitamin B_{12} supplement	. . .	. . .	6-10
Total	2017+	2017+	1999+

* Aureomycin, bacitracin, penicillins, and terramycin are added to starter mashes for the purpose of stimulating growth in young turkeys. Two arsonic compounds are also being used commercially in starter mashes as growth stimulants. The quantity of antibiotic as well as arsonic compound added to a starter mash should be governed by the recommendations of the manufacturer.

Feeding Suggestions

1. Self-feed the starting mash without grains for 8 weeks.
2. After the eighth week begin self-feeding cracked yellow corn and whole oats in separate feed hoppers. Gradually replace the starting mash with growing mash. Complete the change by the end of the tenth week.
3. Feed the growing mash with grains until the turkeys are marketed.
4. Self-feed crushed oystershells or limestone to supply additional calcium to the growing and breeding turkeys.
5. The growing and breeding turkeys should have access to insoluble

ONTARIO AGRICULTURAL COLLEGE. (S. J. Slinger, W. F. Pepper, and J. R. Cavers, O.A.C. Turkey Feed Formulas, O.A.C. Circular 141, revised, January, 1954.)

Starter. This mash contains about 27 per cent protein (N × 6.25). It is made to be fed as an all-mash ration for the first 4 weeks. It will, however, give good results if fed with a free-choice supply of grain after 4 weeks and continuing to 8 weeks of age.

Grower Mash (4 to 8 weeks). This mash contains about 26 per cent protein (N × 6.25). As an alternative to using the starter plus grain from 4 to 8 weeks, this mash may be given as an all-mash ration.

Grower Mash (8 to 24 weeks). This mash contains about 20 per cent protein (N × 6.25). It should be fed with a free-choice supply of grain. This mash and the grower concentrate are formulated for confined birds. If used for birds on range, the dehydrated alfalfa and vitamin A and D concentrates may be reduced by one-half.

Grower Concentrate (8 to 24 weeks). This concentrate when mixed in the proportion of 100 pounds of concentrate to 200 pounds of ground grains — wheat, corn, oats, and barley — will contain about 19 per cent protein (N × 6.25). Greater efficiency of feed utilization will result from mixing the concentrate with ground grains than from feeding the concentrate as such and a free-choice supply of whole grains. The resultant 19 per cent protein mash should be fed with a free-choice supply of grain.

Breeder Mash. This mash contains about 20 per cent protein (N × 6.25). It should be fed in the proportion of 50 parts of mash to 50 parts of grain or 60 parts of mash to 40 parts of grain. The latter ratio is superior during the period of heaviest production. Oystershell or other suitable source of calcium should be freely accessible to the breeders when fed this ration.

Turkey Broiler Finishing Mash. This mash contains about 19 per cent protein (N × 6.25). It is designed as an all-mash ration for turkey broilers the last 6 weeks before marketing. The turkey starter mash (0 to 4 weeks) is satisfactory for the

---

hard grit or gravel when cracked and whole grains are fed. Crushed granite, quartz, and feldspar are examples of hard grit. These materials are preferable to crushed limestone and oystershells for grinding the feed in the gizzard.

6. For the purpose of utilizing more home-grown grains, the 28 per cent crude protein growing mash is preferable to one containing less crude protein.

O.A.C. TURKEY FEED FORMULAS

Ingredient	Turkey Starter Mash (0-4 wk.) lb.	Turkey Grower Mash (4-8 wk.) lb.	Turkey Grower Mash (8-24 wk.) lb.	Grower Concentrate (8-24 wk.) lb.	Turkey Breeder Mash lb.	Turkey Broiler Finishing Mash lb.
Ground wheat	500	500	640	. . .	600	900
Ground yellow corn	300	200	200	. . .	200	500
Pulverized oats	. . .	100	200	. . .	200	. . .
Ground barley	. . .	100	200	. . .	165	. . .
Dehydrated alfalfa meal (100,000 I.U. of vitamin A/lb.) or cereal grass	100	100	120	270	200	50
Fish meal (65% protein)	50	40	20	70	80	50
Meat meal (50% protein)	40	40	40	100	40	40
Dried buttermilk or skimmilk	40	40	40	100	70	40
Soybean oil meal (44% protein)	840	750	425	1200	300	320
Tallow or grease*	20	20	20	30	20	20
Ground limestone	30	30	30	70	50	30
Steamed bonemeal or equivalent	65	65	50	125	55	40
Iodized salt	10	10	10	25	15	5
Vitamin A oil (10,000 I.U./gm.)	1	1	1	3	2	1
Dry vitamin D_3 (1,650 I.C.U./gm.)	2	2	2	5	4	2
Manganese sulfate (feed grade)	0.3	0.3	0.4	1.25	0.5	0.3
DL Methionine (feed grade)	0.5	0.5	. . .	. . .	. . .	0.5
	gm.	gm.	gm.	gm.	gm.	gm.
Riboflavin	3	3	3	8	4	3
Niacin	15	15	15	35	. . .	15
d-alpha-tocopheryl acetate	5	5	5	12	5	. . .
Antibiotic†	4-10	4-10	4-10	10-35	6-20	4-10
Arsonic acid‡	45-90	45-90	45-90	110-220	. . .	45-90
	mg.	mg.	mg.	mg.	mg.	mg.
Vitamin B_{12}	3	3	3	8	6	3
Calculated analysis	%	%	%	%	%	%
Min. crude protein	27.1	25.6	20.1	35.3	20.0	19.1
Min. crude fat	2.8	2.9	3.3	3.0	3.5	3.4
Max. crude fiber	5.2	5.7	6.0	7.6	6.6	3.7
Calcium	1.9	1.9	1.6	3.9	2.3	1.5
Total phosphorus	1.0	1.0	0.8	1.5	0.9	0.8
Inorganic phosphorus	0.68	0.67	0.54	1.24	0.66	0.52

* Tallow or grease should not be used unless it has been stabilized with suitable antioxidants and tested for stability.

† The levels suggested for antibiotics are in terms of the salts of the antibiotics. If penicillin is the antibiotic, use the lower level. If aureomycin, terramycin, or bacitracin are used, the higher levels should be employed.

‡ It is recommended that either 3-nitro, 4-hydroxyphenylarsonic acid, at the lower levels shown, or arsanilic acid, at the higher levels, be included.

feeding of turkey broilers up until the time they are changed to this finishing mash. When used for starting turkey broilers it is recommended that the starter mash be used as an all-mash diet right up until the time of changing to the finishing mash and that the change to the finishing mash be made gradually over a period of about 3 days.

Substitutions. Equal parts of wheat shorts and wheat bran may replace ground barley. Dried whey may replace dried buttermilk or dried skimmilk. For every 40 pounds of dried milk replaced with dried whey, increase the amount of soybean oil meal by 30 pounds and reduce the ground wheat by 30 pounds. Steamed bonemeal may be replaced by defluorinated rock phosphate. Other calcium and phosphorus carriers may be used if replacement is made on the basis of calcium and phosphorus content. Vitamin A oil may be replaced by dry vitamin A products on an equal unitage basis. Manganese sulfate may be replaced by other manganese carriers to supply equal levels of manganese. Ground limestone may be replaced by calcium carbonate.

TEXAS. (Agricultural and Mechanical College of Texas, 1954.)

TEXAS TURKEY RATIONS

Ingredients	Turkey Starter All-Mash %	Turkey Grower All-Mash %	Turkey Fattener All-Mash %	Turkey Laying Mash All-Mash %
Ground milo	20	30	35 1/2	40
Ground yellow corn	17 1/2	20 1/2	25	19 1/2
Wheat gray shorts	5	5	5	5
Soybean oil meal (44% protein)	38*	25*	20*	15
Fish meal (60% protein)	6	5	5	6
Dried whey	3	3	3	3
Dehydrated alfalfa leaf meal	5	6	6	6
Steamed bonemeal or equivalent phosphorus supplement	3	3	3	3
Ground limestone or oystershell	2	2	2	2
Salt	1/2	1/2	1/2	1/2
Supplements†				

* Eight per cent of the soybean oil meal may be replaced by 8 per cent of cottonseed meal meeting the following quality specifications: (1) containing no more than 0.1 per cent free gossypol; (2) should have a nitrogen solubility of at least, 70 per cent in 0.02 sodium hydroxide.

† To be added per ton of feed:

1. Manganese sulfate, 1/2 pound
2. Antibiotics: Use either 10 grams of aureomycin, 10 grams of bacitracin, 10 grams of terramycin, or 4 grams of penicillin. A combination of two, three, or four of the antibiotics may be used. In making up the combination, use a proportionate part of the above given levels on a per ton basis.
3. Vitamin A: 6,000,000 International units. Any source of vitamin A available may be used just so the total number of units added per ton is that given.
4. Vitamin D_3: 2,000,000 International chick units.
5. B vitamins:

    4 grams riboflavin
    10 grams calcium pantothenate (Dextrorotatory)
    40 grams niacin
    800 grams choline chloride

It will probably be necessary to obtain choline chloride in the dry form as a 25 per cent supplement.

6. Vitamin B_{12}: 6 milligrams.
7. Methionine: 1 pound
8. Arsonic acids: Add level according to manufacturer's recommendations (add to starting and growing rations only).

These supplements will be added to the starting, growing, and fattening rations as given. The choline chloride and the methionine may be eliminated from the laying ration.

WASHINGTON. (Washington Poultry Feed Formulas, Poultry Science Department, State College of Washington, Ext. Mimeo. 1186, 1185, and 1184, 1954.)

TURKEY STARTER MASHES

Ingredients	1 %	2 %	3 %	4 %	5 %	6 %
Ground yellow corn or milo*	40.2	37.2	37.2	43.7	40.0	41.5
Soybean oil meal (44% protein)	46.5	46.0	42.0	40.0	39.7	37.2
Fish meal (70% protein)	5.0	5.0	5.0	5.0	5.0	10.0
Meat and bonemeal (50% protein)	...	...	...	5.0	5.0	...
Dehydrated alfalfa or grass (carotene, 12 mg./100 gm.)	2.5	2.5	2.5	2.5	2.5	2.5
Dried brewers' yeast	...	...	4.0	...	...	...
Dried whey	...	4.0	4.0	...	4.0	4.0
Salt (iodized, fine)	0.3	0.3	0.3	0.3	0.3	0.3
Limestone or shell flour	2.0	2.0	2.0	2.0	2.0	2.0
Steamed bonemeal or defluorinated phosphate	3.5	3.0	3.0	1.5	1.5	2.5
Add the following to each ton of feed						
Vitamin A, millions of I.U.	3.5	3.5	3.5	3.5	3.5	3.5
Vitamin D_3, millions of I.C.U.	1.2	1.2	1.2	1.2	1.2	1.2
Riboflavin, gm.	1.6	0.6	...	1.5	0.6	0.5
Calcium pantothenate, gm.	2.6	1.0	...	3.0	1.4	1.5
Choline chloride, lb.	1.0	1.0	1.0	1.0	1.0	1.0
Methionine, lb.	1.0	1.0	1.0	1.0	1.0	1.0
Manganese sulfate lb. (100% pure)	0.4	0.4	0.4	0.4	0.4	0.4
Antibiotic†						

Suggested analysis: protein, 28 per cent; calcium, 2.0 per cent; phosphorus, 1.0 per cent; vitamin A, 4000 International units per pound, vitamin D_3, 600 International chick units per pound, and riboflavin, 2 milligrams per pound.

These mashes may also be used for turkey fryers. The suggested method of feeding follows: During the first 3-4 weeks feed as crushed pellets or crumbled feed. After this feed intermediate size (1/8 inch) pellets. If feather picking develops, mix pellets and mash. After the poults are 6 weeks of age small amounts of cracked or whole grain may be placed with the feed to accustom the turkeys to grain. Feed granite or silica grit of the proper size one day each week.

* Up to 15.0 per cent of ground wheat, ground barley, or finely ground oats may be used to replace an equivalent amount of corn or milo; however, such substitutions will decrease feed efficiency.

† If using diamine or procaine penicillin, use at rate of 3 grams per ton. If using aureomycin, bacitracin or terramycin, use at rate of 10 grams per ton.

TURKEY DEVELOPER MASHES
(8 weeks to maturity)

Ingredients	1 %	2 %	3 %	4 %	5 %
Ground grains*	61.5	49.0	45.0	47.0	55.0
Wheat mixed feed (millrun)*	...	10.0	10.0	10.0	...
Fishmeal (70% protein)	5.0	2.0	...	...	5.0
Meat and bonemeal (50% protein)	...	3.0	...	5.0	...
Soybean oil meal (44% protein)	23.0	20.0	28.0	22.0	14.0
Cottonseed meal (43% protein)	...	...	...	...	10.0
Dehydrated alfalfa or grass (carotene, 12 mg./100 gm.)	5.0	10.0	10.0	10.0	10.0
Limestone or shell flour	2.0	3.0	3.0	4.0	4.0
Steamed bonemeal or defluorinated phosphate	3.5	2.0	3.0	1.0	1.0
Salt (iodized, fine)	1.0	1.0	1.0	1.0	1.0
Add the following to each ton of feed					
Vitamin D_3, millions of I.C.U.	1.2	1.2	1.2	1.2	1.2
Riboflavin (gm.)	1.7	...	...	...	...
Manganese sulfate, lb., (100% pure)	0.4	0.4	0.4	0.4	0.4
Antibiotic†					

Suggested analysis: protein, 20.0 per cent; calcium, 2.0 per cent; phosphorus, 1.0 per cent; vitamin A, 4000 International units per pound; vitamin D_3, 600 International chick units per pound; riboflavin, 2 mg. per pound.

The suggested method of feeding follows: Feed the mash or pellets and whole grain free choice during the entire growing period. Feed granite or silica grit one day each week.

*Ground corn, milo, wheat, barley, or oats may be used singly or in any combination with 0-10 per cent millrun as long as the combined amounts of barley, oats, and millrun do not exceed 35 per cent of the mash.

†If using diamine or procaine penicillin use at rate of 3 grams per ton. If using aureomycin, bacitracin, or terramycin use at rate of 10 grams per ton.

TURKEY BREEDER MASHES AND COMPLETE RATIONS

Ingredients	1 %	2 %	3 %	4 %	5 %
Ground grains*	63.2	53.2	61.2	49.4	29.4
Wheat mixed feed (millrun)*	10.0	15.0	10.0	. . .	15.0
Dehydrated alfalfa or grass (12 mg. carotene/100 gm.)	5.0	10.0	5.0	10.0	20.0
Soybean oil meal (44% protein)	12.0	10.0	9.0	22.0	18.0
Meat and bonemeal (50% protein)	. . .	2.0	. . .	8.0	. . .
Fish meal (70% protein)	4.0	2.0	4.0	. . .	5.0
Dried whey	. . .	2.0	. . .	4.0	4.0
Limestone or shell flour	3.5	3.5	3.5	3.0	3.0
Steamed bonemeal or defluorinated phosphate	2.0	2.0	2.0	3.0	5.0
Salt (iodized)	0.3	0.3	0.3	0.6	0.6
Wheat germ meal	. . .	. . .	5.0	. . .	. . .
Add the following to each ton of feed					
Vitamin A, millions of I.U.	1.0	. . .	1.0	2.0	. . .
Vitamin D_3 millions of I.C.U.	1.0	1.0	1.0	2.0	2.0
Vitamin B_{12}, (mg.)	. . .	3.0	. . .	6.0	. . .
Alpha tocopheryl acetate (gm.)	20.0	10.0	. . .	20.0	. . .
Manganese sulfate, lb. (100% pure)	0.25	0.25	0.25	0.5	0.5
Calcium pantothenate (gm.)	10.0	5.0	10.0	16.0	10.0
Riboflavin (gm.)	2.0	1.5	2.0	3.5	1.0

Suggested analysis: Rations 1 and 2, protein, 16.0 per cent; calcium, 2.0 per cent; phosphorus, 1.0 per cent; vitamin A, 4000 International units per pound; vitamin D_3, 600 International chick units per pound; riboflavin, 2 milligrams per pound. Rations 4 and 5, protein, 20 per cent; calcium, 3.0 per cent; phosphorus 1.5 per cent; vitamin A, 6700 International units per pound; vitamin D_3, 1000 International chick units per pound; riboflavin, 3 milligrams per pound.

Rations 1, 2, and 3 are complete rations and should be fed as mash crumbles or pellets. Rations 4 and 5 are to be fed with grain free choice on the basis of 60 per cent mash and 40 per cent grain.

Limestone grit or shell should be available at all times. Feed granite or silica grit 1 day each week.

*Ground corn, milo, wheat, barley, or oats may be used singly or in combination with 0-15 per cent millrun as long as the combined amounts of barley, oats, and millrun do not exceed 35 per cent of the mash. When the total of millrun, oats, and barley is over 30 per cent, the feed should be pelleted.

WISCONSIN. (University of Wisconsin, 1954.)

WISCONSIN RATIONS FOR TURKEYS

	Starting lb.	Rations lb.	Growing lb.	Rations* lb.	Breeder Rations lb.
Ground yellow corn	210	160	295	295	365
Ground oats	50	50	50	50	100
Wheat bran	50	50	50	50	100
Wheat middlings	50	50	50	50	100
Alfalfa meal	50	50	...	...	100
Meat scrap	100	100	...	50	50
Soybean oil meal	400	400	480	420	150
Fish meal	...	...	...	...	25
Chick size oystershell	20	20	20	20	...
Granite grit	10	10	...	...	...
Special steam bone-meal	20	20	50	40	...
Iodized salt	5	5	5	5	5
Dried whey fortified	...	50	...	...	...
Fish solubles	30	30	...	...	...
300 D feeding oil or powder†	4	4	No	No	5
2000 A feeding oil	2	2	...	...	2
Manganese sulfate (feeding grade)	1/4	1/4	1/4	1/4	1/4
Riboflavin	1 1/2 gm.	...	No	No	1 1/2 gm.
Antibiotic feed supplement‡	Yes	Yes	No	No	...

*With good pasture, free access to grains.
†Based on International chick units.
‡Use according to manufacturer's directions.

SECTION VI. RATIONS FOR DUCKS

CORNELL. (1954.) The duck starting ration is fed as 9/64-inch pellets for the first 2 to 3 weeks. The duck growing ration is fed as 13/64-inch pellets to follow the starting ration. It may be fed until the ducklings are marketed or may be followed by duck fattener for the last 2 weeks before marketing. The duck breeding ration is fed as 13/64-inch pellets. The mature birds should also be given access to oystershell.

CORNELL DUCK RATIONS

Ingredients	Starter lb.	Grower lb.	Breeder lb.
Corn meal	720	675	580
Wheat standard middlings	300	200	300
Wheat flour middlings	300	300	300
Wheat, ground whole	. . .	200	100
Oats, pulverized	200	200	200
Fish meal (60% protein)	100	50	50
Fish solubles (50% solids)	. . .	. . .	50
Meat scrap (50% protein)	50	100	100
Soybean meal (44% protein)	100	50	50
Alfalfa meal (17% protein)	60	60	100
Yeast, dried brewers'	. . .	. . .	40
Whey, dried	50	50	60
Distillers' solubles, dried	50	50	. . .
Limestone, ground	40	40	60
Dicalcium phosphate	20	15	. . .
Salt, iodized	6	6	6
Vitamin A supplement (4000 A/gm.)	2	2	2
D-activated animal sterol (1500 D/gm.)	1	1	1
Riboflavin supplement (3500-4000 mg/lb.)	0.5	0.5	0.5
Manganese sulfate	0.5	0.5	0.5
Niacin, pure	(30 gm.)	(30 gm.)	(30 gm.)
Vitamin E supplement to supply	. . .	. . .	(5 gm.)
Calculated Analysis:	%	%	%
protein	17.5	16.0	17.5
fat	4.25	4.0	4.0
fiber	4.75	4.5	5.0
calcium	1.65	1.70	2.0
phosphorus	0.95	0.86	0.8

CORNELL RATIONS FOR LAYING DUCKS

(L. M. Hurd and K. F. Hilbert, Duck growing, Cornell Bul. 345, revised, 1948.)

Mashes*

Ingredients	Layer Rations 1	2	3	4
	lb.	lb.	lb.	lb.
Yellow corn meal	500	475	475	450
Wheat bran	300	300	300	300
Wheat standard middlings	200	200	200	200
Wheat red dog flour	300	300	300	300
Ground oats, low fiber	200	200	200	200
Soybean meal	150	150	150	150
Meat scrap (55% protein)†	150	100	125	150
Dehydrated alfalfa meal (17% protein)	120	120	120	120
Dried skimmilk	...	50	...	...
Dried buttermilk	...	...	50	...
Dried whey	...	...	...	50
Pulverized limestone	70	70	70	70
Salt	10	10	10	10
Vitamin D from fish oil, feeding oil, or activated animal sterols A.O.A.C. units per pound.‡	650	650	650	650

* To be fed at the rate of 2 parts of mash to 1 part of grain.
† Fish meal may be substituted entirely, or in part, for meat scrap.
‡ Vitamin D may be omitted from the mash when the ducks run outdoors daily.

Grain Mixtures

Ingredients	Modifications 1	2	3	4	5
	lb.	lb.	lb.	lb.	lb.
Cracked yellow corn	50	65	40	40	40
Wheat	50	35	40	40	40
Heavy oats	...	...	20	10	10
Barley	...	...	...	10	...
Buckwheat	...	...	...	...	10

HARPER ADAMS AGRICULTURAL COLLEGE (ENGLAND). Rations for Table Ducklings. (V. K. Tallent, The production of table ducklings, Harper Adams Utility Poultry Jour., 17:357, 1931-1932.)

Ingredients	Starter, First Week, lb.	Grower, 2-7 Weeks, lb.	Fattener for 2 Weeks, lb.
Barley meal	20	40	120 of either
Sussex ground oats	20	40	or a mixture of both
Wheat bran	20	30	. . .
Wheat middlings	40	60	40
Dried milk	10	. . .	. . .
Meat and bonemeal	. . .	20	30
Cod liver oil	2%	. . .	. . .

Developing Rations for Ducks for Eggs. (Duck Notes, Harper Adams Utility Poultry Jour., 13:318 1927-28.)

One to four weeks: 4 or 5 meals daily of a mash made up of 1 part of biscuit meal and equal parts of thirds and Sussex ground oats.

One to two months: 3 meals a day of a mash made up of 1 part of bran and equal parts of Sussex ground oats, maize meal, and thirds, with 1/2 part of fish meal.

Two to four months: 3 meals of a mash made up of 1 part of bran, 3 parts of sharps, 1 part of Sussex ground oats, 1 part of maize meal, and 1/2 part of fish meal.

After 4 months: Feed 2 meals of the above mash, plus grain, at night. The grain can be made up of wheat and kibbled maize.

Ration for Laying Ducks. (The feeding and management of the laying duck, Harper Adams Utility Poultry Jour., 18:597, 1933.) This ration was fed at the Egg Laying Trials for ducks. The grain feed, of which they get 2 ounces per bird daily, consists in parts by weight of 2 wheat, 1 best clipped white oats, 1 cracked maize, and $^1/_{16}$ cracked green peas. The mash ration, in parts dry weight, of which 4 ounces per duck is allowed daily, consists of 3 sharps, 2 Sussex ground oats, 2 maize meal, 1 bran, 1 fish meal, and 1 alfalfa meal.

STATE INSTITUTE OF APPLIED AGRICULTURE, Farmingdale, L. I., New York. (Rations for ducks, Dept. of Poultry, Stencil 1303.)

MASHES FOR MATURE DUCKS

Ingredients	1 lb.	2 lb.
Yellow corn meal	350	300
Wheat bran	200	200
Wheat standard middlings	. . .	100
Second clear flour	125	125
Meat scrap (50% protein)	100	50
Pulverized oats	100	100
Dried skimmilk	50	25
Alfalfa leaf meal	50	50
White fish meal	25	50

DUCK STARTING AND GROWING MASHES
(These mixtures are to be fed from the time the ducklings are a day old until they are marketed.)

Ingredients	1 lb.	2 lb.	3 lb.	4 lb.
Yellow corn meal	300	300	375	500
Wheat flour middlings	200	100	. . .	. . .
Red dog flour	. . .	. . .	100	50
Wheat bran	100	150	300	200
Second clear flour	50	150	. . .	. . .
Dried skimmilk	100	. . .	75	50
Pulverized oats	100	100	. . .	50
Meat scrap (50% protein)	50	100	100	100
White fish meal	50	50	. . .	. . .
Alfalfa leaf meal	50	50	50	50

Fattening Mash. This mixture is designed for those who want to use a special fattening mash. It may be fed 2 to 3 weeks before the ducklings are marketed. It may follow any of the starting and growing mashes.

	Pounds
Yellow corn meal	500
Wheat bran	150
Second clear flour	125
Pulverized oats	100
Dried skimmilk	50
Meat scrap (50% protein)	50
White fish meal	25

SECTION VII. USING LOCAL GRAIN FOR POULTRY

CORNELL. (New York State College of Agriculture at Cornell University, Department of Poultry Husbandry, Ext. Stencil 194, 1951, and 224, 1953.)

Local grain supplies such as oats, wheat, corn, barley, buckwheat, and rye can be used in poultry feeding in the following ways:

1. Scratch grain mixtures.
2. Combined in ground form with a "mixing mash" or mash concentrate to form a complete poultry mash.
3. Used by the feed manufacturer directly as an ingredient in a formula feed.

Scratch Grain Mixtures. Mash mixtures are usually designed to be fed with grain, by any of a variety of feeding systems, so that about equal amounts of mash and the grain mixture are consumed daily. The simplest way of using home-grown or local grain is to incorporate it in the scratch grain mixture; in fact, unless a farmer has more grain available than is required to meet the need for the scratch grain part of his feeding program, it is usually uneconomical for him to use it in any other way. The feed dealer can also use locally purchased grain to supply a large part of his scratch grain volume. The amounts and proportions of various grains available vary with regions. A single grain mixture will not meet the conditions of all areas, nor will the same mixture always be adaptable to the local supply situation. For this reason, the following table (A) shows suggested maximum usage levels of various grains per ton of mixture, rather than grain mixture formulas as such.

TABLE A. SUGGESTED GRAIN USAGE LEVELS FOR SCRATCH MIXTURES.

Grain	Maximum usage level per ton of scratch mixture lb.
Corn (whole or cracked)	1500
Wheat	1500
Oats, heavy	800
Oats, light	500
Barley	800
Buckwheat	400

Experience has shown it to be more generally satisfactory to use a mixture of grains than a single grain. In order to maintain a high level of available energy and digestibility in the grain mixture, it is suggested that at least half of it should be made up of corn and/or wheat, and not more than half of it from oats, barley, and/or buckwheat. Rye is unpalatable to poultry, and is not readily consumed in grain mixtures.

It has become a common practice to use cracked corn in poultry scratch mixtures. It is, of course, important to use cracked corn in the scratch mixture provided for young growing birds. However, whole corn can be used satisfactorily for growing birds after they are 10 to 12 weeks of age, and for pullets and hens. It is most satisfactory to begin feeding whole corn during the growing period so that the birds are accustomed to eating whole corn before they enter the laying houses. If the birds have been accustomed only to cracked corn during the growing period and it is desired to shift them to whole corn after they have entered egg production, it is best to shift gradually in order to avoid a sudden decrease in feed consumption.

In some areas facilities for shelling corn may not be readily available, and it would be desirable to feed corn on the cob. This can be done easily by giving cob corn in the morning in the litter and at night feeding a scratch mixture that has a low proportion or no corn in it. It would be best to weigh the cob corn as fed in order to follow the amount eaten and be able to control grain consumption. The cob will constitute about 1/5 the weight of cob corn. Normally about half of the total feed intake of mature birds will be scratch grain, amounting to about 12 to 15 pounds per 100 birds per day; feeding 7½ pounds of cob corn per day will supply 6 pounds of shell corn, which would be about half of the scratch feed requirement of the birds. This can be adjusted according to season, egg production, and the proportion of corn desired in the scratch portion of the diet.

Formulation of Mixing Mashes. The utilization of local grains in the mash part of the ration is simplified by the use of a so-called "mixing mash." Such mixtures are essentially the nongrain part of a complete poultry ration, designed to be combined in a definite proportion with ground grains.

Tables I and II show the recommended formula patterns and required nutrient content of mixing mashes. Tables III to VII show examples of mixing mash formulas compounded according to the recommended patterns to meet the nutrient requirements.

General considerations covering the choice of ingredients within the ingredient classes are discussed below. (The tables appear at the end of the Appendix.)

Vegetable Proteins. Soybean meal and other vegetable protein supplements are the most plentiful protein sources available for poultry feeding. They can be used to supply most of the supplementary protein needed in poultry mashes. Soybean meal, the ingredient of this class available in greatest supply, can be used alone or in combination with corn gluten meal or peanut meal. Corn gluten and peanut meal should not make up more than 1/4 the total of this class of ingredients used in a mash. Cottonseed meal can be used similarly in combination with soybean meal in mashes for growing birds but should be avoided in rations for hens. Linseed meal cannot be recommended for use in any poultry ration because of its growth-retarding effect.

Animal Proteins. These products serve as sources of protein, minerals, vitamin B_{12}, and at least one other still unidentified nutrient. The minimum levels recommended for starter, confinement grower, and breeder mashes are the amounts needed to aid in supplying the unknown nutrient(s). The lower recommended figure refers to the minimum level of fish products when used alone; the higher figure indicates the approximate level of meat scrap when used alone. A combination of products appears to be preferable. Depending upon cost and availability, levels higher than the indicated minimum amounts can be used in all poultry mashes; the amounts of protein, calcium, phosphorus, and vitamin B_{12}, contributed by the animal products, will accordingly determine the amounts of these nutrients needed from other sources.

The recommended levels of vitamin B_{12}, indicated in the table showing required composition of poultry mashes, refer to the amounts supplied by fish products, meat scrap, and vitamin B_{12} supplements. It is desirable to know the B_{12} content of the particular fish and meat products used, and this may be determined by microbiological assay. When such analytical values are not available, an approximation of the B_{12} content of the mash may be calculated by assigning values of 40 micrograms of vitamin B_{12} per pound of fish meal, 70 micrograms per pound of fish solubles, and 15 micrograms per pound of meat scrap.

Other B-Vitamin Carriers. Included in this class of feedstuffs are dried milk products, dried yeast, dried distillers' solubles, and fermentation solubles. These ingredients are valuable sources of many of the known B-complex vitamins.

The levels recommended are intended to aid in supplying the unknown nutrient(s) referred to above. Because it appears likely that more than one unidentified nutrient may be required in the ration, it is considered wise to use these carriers in combination with animal proteins.

Dehydrated Alfalfa Meal. This product is an important source of vitamin A activity and contributes materially to the protein and riboflavin content of a mash, but it is desirable to limit its use because of its low available energy value. It is, therefore, necessary to use a high-quality meal in order to supply sufficient vitamin A activity at the low-usage levels recommended. As shown in the formula examples, using alfalfa meal containing 100,000 units of vitamin A activity per pound at a level of 250 pounds per ton will meet the requirement for vitamin A in laying and breeding rations if yellow corn makes up approximately half of the grain used in the mash and in the scratch grain mixture. If the alfalfa meal available does not contain sufficient vitamin A activity to meet the requirement at the feeding levels recommended, additional vitamin A should be supplied in another form, such as a vitamin feeding oil, rather than by exceeding the recommended alfalfa meal levels.

Calcium and Phosphorus Supplements. The phosphorus re-requirements are shown both as total phosphorus and "available phosphorus." The available phosphorus content of a mash is the amount supplied by the animal products and the inorganic supplements (bonemeal, defluorinated phosphate, etc.) <u>plus</u> 30 per cent of the rest of the phosphorus of the mash. Calculating available phosphorus gives a more accurate appraisal of the phosphorus value of a mash than does the total phosphorus content.

The phosphorus sources listed in the pattern table are essentially equivalent in the availability of their phosphorus. In choosing a phosphorus supplement, care should be taken to insure that the product is intended for poultry feeding and has a sufficiently low content of fluorine.

The calcium levels recommended for layer and breeder mashes, shown in the table on required nutrient composition, do not meet the total requirement of hens for egg production. Experimental studies have shown that it is undesirable to use a calcium level in the mash sufficiently high to meet this requirement. These rations, therefore, should be supplemented by giving the hens free access to oystershell or some other calcium supplement. It is also advisable to feed such calcium supplements free choice in addition to growing mash.

Vitamin D. The recommended vitamin D levels are shown in International chick units, based on the new vitamin D_3 standard now in official use. Feeding oils and D-activated animal sterols are equally effective sources of vitamin D, unit for unit.

Other Riboflavin and B_{12} Sources. Riboflavin supplements and vitamin B_{12} supplements of guaranteed vitamin content are generally available and can be highly useful in meeting the requirements for these vitamins. The levels of other vitamin-rich feedstuffs in the formula, particularly when amounts greater than the minimum levels are supplied, will determine whether and in what amounts special vitamin supplements should be used.

Use of Mixing Mashes. The mixing mashes allow a wide degree of flexibility in the choice and proportion of grains that can be combined with them. The main considerations involved in choosing the grains are to maintain a sufficiently high level of productive energy (Table VIII) and over-all digestibility together with suitable texture and palatability.

Table B presents suggested maximum usage levels of the common grains per ton of finished mash mixture. Here again it is generally preferable to employ two or more grains rather than a single grain. Because of their high-energy value, corn and/or wheat should constitute at least half of the grain used; conversely, the lower-energy grains should not comprise a total of more than half the grain used.

To make an adequate mash for a particular purpose, the proper mixing mash must be used. In other words, a layer

TABLE B. SUGGESTED GRAIN USAGE LEVELS FOR MASH MIXING

Ground grain	Maximum level per ton lb.	Suggested combinations for use with mixing mashes. (1200 lb. ground grain to be mixed with 800 lb. mixing mash)					
Corn meal	1000	800	...	600	800	800	600
Corn and cob meal	800	...	800	...	...	...	...
Wheat (coarse, ground, or crushed)	1000	200	400	...	...	...	200
Oats, heavy	600	200	...	600	...	...	200
Oats, light	400	...	...	...	400	...	...
Barley	600	...	...	...	...	200	...
Buckwheat	400	...	...	...	...	...	200
Rye (finely ground)	400	...	...	...	...	200	...

mash cannot be made by combining grain with a mixing mash designed to make a starter. Nor is there any simple way that one type of ration can always be converted to another.

The starter mash is intended to be used as an all-mash ration. To use this formula for broilers, it will be advisable to use corn gluten meal to obtain the pigmentation desirable in meat birds; a level of 125 pounds per ton of mixing mash will result in 50 pounds per ton of broiler mash.

The grower, layer, and breeder mashes produced by the respective mixing mashes are 20 per cent protein mashes intended to be fed with approximately equal grain intake according to the usual feeding systems.

Grain-Based Mash Formulas. Use of a large proportion of local grain as ingredients in a mash formula, either in branded feeds or through custom mixing, is a third alternative. Such a procedure requires the development of balanced formulas such as those presented in the circular on poultry rations.

The suggested usage levels of ground grain summarized in Table B for mixing mashes apply directly to this method of mixing as well. Examples of grain-based layer mashes are shown in Table IX to illustrate the wide range of grain proportions that can be used. Other types of rations similarly based on various proportions of local grains can be formulated to meet the specific requirements of growing or breeding chickens by following the recommendations summarized in the circular on poultry rations.

TABLE I. RECOMMENDED FORMULA PATTERNS FOR POULTRY MIXING MASHES

Ingredients	Starter or Broiler (All-Mash) lb./ton	Growers (With grain) Confinement lb./ton	Growers (With grain) Pasture lb./ton	Layer (With grain) lb./ton	Breeder (With grain) lb./ton
Wheat or wheat by-products	0-400	0-200	0-300	0-100	0-100
Vegetable proteins (soybean meal, corn gluten meal, peanut meal)	800-1000	800-1000	1200-1400	1000-1200	700-900
Animal proteins, minimum levels (Fish meal, fish solubles, meat scrap)	125-250	125-250	. . .	. . .	250-400
Other B-vitamin carriers (dried milk products, dried yeast, distillers' dried solubles, fermentation solubles	250	250	. . .	. . .	250-400
Dehydrated alfalfa meal	125-250	250	. . .	250-400	250-400
Additional riboflavin* (if needed)	+	+	−	+	+
Additional vitamin B_{12}* (if needed)	+	+	−	−	+
Additional vitamin A* (if needed)	+	+	−	+	+
Vitamin D_3 (feeding oils or D-activated animal sterols)	+	+	−	+	+
Calcium and phosphorus supplements (steamed bonemeal, dicalcium phosphate, defluorinated phosphate, limestone)	75-125	200-250	250-300	250-300	200-250
Salt	15	25	50	50	50
Manganese sulfate	1	1.2	1.2	1.2	1.2

* Refers to the use of riboflavin supplements, vitamin B_{12} supplements, and vitamin A sources of guaranteed vitamin content, or other vitamin-rich feedstuffs when the formula is otherwise deficient in any of these nutrients.

TABLE II. REQUIRED NUTRIENT CONTENT OF MIXING MASHES

Nutrient	Starter or Broiler (All-Mash)	Growers (with grain) Confinement	Growers (with grain) Pasture	Layer (With grain)	Breeder (With grain)
Protein, %	32	32	32	32	32
Calcium, %	2.5–3.5	4–5	4–5	5–6	5–6
Phosphorus					
Total, %	1.1	1.8	1.8	2.5	2.5
Available, %	0.9	1.6	1.6	1.8	1.8
Riboflavin, mg./lb.	3.3	2.5	...	2.5	4.5
Vitamin B_{12}, μg/lb.	4	4	...	...	8
Vitamin D, I.C.U./lb.	340	675	...	1,700	1,700
Vitamin A, I.U./lb.					
If no corn used	5,000	10,000	...	16,500	16,500
If 50% of grain in mash and scratch is corn	3,500	6,000	...	12,500	12,500

TABLE III. EXAMPLES OF MIXING MASHES, STARTER OR BROILER MASHES

	lb./ton	lb./ton	lb./ton	lb./ton
Wheat flour (or standard) middlings	350	360	225	210
Soybean meal	900	900	750	800
Corn gluten meal	...	...	250	...
Peanut meal	...	...	...	250
Fish meal	125	250	...	...
Fish solubles	...	...	125	...
Meat scrap	125	...	125	250
Corn dried distillers' solubles	125	...	250	...
Dried whey	125	125	...	250
Dried brewers' yeast	...	125	...	...
Dehydrated alfalfa meal	125	125	125	125
Riboflavin supplement to supply (mg. riboflavin)	1250 mg.	...	1400 mg.	...
Vitamin B_{12} supplement to supply (mg. B_{12})	3 mg.	...	...	5 mg.
D-activated animal sterols (1500 I.C.U./gm.)	2	2	2	2
or				
Vitamin feeding oil (300 D, 1500 A)	10	10	10	10
Steamed bonemeal	35	35	60	25
Limestone	70	70	75	75
Salt (iodized)	15	15	15	15
Manganese sulfate (65% feeding grade)	1	1	1	1
Protein, %	34	36	34	34
Calcium, %	3	2.8	3.1	3.3
Phosphorus: total %	1.3	1.3	1.3	1.3
available %	0.9	0.9	0.9	0.9
Vitamin A,* I.U./lb.	6250	6250	6250	6250
Vitamin D, I.C.U./lb.	680	680	680	680
Riboflavin, mg./lb.	3.3	3.3	3.3	3.3
Vitamin B_{12},† μg/lb.	5	5	5	4

* Assuming use of alfalfa meal containing 100,000 International units vitamin A activity and no vitamin feeding oil.

† From animal proteins and vitamin B_{12} supplement.

TABLE IV. EXAMPLES OF MIXING MASHES, CONFINEMENT GROWER MASHES

	lb./ton	lb./ton	lb./ton	lb./ton
Wheat flour (or standard) middlings	120	225	. . .	. . .
Soybean meal	900	775	750	785
Corn gluten meal	. . .	. . .	250	. . .
Peanut meal	. . .	. . .	. . .	250
Fish meal	125	250	. . .	. . .
Fish solubles	. . .	. . .	125	. . .
Meat scrap	125	. . .	125	250
Corn dried distillers' solubles	250	. . .	125	. . .
Dried whey	. . .	125	125	250
Dried brewers' yeast	. . .	125	. . .	. . .
Dehydrated alfalfa meal	250	250	250	250
Vitamin B_{12} supplement to supply (mg. B_{12})	3 mg.	. . .	. . .	6 mg.
D-activated animal sterols (1500 I.C.U./gm.)	2	2	2	2
or				
Vitamin feeding oil (300 D, 1500 A)	10	10	10	10
Steamed bonemeal	150	150	175	140
Limestone	50	75	50	50
Salt (iodized)	25	25	25	25
Manganese sulfate (65% feeding grade)	1.2	1.2	1.2	1.2
Protein, %	34	34	33	34
Calcium, %	4.3	4.5	4.4	4.5
Phosphorus: total, %	2.0	1.9	1.9	1.9
available, %	1.6	1.6	1.6	1.6
Vitamin A,* I.U./lb.	12,500	12,500	12,500	12,500
Vitamin D, I.C.U./lb.	680	680	680	680
Riboflavin, mg./lb.	2.5	3.6	3.4	3.7
Vitamin B_{12},† μg./lb.	5	5	5	5

* Assuming use of alfalfa meal containing 100,000 International units vitamin A activity and no vitamin feeding oil.

† From animal proteins and vitamin B_{12} supplement.

TABLE V. EXAMPLES OF MIXING MASHES, PASTURE GROWER MASHES

	lb./ton	lb./ton	lb./ton	lb./ton
Wheat flour (or standard) middlings	300	225	225	450
Soybean meal	1350	1050	1050	1000
Corn gluten meal	. . .	250	. . .	. . .
Peanut meal	. . .	. . .	250	. . .
Fish meal	. . .	. . .	. . .	125
Meat scrap	. . .	. . .	. . .	125
Corn dried distillers' solubles	. . .	125	. . .	. . .
Dried whey	. . .	. . .	125	. . .
Steamed bonemeal	225	225	225	150
Limestone	75	75	75	100
Salt (iodized)	50	50	50	50
Manganese sulfate (65% feeding grade)	1.2	1.2	1.2	1.2
Protein, %	33	34	33	35
Calcium, %	4.7	4.7	4.8	5.0
Phosphorus: total, %	2.0	2.0	2.0	1.9
available, %	1.6	1.6	1.6	1.6

TABLE VI. EXAMPLES OF MIXING MASHES, LAYER MASHES

	lb./ton	lb./ton	lb./ton	lb./ton
Wheat flour (or standard) middlings	500	100	125	30
Soybean meal	1,100	1,030	950	1,000
Corn gluten meal	...	...	...	125
Peanut meal	...	250	...	...
Fish meal	...	...	125	125
Meat scrap	250	...	125	...
Corn distillers' dried solubles	...	...	125	...
Dried whey	...	...	...	125
Dehydrated alfalfa meal	250	250	250	250
Riboflavin supplement to supply (mg. riboflavin)	1,000 mg.	1,000 mg.	500 mg.	...
D-activated animal sterols (1500 I.C.U./gm.)	5	5	5	5
or				
Vitamin feeding oil (300 D, 1500 A)	25	25	25	25
Steamed bonemeal	225	250	200	225
Limestone	50	70	50	70
Salt (iodized)	50	50	50	50
Manganese sulfate (65% feeding grade)	1.2	1.2	1.2	1.2
Protein, %	34	34	35	34
Calcium, %	5.6	5.2	5.5	5.2
Phosphorus; total, %	2.4	2.1	2.2	2.1
available, %	2.0	1.8	1.9	1.8
Vitamin A,* I.U./lb.	12,500	12,500	12,500	12,500
Vitamin D, I.C.U./lb.	1,700	1,700	1,700	1,700
Riboflavin, mg./lg.	2.5	2.5	2.5	2.7

* Assuming use of alfalfa meal containing 100,000 International units vitamin A activity and no vitamin feeding oil.

TABLE VII. EXAMPLES OF MIXING MASHES, BREEDER MASHES

	lb./ton	lb./ton	lb./ton	lb./ton
Soybean meal	820	700	700	635
Corn gluten meal	...	125	...	...
Peanut meal	...	...	...	125
Fish meal	200	250	...	...
Fish solubles	...	...	200	...
Meat scrap	200	...	200	350
Corn distillers' dried solubles	125	...	250	200
Dried whey	125	225	100	200
Dried brewers' yeast	...	125	...	...
Dehydrated alfalfa meal	250	250	250	250
Riboflavin supplement to supply (mg. riboflavin)	3,000 mg.	700 mg.	1,000 mg.	1,600 mg.
Vitamin B_{12} supplement to supply (mg. B_{12})	7 mg.	8 mg.	...	12 mg.
D-activated animal sterols (1500 I.C.U./gm.)	5	5	5	5
or				
Vitamin feeding oil (300 D, 1500 A)	25	25	25	25
Steamed bonemeal	150	180	175	140
Limestone	75	50	75	50
Salt (iodized)	50	50	50	50
Manganese sulfate (65% feeding grade)	1.2	1.2	1.2	1.2
Protein, %	34	34	32	33
Calcium, %	5.4	4.7	5.2	5.5
Phosphorus, total, %	2.2	2.1	2.1	2.1
available, %	1.9	1.8	1.8	1.8
Vitamin A,* I.U./lb.	12,500	12,500	12,500	12,500
Vitamin D, I.C.U./lb.	1,700	1,700	1,700	1,700
Riboflavin, mg./lb.	4.5	4.5	4.5	4.5
Vitamin B_{12},† μg./lb.	9	8	8	8

* Assuming use of alfalfa meal containing 100,000 International units vitamin A activity and no vitamin feeding oil.

† From animal proteins and vitamin B_{12} supplement.

TABLE VIII. RELATIVE PRODUCTIVE ENERGY CONTENT OF SOME COMMON GRAINS AND GRAIN PRODUCTS.

	Productive energy* Calories per pound
High energy feedstuffs	
Corn	1145
Milo	1144
Kaffir grain	1076
Wheat	1024
Wheat red dog flour	1020
Medium energy feedstuffs	
Corn and cob meal	920
Heavy oats	817
Barley	811
Rye	810
Wheat flour middlings	720
Low energy feedstuffs	
Buckwheat	700
Light oats	642
Wheat standard middlings	581
Wheat bran	478

* From Texas Agr. Expt. Sta. Bull. 678 (1946) by G. S. Fraps.

TABLE IX. EXAMPLES OF GRAIN-BASED LAYER MASHES (TO BE FED WITH EQUAL GRAIN INTAKE)

	lb./ton	lb./ton	lb./ton	lb./ton	lb./ton
Corn meal	1000	900	800	300	600
Wheat (coarse, ground, or crushed)	200	. . .	. . .	600	. . .
Ground oats	. . .	300	200	300	600
Ground barley	. . .	. . .	200	. . .	. . .
Soybean meal	500	500	470	450	450
Meat scraps	100	100	100	100	100
Alfalfa meal	100	100	100	100	100
Steamed bonemeal	90	90	90	100	100
Limestone	20	20	20	20	20
Salt	20	20	20	20	20
Manganese sulfate	0.5	0.5	0.5	0.5	0.5
D-activated animal sterol	2	2	2	2	2
or					
Vitamin feeding oil (300 D, 1500 A)	10	10	10	10	10
Riboflavin supplement to supply (mg. riboflavin)	300 mg.	300 mg.	300 mg.	300 mg.	300 mg.

INDEX

9 780972 177023

36277285R00362

Made in the USA
Lexington, KY
12 October 2014

Best Practices in Child and Adolescent Behavioral Health Care

Series Editor

Fred R. Volkmar
Yale University
New Haven, CT, USA

Best Practices in Child and Adolescent Behavioral Health Care series explores a range of topics relevant to primary care providers in managing a broad range of child and adolescent mental health problems. These include specific disorders, such as anxiety; relevant topics in related disciplines, including psychological assessment, communication assessment, and disorders; and such general topics as management of psychiatric emergencies. The series aims to provide primary care providers with leading-edge information that enables best-care management of behavioral health issues in children and adolescents. The volumes published in this series provide concise summaries of the current research base (i.e., what is known), best approaches to diagnosis and assessment, and leading evidence-based management and treatment strategies. The series also provides information and analysis that primary care providers need to understand how to interpret and implement best treatment practices and enable them to interpret and implement recommendations from specialists for children and effectively monitor interventions.

More information about this series at http://www.springer.com/series/15955

Giacomo Vivanti
Kristen Bottema-Beutel
Lauren Turner-Brown
Editors

Clinical Guide to Early Interventions for Children with Autism

Springer

Editors
Giacomo Vivanti
AJ Drexel Autism Institute
Drexel University
Philadelphia, PA, USA

Kristen Bottema-Beutel
Lynch School of Education
and Human Development
Boston College
Chestnut Hill, MA, USA

Lauren Turner-Brown
UNC TEACCH Autism Program
The University of North Carolina School
of Medicine
Chapel Hill, NC, USA

ISSN 2523-7128 ISSN 2523-7136 (electronic)
Best Practices in Child and Adolescent Behavioral Health Care
ISBN 978-3-030-41159-6 ISBN 978-3-030-41160-2 (eBook)
https://doi.org/10.1007/978-3-030-41160-2

This Springer imprint is published by the registered company Springer Nature Switzerland AG
The registered company address is: Gewerbestrasse 11, 6330 Cham, Switzerland

Series Editor Preface

It is my great pleasure to write an introduction to this much needed book. Nearly 20 years ago, it was my privilege to serve as one of the authors of the ground breaking report from the National Research Council on *Educating Children with Autism* (National Research Council, 2001). At that time, the field was in its infancy with about ten programs around the United States that each had at least one published study on the efficacy of their intervention program for young children with autism. Of course, at the time, the "young child" with autism was usually 4 years of age, sometimes three, and rarely two or under. That situation has, fortunately, now changed with much greater interest being focused on infant siblings and at-risk populations leading to much earlier identification of cases and risk for autism. Greater urgency has also arisen since it now appears that, with early intervention, some students are improving substantially and indeed, many now go to college (Magiati & Howlin, 2019). The body of evidence-based research on treatment has also increased substantially (Odom, Morin, Savage, & Tomaszewski, 2019; Reichow & Barton, 2014). Unfortunately, this substantial body of work has often not been translated into usable form for health care providers and early educators. This volume is intended to address just this need.

The first chapter provides a very helpful overview of changes over time in our conception of autism and its treatment. The second chapter helps us understand the quality of evidence as we evaluate treatments. The third reviews the nature of evidence-based treatments. The fourth chapter addresses understanding the basic social communication problems in autism and is followed by a chapter review the restricted repetitive behaviors that are also ubiquitous to the autism spectrum. The next set of chapters address the major treatment models: ABA, naturalistic methods, and the pioneering Division TEACCH program. The final chapters focus on helping to understand the problem of matching children to treatment programs (a frequent problem in the country as schools often will have one program that may not necessarily be right for a given child). The final two chapters of the book address issues of early intervention and social policy—a growing concern around the world as more awareness of autism and the importance of instituting effective treatments has grown so dramatically.

The authors and their chapters truly represent the entire range of scientifically based disciplines involved in research and clinical practice in early intervention in autism. They include clinical psychologists, behavior analysts, and special educators—all of whom bring complementary perspective to an area that has sadly often been divided into factions that may have little interaction with each other. In all, this is a profoundly helpful and much needed book. It is a great pleasure for me to introduce it.

Irving B. Harris Professor of Child Psychiatry
Pediatrics and Psychology
Yale University School of Medicine
New Haven, CT, USA

Fred R. Volkmar

References

Magiati, I., & Howlin, P. (2019). Adult life for people with autism spectrum disorders. In F. R. Volkmar (Ed.), *Autism and pervasve developmental disorders* (pp. 220–248). Cambridge, UK: Cambridge University Press.

National Research Council. (2001). *Educating young children with autism*. Washington, DC: National Academy Press.

Odom, S. L., Morin, K., Savage, M., & Tomaszewski, B. (2019). Behavioral and educational interventions. In F. Volkmar (Ed.), *Autism and the pervasive developmental disorders* (3rd ed., pp. 176–190). Cambridge: Cambridge University Press.

Reichow, B., & Barton, E. E. (2014). Evidence-based psychosocial interventions for individuals with autism spectrum disorders. In *Handbook of autism and pervasive developmental disorders, Volume 2: Assessment, interventions, and policy* (4th ed., pp. 969–992). Hoboken, NJ: Wiley.

Acknowledgments

The authors would like to express their thanks to the children and families; they had the privilege to work within research studies and clinical practice.

Giacomo Vivanti would like to acknowledge the contribution of Jessica Day-Watkins and Shana Attar in discussing and formulating early ideas for Chaps. 5 and 8, respectively.

Lauren Turner-Brown would like to acknowledge Samantha Scott for contributing photo examples presented in Chapter 7.

Contents

Contributors

Kristen Bottema-Beutel Lynch School of Education and Human Development, Boston College, Chestnut Hill, MA, USA

Shannon Crowley Lynch School of Education and Human Development, Boston College, Chestnut Hill, MA, USA

Josephine Cuda Lynch School of Education and Human Development, Boston College, Chestnut Hill, MA, USA

MaryKate Frisch UNC TEACCH Autism Program, The University of North Carolina School of Medicine, Chapel Hill, NC, USA

Kara Hume School of Education, The University of North Carolina at Chapel Hill, Chapel Hill, NC, USA

So Yoon Kim Lynch School of Education and Human Development, Boston College, Chestnut Hill, MA, USA

Pamela Paragas AJ Drexel Autism Institute, Drexel University, Philadelphia, PA, USA

Melanie Pellecchia Department of Psychiatry, Perelman School of Medicine, University of Pennsylvania, Philadelphia, PA, USA

Rachel Sandercock The University of North Carolina at Chapel Hill, Chapel Hill, NC, USA

Lauren Turner-Brown UNC TEACCH Autism Program, The University of North Carolina School of Medicine, Chapel Hill, NC, USA

Giacomo Vivanti AJ Drexel Autism Institute, Drexel University, Philadelphia, PA, USA

Hongxuan Nicole Zhong AJ Drexel Autism Institute, Drexel University, Philadelphia, PA, USA

About the Editors

Giacomo Vivanti, Ph.D. is an Associate Professor at the AJ Drexel Autism Institute, Drexel University, Philadelphia, PA, USA, and an Honorary Research Fellow at the Olga Tennison Autism Research Centre at La Trobe University, Melbourne, Australia. His research and clinical work focus on early learning and intervention for children with Autism. Dr. Vivanti is an Associate Editor of the *Journal of Autism and Developmental Disorders* and a member of the Editorial Board of the *Journal of Early Intervention*. He is the author of over 50 peer-reviewed scientific articles on autism.

Kristen Bottema-Beutel, Ph.D. is an Associate Professor in the Lynch School of Education and Human Development (LSEHD) at Boston College, Chestnut Hill, MA, USA. Her research focuses on social and language development, and social interaction dynamics in autistic people across the life span. Dr. Bottema-Beutel is the director of the specialization in autism spectrum disorder at LSEHD, a program that prepares future special educators to support autistic students. She has written or co-written more than 30 peer-reviewed articles relevant to autism and other special education topics.

Lauren Turner Brown, Ph.D. served as the Assistant Director of the UNC TEACCH Autism Program for 5 years and Assistant Professor in the Department of Psychiatry at the University of North Carolina at Chapel Hill. She conducted research on early identification and intervention for children with autism spectrum disorder and published over 30 peer-reviewed articles on the topic of ASD. Dr. Turner-Brown is currently in private practice in Chapel Hill, NC, and an Adjunct Assistant Professor at UNC.

Chapter 1
Autism and Autism Treatment: Evolution of Concepts and Practices from Kanner to Contemporary Approaches

Giacomo Vivanti

Autism spectrum disorder (ASD) is a developmental disorder that requires lifelong support. As is often the case for conditions of uncertain etiology, many intervention approaches for ASD exist, only a minority of which have been empirically validated. Evidence-supported early interventions can result in substantial improvements in language, cognitive, social, and adaptive functioning, holding the potential to promote positive long-term outcomes, mitigate lifespan disability, reduce societal costs, and improve personal well-being and productivity of individuals with ASD and their families.

However, advising families in search for the best intervention to help their young children with ASD is challenging, due to the proliferation of intervention options and the heterogeneity of intervention needs within the ASD population. Additional elements of complexity include the striking variability in treatment response, with even the most established interventions producing different levels of success across individuals and contexts, as well as challenges with access to services and the financial impacts on families (Nahmias et al., 2019; Vivanti et al., 2014). Finally, scientific and philosophical divergences across the scientific community, advocacy groups, and practitioners further contribute to a difficult terrain for navigating intervention options. The aim of this book is to provide practical information to navigate this chaotic landscape, starting with an analysis of how knowledge and concepts about ASD and ASD treatment have evolved over the past decades.

G. Vivanti, PhD (✉)
AJ Drexel Autism Institute, Drexel University, Philadelphia, PA, USA
e-mail: gv89@drexel.edu

G. Vivanti et al. (eds.), *Clinical Guide to Early Interventions for Children with Autism*, Best Practices in Child and Adolescent Behavioral Health Care,
https://doi.org/10.1007/978-3-030-41160-2_1

From Kanner to the DSM-5: Evolution of the Diagnostic Concept of Autism and Current Diagnostic Issues

The diagnostic concept of autism was originally formulated in 1943 by an Austrian psychiatrist of Ukrainian origin, Leo Kanner. In his seminal report (1943), Kanner described 11 children affected by what he defined as "autistic disturbances of affective contact," a syndrome characterized by diminished or absent interest in other people, reduced social communication, and a striking "insistence on sameness." Although clinical reports of children with similar characteristics were published before Kanner's report (e.g., De Sanctis, 1906; Klein, 1930/1975; Ssucharewa, 1926), or at around the same time (most notably by Hans Asperger; 1944), Kanner's conceptualization of autism as a distinct clinical syndrome characterized by early onset social communication abnormalities and behavioral rigidity has proven the most influential and enduring.

The validity of autism as a distinct diagnostic entity separate from schizophrenia, language disorders, or general intellectual disability has been supported by subsequent research (Volkmar & McPartland, 2014). Five decades after Kanner's original description, autism was described in a report of the National Institute of Health Autism Working Group as "one of the most reliable diagnoses in psychiatric or developmental research" (Bristol et al., 1996). Following Kanner's first report, the diagnostic definitions of autism in subsequent decades have continued to include the notions of early emerging impairments in social communication (with a discrepancy between social and nonsocial abilities and deficits encompassing both verbal and nonverbal communication) as well as insistence on sameness/resistance to change. Despite this continuity, numerous shifts in the conceptualization and operationalization of autism have occurred, reflecting cultural changes as well as research advances.

In the decades after Kanner's report, the concept of autism was considered by most scholars to be overlapping with childhood psychosis or schizophrenia, with the terms "psychotic" and "autistic" being used interchangeably in research and practice throughout the 1950s, 1960s, and 1970s. Following research by Rutter (1972) and others documenting critical differences between autism and schizophrenia, autism was first included as a separate diagnostic category in the third edition of the *Diagnostic and Statistical Manual of Mental Disorders* in 1980, under the definition of "infantile autism" (DSM-III, APA, 1980). This was later changed to "autistic disorder" in 1987 in the revised edition (DSM-III-TR, APA, 1987). Asperger's disorder, a related diagnostic category described as being characterized by higher intellectual functioning and better language abilities compared to autistic disorder, was added in the fourth edition of the *DSM* (DSM-IV, APA, 1994) as part of five mutually exclusive diagnostic subcategories under the umbrella diagnosis of "pervasive developmental disorders" (APA, 1994). This category also included Rett syndrome, childhood disintegrative disorder, and pervasive developmental disorder—not otherwise specified.

In 2013, the DSM-5 grouped the diagnostic criteria for autism in two clusters that are reminiscent of Kanner's original description: "social communication deficits" and "fixated interests and repetitive behaviors." Additionally, the different subtypes of autism defined by mutually exclusive subcategories used in the previous DSM editions were replaced by a single diagnostic label, "autism spectrum disorder" (ASD). This conceptualization reflects the homogeneity in the core impairments, as well as the continuum of variability in the presentation of the clinical features (i.e., the notion of autism as a "spectrum," originally introduced by Wing and Gould in 1979). Additionally, the DSM-5 includes designations for the level of severity for each symptom cluster (on a 3-point scale ranging from "requiring support" to "requiring very substantial support") as well as relevant clinical "specifiers," including language and cognitive ability levels.

The terms autism and autism spectrum disorder (ASD) are now used interchangeably. The term "Asperger," while no longer used clinically, continues to be present in the mainstream vocabulary, most frequently as a cultural identity concept (e.g., "Asperger culture" or "Aspie culture"; Giles et al., 2014). The terms "high functioning" and "low functioning" autism are not formal diagnostic concepts, but are colloquially used in clinical practice to describe individuals with ASD with less severe versus more severe symptomatology and/or cognitive impairment. Importantly, however, both the DSM-5 and the autistic community suggest that "low support needs" and "high support needs" are more accurate and less stigmatizing, as functioning is often proportional to the amount of support provided.

As no biological marker for ASD has been validated to date, ASD diagnosis is based on the ascertainment of the behavioral manifestations listed in the DSM-5, or other formal classification systems such as the International Classification of Diseases (World Health Organization, 1993), which is largely overlapping with the DSM definition. When diagnostic referral occurs in childhood, this is achieved through a combination of direct observation and parent reports focused on the child's developmental history, often supported by standardized protocols such as the Autism Diagnostic Observation Schedule (ADOS; Lord et al., 2012) and the Autism Diagnostic Interview (ADI-R; Le Couteur, Lord, & Rutter, 2003).

In most cases, a diagnosis of ASD can be made at 18–24 months, although some children might not be fully symptomatic until 36 month and, more rarely, until school age (Lord et al., 2018; Ozonoff et al., 2018). Once a diagnosis is made, it is generally stable, (Ozonoff et al., 2015; Talbott & Rogers, 2016; Zwaigenbaum et al., 2015). However, cases of children who lose their ASD diagnosis at school age have been reported, although the frequency and nature of this phenomenon remain unclear (Fein et al., 2013; Moulton et al., 2016).

Epidemiology

ASD was once considered a rare disorder, with estimates in the 1960s suggesting 4–5 cases in 10,000. Currently, however, ASD is considered to occur in about 1:59 cases (Baio et al., 2018). While the steady rise in the prevalence of ASD in the last decades has been described by some as an "autism epidemic," it is still debated whether the changes in prevalence rates reflect a true increase in ASD cases. Factors such as the progressive broadening of the diagnostic criteria, improvements in diagnostic procedures, and increased awareness as well as the changes in policies for access to services might have contributed to the apparent "epidemic."

The sex ratio (male:female) is 4.3:1, but there is suggestion that females are more likely to remain undiagnosed (Bargiela et al., 2016; Giarelli et al., 2010). In the United States, there is evidence of ethnic and racial disparities in the identification of ASD (Durkin et al., 2017; Mandell et al., 2009). Little is known about other parts of the world in this respect.

Clinical Characteristics

Autism is a developmental disorder originating in infancy. Behavioral manifestations of ASD are affected by and affect the developmental level of the individual (verbal ability and mental age), and the way symptoms manifest themselves at different times is also influenced by the child's chronological age, history of interaction with the environment (including intervention history), and the presence of co-occurring conditions.

Early clinical presentations of ASD as well as changes in the symptomatology over the course of the lifespan are reviewed below.

Social Communication and Social Interaction

Impaired social communication and social interaction are a defining feature of ASD (Carter et al., 2005; see Chap. 3). While early abnormalities in the social domain have been documented as early as the first 6 months of life (Jones & Klin, 2013; Chawarska et al., 2013), in most cases social symptoms become fully manifest during the second year, with research showing that by 18 months of age children with ASD show reduced eye contact (Chawarska et al., 2014); reduced responsivity to human voices, including to their name being called (Miller et al., 2017); reduced interest in observing social scenes (Chawarska et al., 2013); and reduced frequency of imitation (Vivanti & Hamilton, 2014) as well as impairments in joint attention (i.e., the ability to shift attention between a referent and a social partner; Adamson, 1995; Scaife & Bruner, 1975). Joint attention behaviors that are reduced or absent in ASD include using gestures and eye contact to direct another person's attention to an object or event (e.g., looking at the caregiver and pointing to a butterfly), as well as using others' gaze and head turns to identify the target of their attention (e.g., looking at a flower that the caregiver is pointing to). These behaviors, referred to as initiation and response to joint attention, respectively, are linked to subsequent communicative, social–emotional, and cognitive development in typical and atypical development (Bottema-Beutel, 2016; Mundy, 2016). Children with ASD show deficits in both initiation and response to joint attention (Sigman, 1998; Jones et al., 2014), with more pronounced impairments in the initiation component (Mundy, 2011). Recent research has documented that 10-month-old infants later diagnosed with ASD show fewer episodes of initiation of joint attention compared to their peers (Nystrom et al., 2019).

Importantly, many children with ASD show behaviors that are consistent with a classification of "secure attachment" with their caregivers, such as responding differently to caregivers as compared to strangers (Kasari et al., 1993; Sigman & Ungerer, 1984), seeking and maintaining proximity with caregivers after separation (Sigman & Mundy, 1989), engaging in more proximity-seeking behaviors toward their caregiver, and engaging in fewer explorative behaviors in the presence of a stranger (Dissanayake & Crossley, 1996). The presence of these social and affective manifestations toward caregivers may contribute to lower than expected referrals for evaluations by physicians even after a child screens as being at risk for ASD (Pierce et al., 2011). However, proximity-seeking behaviors with caregivers in children with ASD may be less frequent, less sustained, or less conducive to rich social exchanges (Vivanti & Nuske, 2017). Young children with ASD also show diminished engagement in social play routines such as peekaboo (Bolton et al., 2012), as well as reduced pretend and imaginative play (e.g., Barbaro & Dissanayake, 2013).

Additional features include reduced interest in and engagement with peers (McGee et al., 1997), reduced responsivity to others' emotions (Hutman et al., 2010), difficulties interpreting other people's behavior (such as incorrectly predicting behavior based on their own knowledge, rather than others' knowledge; Baron-Cohen, 1995; Senju, 2012), and fewer expressions of pleasure during social interactions (Wan et al., 2013). In many cases, children with ASD do initiate and respond to social contact but their interactions are idiosyncratic or "on their terms" (e.g., approaching unknown people to do "high five" multiple times; Rapin, 2002).

Spoken language is often delayed—and in approximately 25–30% of cases never develops (Tager-Flusberg & Kasari, 2013). While delayed or absent verbal communication does not discriminate ASD from other conditions, a distinctive feature of children with ASD is a lack of attempt to compensate speech deficits with gestures or other forms of nonverbal communication. Abnormal speech patterns, odd words or phrases, echolalia, and unusual tone or pitch in vocalizations or words are other distinctive characteristics of early language in ASD and may persist throughout the lifespan (Kim et al., 2014). Many children with ASD show an increase in their use of communicative speech from childhood to adolescence and adulthood, although the social use and social understanding of communication (pragmatics) is likely to remain impaired. For example, children with ASD might fail to understand others' communication when the communicative intent differs from the literal meaning of a sentence (e.g., irony and sarcasm; Happé, 1994).

Similarly, social and communicative deficits may manifest differently at different developmental stages and in different contexts. At school age, as the child is exposed to increasingly complex social demands, deficits in developing, maintaining, and understanding relationships with peers (such as friendship) become more relevant. Many individuals with ASD learn coping strategies to adapt to their social environment, but social symptoms typically continue to persist throughout the lifespan. For example, in adolescence and adulthood, social interactions may increase in frequency but retain a qualitative impairment (stilted, exaggerated, or "socially awkward" behavior). For many individuals with ASD interest in social contact increases during adolescence and adulthood, including the desire to have friends and romantic relationships, and difficulties with accomplishing these social goals might cause frustration and affect well-being (Sperry & Mesibov, 2005). Experiencing the social world as indecipherable, frustrating, or rejecting can lead individuals with ASD to "give up" on social interactions, which leads to fewer opportunities for developing social skills, further limiting social opportunities and exacerbating social difficulties. See Chap. 3 for an in-depth overview of social communication development and intervention in ASD.

Restricted, Repetitive Patterns of Behavior, Interests, or Activities

Repetitive and restricted behaviors (RRBs) are a heterogeneous group of symptoms characterized by rigidity and resistance to change. These symptoms include behaviors characterized by stereotyped or repetitive movements (such as hand-flapping and repetitive use of objects) or repetitive speech (echolalia and idiosyncratic phrases) and restricted, fixated interests that are unusual in their intensity or focus (such as strong attachments to a specific object, circumscribed or perseverative interests, and excessive focus on one conversation topic). Other features of ASD that fall within this domain are the "insistence on sameness" originally described by Kanner (such as the desire to watch the same episode of a TV show repeatedly or to eat the same food every day) and the rigid adherence to routines or rituals (e.g., singing the song "five little monkeys" while lining up five objects every morning at childcare). Seeking of specific sensations (such as deep pressure), unusual sensory interests (such as peering at or smelling objects), and hyper- or hyporeactivity to sensory inputs (e.g., experiencing everyday sounds as being excessively loud or imperceptible) are also classified as RRBs.

RRBs appear to emerge during infancy and persist across the lifespan, although they might manifest differently at different ages, and their prevalence and severity are extremely variable in the ASD population (Ozonoff et al., 2008; Uljarević et al., 2017). Unlike social symptoms, RRBs are not a distinctive feature of ASD, as some types of repetitive behaviors are observed in intellectual disabilities, psychiatric disorders, neurological conditions, and other clinical conditions with sensory deficits, as well as in typically developing toddlers (Evans et al., 1997). However, individuals with ASD appear to engage in RRBs more frequently compared to those with other conditions, and their RRBs are expressed across a wider range of behaviors (Leekam, Prior, & Uljarevic, 2011).

Several criteria have been proposed to classify RRBs into specific subtypes, such the distinction between lower order (which include finger flicking, body rocking, and hand flapping) and higher order RRBs (including circumscribed interests and fascinations/preoccupations for particular topics, such as trains, wasps, or the French Revolution; Bodfish, 2007) as well as the distinction between repetitive sensory-motor (such as motor body mannerisms, repetitive use of objects, and unusual sensory interests), and "insistence on sameness" behaviors (including rituals and resistance to change; Richler et al., 2007; Prior & Macmillan, 1973). Rather than being mutually exclusive, the proposed subtypes appear to be characterized by permeable boundaries, with cognitive and language functioning influencing the manifestations of different RRBs (Leekam et al., 2011). For example, repetitive use of objects (e.g., spinning the wheels of a toy car) or motor stereotypies such as finger flicking or hand flapping are more likely to occur in children with ASD with lower versus higher cognitive functioning, whereas circumscribed interests are more prevalent in individuals with normative IQ (Bishop, Richler, & Lord, 2006). There is emerging evidence that repetitive behaviors might decrease in frequency and severity with age, independently of the cognitive level, with the exception of stereotyped movements that tend to be more persistent in individuals with co-occurring autism and intellectual disability (Esbensen, Seltzer, Lam, & Bodfish, 2009). See Chap. 4 for a detailed review on the nature and treatment of RRBs in ASD.

Gender Differences in Clinical Presentation

Research on gender differences in ASD phenotypes has mixed evidence, partly because fewer female participants have been involved in research studies compared to males. Evidence from large twin studies suggests that males may require greater familial etiologic load to manifest the ASD phenotype (Robinson et al., 2013). Consistent with this notion, a more severe presentation has been reported in females compared to males (Christensen et al., 2016; Lord & Schopler, 1985) and the sex ratio has been reported to be <2:1 in more severely impaired cases (Loomes et al., 2017). There is some evidence of increased social interest and approach in females versus males as well as female superiority in executive function and visuospatial processing tasks (Bölte et al., 2011; Dean, Harwood & Kasari, 2017; Harrop et al., 2018; Koyama et al., 2009)—however, counterevidence exists (see Ferri, Abel, & Brodkin, 2018, for a recent review). It is possible that gender differences in behaviors related to ASD diagnosis (e.g., social approach) and camouflage of autistic symptoms (i.e., imitation of neurotypical peers to mask ASD symptoms) may result in under- or misdiagnosing among females on the milder end of the spectrum (Mandy et al., 2012), although more research is needed to corroborate this notion.

Co-Occurring Conditions

Autism frequently co-occurs with other developmental, psychiatric, or medical conditions, which might exacerbate the symptoms, aggravate impairment, and complicate diagnosis and treatment. Intellectual disability, which was once thought to be present in most individuals with ASD, is now estimated to occur in 30–50% of children diagnosed with ASD (Charman et al., 2011; Christensen et al., 2018; Postorino et al., 2016; Rydzewska et al., 2018). This change might reflect advances in early detection and improved access to early intervention, as well as increased awareness and diagnostic expertise improving the identification of ASD symptoms in individuals without intellectual disability. While cognitive functioning and ASD symptomatology are conceptually distinct constructs, recent research suggests that children with more severe ASD symptoms are more likely to have co-occurring cognitive impairments (Gotham, Pickles, & Lord, 2012; Vivanti et al., 2013), potentially reflecting a link between barriers to social learning posed by severe social/communicative impairments and developmental delays (Vivanti, Dawson, & Rogers, 2017).

The extreme heterogeneity in intellectual functioning within the ASD population, ranging from severe intellectual disability to above average IQ, results in different challenges and priorities with regards to intervention. Additionally, such variation can be a source of confusion for families, especially those with more cognitively impaired children, who might fail to see the connection between the needs of their children and those expressed by cognitively able individuals with ASD (e.g., self-advocates with ASD who emphasize intelligence as a key feature of ASD and challenge the utility of interventions focused on "normalizing" behavior; Cascio, 2012).

Additionally, ASD co-occurs with several psychiatric disorders (including anxiety, obsessive-compulsive disorder, depression, attention-deficit hyperactivity disorder [ADHD], and oppositional-defiant disorder) more frequently compared to rates in the general population (Rydzewska et al., 2018; Simonoff et al., 2013). The high frequency of mental health difficulties in ASD might reflect (1) shared pathophysiology (i.e., what causes ASD also causes or increases the risk for the comorbid condition); (2) the downstream consequence of growing up with ASD (e.g., coping with social demands that exceed processing capacity, peer rejection, and other negative life experiences stemming from the stigma associated with ASD symptoms); (3) shared symptom domains or overlapping diagnostic criteria; or (4) an interplay between these different factors (Postorino et al., 2017; Uljarevic et al., 2016). Additionally, ASD co-occurs at a higher rate than the typical population with tics and Tourette Syndrome (Canitano & Vivanti, 2007; Kalyva et al., 2016), sleeping disturbances (Souders et al., 2017), eating disorders and restricted and rigid food choices (Sharp et al., 2013), gastrointestinal issues (Holingue et al., 2018), elimination problems (Gorrindo et al., 2012), and most notably, epilepsy, which might be present in up to 25% of the ASD population and is more frequently present in females and more cognitively impaired individuals (Jeste & Tuchman, 2015; Volkmar & Wiesner, 2017).

Etiology

Genetic factors play a critical role in the etiology of ASD, with recent research indicating that approximately 80% of ASD risk is heritable (Bai et al., 2019; Tick, Bolton et al., 2016). Twin and family studies suggest that siblings of children with ASD have a 20–50-fold increased risk of having ASD compared to the general population, and the risk is increased for those with more than one sibling with ASD, while the concordance rate in identical twins is up to 90% (Colvert, Tick et al., 2015; Rutter, 2000). Research has pointed to a large number of common and rare genetic variants associated with ASD risk, but none of them accounts for more than a minority of cases, suggesting that the risk of developing ASD might be predominantly related to the additive contributions from common and rare variants that, individually, are not sufficient to cause the condition (Arnett, Trinh, & Bernier, 2019; Ramaswami & Geschwind, 2018; Weiner et al., 2017).

While this body of research indicates that ASD is one of the most heritable neurodevelopmental conditions, the lack of complete concordance in monozygotic twins indicates that nongenetic factors also contribute to ASD. Environmental factors that have been associated with increased risk for ASD include advanced maternal age (≥40 years) and paternal age (≥50 years; Lyall et al., 2017) as well as preterm birth (Lampi et al., 2012). Additionally, there is some indication that short interpregnancy intervals (<24 months; Zerbo et al., 2015) and maternal hospitalization during pregnancy (Lyall et al., 2017) might be associated with the risk for ASD, although more research is needed to corroborate these initial findings.

The hypotheses that ASD could be caused by vaccines or poor parenting have been repeatedly tested and unequivocally disconfirmed (Capps, Sigman, & Mundy, 1994; Lord et al., 2018; Parker, Schwartz, Todd, & Pickering, 2004; Ventola et al., 2017).

Neurocognitive Models of ASD

While the nature of the neurocognitive processes underlying the ASD phenotype remains unclear, several theoretical models have been proposed. Historically, these have included (a) the notion that ASD symptoms reflect difficulties in the ability to attribute mental states to others, or "theory of mind" (Baron-Cohen, Leslie, & Frith, 1985), (b) the "weak central coherence" account, i.e., a detail-focused processing style, whereby information is processed in terms of constituent parts, rather than global meanings (Frith & Happé, 1994), and (c) deficits in executive functioning which causes difficulties in the flexible organization of behavior across social and nonsocial domains (Ozonoff, 1997). While each of these accounts have contributed critical insight on several phenomena related to ASD, none of them is universally considered to provide a satisfactory account for constellation of features observed in ASD (Frith, 2012).

More recently, theoretical models have been steering away from "single deficit" explanations to focus on the developmental pathways that lead from early risk factors to specific features of ASD (Vivanti, Yerys & Salomone, 2019). Recent accounts informed by longitudinal research on infants at risk for ASD include the notion that social symptoms reflect the downstream consequence of early disruptions in the reflexive, orienting mechanisms that drive newborns' attention toward social stimuli (Di Giorgio et al., 2016), or, alternatively, disruptions in the developmental transition from reflexive orienting to volitional attentional engagement with the social world that occurs during the first 6 months of life (Klin et al., 2015; Shultz et al., 2018). Diminished attentional engagement with social stimuli has been proposed to originate either from domain-specific abnormalities in social–cognitive processing (whereby social stimuli are not experienced as meaningful or interpretable; Leekam, 2016), diminished social motivation (whereby social stimuli are not experienced as rewarding; Chevallier et al., 2012; Mundy, 1995), or widespread nonspecific abnormalities that disrupt social processing because of the inherent complexity and unpredictability of social stimuli compared to nonsocial aspects of the environment (Minshew & Goldstein, 1998; Johnson, 2017). Research does not provide unequivocal support to any of these explanations, with some findings pointing to widespread network abnormalities in infants with ASD, and other research pointing to specific abnormalities within the social brain network, including atypical brain activity in response to social versus nonsocial stimuli and rewards (Pelphrey et al., 2014).

While the causal pathways in ASD remain unclear, these converging lines of inquiry suggest that an altered engagement with social stimuli during early sensitive periods might affect neural specialization and behavioral expertise in the social domain, thus exacerbating initial abnormalities in an iterative fashion (i.e., as children with ASD are less engaged with the social world due to initial biological constraints, they have fewer opportunities to learn and practice social and communication skills, thus failing to build a behavioral repertoire from social experience). A corollary of this developmental perspective is that targeted intervention during early sensitive periods has the potential to mitigate or, according to some scholars, prevent this escalating deviance from typical social development (Dawson, 2008; Vivanti, Dawson, & Rogers, 2017). This topic will be the focus of the remainder of the chapter and of this manual.

Treatment for Autism Spectrum Disorder: Evolution of Concepts and Principles

No pharmacological treatment has been shown to address the core symptoms of ASD, and currently recommended approaches to early intervention for ASD rely on various applications of behavioral, developmental, and special education principles (Lord et al., 2018; Volkmar et al., 2014). The historical evolution of early intervention for ASD is marked by the influence of the different theoretical frameworks that have been prominent within disciplines concerned with ASD at different stages.

Influences from Psychodynamic Theory

The earliest approaches to ASD intervention, in the 1950s and 1960s, were predominantly informed by psychodynamic theory, and in particular by the notions that mother–child dynamics play a critical role in psychopathology (Freud, 1911), and that autistic symptoms are the consequence of inadequate parenting (Bettelheim, 1967; Green & Schecter, 1957; Kanner & Eisenberg, 1956; but see Anna Freud, 1969/2015 for a dissenting voice within the psychoanalytic community). Interventions derived from this framework included psychodynamic psychotherapy to the child and the child's mother, as well as "parentectomy," which involved the separation of children from their supposedly unloving families and their placement in psychiatric residential institutions. The psychodynamic approach to ASD was discredited in the following decades both because of unsatisfactory scientific support and ethical considerations, although various elaborations of the same theoretical framework continued to be perpetuated throughout the 1990s (e.g., Tustin, 1991) and continue to be influential in many countries (Severson, Aune, Jodlowski & Osteen 2008).

Influences from Applied Behavior Analysis

In the mid-1960s, applied behavior analysis (ABA; Baer, Wolf, & Risley, 1968) became a major influence on ASD intervention as Ferster (1964) and Lovaas (1968) and other ABA pioneers introduced the use of practices based on operant conditioning (Skinner, 1953) in the field of ASD. A key concept introduced by the ABA work is the notion that the behavior of children with ASD obeys the same laws that shape learning in typical development (Ferster & DeMyer, 1961; Lovaas & Smith, 1989; Mayville & Mulick, 2011), whereby behaviors followed by a positive consequence (reinforcement) strengthen and are more likely to be produced when the stimulus that triggered the behavior (antecedent) is presented, while those followed by a negative consequence result in an opposite effect. A critical corollary of this notion is that specific behaviors can be encouraged or discouraged through a careful manipulation of antecedents and consequences. Additional influential elements introduced by ABA include the emphasis on unambiguous operational definitions of intervention goals and targets (i.e., promoting the acquisition of clearly defined desirable behaviors and discouraging clearly defined maladaptive behaviors), and the use of empirical data as the platform for decision making and evaluation of outcomes. Early applications of these principles included procedures that have largely been abandoned because of ethical and scientific considerations, such as the use of electric shocks to induce behavior modifications as described by Lovaas and colleagues (1965), which was later defined by Lovaas as "a mistake based on erroneous beliefs" (Lovaas, 1989). Nevertheless, the shift in focus from the psychoanalytic emphasis on unobservable unconscious dimensions to the data-driven observation and manipulation of well-defined behaviors provided the infrastructure for most contemporary approaches to ASD interventions, becoming the foundation for the highly structured approaches known as discrete trial teaching (Lovaas, 1981), as well as subsequent applications of ABA (Schreibman et al., 2015), including the early intervention approach known as early intensive behavioral intervention (EIBI; see Chap. 5).

Influences from Developmental Psychology

The application of concepts from developmental psychology in the field of ASD became another major influence in ASD early intervention practices starting in the 1980s. A concept introduced by developmental literature that became relevant to ASD intervention is constructivism (Bruner, 1978; Montessori, 1912; Piaget, 1929; Vygotsky, 1930–1934/1978), i.e., the notion that skill acquisition during early development is built on the child's active, self-directed engagement with a stimulating physical and social environment, with knowledge gained at specific developmental stages supporting the transition to more advanced developmental stages which enable the acquisition of complex skills. The adult's role in this context is to facilitate skill acquisition through scaffolding (Bruner, 1978), i.e., supporting the engagement of the child in joint routines that build upon the child's initiative and current knowledge to generate opportunities to gain more advanced knowledge (a concept analogous to the construct of 'zone of proximal development', formulated by Vygotsky in the 1930s; Vygotsky, 1930–1934/1978). For example, during shared storybook reading routines, adults scaffold the child's acquisition of new knowledge by establishing a joint focus (the illustrations in the book), highlighting the relationship between the words, images, and emotions associated with the events in the story, eliciting children's verbal and nonverbal responses (i.e., emotional expressions, gestures, words) through pauses and questions, and providing feedback, such as asking for clarification or recasting the child's utterances (Ninio & Bruner, 1978). Pivotal skills in the domains of communication, joint attention, and imitation that are learned during joint activities provide the foundation for engagement in more complex social exchanges, which, in turn, enable the acquisition of further knowledge. A critical corollary of this framework is that advances in some pivotal or prerequisite skills will facilitate the acquisition of more advanced skills.

These concepts from developmental literature became increasingly influential in ASD intervention as research started to show that developmental sequences of skill acquisition in children with ASD appear to follow the same path observed in those with typical development. For example, development of verbal language is predicted by joint attention skills both in typical children and in those with ASD, and improvements in joint attention result in language improvements (Bottema-Beutel, 2016; Kasari, Sigman, Mundy, & Yirmiya, 1990; Sigman et al., 1999; Whalen, Schreibman, & Ingersoll, 2006). Developmental concepts that continue to be prominent in ASD early intervention include the use of "developmentally appropriate" treatment targets and procedures (e.g., teaching developmental prerequisite to facilitate acquisition of more complex skills), the involvement of families and daily routines as a privileged context for learning, and the focus on scaffolding over didactic teaching to promote skill acquisition in early development (Rogers, 1999; Schreibman et al., 2015).

Influences from Neuroscience

Starting from the late 1990s, ASD intervention has been influenced by social neuroscience research in typical development and ASD—i.e., the study of how social information and social experiences shape and are shaped by brain development (Lieberman, 2007). A notion from this field that is of prominent relevance in ASD early intervention is that the neural infrastructure of human sociability relies on an "experience-expectant" process. This means that "hardwired" brain mechanisms bias children to actively seek out opportunities for social engagement during early development. These early social experiences, in turn, provide the input needed for the brain to become specialized in social information processing, which then enables participation in and learning from more sophisticated social interactions (Brownell, 2013; Sullivan, Stone, & Dawson, 2014).

While research in this area is in its infancy, several interconnected brain areas and circuitries involved in this iterative process have been identified. This includes social–cognitive structures responsible for the quick processing of social–emotional cues such as gaze direction and emotional expressions (Frith & Frith, 2010), the social reward system, which underpins the experience of pleasure associated with social interaction (Dolen, Darvishzadeh, Huang, & Malenka, 2013), and the mirror neuron system (Rizzolatti & Sinigaglia, 2008). The mirror neuron system consists of a set of brain regions that activate during action execution as well as during the observation of the same action. This mechanism is thought to enable the observer to understand others' actions and emotions as if she/he would be doing a similar action or experiencing the same emotion, thus facilitating the processing of shared experiences. While the translation of neuroscientific findings into treatment practices is in the very early stages, the influence of social neuroscience perspectives on intervention includes the emphasis on engaging the child in typical social routines during early critical periods of brain plasticity, increasing the reward value of social exchanges, and supporting the child to register the correspondences between his/her and others' actions during shared experiences (Rogers, Vivanti, & Rocha, 2017; Vivanti & Rogers, 2014).

Influences from Implementation Science

A more recent influence on ASD early intervention is the emerging field of implementation science, which studies the factors that facilitate adoption and successful implementation of interventions in the "real world" (Eccles et al., 2009; Green, 2012). This field focuses on features such as organizational systems of the context in which interventions take place, as well as beliefs, cultures, and the "buy-in" of professionals involved in the intervention. A critical notion derived from this research is that the commitment to use intervention techniques and implement them as intended is not only dependent on the level of evidence supporting the intervention, but also on the perceived fit between features of the intervention and stakeholder attitudes (whether they think that using the intervention is the right thing to do), norms (the extent with which they feel they are expected to use the intervention, or believe that their peers are using it), self-efficacy, and the perception of the cost-benefit of adding new approaches to their standard practice. These factors will affect the initial uptake of the intervention, maintenance over time, and the degree of integrity to which it is delivered, thus affecting intervention outcomes. Recent early intervention practices for ASD influenced by implementation science include the introduction of participatory research methods, in which administrators', practitioners', and end users' resources and preferences are examined and taken into consideration from the early stages of designing and piloting new interventions (Dingfelder & Mandell, 2011; Locke et al., 2016; Smith et al., 2007).

Influences from the Neurodiversity Framework

A recent societal influence that has affected debate on intervention for ASD is the concept of neurodiversity, which refers to the notion that neurological differences are to be recognized and respected as any other human variations (den Houting, 2019; Baron-Cohen, 2017), rather than being seen as indicators of a pathology to be corrected or eradicated. Some self-advocates with ASD who adopt this perspective question the need for curing or "normalizing" autism, arguing that the goal of increasing "desirable" and decreasing "undesirable" behaviors in intervention reflects the parameters of what is desirable or undesirable set by a "neurotypical" majority. Further, this approach to treatment has been criticized as being designed to achieve conformity at the expenses of diversity, rather than serving the best interest of those with ASD. According to this perspective, ASD is a way of being in the world, or a culture, which requires support and appreciation, rather than prevention or treatment (Norbury & Sparks, 2013; see also Mesibov, Shea, & Schopler, 2004, for an early application of the concept of autism as a culture for treatment).

Importantly, other advocacy groups are not opposed to the idea of intervention per se, but emphasize the importance of practices aimed at increasing opportunities for self-determination and eliminating environmental and social barriers to civil rights and inclusion in individuals in the autism spectrum. While the positions expressed by neurodiversity advocates are multifaceted and highly debated, especially in the context of the heterogeneity of intervention needs within the ASD population, there is a growing focus on researching treatment methods and outcomes that include preferences and perspectives of individuals with ASD (Pellicano & Stears, 2011; Vivanti, 2020).

Conclusions

Despite the tremendous increase in research in the past decades, many aspects of ASD continue to remain enigmatic. As it has become clear that ASD does not result from a single disruption or etiological pathway, the challenge for early intervention research is to derive practical knowledge from the examination of the interplay between biological, neuropsychological, and environmental factors underlying the heterogeneous and seemingly unrelated clusters of symptoms and associated features that characterize the autism spectrum. Additionally, issues on appreciation of diversity, human rights, and self-determination are increasingly stimulating societal debate and challenging the established intervention paradigms. Despite these challenges, it can be concluded that the current landscape of early intervention for ASD has been shaped by progression from the widespread use of unethical and unsupported treatments to the increasing appreciation and integration of evolving scientific knowledge and more inclusive views on ASD.

While no area of early intervention for ASD is free from debate, and divergences among different schools of thought continue to exist, early interventions for ASD that have proven to be effective converge around a set of key features. These include the engagement of the child in a planned educational/psychosocial intervention that (1) starts early in life, (2) is developmentally appropriate, (3) is implemented throughout the child's day, (4) uses well-defined instructional strategies to target the core features of autism and address functional/adaptive skills, (5) includes systematic assessment procedures to define individualized sets of goals tailored to the individual child's profile of strength and needs, (6) includes a data collection system to monitor progress, and (7) involves caregivers in establishing treatment goals and delivering intervention strategies. Within this framework, different interventions exist, which will be described in detail in the following chapters.

References

Adamson, L. B. (1995). *Communication development during infancy*. Madison, WI: Brown & Benchmark Publishers.

APA. (1980). *Diagnostic and statistical manual (DSM-III)*. Washington, DC: APA.

APA. (1994). *Diagnostic and statistical manual of mental disorders (DSM-IV)*. Washington, DC: APA.
Arnett, A. B., Trinh, S., & Bernier, R. A. (2019). The state of research on the genetics of autism spectrum disorder: Methodological, clinical and conceptual progress. *Current Opinion in Psychology, 27*, 1–5.
Asperger, H. (1944). Die "autistichen Psychopathen" im Kindersalter. *Archiv für Psychiatrie und Nervenkrankheiten, 117*, 76–136.
American Psychiatric Association [APA] (1987). Diagnostic and statistical manual of mental disorders (3rd ed., rev.). Washington, DC: Author.
Bai, D., et al. (2019). Association of genetic and environmental factors with autism in a 5-country cohort. *JAMA Psychiatry, 76*, 1035. https://doi.org/10.1001/jamapsychiatry.2019.1411
Baio, J., Wiggins, L., Christensen, D. L., Maenner, M. J., Daniels, J., Warren, Z., … Durkin, M. S. (2018). Prevalence of autism spectrum disorder among children aged 8 years—Autism and developmental disabilities monitoring network, 11 sites, United States, 2014. MMWR Surveillance Summaries, 67(6), 1. doi:https://doi.org/10.15585/mmwr.ss6706a1
Bargiela, S., Steward, R., & Mandy, W. (2016). The experiences of late-diagnosed women with autism spectrum conditions: An investigation of the female autism phenotype. *Journal of Autism and Developmental Disorders, 46*(10), 3281–3294.
Baron-Cohen, S. (1995). *Mindblindness: An essay on autism and theory of mind*. Cambridge, MA: MIT Press.
Baron-Cohen, S. (2017). Editorial perspective: Neurodiversity–a revolutionary concept for autism and psychiatry. *Journal of Child Psychology and Psychiatry, 58*(6), 744–747.
Baron-Cohen, S., Leslie, A. M., & Frith, U. (1985). Does the autistic child have a "theory of mind"? *Cognition, 21*(1), 37–46. https://doi.org/10.1016/0010-0277(85)90022-8
Bettelheim, B. (1967). *Empty fortress*. New York, NY: The Free Press.
Bishop, S. L., Richler, J., & Lord, C. (2006). Association between restricted and repetitive behaviors and nonverbal IQ in children with autism Spectrum disorders. *Child Neuropsychology, 12*(4–5), 247–267. https://doi.org/10.1080/09297040600630288
Bodfish, J. W. (2007). Stereotypy, self-injury, and related abnormal repetitive behaviors. In J. W. Jacobson, J. A. Mulick, & J. Rojahn (Eds.), *Handbook of intellectual and developmental disabilities* (pp. 481–505). New York, NY: Springer.
Bölte, S., Duketis, E., Poustka, F., & Holtmann, M. (2011). Sex differences in cognitive domains and their clinical correlates in higher-functioning autism spectrum disorders. *Autism, 15*(4), 497–511.
Bottema-Beutel, K. (2016). The relationship between joint attention and language in autism spectrum disorder and typical development: A systematic review and meta-regression analysis. *Autism Research, 9*(10), 1021–1035.
Bristol, M. M., Cohen, D. J., Costello, E. J., Denckla, M., Eckberg, T. J., Kallen, R., … Spence, M. A. (1996). State of the science in autism: Report to the National Institutes of Health. *Journal of Autism and Developmental Disorders, 26*(2), 121–154. https://doi.org/10.1007/Bf02172002
Bruner, J. S. (1978). The role of dialogue in language acquisition. In A. Sinclair, R. Larvella, & W. J. M. Levelt (Eds.), *The child's conception of language*. New York, NY: Springer-Verlag.
Baer, D. M., Wolf, M. M., & Risley, T. R. (1968). Some current dimensions of applied behavior analysis 1. *Journal of applied behavior analysis, 1*(1), 91–97.
Barbaro, J., & Dissanayake, C. (2013). Early markers of autism spectrum disorders in infants and toddlers prospectively identified in the Social Attention and Communication Study. *Autism, 17*(1), 64–86.
Bolton, P. F., Golding, J., Emond, A., & Steer, C. D. (2012). Autism spectrum disorder and autistic traits in the Avon Longitudinal Study of Parents and Children: precursors and early signs. *Journal of the American Academy of Child & Adolescent Psychiatry, 51*(3), 249–260.
Brownell, C. A. (2013). Early development of prosocial behavior: *Current perspectives. Infancy, 18*(1), 1–9.

Capps, L., Sigman, M., & Mundy, P. (1994). Attachment security in children with autism. *Development and Psychopathology, 6*(02), 249–261. https://doi.org/10.1017/S0954579400004569

Carter, A., Ornstein Davis, N., Klin, A., & Volkmar, F. (2005). Social development in autism. In F. Volkmar, P. Rhea, A. Klin, & D. Cohen (Eds.), *Handbook of autism and pervasive developmental disorders* (Vol. 1, 3rd ed., pp. 312–334). Hoboken, NJ: Wiley.

Canitano, R., & Vivanti, G. (2007). Tics and Tourette syndrome in autism spectrum disorders. *Autism, 11*(1), 19-28.

Cascio, M. A. (2012). Neurodiversity: Autism pride among mothers of children with autism spectrum disorders. *Intellectual and Developmental Disabilities, 50*(3), 273–283.

Charman, T., Pickles, A., Simonoff, E., Chandler, S., Loucas, T., & Baird, G. (2011). IQ in children with autism spectrum disorders: Data from the special needs and autism project (SNAP). *Psychological Medicine, 41*(3), 619–627.

Chawarska, K., Macari, S., & Shic, F. (2013). Decreased spontaneous attention to social scenes in 6-month-old infants later diagnosed with autism spectrum disorders. *Biological Psychiatry, 74*(3), 195–203.

Chawarska, K., Shic, F., Macari, S., Campbell, D. J., Brian, J., Landa, R., ... Young, G. S. (2014). 18-month predictors of later outcomes in younger siblings of children with autism spectrum disorder: A baby siblings research consortium study. *Journal of the American Academy of Child & Adolescent Psychiatry, 53*(12), 1317–1327.

Chevallier, C., Kohls, G., Troiani, V., Brodkin, E. S., & Schultz, R. T. (2012). The social motivation theory of autism. *Trends in Cognitive Sciences, 16*(4), 231–239. https://doi.org/10.1016/j.tics.2012.02.007

Christensen, D. L., Bilder, D. A., Zahorodny, W., et al. (2016). Prevalence and characteristics of autism Spectrum disorder among 4-year-old children in the autism and developmental disabilities monitoring network. *Journal of Developmental and Behavioral Pediatrics, 37*(1), 1–8.

Christensen, D. L., Braun, K. V. N., Baio, J., Bilder, D., Charles, J., Constantino, J. N., ... Lee, L. C. (2018). Prevalence and characteristics of autism spectrum disorder among children aged 8 years—Autism and developmental disabilities monitoring network, 11 sites, United States, 2012. *MMWR Surveillance Summaries, 65*(13), 1.

Colvert, E., Tick, B., McEwen, F., Stewart, C., Curran, S. R., Woodhouse, E., ... Ronald, A. (2015). Heritability of autism spectrum disorder in a UK population-based twin sample. *JAMA Psychiatry, 72*(5), 415–423.

Dawson, G. (2008). Early behavioral intervention, brain plasticity, and the prevention of autism spectrum disorder. *Development and Psychopathology, 20*, 775–803.

den Houting, J. (2019). Neurodiversity: An insider's perspective. Autism: the international *Journal of research and practice, 23*(2), 271.

De Sanctis, S. (1906). Sopra alcune varieta' della demenza precoce. *Rivista Sperimentale de Freniatria e di Medicina Legale, 32*, 141–165.

Dean, M., Harwood, R., & Kasari, C. (2017). The art of camouflage: Gender differences in the social behaviors of girls and boys with autism spectrum disorder. *Autism, 21*(6), 678–689.

Dingfelder, H. E., & Mandell, D. S. (2011). Bridging the research-to-practice gap in autism intervention: An application of diffusion of innovation theory. *Journal of Autism and Developmental Disorders, 41*(5), 597–609.

Durkin, M. S., Maenner, M. J., Baio, J., Christensen, D., Daniels, J., Fitzgerald, R., ... Wingate, M. S. (2017). Autism spectrum disorder among US children (2002–2010): Socioeconomic, racial, and ethnic disparities. *American Journal of Public Health, 107*(11), 1818–1826.

Di Giorgio, E., Frasnelli, E., Salva, O. R., Scattoni, M. L., Puopolo, M., Tosoni, D., ... & Vallortigara, G. (2016). Difference in visual social predispositions between newborns at low- and high-risk for autism. *Scientific reports, 6*(1), 1–9.

Dissanayake, C., & Crossley, S. A. (1996). Proximity and sociable behaviours in autism: Evidence for attachment. *Journal of child psychology and psychiatry, 37*(2),149–156.

Dölen, G., Darvishzadeh, A., Huang, K. W., & Malenka, R. C. (2013). Social reward requires coordinated activity of nucleus accumbens oxytocin and serotonin. *Nature, 501*(7466), 179–184.
Eccles, M. P., Armstrong, D., Baker, R., Cleary, K., Davies, H., Davies, S., … Logan, S. (2009). An implementation research agenda. *Implementation Science, 4*(1), 18.
Esbensen, A., Seltzer, M., Lam, K. L., & Bodfish, J. (2009). Age-related differences in restricted repetitive behaviors in autism Spectrum disorders. *Journal of Autism and Developmental Disorders, 39*(1), 57–66. https://doi.org/10.1007/s10803-008-0599-x
Evans, D. W., Leckman, J. F., Carter, A., Reznick, J. S., Henshaw, D., King, R. A., & Pauls, D. (1997). Ritual, habit, and perfectionism: The prevalence and development of compulsive-like behavior in Normal Young children. *Child Development, 68*(1), 58–68. https://doi.org/10.1111/j.1467-8624.1997.tb01925.x
Fein, D., Barton, M., Eigsti, I.-M., Kelley, E., Naigles, L., Schultz, R. T., … Tyson, K. (2013). Optimal outcome in individuals with a history of autism. *Journal of Child Psychology and Psychiatry, 54*(2), 195–205. https://doi.org/10.1111/jcpp.12037
Ferri, S. L., Abel, T., & Brodkin, E. S. (2018). Sex differences in autism spectrum disorder: A review. *Current Psychiatry Reports, 20*(2), 9.
Ferster, C. B. (1964). Positive reinforcement and behavioral deficits of autistic children. In *Conditioning techniques in clinical practice and research* (pp. 255–274). Berlin, Heidelberg: Springer.
Ferster, C. B., & DeMyer, M. K. (1961). The development of performances in autistic children in an automatically controlled environment. *Journal of Chronic Diseases, 13*(4), 312–345.
Freud, A. (1969/2015). *Selected writings*. London: Penguin.
Freud, S. (1911). Formulations on the two principles of mental functioning. *The Standard Edition of the Complete Psychological Works of Sigmund Freud, XII*, 1911–1913.
Frith, U. (2012). Why we need cognitive explanations of autism. *The Quarterly Journal of Experimental Psychology, 65*(11), 2073–2092. https://doi.org/10.1080/17470218.2012.697178
Frith, U., & Happé, F. (1994). Autism: Beyond "theory of mind". *Cognition, 50*(1–3), 115–132. https://doi.org/10.1016/0010-0277(94)90024-8
Frith, U., & Frith, C. (2010). The social brain: allowing humans to boldly go where no other species has been. Philosophical Transactions of the Royal Society B: *Biological Sciences, 365*(1537), 165–176.
Giarelli, E., Wiggins, L. D., Rice, C. E., Levy, S. E., Kirby, R. S., Pinto-Martin, J., & Mandell, D. (2010). Sex differences in the evaluation and diagnosis of autism spectrum disorders among children. *Disability and Health Journal, 3*(2), 107–116.
Giles, D. C. (2014). 'DSM-V is taking away our identity': The reaction of the online community to the proposed changes in the diagnosis of Asperger's disorder. *Health, 18*(2), 179–195.
Gorrindo, P., Williams, K. C., Lee, E. B., Walker, L. S., McGrew, S. G., & Levitt, P. (2012). Gastrointestinal dysfunction in autism: Parental report, clinical evaluation, and associated factors. *Autism Research, 5*(2), 101–108.
Gotham, K., Pickles, A., & Lord, C. (2012). Trajectories of autism severity in children using standardized ADOS scores. *Pediatrics, 130*(5), e1278–e1284.
Green, J. (2012). Editorial: Science, implementation, and implementation science. *Journal of Child Psychology and Psychiatry, 53*, 333–336.
Green, M. R., & Schecter, D. E. (1957). Autism and symbiotic disorders in three blind children. *Psychiatric Quarterly, 31*(4), 628–646.
Happé, F. G. (1994). An advanced test of theory of mind: Understanding of story characters' thoughts and feelings by able autistic, mentally handicapped, and normal children and adults. *Journal of Autism and Developmental Disorders, 24*(2), 129–154.
Harrop, C., Jones, D., Zheng, S., Nowell, S. W., Boyd, B. A., & Sasson, N. (2018). Sex differences in social attention in autism spectrum disorder. *Autism Research, 11*(9), 1264–1275.
Holingue, C., Newill, C., Lee, L. C., Pasricha, P. J., & Daniele Fallin, M. (2018). Gastrointestinal symptoms in autism spectrum disorder: A review of the literature on ascertainment and prevalence. *Autism Research, 11*(1), 24–36.

Hutman, T., Rozga, A., DeLaurentis, A., et al. (2010). Response to distress in infants at risk for autism: A prospective longitudinal study. *Journal of Child Psychology and Psychiatry, 51*(9), 1010–1020.

Jeste, S. S., & Tuchman, R. (2015). Autism spectrum disorder and epilepsy: Two sides of the same coin? *Journal of Child Neurology, 30*(14), 1963–1971.

Johnson, M. H. (2017). Autism as an adaptive common variant pathway for human brain development. *Developmental Cognitive Neuroscience, 25*, 5–11.

Jones, E. J. H., Gliga, T., Bedford, R., Charman, T., & Johnson, M. H. (2014). Developmental pathways to autism: A review of prospective studies of infants at risk. *Neuroscience & Biobehavioral Reviews, 39*, 1–33. https://doi.org/10.1016/j.neubiorev.2013.12.001

Jones, W., & Klin, A. (2013). Attention to eyes is present but in decline in 2–6-month-old infants later diagnosed with autism. *Nature, 504*(7480), 427–431.

Kalyva, E., Kyriazi, M., Vargiami, E., & Zafeiriou, D. I. (2016). A review of co-occurrence of autism spectrum disorder and Tourette syndrome. *Research in Autism Spectrum Disorders, 24*, 39–51.

Kanner, L. (1943). Autistic disturbances of affective contact. *The Nervous Child, 2*(3), 217–250.

Kanner, L., & Eisenberg, L. (1956). Early infantile autism: Childhood schizophrenia symposium. *American Journal of Orthopsychiatry, 26*, 556–564.

Kim, S. H., Paul, R., Tager-Flusberg, H., & Lord, C. (2014). Language and communication in autism. In F. Volkmar, R. Paul, S. Rogers, & K. Pelphrey (Eds.), *Handbook of autism and pervasive developmental disorders* (4th ed.). New York: Wiley.

Klein, M. (1930/1975). The importance of symbol formation in the development of the ego. In M. Klein (Ed.), *Love, guilt and reparation and other works 1921–1945* (pp. 219–232).

Klin, A., Shultz, S., & Jones, W. (2015). Social visual engagement in infants and toddlers with autism: Early developmental transitions and a model of pathogenesis. *Neuroscience and Biobehavioral Reviews, 50*, 189–203.

Koyama, T., Kamio, Y., Inada, N., & Kurita, H. (2009). Sex differences in WISC-III profiles of children with high-functioning pervasive developmental disorders. *Journal of Autism and Developmental Disorders, 39*(1), 135.

Kasari, C., Sigman, M., & Yirmiya, N. (1993). Focused and social attention of autistic children in interactions with familiar and unfamiliar adults: A comparison of autistic, mentally retarded, and normal children. *Development and Psychopathology, 5*(3), 403–414.

Kasari, C., Sigman, M., Mundy, P., & Yirmiya, N. (1990). Affective sharing in the context of joint attention interactions of normal, autistic, and mentally retarded children. *Journal of autism and developmental disorders, 20*(1), 87–100.

Lampi, K. M., Lehtonen, L., Tran, P. L., Suominen, A., Lehti, V., Banerjee, P. N., … Sourander, A. (2012). Risk of autism spectrum disorders in low birth weight and small for gestational age infants. *The Journal of Pediatrics, 161*(5), 830–836.

Le Couteur, A., Lord, C., & Rutter, M. (2003). *The autism diagnostic interview–Revised (ADI-R)*. Los Angeles, CA: Western Psychological Services.

Leekam, S. R., Prior, M. R., & Uljarevic, M. (2011). Restricted and repetitive behaviors in autism spectrum disorders: A review of research in the last decade. *Psychological Bulletin, 137*(4), 562–593.

Leekam, S. (2016). Social cognitive impairment and autism: what are we trying to explain?. Philosophical Transactions of the Royal Society B: *Biological Sciences, 371*(1686), 20150082.

Lieberman, M. D. (2007). Social cognitive neuroscience: A review of Core processes. *Annual Review of Psychology, 58*(1), 259–289.

Locke, J., Beidas, R. S., Marcus, S., Stahmer, A., Aarons, G. A., Lyon, A. R., … Mandell, D. S. (2016). A mixed methods study of individual and organizational factors that affect implementation of interventions for children with autism in public schools. *Implementation Science, 11*, 135.

Loomes, R., Hull, L., & Mandy, W. P. L. (2017). What is the male-to-female ratio in autism Spectrum disorder? A systematic review and meta-analysis. *Journal of the American Academy of Child and Adolescent Psychiatry, 56*(6), 466–474.

Lord, C., Elsabbagh, M., Baird, G., & Veenstra-Vanderweele, J. (2018). Autism spectrum disorder. *The Lancet, 392*, 508.

Lord, C., Rutter, M., DiLavore, P. C., Risi, S., Gotham, K., & Bishop, S. (2012). *Autism diagnostic observation schedule, second edition (ADOS-2)*. Torrance, CA: Western Psychological Services.

Lord, C., & Schopler, E. (1985). Brief report: Differences in sex ratios in autism as a function of measured intelligence. *Journal of Autism and Developmental Disorders, 15*(2), 185–193.

Lovaas, O. I., Schaeffer, B., & Simmons, J. Q. (1965). Building social behavior in autistic children by use of electric shock. *Journal of Experimental Research in Personality*.

Lovaas, O. I. (1968). Some studies on the treatment of childhood schizophrenia. In *Research in psychotherapy conference, 3rd, may–June* (p. 1966). Chicago, IL: American Psychological Association.

Lovaas, O. I. (1981). *The me book: Teaching developmentally disabled children*. Austin, TX: PRO-ED.

Lovaas, O. I. (1989). Concerns about misinterpretation and placement of blame. *American Psychologist, 44*(9), 1243–1244.

Lovaas, O. I., & Smith, T. (1989). A comprehensive behavioral theory of autistic children: Paradigm for research and treatment. *Journal of Behavior Therapy and Experimental Psychiatry, 20*(1), 17–29.

Lyall, K., Croen, L., Daniels, J., Fallin, M. D., Ladd-Acosta, C., Lee, B. K., … Windham, G. C. (2017). The changing epidemiology of autism spectrum disorders. *Annual Review of Public Health, 38*, 81–102.

Mandell, D. S., Wiggins, L. D., Carpenter, L. A., Daniels, J., DiGuiseppi, C., Durkin, M. S., … Kirby, R. S. (2009). Racial/ethnic disparities in the identification of children with autism Spectrum disorders. *American Journal of Public Health, 99*(3), 493–498. https://doi.org/10.2105/ajph.2007.131243

Mandy, W., Chilvers, R., Chowdhury, U., et al. (2012). Sex differences in autism spectrum disorder: Evidence from a large sample of children and adolescents. *Journal of Autism and Developmental Disorders, 42*(7), 1304–1313.

Mayville, E. A., & Mulick, J. A. (2011). *Behavioral foundations of effective autism treatment*. New York: Sloan Pub.

McGee, G. G., Feldman, R. S., & Morrier, M. J. (1997). Benchmarks of social treatment for children with autism. *Journal of Autism and Developmental Disorders, 27*(4), 353–364.

Mesibov, G. B., Shea, V., & Schopler, E. (2004). *The TEACCH approach to autism spectrum disorders*. New York, NY: Springer Science & Business Media.

Minshew, N. J., & Goldstein, G. (1998). Autism as a disorder of complex information processing. *Mental Retardation and Developmental Disabilities Research Reviews, 4*(2), 129–136. https://doi.org/10.1002/(sici)1098-2779

Montessori, M. (1912). *The Montessori method*. New York: Stokes.

Moulton, E., Barton, M., Robins, D. L., Abrams, D. N., & Fein, D. (2016). Early characteristics of children with ASD who demonstrate optimal progress between age two and four. *Journal of Autism and Developmental Disorders, 46*(6), 2160–2173.

Mundy, P. (1995). Joint attention and social-emotional approach behavior in children with autism. *Development and Psychopathology, 7*(1), 63–82.

Mundy, P. (2011). The social behavior of autism: A parallel and distributed information processing perspective. In D. G. Amaral, G. Dawson, & D. H. Geschwind (Eds.), *Autism Spectrum disorders* (pp. 149–171). New York, NY: Oxford University Press.

Mundy, P. (2016). *Autism and joint attention: Development, neuroscience, and clinical fundamentals*. New York: Guilford Publications.

Miller, M., Iosif, A. M., Hill, M., Young, G. S., Schwichtenberg, A. J., & Ozonoff, S. (2017). Response to name in infants developing autism spectrum disorder: a prospective study. *The Journal of pediatrics, 183*, 141–146.

Nahmias, A. S., Pellecchia, M., Stahmer, A. C., & Mandell, D. S. (2019). *Effectiveness of community-based early intervention for children with autism spectrum disorder: A meta-analysis*. Journal of Child Psychology and Psychiatry (Vol. 60, p. 1200).

Ninio, A., & Bruner, J. (1978). The achievement and antecedents of labeling. *Journal of Child Language, 5*, 1–15.

Norbury, C. F., & Sparks, A. (2013). Difference or disorder? Cultural issues in understanding neurodevelopmental disorders. *Developmental Psychology, 49*(1), 45–58. https://doi.org/10.1037/a0027446

Nyström, P., Thorup, E., Bölte, S., & Falck-Ytter, T. (2019). Joint attention in infancy and the emergence of autism. *Biological Psychiatry, 86*, 631. https://doi.org/10.1016/j.biopsych.2019.05.006

Ozonoff, S. (1997). Components of executive function in autism and other disorders. In *Autism as an executive disorder* (pp. 179–211). Oxford: Oxford University Press.

Ozonoff, S., Macari, S., Young, G. S., Goldring, S., Thompson, M., & Rogers, S. J. (2008). Atypical object exploration at 12 months of age is associated with autism in a prospective sample. *Autism, 12*(5), 457–472.

Ozonoff, S., Young, G. S., Brian, J., Charman, T., Shephard, E., Solish, A., & Zwaigenbaum, L. (2018). Diagnosis of autism spectrum disorder after age 5 in children evaluated longitudinally since infancy. *Journal of the American Academy of Child & Adolescent Psychiatry, 57*(11), 849–857.

Ozonoff, S., Young, G. S., Landa, R. J., Brian, J., Bryson, S., Charman, T., … Iosif, A. M. (2015). Diagnostic stability in young children at risk for autism spectrum disorder: A baby siblings research consortium study. *Journal of Child Psychology and Psychiatry, 56*(9), 988e998.

Parker, S. K., Schwartz, B., Todd, J., & Pickering, L. K. (2004). Thimerosal-containing vaccines and autistic Spectrum disorder: A critical review of published original data. *Pediatrics, 114*(3), 793–804. https://doi.org/10.1542/peds.2004-0434

Pellicano, E., & Stears, M. (2011). Bridging autism, science and society: Moving toward an ethically informed approach to autism research. *Autism Research, 4*(4), 271–282. https://doi.org/10.1002/aur.201

Pelphrey, K. A., Yang, D. Y.-J., & McPartland, J. C. (2014). Building a social neuroscience of autism spectrum disorder. In S. Anderson & D. Pine (Eds.), *The neurobiology of childhood* (pp. 215–233). New York, NY: Springer.

Piaget, J. (1929). *The child's conception of the world*. Ithaca, New York: Routledge & K. Paul.

Postorino, V., Fatta, L. M., Sanges, V., Giovagnoli, G., De Peppo, L., Vicari, S., & Mazzone, L. (2016). Intellectual disability in autism spectrum disorder: Investigation of prevalence in an Italian sample of children and adolescents. *Research in Developmental Disabilities, 48*, 193–201.

Postorino, V., Kerns, C., Vivanti, G., Bradshaw, J., Siracusano, M., & Mazzone, L. (2017). Anxiety disorders and obsessive-compulsive individuals with autism spectrum disorder. *Current Psychiatry Reports, 19*(12), 92. https://doi.org/10.1007/s11920-017-0846-y

Prior, M., & Macmillan, M. B. (1973). Maintenance of sameness in children with Kanner's syndrome. *Journal of Autism and Childhood Schizophrenia, 3*(2), 154–167.

Pierce, K., Conant, D., Hazin, R., Stoner, R., & Desmond, J. (2011). Preference for geometric patterns early in life as a risk factor for autism. *Archives of general psychiatry, 68*(1), 101–109.

Ramaswami, G., & Geschwind, D. H. (2018). Genetics of autism spectrum disorder. *Handbook of Clinical Neurology, 147*, 321–329.

Rapin, I. (2002). Diagnostic dilemmas in developmental disabilities: Fuzzy margins at the edges of normality. An essay prompted by Thomas Sowell's new book: The Einstein syndrome. *Journal of Autism and Developmental Disorders, 32*(1), 49–57.

Richler, J., Bishop, S. L., Kleinke, J. R., & Lord, C. (2007). Restricted and repetitive behaviors in young children with autism spectrum disorders. *Journal of Autism and Developmental Disorders, 37*, 73–85.

Robinson, E. B., Lichtenstein, P., Anckarsäter, H., Happé, F., & Ronald, A. (2013). Examining and interpreting the female protective effect against autistic behavior. *Proceedings of the National Academy of Sciences, 110*(13), 5258–5262. https://doi.org/10.1073/pnas.1211070110

Rogers, S. J., & Talbott, M. R. (2016). Early identification and early treatment of autism spectrum disorder. *International Review of Research in Developmental Disabilities, 50*, 233–275.

Rutter, M. (1972). Childhood schizophrenia reconsidered. *Journal of Autism and Childhood Schizophrenia, 2*(3), 315–337.

Rutter, M. (2000). Genetic studies of autism: From the 1970s into the millennium. *Journal of Abnormal Child Psychology, 28*(1), 3–14. https://doi.org/10.1023/A:1005113900068

Rydzewska, E., Hughes-McCormack, L. A., Gillberg, C., Henderson, A., MacIntyre, C., Rintoul, J., & Cooper, S. A. (2018). Prevalence of long-term health conditions in adults with autism: Observational study of a whole country population. *BMJ Open, 8*(8), e023945.

Rizzolatti, G., & Sinigaglia, C. (2008). Mirrors in the brain: How our minds share actions and emotions. Oxford University Press, USA.

Rogers, S. J., Vivanti, G., & Rocha, M. (2017). Helping young children with autism spectrum disorder develop social ability: The Early Start Denver Modelapproach. In Leaf, J. (Ed) Handbook of social skills and autism spectrum disorder (pp. 197–222). Springer, Cham.

Rogers, S. J. (1999). Intervention for young children with autism: From research to practice. *Infants & Young Children, 12*(2), 1–16.

Scaife, M., & Bruner, J. S. (1975). The capacity for joint visual attention in the infant. *Nature, 253*(5489), 265–266.

Senju, A. (2012). Spontaneous theory of mind and its absence in autism spectrum disorders. *The Neuroscientist, 18*(2), 108–113.

Sharp, W. G., Berry, R. C., McCracken, C., Nuhu, N. N., Marvel, E., Saulnier, C. A., … Jaquess, D. L. (2013). Feeding problems and nutrient intake in children with autism spectrum disorders: A meta-analysis and comprehensive review of the literature. *Journal of Autism and Developmental Disorders, 43*(9), 2159–2173.

Sigman, M. (1998). Change and continuity in the development of children with autism. *The Journal of Child Psychology and Psychiatry and Allied Disciplines, 39*(6), 817–827.

Sigman, M., & Mundy, P. (1989). Social attachments in autistic children. *Journal of the American Academy of Child and Adolescent Psychiatry, 28*(1), 74–81.

Sigman, M., & Ungerer, J. A. (1984). Cognitive and language skills in autistic, mentally retarded, and normal children. *Developmental Psychology, 20*(2), 293.

Simonoff, E., Jones, C. R. G., Baird, G., Pickles, A., Happé, F., & Charman, T. (2013). The persistence and stability of psychiatric problems in adolescents with autism spectrum disorders. *Journal of Child Psychology and Psychiatry, 54*(2), 186–194. https://doi.org/10.1111/j.1469-7610.2012.02606.x

Smith, T., Scahill, L., Dawson, G., Guthrie, D., Lord, C., Odom, S., … Wagner, A. (2007). Designing research studies on psychosocial interventions in autism. *Journal of Autism and Developmental Disorders, 37*(2), 354–366. https://doi.org/10.1007/s10803-006-0173-3

Souders, M. C., Zavodny, S., Eriksen, W., Sinko, R., Connell, J., Kerns, C., … Pinto-Martin, J. (2017). Sleep in children with autism spectrum disorder. *Current Psychiatry Reports, 19*(6), 34.

Sperry, L. A., & Mesibov, G. B. (2005). Perceptions of social challenges of adults with autism spectrum disorder. *Autism, 9*(4), 362–376.

Ssucharewa, G. E. (1926). Die schizoiden Psychopathien im Kindesalter. *Monatsschrift für Psychiatrie und Neurologie, 60*, 235–261.

Schreibman, L., Dawson, G., Stahmer, A. C., Landa, R., Rogers, S. J., McGee, G. G., ... & McNerney, E. (2015). Naturalistic developmental behavioral interventions: Empirically validated treatments for autism spectrum disorder. *Journal of autism and developmental disorders, 45*(8), 2411–2428.

Severson, K. D., Aune, J. A., Jodlowski, D., & Osteen, M. (2008). Autism and representation. New York: Routledge

Shultz, S., Klin, A., & Jones, W. (2018). Neonatal transitions in social behavior and their implications for autism. *Trends in cognitive sciences, 22*(5), 452–469.

Sigman, M., Ruskin, E., Arbelle, S., Corona, R., Dissanayake, C., Espinosa, M., ... & Robinson, B. F. (1999). Continuity and change in the social competence of children with autism, Down syndrome, and developmental delays. *Monographs of the society for research in child development*, i-139.

Skinner, B. F. (1953). Science and human behavior: Simon and Schuster.

Sullivan, K., Stone, W. L., & Dawson, G. (2014). Potential neural mechanisms underlying the effectiveness of early intervention for children with autism spectrum disorder. *Research in Developmental Disabilities, 35*(11), 2921–2932.

Tager-Flusberg, H., & Kasari, C. (2013). Minimally verbal school-aged children with autism spectrum disorder: The neglected end of the spectrum. *Autism Research, 6*(6), 468–478.

Tick, B., Bolton, P., Happé, F., Rutter, M., & Rijsdijk, F. (2016). Heritability of autism spectrum disorders: A meta-analysis of twin studies. *Journal of Child Psychology and Psychiatry, 57*(5), 585–595.

Tustin, F. (1991). Revised understandings of psychogenic autism. *International Journal of Psycho-Analysis, 72*, 585–591.

Uljarević, M., Baranek, G., Vivanti, G., Hedley, D., Hudry, K., & Lane, A. (2017). Heterogeneity of sensory features in autism spectrum disorder: Challenges and perspectives for future research. *Autism Research, 10*(5), 703–710.

Uljarevic, M., Nuske, H., & Vivanti, G. (2016). Anxiety in autism Spectrum disorder. In B. Vitiello & L. Mazzone (Eds.), *Psychiatric symptoms and comorbidities in autism spectrum disorder* (pp. 21–38). New York, NY: Springer.

Vivanti, G., Dawson, G., & Rogers, S. J. (2017). Early learning in autism. In Implementing the group-based early start Denver model for preschoolers with autism (pp. 1–12). Cham: Springer International Publishing.

Vivanti, G., Dissanayake, C., Zierhut, C., Rogers, S. J., & Victorian ASELCC Team (2013). Brief report: Predictors of outcomes in the early start Denver model delivered in a group setting. *Journal of Autism and Developmental Disorders, 43*(7), 1717–1724.

Vivanti, G., & Hamilton, A. F. (2014). Imitation in autism spectrum disorders. In F. Volkmar, R. Paul, S. Rogers, & K. Pelphrey (Eds.), The handbook of autism and developmental disorders (pp. 278–301). New York: Wiley.

Vivanti, G., & Nuske, H. J. (2017). Autism, attachment, and social learning: Three challenges and a way forward. *Behavioural Brain Research, 325*, 251–259.

Vivanti, G., Prior, M., Williams, K., & Dissanayake, C. (2014). Predictors of outcomes in autism early intervention: Why don't we know more? *Frontiers in Pediatrics, 2*, 58.

Vivanti, G., & Rogers, S. J. (2014). Autism and the mirror neuron system: Insights from learning and teaching. *Philosophical Transactions of the Royal Society of London. Series B, Biological Sciences, 369*(1644), 20130184–20130184.

Vivanti, G., Yerys, B., & Salomone, E. (2019). Psychological factors in autism spectrum disorder. In F. Volkmar (Ed.), *Autism and pervasive developmental disorders*. Cambridge: Cambridge University Press.

Vivanti, G. (2020). Ask the Editor: What is the Most Appropriate Way to Talk About Individuals with a Diagnosis of Autism?. *Journal of Autism and Developmental Disorders, 50*(2), 691–693.

Volkmar, F., Siegel, M., Woodbury-Smith, M., King, B., McCracken, J., State, M., & Child, A. A. (2014). Practice parameter for the assessment and treatment of children and adolescents with autism spectrum disorder. *Journal of the American Academy of Child & Adolescent Psychiatry, 53*(2), 237–257.

Volkmar, F. R., & McPartland, J. C. (2014). From Kanner to DSM-5: Autism as an evolving diagnostic concept. *Annual Review of Clinical Psychology, 10*, 193–212.

Volkmar, F. R., & Wiesner, L. (2017). *Essential clinical guide to understanding and treating autism*. Hoboken, NJ: Wiley.
Vygotsky, L. (1930–1934/1978). Vygotsky, L. S. (1978). *Mind in society: The development of higher psychological processes* (A. R. Luria, M. Lopez-Morillas & M. Cole [with J. V. Wertsch], Trans.) Cambridge, Mass.: Harvard University Press.
Ventola, P., Lei, J., Paisley, C., Lebowitz, E., & Silverman, W. (2017). Parenting a child with ASD: Comparison of parenting style between ASD, anxiety, and typical development. *Journal of autism and developmental disorders, 47*(9), 2873–2884.
Wan, M. W., Green, J., Elsabbagh, M., et al. (2013). Quality of interaction between at-risk infants and caregiver at 12–15 months is associated with 3-year autism outcome. *Journal of Child Psychology and Psychiatry, 54*(7), 763–771.
Weiner, D. J., Wigdor, E. M., Ripke, S., Walters, R. K., Kosmicki, J. A., Grove, J., … Werge, T. (2017). Polygenic transmission disequilibrium confirms that common and rare variation act additively to create risk for autism spectrum disorders. *Nature Genetics, 49*(7), 978.
Whalen, C., Schreibman, L., & Ingersoll, B. (2006). The collateral effects of joint attention training on social initiations, positive affect, imitation, and spontaneous speech for young children with autism. *Journal of Autism and Developmental Disorders, 36*(5), 655–664.
Wing, L., & Gould, J. (1979). Severe impairments of social interaction and associated abnormalities in children: Epidemiology and classification. *Journal of Autism and Developmental Disorders, 9*(1), 11–29.
World Health Organization (1993) *The ICD-10 classification of mental and behavioural disorders: Diagnostic criteria for research*. Retrieved from http://apps.who.int/iris/handle/10665/37108.
Zerbo, O., Yoshida, C., Gunderson, E. P., Dorward, K., & Croen, L. A. (2015). Interpregnancy interval and risk of autism Spectrum disorders. *Pediatrics, 136*(4), 651.
Zwaigenbaum, L., Bryson, S. E., Brian, J., Smith, I. M., Roberts, W., Szatmari, P., … Vaillancourt, T. (2015). Stability of diagnostic assessment for autism spectrum disorder between 18 and 36 months in a high-risk cohort. *Autism Research, 9*, 790. https://doi.org/10.1002/aur.1585

Chapter 2
Criteria to Evaluate Evidence in Interventions for Children with Autism

Lauren Turner-Brown and Rachel Sandercock

Introduction

What is the best intervention for a child with autism? This question has been asked by parents, professionals, and researchers for decades. Many voices answer this question, insisting that approach A can cure ASD, that approach B is useless, and approach C is harmful. At the same time, others insist that approach A is harmful, approach B is the best for everyone, and approach C is useless. The challenge for parents and professionals asking this question is knowing who to believe and how to interpret claims. Fortunately, considerable research and rigorous reviews of that research exist to help in the process. The results of this research have shown that there is not one answer to the question asked. In this chapter, we introduce common terminology for different treatment approaches, ways their strength of evidence have been tested, and guidance on how to interpret research findings on early intervention for children with ASD.

Evaluating Research

Several groups have reviewed literature on autism interventions in an attempt to establishing which approaches are effective (and which approaches are ineffective). Examples of reviews include the National Standards Project (NSP) and the National

L. Turner-Brown (✉)
UNC TEACCH Autism Program, The University of North Carolina School of Medicine, Chapel Hill, NC, USA
e-mail: ltb@laurenturnerbrownphd.com

R. Sandercock
The University of North Carolina at Chapel Hill, Chapel Hill, NC, USA

G. Vivanti et al. (eds.), *Clinical Guide to Early Interventions for Children with Autism*, Best Practices in Child and Adolescent Behavioral Health Care,
https://doi.org/10.1007/978-3-030-41160-2_2

Professional Development Center on Autism Spectrum Disorder (NPDC), as well as reviews by the Centers for Medicare and Medicaid Services, Cochrane reviews, and the Agency for Healthcare Research and Quality (Mandell, Young, Corea, & Kimani, 2010; National Autism Center, 2009; Reichow, Hume, Barton, & Boyd, 2018; Warren et al., 2012; Wong et al., 2015). In addition to these agencies and organizations, recent reviews have also been conducted by French & Kennedy (2018) and Smith & Iadarola (2015). These reviews utilized varying criteria to evaluate evidence in the literature, with some more stringent than others, and classified intervention approaches according to the amount or strength of support determined to exist in the literature. In general, strength of evidence is determined by evaluating the *risk of bias*, i.e., the risk that a study might over- or underestimate the true intervention effect. For example, our confidence that a study provides an unbiased (and therefore credible) documentation of intervention effects is reduced when clinicians assessing intervention outcomes are aware of which intervention the participants have received, when many participants discontinue their intervention and their outcomes are not assessed, when researchers report results from some but not all outcome measures (i.e., selective outcome reporting), or when additional factors that might affect participants' outcomes are not taken into account (e.g., participants receiving additional interventions). A variety of research approaches exist to address these risks, such as "blinding" assessors, randomly allocating participants to intervention or control conditions and reporting all outcome measures for all participants even when they decide to discontinue the intervention before all the planned sessions are concluded. Box 2.1 reports common research designs to evaluate intervention effectiveness, including relevant terminology and implications for risk of bias (Barker, Pistrang, & Elliott, 2016).

Box 2.1: Key Terminologies for Intervention Research

Independent variable: The treatment or intervention that is varied by the experimenter.

Dependent variable: The measure of the independent variable's effect; in other words, the outcome measure or behaviors/skills that are changed by the intervention. (e.g., expressive language skills or frequency of aggressive behavior).

Efficacy: The performance of an intervention under ideal and controlled circumstances.

Effectiveness: The performance of an intervention under "real-world" conditions (e.g., when tested by various groups in various settings, including community settings).

Fidelity: The degree to which the intervention is delivered as described. (e.g., How well did the therapist adhere to the intended implementation of an intervention in each session?)

Intention-to-treat analysis: A conservative design approach whereby participants are compared within the groups to which they were initially randomized, independently of variations such as participants dropping out or receiving additional services. This approach protects from the risk of selectively reporting outcomes for participants who were satisfied with the intervention progress, thus inflating the intervention effect.

Quasi-experimental design: Research design that does not use random assignment to determine intervention and nonintervention groups; groups instead may be determined by naturally formed or preexisting conditions (e.g., students already attending schools A and B).

Randomized clinical trials (RCT): An experimental design that randomly assigns participants to the experimental groups or conditions (i.e., receiving the intervention vs. the control group) so that the groups will then be equivalent except for the experimental manipulation, allowing researchers to infer causality about any relationships found between an intervention and subsequent outcomes. Although this design does not eliminate external factors that contribute to variance, it eliminates the risk of a systematic bias in favor of one group through randomization.

Reliability: The degree of consistency and reproducibility of the measurement, across raters (interrater reliability) or repeated administrations (test–retest reliability); in other words, the extent to which you achieve equivalent results each time when repeating measurement in different ways.

Validity: The degree to which a tool (such as questionnaire or test) measure what it is intended to measure.

Single case/single-subject design: A research design using single participants or small groups of participants who serve as their own control to measure the effects of an intervention; outcomes are measured within-subjects (e.g., child before and after intervention begins) rather than between-subjects (e.g., comparing changes in one group that received intervention to another group that received different interventions).

Waitlist control design: A research design in which participants are either assigned to the experimental group, in which they receive an intervention immediately, or are placed on a waiting list to receive the intervention once the experimental group has completed it.

Despite the plethora of approaches used to minimize the risk that study results do not reflect true intervention effects, it is virtually impossible to eliminate all possible "confound factors" when measuring treatment outcomes, making it necessary to establish what could be considered "acceptable" versus unacceptable risks of bias in intervention evaluation research.

Notably, there is no universal consensus within the field of ASD early intervention as to what criteria should be used to evaluate the strength of evidence and determine the impact of risk of bias on the estimates of intervention effects (Vivanti et al., 2018). For example, earlier reviews of intervention approaches included single-subject or case series designs (e.g., Rogers & Vismara, 2008; see

Box 2.1 for a definition of single-subject design studies), while more recent reviews tend to exclude studies that do not have clear group comparison designs (e.g., Smith & Iadarola, 2015). While excluding single-subject designs may be more rigorous from a research methodology standpoint, many in the field take issue with this approach as the heterogeneous nature of ASD has historically lent itself to a wide body of research based on individual subjects.

Agency	Publication year	Type of review
National Research Council	2001	Broad review yielded general recommendations for types and amounts of intervention for young children with ASD.
National Standards Project	2009, 2015	Categorized interventions as *Emerging, Established,* or *Unestablished.*
National Professional Development Center	2010, 2014	Funded by Department of Education; most recently identified 24 practices as having sufficient research to be considered *evidence-based practices.*
Cochrane Reviews	Multiple	Mission to promote evidence-informed health decision-making by producing systematic reviews of research evidence. Multiple reviews on ASD treatments, including complementary treatments, medications, and behavioral interventions. For young children, one review on early intensive behavioral intervention and parent-mediated interventions.
Center for Medicare and Medicaid	2011	A review provided information to Medicaid about evidence base for a range of interventions for ASD, categorizing them as established, emerging, and unestablished.
Agency for Healthcare Research and Quality	Multiple	Comprehensive reviews of behavioral, complementary, and alternative medicine (CAM) and sensory interventions for children with ASD.

For example, the NPDC labeled an intervention approach as being an evidence-based practice if the following criteria were met in their review: at least two high-quality experimental or quasi-experimental group design articles by at least two different researchers/groups, or at least five high-quality single-subject (SS) articles by at least three different researchers with at least 20 participants across all studies, or a combination of one or more high-quality quasi-experimental or experimental group designs AND three or more high-quality SS designs by two or more researchers. Using these criteria, the NPDC identified 27 evidence-based practices (EBPs) and provided a summary table that shows for which areas of development and for which age the practices have enough evidence. Other criteria, such as the grading of recommendations assessment, development, and evaluation (GRADE system), used by the World Health Organization and Cochrane Reviews are more stringent and classifies studies that do not use randomization as at high risk of bias (see the recent review on autism early intensive behavioral intervention by Reichow et al., 2018). While each reviewing agency varied slightly in the specific criteria for setting up a practice as "evidence based," or "established," there is considerable overlap in the resulting lists of approaches with strongest research support.

These reviews are excellent places to familiarize oneself with established or promising intervention approaches. However, they exist at a certain time point and are not "living" documents. Thus, an approach may not be on the list of established practices simply because the research on that approach was conducted more recently than the review. While the number of high-quality, large studies exploring interventions for ASD is larger than for other neurodevelopmental disorders (Kasari, Gulsrud, Paparella, Hellemann, & Berry, 2015) there are considerably fewer group design studies in ASD in comparison to other mental health conditions in children. Thus, decisions about what works for children with ASD are being made based on less research than other conditions (see McGrew, Ruble, & Smith, 2016 for additional commentary).

Factors of Experimental Rigor

While the amount of research on an intervention is an important consideration, it is also important to consider the methodological strength of the existing studies when evaluating an intervention approach. This requires first assessing the research design of the studies on a particular intervention. Research design reflects the degree to which experimental control was demonstrated, which is tied to the number of participants and/or groups involved and the type of design that was used.

Importantly, however, different methodological approaches are relevant at different stages of treatment development and evaluation. The key stages in research on interventions for individuals with ASD are as follows: (a) formulation and systematic application of a new intervention technique, (b) developing a manual and research plan for evaluation of intervention across sites, (c) *randomized clinical trials* (RCT), and (d) community effectiveness studies (Smith et al., 2007; Vivanti et al., 2018). This process aims to progress steadily across a continuum of evaluation strategies, from efficacy to effectiveness trials. *Efficacy* refers to the performance of an intervention under ideal and control circumstances, while *effectiveness* refers to its performance under "real-world" conditions (Singal, Higgins, & Waljee, 2014).

The first stage in this progression aims to demonstrate that an intervention technique has the potential for therapeutic benefit. At this stage, a series of *singe-case designs* may be an appropriate approach, particularly for interventions that require significant resources or comprise novel approaches. The second and third stages focus on standardizing an intervention and then implementing the intervention in highly controlled RCTs. While efficacy studies optimize the likelihood of detecting the effects of an intervention, the use of carefully selected subject and clinicians paired with significant research oversight limits generalizability to the community. Thus, the fourth stage assesses the effectiveness of an intervention when implemented by competent clinicians in real-world settings. Finally, the last stage of intervention studies addresses the challenge of implementing findings by translating research into actual policy or practice. Additional details about these approaches follow (Fig. 2.1).

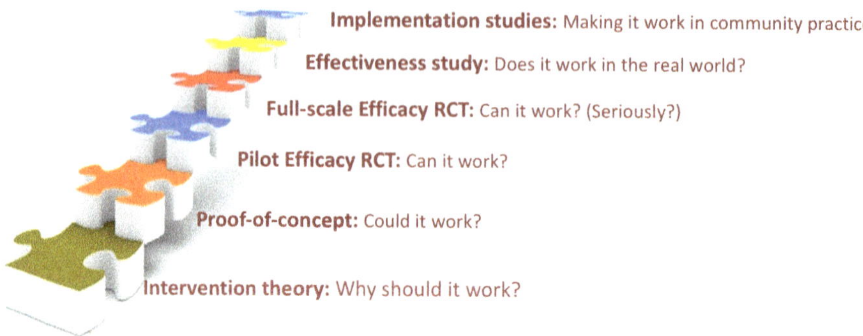

Fig. 2.1 Hierarchy of steps and associated costs of intervention, implementation, and evaluation (based on Vivanti et al., 2018). Each step is illustrated in Box 2.2

Box 2.2: Stages and Processes in Developing, Evaluating, and Implementing Interventions (Adapted from Vivanti et al., 2018)

Interventions are based on intervention *theories* which articulate the rationale for a given approach, including the definition of the hypothesized factors leading to the features being targeted and the putative processes of intervention change (Kazdin, 1999). Subsequently, *proof-of-concept* work using small-scale studies (such as single-subject designs, case series, and pilot-controlled trials) is conducted to examine preliminary evidence in support of the feasibility and potential utility of the approach, including evidence of feasible delivery, acceptability to key stakeholders and end users, as well as preliminary indication of effect in the anticipated direction. With initial support for a model, evaluation typically proceeds to *pilot testing* with larger numbers of participants, and then to *full-scale efficacy trials* with a sufficiently sized sample to establish whether or not the intervention can achieve its hypothesized effects on the target population when implemented in optimal conditions (e.g., by trained clinicians implementing the intervention to a high degree of fidelity). Interventions should then ideally be subject to tests of *effectiveness*, evaluating the extent to which the benefits documented in efficacy trials are maintained when early intervention is implemented in the "real world" (rather than artificial settings, such as highly resourced University labs), by professionals who implement the intervention in the context of the complex needs, the large caseload, and the less resources available in community settings. Finally, *implementation science* addresses how to ensure the successful implementation of the intervention within community settings by systematically examining the barriers and facilitators to adopting the intervention and delivering to a high degree of fidelity.

Research Design

Single-subject designs are tightly controlled studies that explore specific changes in observable behavior when an intervention is introduced and taken away. These designs can be quite useful if results are replicated across different participants, different conditions, and/or different measures of the target outcome(s) (Horner et al., 2005). To ensure that single-subject studies are as methodologically sound as possible, guidelines exist on how to best enact them. For example, it is important to establish a clear baseline period during which the individual receives no intervention to allow for pre-treatment measurement. Maintaining continuous data collection throughout the baseline and intervention periods then allows clear evidence that the intervention leads to changes in the outcome measures. Pre- and posttreatment assessment should also be conducted by someone with no knowledge of whether or not the individual is currently receiving the intervention and who is unaware of the target outcomes (Smith et al., 2007).

A *randomized clinical trial* (RCT; see key terminology) is the most rigorous experimental design, with multiple participant groups randomly assigned to control (i.e., nontreatment) and intervention conditions simultaneously across multiple implementation sites. Random assignment is beneficial as it increases the likelihood that experimental groups are not significantly different from one another at the outset, and thus changes that occur following the start of the intervention can be more confidently assumed to be a direct result of the intervention itself. A *quasi-experimental design* utilizes treatment and control groups but differs from an RCT in that it lacks the element of random assignment. The lack of random assignment in quasi-experimental designs makes it more difficult to assume that the intervention and control groups are similar (e.g., on levels of symptom severity or ability level on the target skill), pretreatment. However, such approaches are often more viable in clinical or community settings. For example, it can be challenging to randomly assign children to schools; thus, this approach is common for research conducted in school settings. *Waitlist control designs* are one type of quasi-experiment that functions well in such settings. Waitlist control designs allow researchers to assign participants to an intervention in accordance to need while maintaining a wait-list of individuals who will serve as the control group while they are not receiving the intervention. Those placed on the waitlist eventually receive the intervention in a later iteration. This approach allows comparisons between groups while also ensuring that all participants receive clinical services.

Measurement

It is next important to consider how the intervention and child outcomes are measured. To provide evidence in support of an intervention, a study must clearly define its *independent variable*—in other words, how the intervention is implemented.

This requires establishing and maintaining adequate levels of adherence to intervention protocols *(i.e., fidelity)* by providers, as well as having a clear system in place to reliably collect data about how those providers implement the intervention. Accurate and reliable measurement of the intervention targets (e.g., language or play or social skills) is even more essential, as outcome data provide the clearest indication of intervention efficacy. This measurement requires strong objective tests or measures. A strong measure should have established *reliability*, meaning it is consistent in what it measures across people and within the items included in the measure. It should also be *valid*, meaning it measures what intends to. For example, a strong measure of language outcomes should accurately measure language skills (as opposed to motor skills) and be consistent (the child's score would be the same if he took the test a week later). Additionally, when members of the study team are measuring outcomes, strong research ensures that the people who are measuring outcomes are not the same people who implemented the intervention (evaluators are *blind*), and, ideally, do not know whether a participant received an intervention or the hypotheses of the study. This control is critical to reducing bias in intervention research.

Many interventions target multiple skill areas. Thus, ensuring that researchers have measured outcomes for all areas targeted or hypothesized to change based on the researcher's *theory of change* is important (see Vivanti et al., 2018; Colombi et al., 2019, for additional information about theoretical perspectives). To demonstrate efficacy, the data collected must effectively capture the target skill or behavior. For example, in a study of an intervention that specifically targets receptive language, measured outcomes must include what language the child understands, as opposed to a measure of the child's vocalizations produced. Often, interventions in ASD aim to change several areas simultaneously (e.g., language, social, and cognitive skills). As such, an intervention may not be equally efficacious for all treatment targets, but we are able to glean from these studies an understanding of what aspects or domains of an intervention are and are not functioning as intended.

Participants

When judging the quality of intervention research, also consider how participants were ascertained. It is important to note whether participant diagnostic categorization aligns with *DSM-5* (American Psychiatric Association, 2013) and/or *ICD-10* (World Health Organization, 1992) criteria. The extent to which comorbidities that were included or excluded from research samples is an additional important consideration. Often, children with common comorbidities, such as epilepsy or intellectual disability, are excluded to create a more homogeneous research sample. However, this is problematic as it may affect how reflective these samples are of a given community or clinic population and fails to provide information about the extent to which children with more treatment needs would benefit from the intervention in question.

Another important question when evaluating intervention research is whether well-established diagnostic tools were used to determine participant eligibility. The *Autism Diagnostic Observation Schedule–2nd Edition* (Lord et al., 2012) and *Autism Diagnostic Interview–Revised* (Rutter, Le Couteur, & Lord, 2003) are typically considered "gold standard" measures for supporting diagnoses of ASD; however, these measures require significant training to administer reliably. Consequently, studies may opt to use diagnostic tools or screeners that require fewer resources. Studies that do not use ADOS-2 or ADI-R may still be very informative about an intervention's utility, but one should be aware that participant diagnostic characterization may be more limited than in studies that include more established assessment tools.

Generalization of intervention effects is also a key consideration. Examining how and to what extent researchers attempted to assess maintenance of effects, postintervention, speaks directly to an intervention's practical utility for a child. Also consider if and how intervention effects were demonstrated across settings, stimuli, responses, or participants. This is particularly relevant given the heterogeneous nature of ASD. While research provides information about whether an intervention works at the group level, these types of studies are not able to account for the individual differences that may come into play for a particular child. By keeping these factors in mind when examining the empirical support for an intervention, it will be easier to differentiate quality research from unsound or misleading research. While many emerging early intervention approaches for ASD may not have a large *quantity* of supporting research, it is as—if not more—important to consider the *quality* of the work that does exist before recommending an intervention.

Targeted Outcomes

Due to the heterogeneity of the diagnosis, ASD poses a unique challenge in determining targeted treatment outcomes, whereas some children may have average or near-average cognitive and language abilities, others may be severely impaired; the severity level of social deficits, restricted interests, and repetitive behaviors also vary widely. The prevalence of comorbid disorders, such as anxiety and ADHD, further complicates the picture. As a result, it is impossible to establish "one size fits all" goals and highlights the importance of considering the heterogeneity of the research sample used to evaluate an intervention. When recommending an intervention to a family, a primary goal should be to meet the demonstrated needs of the child. This requires selecting an intervention that is well matched to the outcomes that would be most beneficial to the child, while also considering the treatment targets the family views as the highest priority. The area of greatest impairment may not always align with the highest priority for a family at a given time point; for example, it may seem that increasing language and communication skills for a nonverbal child would be the most essential treatment target, whereas the caregivers may feel that improving independent play skills so that they are able to attend to siblings or get other tasks done is the most urgent need. It is therefore important to balance the individual needs of the child with the needs of the family.

In studying an intervention, the developmental or behavioral outcomes measured serve as the dependent variable. Developmental outcomes focus on improving functioning in the domains of cognitive ability, communication, social interaction, play, and/or motor skills. Target skills to increase can include communication, higher cognitive function, interpersonal skills, learning readiness, motor skills, personal responsibility, play, self-regulation, joint attention, school readiness skills, and self-help/adaptive behaviors. Interventions may aim to increase skills in a variety of settings, such as home, school, and in the community. These variables may be measured in a variety of ways, including discrete behaviors (e.g., verbalizations, social initiations), standardized assessments (e.g., IQ testing), or parent/teacher behavioral ratings (Wong et al., 2015). While some intervention targets aim to increase developmentally appropriate skills, others aim to improve functioning by decreasing challenging or interfering behaviors (National Autism Center, 2009). Challenging behaviors—such as noncompliance or emotional outbursts—are commonly targeted for decrease; decreasing repetitive behaviors and sensory-seeking or sensory-averse behaviors such as pinching or screaming and covering one's ears may also be goals of intervention (National Autism Center, 2009; Wong et al., 2015).

Finally, some interventions target parents directly, whether to teach parents new skills or to improve parent and/or family well-being (Wong et al., 2015). As parent stress is typically quite high for parents of young children with ASD (Schieve, Blumberg, Rice, Visser, & Boyle, 2007), interventions that either directly target parent well-being or have established evidence to decrease parent stress may be important to consider alongside child outcomes (Kasari et al., 2015).

Individualization and Implementation Factors

Considering the fit for an individual child and the viability of implementation are key determinants in selecting an appropriate intervention. As previously addressed, it is important to select developmentally appropriate outcome targets that suit the needs of an individual child. However, it is also essential to consider the age range for which an intervention is intended, as well as the ages of the participants included in research trials. For children with ASD, developmental age may not always be equivalent to chronological age due to pervasive delays that may be present across domains. As such, consider not only a child's numerical age and the recommended age range for an intervention but also the child's current functioning level. Identifying the baseline skills (e.g., expressive language level) required for a particular intervention is essential to determining best fit. For example, an intervention shown to be effective with children with average to above average cognitive abilities may be less beneficial for a same aged child with far fewer base skills; likewise, an intervention intended for toddlers may also be efficacious for an older child with profound delays. Additionally, the extent to which a treatment style matches chronological age norms should be considered. For example, an intervention that utilizes sensory games or physical contact (e.g., tickling) would not be a good fit for an adolescent, as encouraging these behaviors in an older child would be inappropriate even if the mental age is more closely aligned to an infant/toddler level of functioning.

Accessibility and implementation of an intervention are also key factors. First, recognize that access to a desired treatment may not be equally feasible for all families due to location and/or financial resources. In many cases, the intervention ultimately selected may not be the ideal; however, one should strive to recommend a treatment that is the best possible fit for the desired treatment outcomes within the limitations of access and availability. Also consider the setting in which the family is seeking treatment: is a clinic-, school-, or home-based approach most suited to their needs? If the intention is for an intervention to be moved from the setting in which it was developed into a different setting (e.g., from a clinic setting into a home setting) due to access or family preference, is it important to consider whether or that there is existing evidence to support generalization to the alternative setting (Callahan, Henson, & Cowan, 2008).

The feasibility of implementing an intervention may also be limited by resource and provider constraints. An intervention that requires highly specialized materials or equipment is less likely to be available to most families or community providers (Wong et al., 2015). The required practitioner skill level needed to administer an intervention can also be a barrier. High-quality intervention research often involves carefully trained practitioners with ongoing fidelity checks; while this provides a standard of desired competence, it may be unrealistic to expect the same level of rigorous training in the community. Research that includes generalization in the community provides a better estimate of how an intervention will perform outside of controlled settings. Moreover, it may be difficult to find a practitioner who can implement an intervention if that intervention requires extensive specialized training.

Parent involvement is another important consideration in selecting an intervention. Some interventions may require more or less active involvement from parents than others, and parent commitment to treatment and availability to take part should inform intervention recommendations. For example, an intervention that requires a parent to be present at the same time several days a week may simply not be feasible for many working families. Naturalistic approaches are often considered more "family friendly," as parents can implement strategies during everyday routines, such as meals and playtime (Mcgee & Morrier, 2005; Schreibman et al., 2015). The individual outcome goals will also determine the extent of parent involvement. Parent coaching models targeting challenging behaviors or noncompliance, for example, require the presence of a parent at each treatment session. Interventions built around developmental goals, such as communication or play skills, however, may allow for more flexibility in shaping the amount of parent involvement to fit the needs and availability of an individual family.

Unsupported Treatments

While it is useful to become familiar with up-to-date evidence about interventions, the loudest voices in many communities are proponents of interventions that may have never been studied in any formal way. These approaches are sometimes characterized as complementary and alternative medicine (CAM), and research suggests that between 50% and 92% of children with ASD have tried or are actively using one of these approaches (Hanson et al., 2007; Harrington, Rosen, Garnecho, & Patrick, 2006).

One challenge with CAM or other unsupported approaches is the risk of placebo effect. A classic example in the ASD field is research on the effects of secretin on children with ASD: anecdotal reports from families were highlighted in the media to suggest that the intravenous infusion of synthetic human secretin significantly reduced symptoms of ASD. A double-blind, placebo-control RCT was then conducted and concluded no treatment effects of secretin on a variety of clinical outcomes. The percentage of children who showed significant improvements while in the placebo condition was comparable to those in the treatment condition (Williams et al., 2012). Seeing change in the presence of no treatment seems surprising, but other studies have demonstrated a placebo-like response using parent report measures even in the absence of treatment (Jones, Carberry, Hamo, & Lord, 2017). It is possible that parents' hope for change or additional attention leads to changes in how they report about their child in these studies.

A second challenge with CAM or other unsupported approaches is the safety of children. Many families will try a gluten-free diet based on stories of success from other families affected by ASD. Research studies of this diet have been conducted, and, for the most part, have shown no clinically significant effects of these diets (Piwowarczyk, Horvath, Łukasik, Pisula, & Szajewska, 2018). Yet these studies have also shown that there are no clear adverse effects of taking gluten out of the diet. Thus, the risk is minimal (aside from cost, effort, and potential impact on social opportunities involved in maintaining a strict diet, e.g., preventing a child to join a birthday party where other children are eating the cake as the diet precludes eating cake). In contrast, there are treatments that carry more significant risks to the overall health of children. For example, chelation is a treatment that some claim removes toxins from the blood (e.g., mercury) of children with ASD, and that this toxin removal leads to symptom improvement in the children. Minimal quality research has been conducted and the highest quality study conducted demonstrated no significant treatment effects (James, Williams, Silove, & Stevenson, 2015). Further, there are reports of significant health risks associated with chelation, including death (Brown, Willis, Omalu, & Leiker, 2006).

In one secretin study, 69% of families indicated that they were still interested in trying secretin after learning it was not effective (Sandler et al., 1999). The popularity of unsupported treatments is due in part to the fact that the precise etiology of ASD is still unclear, driving the spread of possible theories and corresponding remedies. The complex nature of ASD also creates many areas of need, which may drive caregivers to seek treatments beyond what supported interventions are able to address (Smith & Wick, 2008). Additionally, caregivers may hear more about unsupported treatments than about evidence-based interventions, particularly through anecdotal channels, such as social media. Often, these treatment approaches are paired with words like "cure" or "healing," which understandably draw in families who are desperate for answers. Novel unsupported treatments often receive more media attention, as well, and the sense of being antagonized by the "establishment" may help to fuel emotionally engaging and persuasive elements of these treatments (Smith, 2015). If the treatment offers hope for improvement, families may want to try it. Therefore, physicians must be able to speak knowledgeably about these unconventional treatments, especially if those treatments may pose significant risk of injury or death (Harrington et al., 2006).

Conclusion

In summary, there are great resources available for professionals and/or parents to read and explore that provide information about evidence-based intervention approaches and how to implement them. Paying attention to the methods a program uses to evaluate its effects (e.g., type of study, what outcomes were measured, etc.) can help one distinguish between an approach that is popular but likely not effective and one that may have a real chance to change outcomes for a child. While there is a growing body of research on what works for children with ASD, the field continues to fall behind other mental health conditions in terms of the number of large, high-quality studies of different approaches. The individual differences in children with ASD can contribute to challenges establishing firm evidence that an approach is effective for such a diverse group of individuals. Therefore, attending to both quantity and quality of research on an approach and the outcomes that seem most relevant to a child and family are all critical. Finally, in addition to reading literature and examining evidence, it is critical to listen to families about their preferences and make efforts to align recommendations to those preferences. The high rate with which families seek unsupported treatments highlights the impact of sharing success stories in addition to scientific findings.

References

American Psychiatric Association. (2013). *Diagnostic and statistical manual of mental disorders* (5th ed.). Arlington, VA: American Psychiatric Publishing.

Barker, C., Pistrang, N., & Elliott, R. (2016). *Research methods in clinical psychology* (3rd ed.). West Sussex, UK: John Wiley and Son, Ltd..

Brown, M. J., Willis, T., Omalu, B., & Leiker, R. (2006). Deaths resulting from hypocalcemia after administration of edetate disodium: 2003–2005. *Pediatrics, 118*(2), e534–e536. https://doi.org/10.1542/peds.2006-0858

Callahan, K., Henson, R. K., & Cowan, A. K. (2008). Social validation of evidence-based practices in autism by parents, teachers, and administrators. *Journal of Autism and Developmental Disorders, 38*(4), 678–692. https://doi.org/10.1007/s10803-007-0434-9

Colombi, C., Vivanti, G., & Rogers, S. (2019). Evidenced-based practices. In R. Rieske (Ed.), *Handbook of interdisciplinary treatments for autism spectrum disorder*. Cham: Autism and Child Psychopathology Series. Springer.

French, L., & Kennedy, E. M. M. (2018). Annual research review: Early intervention for infants and young children with, or at-risk of, autism spectrum disorder: A systematic review. *Journal of Child Psychology and Psychiatry, 59*(4), 444–456. https://doi.org/10.1111/jcpp.12828

Hanson, E., Kalish, L. A., Bunce, E., Curtis, C., McDaniel, S., Ware, J., & Petry, J. (2007). Use of complementary and alternative medicine among children diagnosed with autism spectrum disorder. *Journal of Autism and Developmental Disorders, 37*(4), 628–636. https://doi.org/10.1007/s10803-006-0192-0

Harrington, J. W., Rosen, L., Garnecho, A. N. A., & Patrick, P. a. (2006). Parental perceptions and use of complementary and alternative medicine practices for children with autistic spectrum disorders in private practice. *Journal of Developmental and Behavioral Pediatrics: JDBP, 27*(2 Suppl), S156–S161. https://doi.org/10.1097/00004703-200604002-00014

Horner, R. H., Carr, E. G., Halle, J., McGee, G., Odom, S., & Wolery, M. (2005). The use of single subject research to identify evidence-based practice in special education. *Exceptional Children, 71*(2), 165–191. https://doi.org/10.1177/001440290507100203

James, S., Williams, K., Silove, N., & Stevenson, S. W. (2015). Chelation for autism spectrum disorder (ASD). *Cochrane Database of Systematic Reviews, 2015*(5), CD010766. https://doi.org/10.1002/14651858.CD010766

Jones, R. M., Carberry, C., Hamo, A., & Lord, C. (2017). Placebo-like response in absence of treatment in children with Autism. *Autism Research, 10*(9), 1567–1572. https://doi.org/10.1002/aur.1798

Kasari, C., Gulsrud, A., Paparella, T., Hellemann, G., & Berry, K. (2015). Randomized comparative efficacy study of parent-mediated interventions for toddlers with autism. *Journal of Consulting and Clinical Psychology, 83*(3), 554–563. https://doi.org/10.1037/a0039080

Kazdin, A. E. (1999). The meanings and measurement of clinical significance. *Journal of Consulting and Clinical Psychology, 67*(3), 332–339.

Lord, C., Rutter, M., Dilavore, P., Risi, S., Gotham, K., & Bishop, S. L. (2012). *Autism diagnostic observation schedule: ADOS-2*. Los Angeles, CA: Western Psychological Services.

Mandell, D., Young, J., Corea, C., & Kimani, J. (2010). Autism spectrum disorders (ASDs) services project. *Centers for Medicare and Medicaid Services*, 1–120. Retrieved from https://www.impaqint.com/sites/default/files/project-reports/Autism_Spectrum_Disorders.pdf.

Mcgee, G. G., & Morrier, M. J. (2005). Preparation of autism specialists. In F. R. Volkmar, R. Paul, A. Klin, & D. Cohen (Eds.), *Handbook of autism and pervasive developmental disorders* (3rd ed.). Hoboken, NJ: John Wiley and Sons.

McGrew, J. H., Ruble, L. A., & Smith, I. M. (2016). Autism spectrum disorder and evidence-based practice in psychology. *Clinical Psychology: Science and Practice, 23*(3), 239–255. https://doi.org/10.1111/cpsp.12160

National Autism Center. (2009). *Findings and conclusions: National standards project, phase 1*. MA: Randolf.

National Autism Center. (2015). *Findings and conclusions: National standards project, phase 2*. MA: Randolf.

National Research Council. (2001). *Educating children with autism*. Washington, DC: National Academy Press.

Piwowarczyk, A., Horvath, A., Łukasik, J., Pisula, E., & Szajewska, H. (2018). Gluten- and casein-free diet and autism spectrum disorders in children: A systematic review. *European Journal of Nutrition, 57*(2), 433–440. https://doi.org/10.1007/s00394-017-1483-2

Reichow, B., Hume, K. A., Barton, E. E., & Boyd, B. A. (2018). Early intensive behavioral intervention (EIBI) for young children with autism spectrum disorder (ASD). *Cochrane Database of Systematic Reviews, 5*, CD009260. https://doi.org/10.1002/14651858.CD009260.pub3

Rogers, S. J., & Vismara, L. A. (2008). Evidence-based comprehensive treatments for early autism. *Journal of Clinical Child and Adolescent Psychology, 37*, 8–38. https://doi.org/10.1080/15374410701817808

Rutter, M., Le Couteur, A., & Lord, C. (2003). Autism diagnostic interview—revised. Los Angeles, CA: Western Psychological Services.

Sandler, A. D., Sutton, K. A., DeWeese, J., Girardi, M. A., Sheppard, V., & Bodfish, J. W. (1999). Lack of benefit of a single dose of synthetic human secretin in the treatment of autism and pervasive developmental disorder. *The New England Journal of Medicine, 341*(24), 1801–1806. Retrieved from http://www.ncbi.nlm.nih.gov/entrez/query.fcgi?cmd=Retrieve&db=PubMed&dopt=Citation&list_uids=10588965.

Schieve, L. A., Blumberg, S. J., Rice, C., Visser, S. N., & Boyle, C. (2007). The relationship between autism and parenting stress. *Pediatrics, 119*(Supplement 1), S114–S121. https://doi.org/10.1542/peds.2006-2089q

Schreibman, L., Dawson, G., Stahmer, A. C., Landa, R., Rogers, S. J., McGee, G. G., … Halladay, A. (2015). Naturalistic developmental behavioral interventions: Empirically validated treatments for autism spectrum disorder. *Journal of Autism and Developmental Disorders, 45*(8), 2411–2428. https://doi.org/10.1007/s10803-015-2407-8

Singal, A. G., Higgins, P. D. R., & Waljee, A. K. (2014). A primer on effectiveness and efficacy trials. *Clinical and Translational Gastroenterology, 5*(2), e45–e44. https://doi.org/10.1038/ctg.2013.13

Smith, T. (2015). The appeal of unvalidated treatments. In R. M. Foxx & J. A. Mulick (Eds.), *Controversial therapies for autism and intellectual disabilities: Fad, fashion, and science in professional practice*. London: Routledge.

Smith, T., & Iadarola, S. (2015). Evidence base update for autism spectrum disorder evidence base update for autism spectrum disorder. *HCAP, 44*(6), 897–922. https://doi.org/10.1080/15374416.2015.1077448

Smith, T., Scahill, L., Dawson, G., Guthrie, D., Lord, C., Odom, S., … Wagner, A. (2007). Designing research studies on psychosocial interventions in autism. *Journal of Autism and Developmental Disorders, 37*(2), 354–366. https://doi.org/10.1007/s10803-006-0173-3

Smith, T., & Wick, J. (2008). Controversial treatments. In K. Chawarska, A. Klin, & F. R. Volkmar (Eds.), *Autism spectrum disorders in infants and toddlers: Diagnosis, assessment, and treatment* (pp. 243–273). New York: Guilford Press.

Vivanti, G., Kasari, C., Green, J., Mandell, D., Maye, M., & Hudry, K. (2018). Implementing and evaluating early intervention for children with autism: Where are the gaps and what should we do? *Autism Research, 11*(1), 16–23. https://doi.org/10.1002/aur.1900

Warren, Z., Veenstra-Vander Weele, J., Stone, W., Bruzek, J. L., Nahmias, A. S., Foss-Feig, J. H., … McPheeters, M. L. (2012). Therapies for children with autism spectrum disorders. *American Family Physician, 85*(9), 878–879.

Williams, K., Wray, J. A., & Wheeler, D. M. (2012). Intravenous secretin for autism spectrum disorders (ASD). *Cochrane Database of Systematic Reviews, 4*, CD003495.

Wong, C., Odom, S. L., Hume, K. A., Cox, A. W., Fettig, A., Kucharczyk, S., … Schultz, R. T. (2015). Evidence-based practices for children, youth, and young adults with autism spectrum disorder: A comprehensive review. *Journal of Autism and Developmental Disorders, 45*(7), 1951–1966. https://doi.org/10.1007/s10803-014-2351-z

World Health Organization. (1992). *International classification of diseases and related health problems (10th rev)*. Geneva, Switzerland: WHO.

Chapter 3
Understanding and Addressing Social Communication Difficulties in Children with Autism

Kristen Bottema-Beutel

Atypical social communication profiles represent one of the two domains that define autism spectrum disorder (ASD). According to the DSM-5 (American Psychiatric Association, 2013; see Chap. 1), the social communication domain involves differences in three areas: (a) social–emotional reciprocity within interpersonal interactions, (b) the use and interpretation of nonverbal communication, and (c) the development and maintenance of relationships with others. This chapter will focus on the developmental trajectory of social communication milestones, and the intervention strategies used to support social communication development in children with ASD.

While all communications are inherently social, *social communication* is a term that refers to instances when communicative repertoires are deployed for the primary purpose of sharing with, and relating to, others. This is distinguished from communication for more instrumental or utilitarian purposes, such as requesting desired items or regulating others' behavior. Social–communication is separated out in nosology of ASD because this form of communication is more impaired in children with ASD as compared to other forms (Shumway & Wetherby, 2009; Wetherby, 2006), and is more difficult to influence via intervention (Yoder et al., 2015). Further, the social dimension of communication in particular is implicated in other aspects of social functioning more broadly (Bottema-Beutel, Kim, & Crowley, 2019). For example, response to joint attention in early childhood is correlated with adult social skills (Gillespie-Lynch et al., 2012). It should however be acknowledged that the line between social and instrumental communication is not always clear cut. Further,

---

The original version of this chapter was revised. The correction to this chapter is available at https://doi.org/10.1007/978-3-030-41160-2_11

K. Bottema-Beutel (✉)
Lynch School of Education and Human Development, Boston College, Chestnut Hill, MA, USA
e-mail: botteabe@bc.edu

G. Vivanti et al. (eds.), *Clinical Guide to Early Interventions for Children with Autism*, Best Practices in Child and Adolescent Behavioral Health Care,
https://doi.org/10.1007/978-3-030-41160-2_3

this distinction becomes less conceptually sound beyond the preschool period when interactions become more complex, and assigning single motives to communicative acts is not always feasible. Still, this distinction is useful for understanding early development in ASD and the features of communication that are most affected.

Characterizing the Social–Communication Domain in ASD

Social communication—and social functioning more broadly—is highly heterogeneous in ASD. In the late 1970s, Lorna Wing described three distinct social profiles that were noted in a survey of children with ASD (Wing & Gould, 1979). She termed these *active-odd, aloof,* and *passive*. Active-odd children often made social overtures, but did so in a way that was atypical and did not always achieve engagement from an interaction partner (e.g., approaching another child multiple times and talking to them about cars, even after they did not express interest). Aloof children tended to avoid social interaction and seemed to have developed a preference for aloneness. Finally, passive children did not seek out interactions with others, but neither did they avoid interactions when they were approached. Since this early characterization, researchers have attempted to more precisely describe features of social communication in ASD with the goal of capturing ASD-distinctive patterns, subgroups within the ASD population, and specific intervention targets.

Social–communication comprises a complex interplay of developmental achievements. There is no universal agreement about the nature and mechanisms of social–communication, and different approaches have been used to investigate this area, with some research focusing on discrete "skills" within the social communication domain, and others using a more holistic, interactional approach (e.g., Hobson, 2007; Sterponi, de Kirby, & Shankey, 2015). Evidence suggests that both conceptualizations may be useful for characterizing social communication in ASD. For example, Bishop and colleagues (2016) used factor analysis to identify two subdomains of social communication; they termed these *basic social communication* and *interaction quality*. Basic social communication refers to more discrete, within-child behavior repertoires, including the use of eye contact, display of emotion using facial expressions, and sharing enjoyment with others. Interaction quality refers to *dyadic* characteristics of interaction, including reciprocity, conversation quality, and the development of rapport within interaction.

However, an overfocus on discrete, piecemeal behaviors can be misleading (although this approach has certainly dominated the ASD literature in the recent past). It is important to remember that, even if identifying isolated behavior is helpful for diagnosing ASD, actual human social interaction does not involve the simple expression and reception of discrete social behaviors. Rather, social interaction is multimodal, contextually situated, and sequential, and an appreciation of these aspects is critical for understanding both the nature of social communication differences in ASD and how best to support children in relation to these differences.

While many professionals who are familiar with the concept of social communication understand multimodality (i.e., the communicative relevance of bodily and gestural actions in addition to spoken language), and the contextual nature of social meanings (i.e., that words will have different meanings in different contexts), they may be less familiar with the sequential nature of interaction. That is, communicative acts project and constrain the subsequent communicative acts of an interaction partner, and are projected and constrained by communicative acts that have come before (Schegloff, 2007). Because of this reality, it is rarely useful to consider communicative behavior as a strictly "within-child" phenomenon that is a direct manifestation of cognitive capacities (Sterponi, de Kirby, & Shankey, 2015). Instead, communicative acts should be considered interactional achievements where all social partners are at least partially implicated in their production (Schegloff, 1982; Sterponi & Fasulo, 2010). For example, echolalia, which is the repetition of the speech of others, was long considered to be nonsocial and emblematic of disengagement with others (Kanner, 1943). However, Sterponi and Shankey (2014), building on Prizant and Duchan's (1981) work, offer a reappraisal of echolalia that illustrates how close analysis of the interactive contexts in which echolalia is produced show that these utterances are often sensitive to the social context, are projected as relevant responses by the child's interaction partners (i.e., interaction partners design their overtures so that an echolalic response the child is known to produce is a suitable response), and responsive to prior utterances. Therefore, echolalia should be considered a communicative resource. Prior to this reconceptualization, echolalia was considered a target for remediation.

A variety of instruments are used to characterize social communication in young children with ASD. Three of the most common are the *Vineland Adaptive Communication Scales* (VABS-II; socialization and communication domains), the *Communication and Symbolic Behavior Scales,* and the *Early Social Communication Scales* (Mundy et al., 2003). During early development, it is important to use instruments that differentiate communication from language, and that differentiate social communication from communication more generally (as do the three instruments just mentioned). See Anagnostou et al., 2015 for an overview of social communication measurement systems that are relevant to the study of ASD.

Social Communication Development in Typical Development and ASD

Prelinguistic Development in TD Children

Social–communication development begins shortly after birth, when infants show a propensity to orient to the social overture of others. Within the first days, infants show preferential looking to faces as compared to other aspects of their environment, and a preference for their mothers' voice as compared to other voices (DeCasper & Fifer, 1980; Frank, Vul, & Johnson, 2009). Eventually, infants begin to respond to adult bids for interaction and develop the ability to temporally coordinate their actions with their caregivers, such as by smiling or cooing in response to caregiver's smiles, vocalizations, and infant directed speech (Abney, Warlaumont, Oller, Wallot, & Kello, 2016). This form of dyadic engagement with a caregiver is termed *primary intersubjectivity* (Trevarthen, 1979), or what Bakeman and Adamson (1984) refer to as *person* engagement. According to Trevarthen, this involves adapting intentional actions to incorporate the intentional actions of interaction partners. As noted by Tomasello (2019), engagement in these "protoconversations" provides a foundation for more advanced cooperative activities, including actual (verbal) conversations and joint activities (e.g., building a lego tower with a peer).

At around 6 months, infants are able to respond to bids for *joint attention* as they begin to shift their attention between a caregiver and an object or event, following a caregiver's directive (Scaife & Bruner, 1975). At around 9 months, infants can direct their caregiver's attention toward interesting objects and events using prelinguistic gestures, vocalizations, and eye gaze (Leekam & Moore, 2001). These joint attention processes mark a progression from *dyadic* to *triadic* interactions that incorporate aspects of the environment into interactional repertoires (Mundy, 2016). Trevarthen (1987) refers to this set of developmental achievements as *secondary intersubjectivity*. Bakeman and Adamson (1984) describe a similar phenomenon, which they term *joint engagement*. They use this term to refer to prolonged interactions between caregivers and children that involve reciprocity within play activities, and shifting attention back and forth to one another at relevant moments within the interaction. The amount of time children spend in this type of engagement with their caregivers increases in the second half of the first year, and into the second year (Bakeman & Adamson, 1984; Carpenter, Nagell, Tomasello, Butterworth, & Moore, 1998). These joint attention and engagement activities set the stage for the onset and continuing development of language, which will be discussed below.

Prelinguistic Development in Children with ASD

Because children are usually not reliably diagnosed with ASD until after their second birthday, it has been challenging for researchers to study the developmental trajectory of early social communication in this population. However, there are at least two strategies for gaining insight into the prediagnostic period in ASD (see Yirmiya & Charman, 2010 for a comprehensive review of this work). The first is to examine home video recordings produced prior to the child's second year. This line of research has shown that a variety of social communication behaviors are reduced in frequency or absent in infants later diagnosed with ASD, joint attention, using and responding to gestures, intentional communication, expressions of emotion, and social orienting to others. These findings have been replicated across several studies using this method. It should however be noted that there are some drawbacks to using home video recordings as a data source, such as a lack of standardization of the measurement context (Yirmiya & Charman, 2010).

The second strategy to studying the early period of ASD development leverages the heritable nature of ASD. That is, 20% of infants who have an older sibling diagnosed with ASD will go on to be diagnosed themselves (Ozonoff et al., 2011). Given the relatively high probability of subsequent diagnosis for infant siblings, researchers can collect data on large groups of these infants and then retain data on participants that do go on to develop ASD for longitudinal analyses (Zwaigenbaum et al., 2007). Given the prospective nature of this method, more sophisticated and standardized data collection techniques have been used as compared to home videos, including eye-tracking technology. Several studies using this technology have found that, prior to the first birthday, infants later diagnosed with ASD attend less to social scenes than do children who are not eventually diagnosed with ASD (Chawarska, Macari, & Shic, 2013; Falck-Ytter, et al., 2018). An early eye-tracking study has also suggested that infant siblings who go on to be diagnosed with ASD show a decline in gaze to their caregiver's eyes from the period between 3 and 6 months, while typically developing infants increase their gaze to caregivers' eyes over the same time period (Jones & Klin, 2013). Additional research has documented that at 10 months, infants later diagnosed with ASD are less likely to initiate joint attention episodes with a social partner when observing an interesting novel event (Nyström et al., 2019). This could mean that early differences in engagement with social stimuli are foundational to the developmental trajectory of ASD. Importantly, children with ASD continue to show differences in gaze patterns throughout early childhood and into adulthood. This includes differences in looking patterns in response to gestures and speech, and atypical gaze shifts to features of the environment and to people when viewing a social scene (Davis & Carter, 2014; Klin, Jones, Schultz, & Volkmar, 2003; see Hamner & Vivanti, 2019, for a review on eye-tracking studies in ASD).

Another early emerging difference in children with ASD is a decreased propensity for imitation as compared to typically developing children (see Vivanti & Hamilton, 2014 for a review). This difference is particularly noteworthy, as imitating others is a resource by which young children engage in reciprocal interactions with caregivers. Indeed, propensity for imitation in children with ASD is highly correlated with overall social functioning (Bottema-Beutel, Kim, & Crowley, 2019), as well as treatment outcomes (Vivanti et al., 2013; Smith, Klorman, & Mruzek, 2015). Children with ASD also show differences in pretend play by the second year and seem to engage in less pretense than their typically developing peers (Barbaro & Dissanayake, 2013). Hobson and colleagues found preliminary evidence that, later in childhood, pretend play is correlated with communication and social interaction (Hobson, Hobson, Malik, Bargiota, & Caló 2013).

These early social communication milestones have received much attention in early developmental research because they appear to differentiate children with ASD from typically developing and intellectually disabled children and/or because they predict later developmental achievements in children with ASD. Interestingly, there is some evidence that early joint engagement processes are even more tightly linked to later developmental milestones, such as language and social functioning, in children with ASD as compared to children who are typically developing (Bottema-Beutel, 2016; Bottema-Beutel, Woynaroski et al., 2019). This could be because children with ASD spend less time jointly engaged with caregivers, which may make each episode more crucial for development (Adamson et al., 2008). It should be noted however, that not all children who receive an ASD diagnosis in early or later childhood show these early social communication differences.

Language and Conversational Development in Typically Developing Children

Starting in the second year, typically developing children incorporate spoken language into their communicative repertoires. This begins with *holophrases*, or one word utterances that are imbued with the meaning of fully formed sentences, and can be used for a variety of interactional and pragmatic purposes. Later in the second year, children begin to combine words together, and eventually develop phrase and sentential speech. During this time, children are also increasingly able to integrate gaze, expression, and emerging vocabulary, and engage in increasingly complex interactions. By the end of the preschool period, children have acquired large vocabularies, and are able to combine words using complex syntactic structures which can be used flexibly across discourse contexts (Tager-Flusberg et al., 2009).

Pragmatics refers to aspects of language as it is actually used (rather than its structural properties), and foregrounds the social context in which language is produced as constitutive of meaning. Pragmatic development is the process by which children learn to formulate their own talk, and understand others' talk, according to the social context. For example, when children incorporate "slang" terms when interacting with peers, but not with their teachers, this would reflect their pragmatic development. This domain of development continues long after the onset of speech (and even into adulthood). Most typically developing children are able to adapt their talk to a variety of contexts by school entry. This includes adaptation in *suprasegmental* features, which are feature beyond simple components of words and syllables, such as speech register, intonation, volume, and tone. Children also learn the mechanics of conversation, such as turn-taking (including speaker allocation and speaker transition), presupposition (i.e., designing turns at talk so that they take into account what a conversation partner already knows), and implicature (i.e., the inferential aspects of talk that are drawn upon when principles of conversation are violated, as occurs with the use of irony). Many pragmatic regularities of talk are culturally specific, and children learn these regularities by participating in interactions with more linguistically competent others (Schieffelin & Ochs, 1986).

Language and Conversational Development in Children with ASD

Well into early childhood, children with ASD continue to display fewer initiations for and responses to joint attention, and spend less time jointly engaged with caregivers than their peers without ASD. Each of these constructs bear concurrent and longitudinal correlations with language development (Adamson et al., 2008; Toth et al., 2006; Yoder, Watson, & Lambert, 2015). The effects of these delays on speech are evident by the second year. Indeed, language delays are an early-emerging concern of caregivers who already have a child diagnosed with ASD (Talbott, Nelson, & Tager-Flusberg, 2015).

The development of spoken language is highly heterogeneous in children with ASD. Some children show no evidence of delay in speech onset while others show delays but eventually develop average or above average lexicons and language skill. Recent estimates suggest that around 25–30% of children diagnosed with ASD do not go on to develop spoken language that can be used flexibly and consistently (Tager-Flusberg, Paul, & Lord, 2005; Tager-Flusberg, 2016; Tager-Flusberg & Kasari, 2013). Some research suggests that once children with ASD do develop spoken language abilities, they use talk for more constrained purposes than children without ASD (Ziatas, Durkin, & Pratt, 2003). After speech onset, children with ASD continue to show atypicalities in nonverbal aspects of communication, including gaze, use of gestures, and facial expressions (for a summary of this research, see Davis & Carter, 2014).

All children with ASD, regardless of language development, show differences in their pragmatic use of language as compared to language–age peers. These differences may become more apparent once children enter preschool, given the increasing complexity of social contexts in early childhood as compared to infancy. Within conversation, children with ASD may show difficulty with presupposition, and appear not to take their conversation partner's prior knowledge into account when formulating their own talk. For example, a child with ASD might begin a narrative without providing sufficient detail to understand the context of the narrative or the specific people involved. Other pragmatic differences include pronominal reversal (e.g., substituting "you" for "I"), overly formal phrasing, topic perseveration, and atypicalities in prosody as well as interpreting prosody in others' speech (summarized in Eigsti, de Marchena, Schuh, & Kelley, 2011, and in Whyte & Nelson, 2015).

Taking an interactional approach, qualitative research in older children and youth suggests that, within conversation, individuals with ASD have difficulty with at least three aspects of talk; interactional coordination, aligning interactional priorities with their conversation partners, and enacting meaning across conversational turns in a way that is consistent with their interlocutors (reviewed in Bottema-Beutel, 2017). Interactional coordination refers to the overall "course of action" that is implemented through conversation, which requires collaboration between interaction partners (e.g., debating, storytelling, affiliating). Similarly, in order for talk to proceed without significant breakdown, interaction partners must maintain at least partially aligned interactional priorities. If, for example, one partner has prioritized listing fine-grained details of a past event during a narrative retelling, and the other partner prioritizes discerning the "moral" or "point" of the story, this may reflect misaligned interactional priorities. Finally, meaning in conversation is not localized to the utterance level; instead, meaning accrues incrementally cross multiple conversational turns. If individuals with ASD are unable to track meaning across an entire stretch of talk, interaction partners may not orient to the overall meaning of the talk in similar ways.

Other research on interactions has suggested that children with ASD may have relatively more difficulty with features of talk that rely on sociocultural meanings, such as interpreting *indexicality* in talk (Ochs et al., 2004). Indexicality refers to meanings beyond semantic properties of words that are unique to social contexts (e.g., deictic expressions such as "Here I am!", where the referent "I" depends on the speaker). Less difficult (although still impaired as compared to children without ASD) is providing *type-fitted* responses to an interaction partner's talk, such as responding to a question with an answer (Capps, Kehres, & Sigman, 1998).

Peer Interactions and Friendships

Most research on peer interactions and relationships in children with ASD has been conducted on children who are of late elementary school age. This research suggests that children with ASD are often isolated from their peers in school contexts, and have fewer reciprocated friendships. They also report spending less time with their friends, and rate their friendships lower in quality than typically developing children (Chamberlain, Kasari, & Rotheram-Fuller, 2007; Kasari, Locke, Gulsrud, & Rotheram-Fuller, 2011; Solomon et al., 2011; also see Petrina et al., 2014 for a review). Importantly, research shows that often children with ASD do desire friendships, and many report having at least one friend (Petrina et al., 2014). Social isolation and fewer friendships may be due at least in part to typically developing peers' perception of children with ASD, rather than conceptual misunderstanding about the nature of friendships (Bottema-Beutel et al., 2019).

Heterogeneity in Social Communication Development in Children with ASD

It is important to note that the developmental trajectories evidenced in children with ASD are far from uniform. As mentioned in Chap. 1, some children show regression in development after appearing to develop along a typical trajectory, and others do not appear to manifest the characteristics of ASD (that are noted by caregivers or professionals) until after the second year (Ozonoff et al., 2018; Yirmiya & Charman, 2010). Ozonoff et al. (2018) studied this complex phenomenon in a prospective, longitudinal study of infant siblings of children with ASD, who had a higher probability of being diagnosed with ASD. Fourteen of the children in this sample were not diagnosed with ASD at age 3 despite multiple screenings, but were eventually diagnosed with ASD in later childhood. The reasons for "missed diagnosis" seemed to vary within children, with some seeming to manifest clearer characteristics of ASD over time, and others seeming to "evolve into impairment" (Ozonoff et al., 2018, p. 856) as social demands increased in later childhood. Fountain, Winter, and Bearman (2012) documented distinct developmental trajectories of social communication with the ASD population. Some children appeared to start out with greater social and communication impairments, but then "bloom" to display relatively less impairment later in childhood. Other children displayed the opposite profile and showed increasing levels of social communication impairment over time, while still other children maintained similar levels of impairment throughout childhood.

Bilingualism and Social Communication Development

Researchers are only beginning to explore issues related to children with ASD who are raised in environments where multiple languages are spoken. However, current research suggests that children with ASD, even those who are significantly delayed in language development, are able to acquire receptive and expressive vocabulary in multiple languages (Dai, Burke, Naigles, Eigsti, & Fein, 2018). In fact, children with ASD may experience some cognitive advantages to being bilingual (Gonzalez-Barrero & Nadig, 2017). This is important to note, because parents are often advised to avoid using their heritage language with their child with ASD, if it differs from the child's language of instruction (Hudry et al., 2018). Qualitative studies of family language practices have documented the difficulties families face when given such advice, as it often means decreasing interactions with their children with ASD (Yu, 2016). This appears to be especially important when caregivers are more fluent in their heritage language as compared to their child's language of instruction.

Addressing Social Communication in ASD

Researchers have begun to identify promising avenues for supporting social communication in young children with ASD, which may be one reason why more children diagnosed with ASD now go on to develop complex language abilities than early estimates suggested (Tager-Flusberg & Kasari, 2013). One of the most promising avenues for early interventions that support social communication outcomes is the facilitation of joint engagement routines (sometimes also called "joint activity routines" or "joint action routines" Ratner & Bruner, 1978). The following paragraphs describe this concept in detail.

Supporting Joint Engagement Routines

Research on typical and atypical development has highlighted the importance of *joint engagement routines* between caregivers and children, or between interventionists and children, for social communication development (Adamson & Bakeman, 1982; Hirsh-Pasek et al., 2015; Rogers, Vivanti & Rocha, 2017). These routines involve repeated interactions between the child and communicative partner involving toys (or other salient aspects of the environment) that are predictable but flexible, and increase in complexity over time. Adults generally follow the child's lead, incorporate play materials that are of especial interest to the child, and cooperate with the child to accomplish a shared goal that provides opportunities to do things together and learn from such experiences (e.g., building a tower with blocks). In this context, child and adult coordinate their actions and share their emotions through gestures, facial expressions, body postures, and reciprocal imitation to communicate, negotiate, and achieve their shared goal (e.g., taking turns in adding blocks to the tower, and smiling to one another to share the suspense when the last block is added to the stack).

Correlational evidence for the utility of joint engagement routines for promoting social communication and language development has been well-documented for both typically developing children and children with ASD (Adamson, Bakeman, Deckner, and Romski 2008; Bakeman & Adamson, 1984; Bottema-Beutel et al., 2014). Further, joint engagement as a dyadic construct appears more highly correlated with later development, such as expressive language, than similar constructs that are measured to reflect discrete behaviors produced by the child (e.g., the number of gestures a child produces to initiate joint attention) (Adamson, Bakeman, Suma, and Robins 2019).

At present, researchers are attempting to maximize the effectiveness of joint engagement routines by identifying the most developmentally important forms of joint engagement, and identifying caregiver/interventionist strategies that increase the likelihood that joint engagement will occur. An especially promising joint engagement format appears to include the following three elements: (a) the child does *not* shift visual attention between the play materials and the adult, (b) it involves reciprocal interactions on toys (e.g., turn taking routines and back-and-forth imitation of actions on objects), and (c) it includes adult's talk about the child's focus of attention (Adamson et al., 2008; Bottema-Beutel et al., 2014; Crandall et al., 2019). This form of joint engagement appears to strike a balance in terms of cognitive demands, in that it does not require the child to shift visual attentional resources between play materials and an adult, but does require reciprocal interaction with the adult via actions on the play materials (Bakeman & Adamson, 1984). The scaffolding that adults provide within this form of engagement may serve as an interactional "template" that allows for reciprocal back-and-forth exchanges (Bottema-Beutel, Lloyd, Watson, and Yoder, 2018). Further, when caregivers talk about the child's focus of attention, children are not required to shift attention to something new in order to connect the talk to the objects or events being referenced. This form of talk appears to be especially facilitative of word learning (McDuffie & Yoder, 2010; Yoder, Watson, & Lambert, 2015). Recent research has also suggested that this kind of engagement may mediate the pathway between children's emerging ability to say words, and their subsequent ability to understand new words (Bottema-Beutel et al., 2018).

Correlational research suggests that adaptive interaction strategies can increase the probability that children will jointly engage with adult interaction partners. This includes providing suggestions about what children can do with the toys they are already playing with (Bottema-Beutel, Lloyd, Watson, & Yoder, 2018). Similarly, children are also more likely to play with toys at their most advanced level when caregivers give suggestions about ways to play with toys (Bottema-Beutel, Malloy, Lloyd, Louick, Watson, & Yoder, 2018). Additionally, engagement in activities that are *emotionally* engaging increase the child's attention and facilitate the appreciation of the partner's social–communicative and emotional facial and bodily cues (e.g., smiling expectantly before blowing bubbles to communicate a feeling of "suspense"; Vivanti & Rogers, 2014). Finally, *mirrored pacing*, which involves an adult imitating children's toy play at moments when children are most likely to attend, also appears to increase the overall duration of joint engagement (Gulsrud, Hellemann, Shire, & Kasari, 2016).

Experimental studies have shown that when trained interventionists facilitate joint engagement routines in children with ASD, participants show increases in both social communication and language, and these increases continue after the intervention has stopped (Kasari, Freeman, & Paparella, 2006; Kasari, Paparella, Freeman, & Jahromi, 2008; see Chap. 6). These findings are important, as they document intervention effects that are developmentally well beyond what is directly taught within the intervention. Social communication can also be improved when caregivers are provided coaching on joint engagement routines, and then implement them within everyday interactions with their children (Green et al., 2010; Kasari, Gulsrud, Wong, Kwon, & Locke, 2010; Pickles et al., 2016; Rogers, Vismara, Wagner, McCormick, Young, & Ozonoff, 2014). Finally, there is evidence of the effectiveness of these types of interventions when they are implemented in community contexts, such as early childcare centers (e.g., Vivanti et al., 2014, 2019), and efforts to improve the accessibility and community implementation of early intervention for children with ASD, especially for families from minoritized groups or low socioeconomic backgrounds, are increasing (Chang, Shire, Shih, Gelfand & Kasari, 2016; Shire et al., 2017).

Supporting Later Social Communication Development

The early intervention period appears to be the time when children are most receptive to the benefits of social communication interventions. For example, longitudinal research has shown that improvement in verbal functioning between age 2 and 3 predicts children's later language development (Anderson et al., 2014; Pickles et al., 2014). Further, children who start intervention at younger ages appear to have better language outcomes (Smith et al., 2015; Vivanti et al., 2019). Still, even children who do participate in early intervention may need continued support in the social communication domain later in childhood and into adulthood.

While research on supporting more advanced pragmatic aspects of language in the preschool period is at its infancy, preliminary evidence suggests that pragmatic aspects of language may be influenced by lexical acquisition; that is, children with more vocabulary also have greater pragmatic skill (Whyte & Nelson, 2015). Importantly, while some pragmatic regularities can effectively be taught as hard and fast rules (e.g., not cursing in class), other areas of pragmatics are much more complex and not entirely rule-bound. This may make direct instruction ineffective for facilitating pragmatic development. While research in this area is still in the early phases, supporting the extent to which children are able to engage in linguistic interactions with peers and adults may indirectly support both lexical acquisition and downstream pragmatic development. Supported peer engagement increases children's opportunities to learn pragmatic aspects of language, and ensures that the skills they do learn are relevant to the interactions they have with their peers (as opposed to a more idealized form of interaction that is more relevant to formal interactions with adults).

Additionally, there is evidence that in young elementary age children, teaching typically developing children to identify and approach socially isolated children improves the social connectedness of children with ASD (Kasari, Rotheram-Fuller, Locke, & Gulsrud, 2012). Facilitating play experiences between children with ASD and their typically developing peers also leads to greater social involvement with peers (Wolfberg, DeWitt, Young, & Nguyen, 2015). Importantly, this approach appears to be more effective than direct social skill instructions for improving social connectedness.

Supporting Children Who Are Nonverbal

For the 25–30% of children with ASD who do not develop spoken language by the preschool period, alternative and augmentative communication (AAC) systems are a critical tool for maximizing participation in social life, and for continuing to facilitate social communication development. These systems can be low-tech, and consist of objects or laminated icons that are used as communicative symbols. They can also be high-tech, such as an iPad equipped with an app that translates icons displayed on the screen to voice output. Such AAC devices can be programmed with language capabilities that are as complex as formal languages, in terms of flexibility and generativity (i.e., infinite combinations of words can be produced). High-tech devices can be expensive and complex to learn. Therefore, the assistance of a trained speech language pathologist who is experienced in supporting families in accessing this technology is critical to ensuring that it is adequately incorporated into the child's communicative repertoire. Some caregivers may be concerned that adopting an AAC device will further delay the onset of speech. In fact, research has shown that the opposite is true; children with ASD often acquire speech as a result of using an AAC device (Kasari et al., 2014).

A popular low-tech approach is the picture exchange communication system (PECS), which involves the use of picture cards that are combined and displayed on a Velcro board, and then exchanged with a communication partner (see also Chap. 7). This intervention uses reinforcement to aid the child in connecting the icons on the cards with their referents (e.g., a card depicting a cookie can be exchanged for an actual cookie, which will reinforce the concept that the cookie icon symbolizes "cookie"). However, there is currently very little evidence to suggest that this approach improves *social* communication in children with ASD; it appears much more useful for teaching requests (Ganz, Earles-Vollrath, Heath, Parker, Rispoli, & Duran, 2012). In contrast, there is some research to suggest that incorporating speech generating AAC devices into joint engagement interventions has measurable effects on children's social communication outcomes (Kasari et al., 2014).

Interventions that Target Developmentally Distal Outcomes

It should be noted that some of the currently available early interventions appear to be more effective in improving aspects of social communication that are proximal to the intervention (i.e., skills that are directly taught or addressed by the intervention) and context bound (i.e., skills that are only demonstrated within contexts very similar to the intervention context, for example saying "hello" in response to a specific prompt and reward system; Yoder et al., 2013). This is concerning, as the practical or developmental benefits for such outcomes are unclear. However, there are several intervention studies that have shown distal (i.e., outcomes that are developmentally beyond what is directly taught or addressed by the intervention) and generalized effects (i.e., outcomes that appear in contexts that are dissimilar to the intervention context) on social communication. These interventions share some important characteristics; they involve joint engagement routines in natural contexts (which are usually play activities), provide a balance between child-centeredness and adult support, support parent and family involvement, maintain a developmental orientation, and address the child's physiological regulation (Bottema-Beutel, Yoder, Woynoroski, & Sandbank, 2014). These types of interventions will be discussed further in subsequent chapters focusing on intervention.

Future Directions for Research

While social communication intervention research has certainly made strides in the last several decades, more well-designed intervention research is needed that can tease apart the active ingredients of early interventions designed to support social communication, and the processes by which these strategies influence broader development in children with ASD. Additional work also needs to be conducted to better understand peer relatedness in children with ASD, and how peer relationships are intertwined with other aspects of social communication development. Finally, the majority of early intervention research designed to impact social communication has been conducted on participant samples that are of European or Euro-American descent and are monolingual English speakers. Given that social communication interventions often involve influencing family interactions, more research will need to be conducted with culturally diverse families, so that intervention strategies can be adapted accordingly (see for example Guiberson & Ferris, 2019).

Conclusion

Social communication involves communication for sharing with and relating to others, and is a core area of impairment in ASD. Differences in social communication are thought to begin early in children's development, and to impact the development of a variety of developmental achievements including language and peer relationships. For young children with ASD, supporting joint engagement routines within adult–child interactions appears to be a promising means to advance children's social communication. Intervention effects from interventions that focus on joint engagement routines are developmentally distal to the intervention procedures, and appear to influence children's generalized behavior. More research is needed on the development of pragmatic language and the formation of friendships, and interventions to support these milestones.

References

Abney, D. H., Warlaumont, A. S., Oller, D. K., Wallot, S., & Kello, C. T. (2016). Multiple coordination patterns in infant and adult vocalizations. *Infancy: The Official Journal of the International Society on Infant Studies, 22*(4), 514–539.

Adamson, L., & Bakeman, R. (1982). Affectivity and reference: Concepts, methods, and techniques in the study of communication development of 6-to 18-month-old infants. *Emotion and Early Interaction*, 213–236.

Adamson, L. B., Bakeman, R., Deckner, D. F., & Romski, M. (2008). Joint engagement and the emergence of language in children with autism and Down syndrome. *Journal of Autism and Developmental Disorders, 39*(1), 84–96.

Adamson, L. B., Bakeman, R., Suma, K., & Robins, D. L. (2019). An expanded view of joint attention: Skill, engagement, and language in typical development and autism. *Child Development, 90*(1), e1–e18.

American Psychiatric Association. (2013). *Diagnostic and statistical manual of mental disorders* (5th ed.). Arlington, VA: American Psychiatric Publishing.

Anagnostou, E., Jones, N., Huerta, M., Halladay, A. K., Wang, P., Scahill, L., … Dawson, G. (2015). Measuring social communication behaviors as a treatment endpoint in individuals with autism spectrum disorder. *Autism, 19*(5), 622–636.

Anderson, D. K., Liang, J. W., & Lord, C. (2014). Predicting young adult outcome among more and less cognitively able individuals with autism spectrum disorders. *Journal of Child Psychology and Psychiatry, 55*(5), 485–494.

Bakeman, R., & Adamson, L. B. (1984). Coordinating attention to people and objects in mother-infant and peer-infant interaction. *Child Development, 55*(4), 1278–1289.

Bishop, S. L., Havdahl, K. A., Huerta, M., & Lord, C. (2016). Subdimensions of social-communication impairment in autism spectrum disorder. *Journal of Child Psychology and Psychiatry, 57*(8), 909–916.

Barbaro, J., & Dissanayake, C. (2013). Early markers of autism spectrum disorders in infants and toddlers prospectively identified in the Social Attention and Communication Study. *Autism, 17*(1), 64–86.

Bottema-Beutel, K., Yoder, P., Hochman, J.M., & Watson, L. (2014). The role of supported joint engagement and parent utterances in language and social communication development in children with autism spectrum disorder. *Journal of Autism and Developmental Disorders, 44*, 2162–2174.

Bottema-Beutel, K., Malloy, C., Cuda, J., Kim, S. Y., & MacEvoy, J. (2019). Responses to vignettes depicting friendship transgressions: Similarities and differences in children with and without autism spectrum disorder. *Journal of Autism and Developmental Disorders, 49*(12), 4709–4720.

Bottema-Beutel, K. (2016). The relationship between joint attention and language in autism spectrum disorder and typical development: A systematic review and meta-regression analysis. *Autism Research, 9*(10), 1021–1035.

Bottema-Beutel, K. (2017). Glimpses into the blind spot: Social interaction and autism. *Journal of Communication Disorders, 68*, 24–34.

Bottema-Beutel, K., Kim, S. Y., & Crowley, S. (2019). A systematic review and meta-regression analysis of social functioning correlates in autism and typical development. *Autism Research, 12*(2), 152–175.

Bottema-Beutel, K., Lloyd, B., Watson, L., & Yoder, P. J. (2018). Bidirectional influences of caregiver utterances and supported joint engagement in children with and without autism spectrum disorder. *Autism Research, 11*, 755–765.

Bottema-Beutel, K., Malloy, C., Cuda, J., Kim, S. Y., & MacEvoy, J. (2019). Responses to vignettes depicting friendship transgressions: Similarities and differences in children with and without autism spectrum disorder. *Journal of Autism and Developmental Disorders, 49*(12), 4709–4720.

Bottema-Beutel, K., Malloy, C., Lloyd, B., Louick, R., Nelson, L. J., Watson, L. R., & Yoder, P. J. (2018). Sequential associations between caregiver talk and child play in autism spectrum disorder and typical development. *Child Development, 89*(3), e157–e166.

Bottema-Beutel, K., Woynaroski, T., Louick, R., Stringer Keefe, E., Watson, L. R., & Yoder, P. J. (2019). Longitudinal associations across vocabulary modalities in children with autism and typical development. *Autism, 23*(2), 424–435.

Bottema-Beutel, K., Yoder, P., Hochman, J. M., & Watson, L. (2014). The role of supported joint engagement and parent utterances in language and social communication development in children with autism spectrum disorder. *Journal of Autism and Developmental Disorders, 44*, 2162–2174.

Bottema-Beutel, K., Yoder, P., Woynoroski, T., & Sandbank, M. (2014). Targeted intervention for social-communication symptoms in preschoolers. In F. R. Volkmar, R. Paul, S. J. Rogers, & K. A. Pelphrey (Eds.), *Handbook of autism and pervasive developmental disorders*. Hoboken, NJ: Wiley.

Capps, L., Kehres, J., & Sigman, M. (1998). Conversational abilities among children with autism and children with developmental delays. *Autism, 2*(4), 325–344.

Carpenter, M., Nagell, K., Tomasello, M., Butterworth, G., & Moore, C. (1998). Social cognition, joint attention, and communicative competence from 9 to 15 months of age. *Monographs of the Society for Research in Child Development, 63*(4), i-174.

Chamberlain, B., Kasari, C., & Rotheram-Fuller, E. (2007). Involvement or isolation? The social networks of children with autism in regular classrooms. *Journal of Autism and Developmental Disorders, 37*(2), 230–242.

Chang, Y. C., Shire, S. Y., Shih, W., Gelfand, C., & Kasari, C. (2016). Preschool deployment of evidence-based social communication intervention: JASPER in the classroom. *Journal of Autism and Developmental Disorders, 46*(6), 2211–2223.

Chawarska, K., Macari, S., & Shic, F. (2013). Decreased spontaneous attention to social scenes in 6-month-old infants later diagnosed with autism spectrum disorders. *Biological Psychiatry, 74*(3), 195–203.

Crandall, M. C., Bottema-Beutel, K., McDaniel, J., Watson, L. R., & Yoder, P. J. (2019). Children with autism spectrum disorder may learn from caregiver verb input better in certain engagement states. *Journal of Autism and Developmental Disorders, 49*, 3102–3112.

Dai, Y. G., Burke, J. D., Naigles, L., Eigsti, I. M., & Fein, D. A. (2018). Language abilities in monolingual-and bilingual-exposed children with autism or other developmental disorders. *Research in Autism Spectrum Disorders, 55*, 38–49.

Davis, N. O., & Carter, A. S. (2014). Social development in autism. In F. R. Volkmar, S. J. Rogers, R. Paul, & K. A. Pelphrey (Eds.), *Handbook of autism and developmental disorders* (4th ed., pp. 312–334). Hoboken, NJ: Wiley.

DeCasper, A. J., & Fifer, W. P. (1980). Of human bonding: Newborns prefer their mothers' voices. *Science, 208*(4448), 1174–1176.

Eigsti, I. M., de Marchena, A. B., Schuh, J. M., & Kelley, E. (2011). Language acquisition in autism spectrum disorders: A developmental review. *Research in Autism Spectrum Disorders, 5*(2), 681–691.

Falck-Ytter, T., Nyström, P., Gredebäck, G., Gliga, T., Bölte, S., Team, E. A. S. E., … Hedenius, M. (2018). Reduced orienting to audiovisual synchrony in infancy predicts autism diagnosis at 3 years of age. *Journal of Child Psychology and Psychiatry, 59*(8), 872–880.

Fountain, C., Winter, A. S., & Bearman, P. S. (2012). Six developmental trajectories characterize children with autism. *Pediatrics, 129*(5), e1112–e1120.

Frank, M. C., Vul, E., & Johnson, S. P. (2009). Development of infants' attention to faces during the first year. *Cognition, 110*(2), 160–170.

Ganz, J. B., Earles-Vollrath, T. L., Heath, A. K., Parker, R. I., Rispoli, M. J., & Duran, J. B. (2012). A meta-analysis of single case research studies on aided augmentative and alternative communication systems with individuals with autism spectrum disorders. *Journal of Autism and Developmental Disorders, 42*(1), 60–74.

Gillespie-Lynch, K., Sepeta, L., Wang, Y., Marshall, S., Gomez, L., Sigman, M., & Hutman, T. (2012). Early childhood predictors of the social competence of adults with autism. *Journal of Autism and Developmental Disorders, 42*(2), 161–174.

Gonzalez-Barrero, A. M., & Nadig, A. S. (2017). Can bilingualism mitigate set-shifting difficulties in children with autism spectrum disorders? *Child Development, 90*(4), 1043–1060.

Green, J., Charman, T., McConachie, H., Aldred, C., Slonims, V., Howlin, P., … Barrett, B. (2010). Parent-mediated communication-focused treatment in children with autism (PACT): A randomised controlled trial. *The Lancet, 375*(9732), 2152–2160.

Guiberson, M., & Ferris, K. P. (2019). Early language interventions for young dual language learners: A scoping review. *American Journal of Speech-language Pathology, 28*(3), 945–963.

Gulsrud, A. C., Hellemann, G., Shire, S., & Kasari, C. (2016). Isolating active ingredients in a parent-mediated social communication intervention for toddlers with autism spectrum disorder. *Journal of Child Psychology and Psychiatry, 57*(5), 606–613.

Hamner, T., & Vivanti, G. (2019). Eye-tracking research in autism spectrum disorder: What are we measuring and for what purposes? *Current Developmental Disorders Reports, 6*(2), 37–44.

Hirsh-Pasek, K., Adamson, L. B., Bakeman, R., Owen, M. T., Golinkoff, R. M., Pace, A., … Suma, K. (2015). The contribution of early communication quality to low-income children's language success. *Psychological Science, 26*(7), 1071–1083.

Hobson, J. A., Hobson, R. P., Malik, S., Bargiota, K., & Caló, S. (2013). The relation between social engagement and pretend play in autism. *British Journal of Developmental Psychology, 31*(1), 114–127.

Hobson, R. P. (2007). Communicative depth: Soundings from developmental psychopatholoy. *Infant Behavior and Development, 30*, 267–277.

Hudry, K., Rumney, L., Pitt, N., Barbaro, J., & Vivanti, G. (2018). Interaction behaviors of bilingual parents with their young children with autism spectrum disorder. *Journal of Clinical Child & Adolescent Psychology, 47*(sup1), S321–S328.

Jones, W., & Klin, A. (2013). Attention to eyes is present but in decline in 2–6-month-old infants later diagnosed with autism. *Nature, 504*(7480), 427.

Kanner, L. (1943). Autistic disturbances of affective contact. *The Nervous Child, 2*, 217–250.

Kasari, C., Freeman, S., & Paparella, T. (2006). Joint attention and symbolic play in young children with autism: A randomized controlled intervention study. *Journal of Child Psychology and Psychiatry, 47*(6), 611–620.

Kasari, C., Gulsrud, A. C., Wong, C., Kwon, S., & Locke, J. (2010). Randomized controlled caregiver mediated joint engagement intervention for toddlers with autism. *Journal of Autism and Developmental Disorders, 40*(9), 1045–1056.

Kasari, C., Kaiser, A., Goods, K., Nietfeld, J., Mathy, P., Landa, R., … Almirall, D. (2014). Communication interventions for minimally verbal children with autism: A sequential multiple assignment randomized trial. *Journal of the American Academy of Child and Adolescent Psychiatry, 53*(6), 635–646.

Kasari, C., Locke, J., Gulsrud, A., & Rotheram-Fuller, E. (2011). Social networks and friendships at school: Comparing children with and without ASD. *Journal of Autism and Developmental Disorders, 41*(3), 533–544.

Kasari, C., Paparella, T., Freeman, S., & Jahromi, L. B. (2008). Language outcome in autism: Randomized comparison of joint attention and play interventions. *Journal of Consulting and Clinical Psychology, 76*(1), 125.

Kasari, C., Rotheram-Fuller, E., Locke, J., & Gulsrud, A. (2012). Making the connection: Randomized controlled trial of social skills at school for children with autism spectrum disorders. *Journal of Child Psychology and Psychiatry, 53*(4), 431–439.

Klin, A., Jones, W., Schultz, R., & Volkmar, F. (2003). The enactive mind, or from actions to cognition: Lessons from autism. *Philosophical Transactions of the Royal Society of London B: Biological Sciences, 358*(1430), 345–360.

Leekam, S. & Moore, C. (2001). The development of attention and joint attention in children with autism. In: Burack JA, Charman T, Yirmiya N, et al. (Eds.), *The Development of Autism: Perspectives from Theory and Research* (pp. 105–129). Mahwah, NJ: Lawrence Erlbaum Associates.

McDuffie, A., & Yoder, P. (2010). Types of parent verbal responsiveness that predict language in young children with autism spectrum disorder. *Journal of Speech, Language, and Hearing Research, 53*(4), 1026–1039.

Mundy, P., Delgado, C., Block, J., Venezia, M., Hogan, A., & Seibert, J. (2003). *Early social communication scales (ESCS)*. Coral Gables, FL: University of Miami.

Mundy, P. C. (2016). *Autism and joint attention: Development, neuroscience, and clinical fundamentals*. New York, NY: The Guilford Press.

Nyström, P., Thorup, E., Bölte, S., & Falck-Ytter, T. (2019). Joint attention in infancy and the emergence of autism. *Biological Psychiatry, 86*(8), 631–638. https://doi.org/10.1016/j.biopsych.2019.05.006

Ozonoff, S., Young, G. S., Brian, J., Charman, T., Shephard, E., Solish, A., & Zwaigenbaum, L. (2018). Diagnosis of autism spectrum disorder after age 5 in children evaluated longitudinally since infancy. *Journal of the American Academy of Child & Adolescent Psychiatry, 57*(11), 849–857.

Ozonoff, S., Young, G. S., Carter, A., Messinger, D., Yirmiya, N., Nwaigenbaum, L., … Stone, W. L. (2011). Recurrence risk for autism spectrum disorders: A Baby Siblings Research Consortium study. *Pediatrics, 128*, e488–e495.

Ochs, E., Kremer-Sadlik, T., Sirota, K. G., & Solomon, O. (2004). Autism and the social world: an anthropological perspective. *Discourse Studies, 6*(2), 147–183.

Petrina, N., Carter, M., & Stephenson, J. (2014). The nature of friendship in children with autism spectrum disorders: A systematic review. *Research in Autism Spectrum Disorders, 8*(2), 111–126.

Pickles, A., Anderson, D. K., & Lord, C. (2014). Heterogeneity and plasticity in the development of language: A 17-year follow-up of children referred early for possible autism. *Journal of Child Psychology and Psychiatry, 55*(12), 1354–1362.

Pickles, A., Le Couteur, A., Leadbitter, K., Salomone, E., Cole-Fletcher, R., Tobin, H., ... & Aldred, C. (2016). Parent-mediated social communication therapy for young children with autism (PACT): long-term follow-up of a randomised controlled trial. *The Lancet, 388*(10059), 2501–2509.

Prizant, B. M., & Duchan, J. F. (1981). The functions of immediate echolalia in autistic children. *Journal of Speech and Hearing Disorders, 46*(3), 241–249.

Ratner, N., & Bruner, J. (1978). Games, social exchange and the acquisition of language. *Journal of Child Language, 5*(03), 391–401.

Rogers, S. J., Vivanti, G., & Rocha, M. (2017). Helping young children with autism spectrum disorder develop social ability: The early start denver model approach. In *Handbook of social skills and autism spectrum disorder* (pp. 197–222). Springer, Cham.

Rogers, S. J., Vismara, L., Wagner, A. L., McCormick, C., Young, G., & Ozonoff, S. (2014). Autism treatment in the first year of life: A pilot study of infant start, a parent-implemented intervention for symptomatic infants. *Journal of Autism and Developmental Disorders, 44*(12), 2981–2995.

Scaife, M., & Bruner, J. S. (1975). The capacity for joint visual attention in the infant. *Nature, 253*, 265–266.

Schegloff, E. A. (1982). Discourse as an interactional achievement: Some uses of 'uh huh' and other things that come between sentences. In D. Tannen (Ed.), *Analyzing discourse: Text and talk* (pp. 71–93). Washington, DC: Georgetown University Press.

Schegloff, E. A. (2007). *Sequence organization in interaction: Volume 1: A primer in conversation analysis*. New York, NY: Cambridge University Press.

Schieffelin, B. B., & Ochs, E. (Eds.). (1986). *Language socialization across cultures (No. 3)*. New York, NY: Cambridge University Press.

Shumway, S., & Wetherby, A. M. (2009). Communicative acts of children with autism spectrum disorders in the second year of life. *Journal of Speech, Language, and Hearing Research, 52*, 1139–1165.

Smith, T., Klorman, R., & Mruzek, D. W. (2015). Predicting outcome of community-based early intensive behavioral intervention for children with autism. *Journal of Abnormal Child Psychology, 43*(7), 1271–1282.

Solomon, M., Buaminger, N., & Rogers, S. J. (2011). Abstract reasoning and friendship in high functioning preadolescents with autism spectrum disorders. *Journal of Autism and Developmental Disorders, 41*(1), 32–43.

Sterponi, L., & Fasulo, A. (2010). "How to go on": Intersubjectivity and progressivity in the communication of a child with autism. *Ethos, 38*(1), 116–142.

Sterponi, L., de Kirby, K., & Shankey, J. (2015). Rethinking language in autism. Autism, 19(5), 517–526.

Sterponi, L., & Shankey, J. (2014). Rethinking echolalia: Repetition as interactional resource in the communication of a child with autism. *Journal of Child Language, 41*(2), 275–304.

Tager-Flusberg, H. (2016). Risk factors associated with language in autism spectrum disorder: Clues to underlying mechanisms. *Journal of Speech, Language, and Hearing Research, 59*, 143–154.

Tager-Flusberg, H., & Kasari, C. (2013). Minimally verbal school-aged children with autism spectrum disorder: The neglected end of the spectrum. *Autism Research, 6*(6), 468–478.

Tager-Flusberg, H., Paul, R., & Lord, C. (2005). Language and communication in autism. In D. J. Cohen & F. R. Volkmar (Eds.), *Handbook of autism and pervasive developmental disorders* (3rd ed., pp. 195–225). New York, NY: Wiley.

Tager-Flusberg, H., Rogers, S., Cooper, J., Landa, R., Lord, C., Paul, R., … Yoder, P. (2009). Defining spoken language benchmarks and selecting measures of expressive language development for young children with autism spectrum disorders. *Journal of Speech, Language, and Hearing Research, 52*(3), 643–652.

Talbott, M. R., Nelson, C. A., & Tager-Flusberg, H. (2015). Diary reports of concerns in mothers of infant siblings of children with autism across the first year of life. *Journal of Autism and Developmental Disorders, 45*, 2187–2199.

Trevarthen, C. (1979). Communication and cooperation in early infancy: A description of primary intersubjectivity. In M. M. Bullowa (Ed.), *Before speech: The beginning of interpersonal communication* (pp. 321–347). New York NY: Cambridge University Press.

Trevarthen, C. (1987). Sharing makes sense: Intersubjectivity and the making of an infant's meaning. In R. Steele & T. Threadgold (Eds.), *Language topics: Essays in honour of Michael Halliday, Vol. 1* (pp. 177–199). Amsterdam: John Benjamins.

Tomasello, M. (2019). Becoming human: A theory of ontogeny. Belknap Press.

Toth, K., Munson, J., Meltzoff, A. N., & Dawson, G. (2006). Early predictors of communication development in young children with autism spectrum disorder: Joint attention, imitation, and toy play. *Journal of Autism and Developmental Disorders, 36*(8), 993–1005.

Vivanti, G., Dissanayake, C., Duncan, E., Feary, J., Capes, K., Upson, S., ... & Hudry, K. (2019). Outcomes of children receiving Group-Early Start Denver Model in an inclusive versus autism-specific setting: A pilot randomized controlled trial. *Autism, 23*(5), 1165–1175.

Vivanti, G., & Rogers, S. J. (2014). Autism and the mirror neuron system: insights from learning and teaching. *Philosophical Transactions of the Royal Society B: Biological Sciences, 369*(1644), 20130184.

Vivanti, G., Dissanayake, C., Zierhut, C., Rogers, S. J., & Victorian ASELCC Team. (2013). Brief report: Predictors of outcomes in the Early Start Denver Model delivered in a group setting. *Journal of Autism and Developmental Disorders, 43*(7), 1717–1724.

Vivanti, G., & Hamilton, A. (2014). Imitation in autism spectrum disorders. In F. Volkmar, R. Paul, S. J. Rogers, & K. A. Pelphrey (Eds.), *The handbook of autism and pervasive developmental disorders* (4th ed., pp. 278–301). New York: Wiley.

Vivanti, G., Paynter, J., Duncan, E., Fothergill, H., Dissanayake, C., Rogers, S. J., & Victorian ASELCC Team. (2014). Effectiveness and feasibility of the Early Start Denver Model implemented in a group-based community childcare setting. *Journal of Autism and Developmental Disorders, 44*(12), 3140–3153.

Wetherby, A. M. (2006). Understanding and measuring social communication in children with autism spectrum disorders. In T. Charman & W. Stone (Eds.), *Social and communication development in autism spectrum disorders: Early identification, diagnosis, and intervention* (pp. 3–34). New York, NY: Guilford Press.

Whyte, E. M., & Nelson, K. E. (2015). Trajectories of pragmatic and nonliteral language development in children with autism spectrum disorders. *Journal of Communication Disorders, 54*, 2–14.

Wing, L., & Gould, J. (1979). Severe impairments of social interaction and associated abnormalities in children: Epidemiology and classification. *Journal of Autism and Developmental Disorders, 9*(1), 11–29.

Wolfberg, P., DeWitt, M., Young, G. S., & Nguyen, T. (2015). Integrated play groups: Promoting symbolic play and social engagement with typical peers in children with ASD across settings. *Journal of Autism and Developmental Disorders, 45*(3), 830–845.

Yirmiya, N., & Charman, T. (2010). The prodrome of autism: Early behavioral and biological signs, regression, peri-and post-natal development and genetics. *Journal of Child Psychology and Psychiatry, 51*(4), 432–458.

Yoder, P., Watson, L. R., & Lambert, W. (2015). Value-added predictors of expressive and receptive language growth in initially nonverbal preschoolers with autism spectrum disorders. *Journal of Autism and Developmental Disorders, 45*(5), 1254–1270.

Yoder, P. J., Bottema-Beutel, K., Woynaroski, T., Chandrasekhar, R., & Sandbank, M. (2013). Social communication intervention effects vary by dependent variable type in preschoolers with autism spectrum disorders. *Evidence-Based Communication Assessment and Intervention, 7*(4), 150–174.

Yu, B. (2016). Bilingualism as conceptualized and bilingualism as lived: A critical examination of the monolingual socialization of a child with Autism in a bilingual family. *Journal of Autism and Developmental Disorders, 46*(2), 424–435.

Ziatas, K., Durkin, K., & Pratt, C. (2003). Differences in assertive speech acts produced by children with autism, Asperger syndrome, specific language impairment, and normal development. *Development and Psychopathology, 15*(1), 73–94.

Zwaigenbaum, L., Thurm, A., Stone, W., Baranek, G., Bryson, S., Iverson, J., … Sigman, M. (2007). Studying the emergence of autism spectrum disorders in high-risk infants: Methodological and practical issues. *Journal of Autism and Developmental Disorders, 37*, 466–480.

Chapter 4
Understanding and Addressing Restricted and Repetitive Behaviors in Children with Autism

Lauren Turner-Brown and MaryKate Frisch

> "In his second year he 'developed a mania for spinning blocks and pans and other round objects.'"
>
> —Kanner, 1943

Introduction

In 1943, Leo Kanner detailed the rigidity and repetitious behaviors of 11 case studies of children who he assumed to have "inborn autistic disturbances of affective contact." One link between Kanner's cases was rigid behaviors and a "strong urge for sameness."Today, an observation of repetitive behaviors in a young child, such as the ones described by Kanner in the quote above, would cause suspicion for the presence of autism spectrum disorder (ASD). Restrictive and repetitive behaviors (RRBs) are key attributes of diagnosis of ASD. The *Diagnostic and Statistical Manual* 5th Edition (DSM-5) divides RRBs into four groups (1) repetitive movements, use of objects, or speech; (2) insistence on sameness, inflexible routines, or ritualized patterns of verbal or nonverbal behaviors; (3) highly restricted interests; and (4) hyper- or hyporeactivity to sensory input or unusual interests (American Psychiatric Association, 2013). RRBs are often further grouped into two categories: low-order behaviors, which include repetitive movements of body and objects and high-order behaviors, which include

The original version of this chapter was revised. The correction to this chapter is available at https://doi.org/10.1007/978-3-030-41160-2_11

L. Turner-Brown (✉)
UNC TEACCH Autism Program, The University of North Carolina School of Medicine, Chapel Hill, NC, USA
e-mail: ltb@laurenturnerbrownphd.com

M. Frisch
UNC TEACCH Autism Program, The University of North Carolina School of Medicine, Chapel Hill, NC, USA

G. Vivanti et al. (eds.), *Clinical Guide to Early Interventions for Children with Autism*, Best Practices in Child and Adolescent Behavioral Health Care,
https://doi.org/10.1007/978-3-030-41160-2_4

restricted interests, insistence of sameness, and ritualized verbal patterns (Turner, 1999). Much of the literature around young children and RRBs focuses on repetitive sensory motor (RSM) behaviors when discussing low-order behaviors and "insistence on sameness" behaviors when discussing high-order behaviors (Bishop et al., 2013; Richler, Huerta, Bishop, & Lord, 2010). Below, we characterize each of these symptoms and how they may present themselves in young children with ASD.

Characterizing RRB Symptoms

RRBs can occur in typical toddler development; therefore, distinguishing between typicality and atypicality relies on categorizing the type, frequency, and intensity of the behavior (American Psychiatric Association, 2013). Differences begin to emerge in the second year of life between the RRBs of typical infants and infants with ASD (Elison et al., 2014; Wolff et al., 2014), and between infants with other developmental delays and those with ASD (Morgan, Wetherby, & Barber, 2008; Watt et al., 2008). RRB symptoms are complex in part because they may interfere with development and also may serve as areas of strength and interest that can facilitate learning in other areas. Below, we describe each symptom in this domain.

Repetitive Movements, Use of Objects, or Speech

Repetitive body movements are characteristic of typical infant development in the first 2 years of life. Babies flap their arms to balance and when expecting an action. In typical development, these repetitive movements decrease significantly by 2 years of age (Shafer, Newell, Lewis, & Bodfish, 2017). However, in young children with ASD, and in children with global developmental delays, they might continue. In addition to flapping, repetitive body movements may also include spinning or pacing, posturing hands or fingers, or full body movements like rocking. These movements may be adaptive during typical infancy by allowing infants to explore their environment and functionally change their behavior as a result. In contrast, children with ASD may not integrate sensory feedback to adapt their movements to environment. Thus, these behaviors become maladaptive and can interfere with learning and play (Shafer et al., 2017). For example, a child who rocks his body as he is learning to crawl may no longer engage in rocking once he has mastered the skill of crawling. In contrast, consider an infant who already knows how to crawl, and while crawling toward a caregiver who has called his name, pauses and rocks back and forth repetitively. This behavior no longer promotes the development of a skill and interferes with the child responding to his parent.

Repetitive use of objects in young children can present itself as simply playing with a toy repeatedly in the same manner. For example, a child might roll a car back and forth on the floor without ever moving outside of a specific area. Another child might hold a spoon and shake it up and down repetitively. In young children, repetition is a learning strategy, so deciding what makes the repetitive use of an object a symptom rather than a strategy is determined through the observation of patterns over time. While a typically developing toddler may open and close the door on a play house multiple times, she or he will move on to other actions after figuring out how the doors and windows work. In contrast, a child with ASD may continue to open and close the doors to the exclusion of other actions with that toy.

Finally, repetitive speech includes echolalia (repeating words others have said) and idiosyncratic phrases. Echolalia can be immediate or delayed. Immediate echolalia may present itself as repeating the question a person has asked (e.g., Mom says, "do you want some juice?" and the child responds, "you want some juice"). Delayed echolalia often presents as a child reciting a phrase she has heard before, either from a person in her environment or a cartoon or commercial he or she watched. For example, upon entering a tunnel on his ride to preschool in the morning, a child always says, "would you could you in the dark?" echoing his parents' reading of a Dr. Seuss book *Green Eggs and Ham*. Some children reverse their pronouns as part of this echolalia, asking for a snack by saying, "you want cracker." Intonation patterns of this speech in young children with ASD stands out as children often echo not only the words, but the exact intonation of the previous speaker each time.

Insistence on Sameness, Inflexible Adherence to Routines, or Ritualistic Behavior

Although insistence on sameness and ritualistic behavior can appear later in life, symptoms may be present in early childhood. For example, a child might insist on eating a particular food (e.g., chips) using a particular plate (e.g., the green one), sitting in a particular chair (e.g., the red one) at each meal. This behavior, by itself, is common in typically developing children between ages 2 and 4 years, when most children become increasingly inflexible as part of normative development (Evans et al., 1997). What distinguishes the behavior in children with ASD is the level of adherence, the degree to which the child becomes upset when the routine is interrupted, and, at times, the idiosyncrasies associated with the routine. To take the same example above, a child with ASD might also only eat one brand of chips and associate a different color plate with a different food s/he eats.

Restricted Interests

Highly restricted interests are often what stand out when meeting an older child or adult with ASD, as they may be able to describe in detail numerous facts about unusual topics such as train schedules or car models. In early childhood, when many children with ASD have not yet developed functional speech, these interests present themselves a bit differently. Rather than talking excessively about a topic, children may play exclusively with one toy (e.g., a toy train) or carry around a particular object (e.g., spoons). At times, these interests can be avenues toward engagement, and highlight strengths of a child with ASD. For example, a child who loves trains may learn to count, distinguish colors, and play creatively through train activities. Parents often see these interests as ways to highlight their child's strengths and interests. For example, a child with a strong interest in dinosaurs may develop this vocabulary for types of dinosaurs ahead of his peers and beyond parents' knowledge. At other times, these interests can interfere with development. For example, a child with restricted interests in trains may become aggressive toward a peer who tries to play with them and may miss other activities in preschool such as singing and art because of exclusive play with trains. Challenging behaviors may result when a child needs to transition away from a preferred toy or when a parent does not bring along the favorite block the child likes to carry.

Hyper- or Hyporeactivity to Sensory Input or Unusual Interests

Atypical sensory reactions and interests are the final symptoms in this category and include both overreaction (hyperreactivity) and underreaction (hyporeactivity). Examples of hyperreactivity include a child covering her ears when she hears loud sounds or refusing to eat foods with certain textures. Examples of hyporeactivity include a child who does not respond when his name is called or does not seem to notice when he is hurt. Along with these types of reactivity, children with ASD might seek sensory input in unusual ways, such as rubbing a fabric in their hands, squeezing objects, mouthing, or chewing beyond the stage when it is developmentally appropriate. While children with a range of developmental disabilities often show hyperreactivity, it is the combination of hyperreactivity with hyporeactivity that is often indicative of a diagnosis of ASD (Ausderau et al., 2014).

In contrast to OCD symptoms, RRBs in ASD frequently do not cause distress, but rather reflect preferred and/or comforting activities. Despite the positive valence, RRBs can lead to distress and even tantrums and aggression when the individual is interrupted or asked to stop the behavior (Klin, Danovitch, Merz, & Volkmar, 2007; Postorino et al., 2017)

Correlates of RRBs

Ability

Some RRB features are associated with ability level. Children who have more significant intellectual disability often display increased RSM such as stereotypies or sensory interests (Bishop, Richler, & Lord, 2006; Lam, Bodfish, & Piven, 2008; Richler et al., 2010). However, this association is less clear in younger children (e.g., under 3 years)—regardless of intellectual ability, many young children with ASD engage in RSM (Bishop et al., 2006). In contrast, insistence on sameness has been shown to be associated with intelligence in the opposite way, with individuals who have higher ability showing higher challenges with insistence on sameness (Bishop et al., 2006; Lam et al., 2008; Richler et al., 2010). In very young children with or at risk for ASD, RRB symptoms are strongly associated, as a whole, with socialization and adaptive behavior abilities (Schertz, Odom, Baggett, & Sideris, 2016; Wolff, Boyd, & Elison, 2016). In addition, there is some evidence that early presence of significantly impairing RRBs is predictive of less optimal outcomes in children with ASD (Troyb et al., 2016).

Age

Before age 2 or 3, it can be challenging to distinguish children with ASD from children with other developmental delays based on the presence of RRBs (Lord, 1995; Stone et al., 1999), especially when observing a child in one setting or asking parents about RRBs. With recorded videos, detailed coding, or specific screening of these behaviors researchers have found that children who develop ASD show more RRBs than their typically developing peers even in the first 2 years of life (Elison et al., 2014; Morgan et al., 2008; Turner-Brown, Baranek, Reznick, Watson, & Crais, 2013; Watt et al., 2008). Thus, the symptoms are present early in life; RSM behaviors seem to decrease over time while insistence on sameness behaviors may increase over time (Richler et al., 2010; Watt et al., 2008).

Sleep

Many children with ASD have some kind of difficulty with sleep, whether it is difficulty falling asleep, staying asleep, or waking (Hollway & Aman, 2011). Decreased sleep is associated with a range of symptoms, including RRBs in children with ASD. In some cases, RRBs may interfere with the process of going to sleep (Richdale & Schreck, 2009). For example, a child may have ritualistic behavior around bedtime that is hard to interrupt. Or, the relationship could go the other way, with decreased sleep leading to increased RRBs (Abel, Schwichtenberg, Brodhead, & Christ, 2018). Some research suggests that decreased sleep is particularly associated with increases in repetitive and stereotyped movements (Hundley, Shui, & Malow, 2016). It is likely that the relationship between RRB and sleep is bidirectional—suggesting that changes in either area may affect the other (Hollway & Aman, 2011).

Gender

In young children with ASD, there do not seem to be differences between males and females and severity of RRB. At older ages findings are mixed, but there is preliminary evidence that RRB symptoms may be worse in males than females (Harrop,

Gulsrud, & Kasari, 2015; Knutsen, Crossman, Perrin, Shui, & Kuhlthau, 2019; Van Wijngaarden-Cremers et al., 2014).

Family Well-Being

Many families become involved in their child's ritualistic behavior—imagine the child who screams whenever he arrives at the park to discover he does not have his train to carry around with him. His caregiver must decide whether to return home to retrieve the train (and prevent screaming in public) or to allow and manage the screaming in hope that the child will calm down quickly. These decisions are challenging in the moment as both have immediate negative consequences for the parent (e.g., screaming or added driving). Making decisions to prevent screaming may inadvertently increase the rigidity the child has around having access to that object. It is not surprising, then, that high levels of parent stress have been documented for children with ASD in numerous studies (see Hayes & Watson, 2013, for a review) and that parent stress is frequently associated with challenging and/or RRBs. Parents find RRBs particularly difficult to manage in their daily lives, even more challenging than communication symptoms (Bishop, Richler, Cain, & Lord, 2007; Lecavalier, Leone, & Wiltz, 2006). When RRBs increase, parent stress may increase (Harrop, McBee, & Boyd, 2016). In addition, increased parent stress can negatively impact outcomes of early intervention (Osborne, McHugh, Saunders, & Reed, 2008).

In sum, RRBs are observable early in a child's life, with atypicalities present as early as 12 months. Some of these behaviors decrease across development, such as RSM behaviors, while insistence on sameness behaviors tends to increase over time, particularly during early childhood (Richler et al., 2010). These changes in patterns of the display of RRBs are mirrored by changes in parent stress; as RRBs decrease, so do parenting stress ratings (Harrop, McBee, et al., 2016). Sleep may play a significant role in RRBs.

Why Do Children Engage in RRBs?

Consider a 2-year-old child who is repetitively lining up his crayons in a precise way. When his brother suggests they play with blocks, he does not look over to see what is going on because the crayons are holding his attention. Thus, he misses the opportunity to engage with his brother and play with something different. When it is time to clean up and move to meal time, he becomes upset because he does not have his line of crayons perfect yet. So, he misses the family meal. Finally, because he is so focused on color arrangement of his crayons, he resists when his mother tries to teach him to color with them. These three examples of missed opportunities highlight some of the negative consequences of RRBs on child learning and development. When asked, his parents might describe this behavior differently, however.

They may see this behavior as a strength, as their son knows all the colors in a 128-pack of crayons and can count to 128 at a really early age.

Why do children with ASD engage in RRBs? Do individuals with ASD have lower social motivation and higher motivation to engage with objects? Or, is their entire brain circuitry dysregulated such that reward is processed differently for both social interaction and engagement with objects? Do children with autism have difficulty shifting their attention from one thing to another leading to extended focus on one activity? Researchers have explored these theories, and found some support for many of them along with differences in both the brain size and function that may contribute to development and maintenance of RRBs (Bodfish, Symons, Parker, & Lewis, 2000; Boyd, McDonough, Rupp, Khan, & Bodfish, 2011; Dichter et al., 2012; Klin, Jones, Schultz, Volkmar, & Cohen, 2002; Pierce, Glad, & Schreibman, 1997; Troyb et al., 2016; Turner, 1999).

While there is no one answer to explain the myriad of RRB manifestations, engagement in RRBs can cause a child to miss potential learning opportunities starting early in development. Thus, early intervention has the potential to increase learning opportunities by addressing RRBs and expanding the range of adaptive skills a child develops.

Effects of Early Intervention on RRBs

A majority of early intervention research has focused on promoting early social communication skills rather than on reducing RRBs. Yet there are several focused interventions that specifically target reduction of RRBs, and a range of comprehensive treatment approaches that aim to reduce RRB among a wide range of other treatment targets (e.g., increase communication). We review findings from both below.

Comprehensive Treatment Models

Despite the growing number of comprehensive treatment models (Lee, Odom, & Loftin, 2007) demonstrating positive effects on cognitive, communication, and adaptive skills, there is less evidence of their effects on RRBs. For example, research on Early Intensive Behavioral intervention (EIBI; see Chap. 5), TEACCH (see Chap. 7), Early Start Denver Model (ESDM; see Chap. 6), and Learning Experiences and Alternate Program for Preschoolers and their Parents (LEAP) has shown limited immediate effects on RRBs, despite positive changes in other areas (e.g., Boyd et al., 2014; Dawson et al., 2010; Reichow, Hume, Barton, & Boyd, 2018). There are many possible reasons for these findings. First, high-quality studies of comprehensive treatment models often measure symptom change in a global way. For example, parents might complete a symptom inventory of all types of RRBs, before and after treatment. If the total score increases, it means there are more behaviors and/or the behaviors are more problematic. If the score decreases, it means that there are fewer behaviors and/or the behaviors are less problematic. While this measure tells a lot about overall severity of RRBs, it may be too broad to detect slight changes in specific RRBs that result from intervention.

A second reason why comprehensive treatment models may not have shown positive effects on RRBs in early childhood is the natural progression of these behaviors. Research has shown that RSM often decreases across early childhood. Thus, detecting a treatment effect on top of natural decreases is challenging. In contrast, insistence on sameness or higher-order RRBs may increase during these years, making it even more challenging to show improvement.

Finally, many comprehensive treatment models are designed to focus primarily on social communication and adaptive functioning. Theoretically, as adaptive skills increase (e.g., a child learns to play with more toys or ask for help), RRBs would decrease as a result. If this theory is valid, it might be the case that RRBs would show a decrease long after an intervention is complete rather than immediately after it ends. Some evidence supports this theory, as a 2-year follow up study of ESDM showed more effects of ESDM on RRB 2 years later than immediately after ESDM was implemented (Estes et al., 2015).

In sum, while the evidence of effects of comprehensive treatment models on RRB is limited, research is ongoing. As stated, these models often emphasize building skills rather than reducing symptoms. Where research has shown more positive effects is when examining focused intervention practices whose specific target is reduction of a specific behavior. We review these below.

Focused Intervention Practices

The principles of applied behavior analysis (ABA) and cognitive behavioral therapy (CBT) underlie the focused approaches shown to reduce RRBs. ABA techniques aim to reduce or increase a specific behavior by changing the contingencies under which the behavior occurs. Behaviors occur in an antecedent–behavior–consequence context (ABC; see Chaps. 1 and 5), and efforts to change behavior focus on modifying either the antecedent or the consequence associated with the behavior. Imagine the situation of a child entering a loud preschool classroom. Upon entering, the child covers his ears and rocks his body. His parent then takes his hands off his ears and says, "hands down." The behavior is covering ears, the antecedent is the loudness in the classroom setting, and the consequence is the physical movement of the child's hands and verbal direction. ABA techniques to reduce these behaviors focus on changing antecedents or consequences. CBT techniques are similar to ABA, but also consider internal states (e.g., thoughts and feelings) in addition to the ABCs of behavior.

In their review of interventions targeting RRBs, Boyd and colleagues organized successful approaches to reducing RRBs into three categories: consequence-based interventions that interrupt the reinforcement provided by an RRB, antecedent-based interventions that reduce the likelihood of the occurrence of an RRB by altering the environment, and antecedent-based interventions that enrich skills or the environment that may consequently affect the presence of RRBs (Boyd, McDonough, & Bodfish, 2012). For simplicity, we group these as (1) preventing RRBs and (2) changing consequences to RRBs below.

Preventing RRB

Several practices have effectively reduced RRBs by aiming to prevent their occurrence; if we know the contexts in which the behavior occurs, we can change the environment to prevent the behavior and/or teach alternative skills to use instead of an RRB. As illustrated in the following sections, using visual schedules and cues, schedule variation, exercise, and functional communication training are all research-supported approaches for reducing RRBs in this way.

Functional communication training (FCT; Kennedy, Meyer, Knowles, & Shukla, 2000) and similar approaches involve teaching an individual a more appropriate skill, such as a communication or play skill that may serve the same function as an RRB. Consider this scenario. A young child flaps his hands often at school. A functional analysis determined that this behavior occurs most often when a teacher gives a demand, such as "time to clean up," suggesting that the function of this stereotyped behavior is avoiding a demand. FCT would then teach this child a more appropriate way to get the same result. For example, a therapist might teach a communicative behavior such as signing "break" to request a break from the demand. Teaching more adaptive skills is effective for reducing stereotypies and self-injurious behavior (Kennedy et al., 2000; Lee et al., 2007; Loftin, Odom, & Lantz, 2008; Rispoli, Camargo, Machalicek, Lang, & Sigafoos, 2014; Tiger, Hanley, & Bruzek, 2008).

A second strategy for preventing RRB is using visual schedules and cues. Visual schedules are a component of the TEACCH Approach (Mesibov, Shea, & Schopler, 2006; see Chap. 7) and involve providing visual cues at the developmental level of the child to let the child know what will happen next. Schedules vary in form (e.g., objects, pictures, and written lists) and length (e.g., what is next, two-step, part day, full day). In the context of RRBs, it can be useful to schedule time for when a child can engage in RRB. For example, showing the child that first he must play outside and then he can play on his tablet with picture cues may reduce attempts to bring the iPad to outdoor play (see Lequia, Machalicek, & Rispoli, 2012, for a review, and see Fig. 4.1 for an example of this type of schedule). Using visual cues about upcoming changes in an activity or routine (Horner, Day, & Day, 2006) may also reduce RRBs. This approach may help a child who asks repeated questions about the weather. Placing a time on the schedule when it is appropriate to discuss the weather may reduce weather-talk at other times of day.

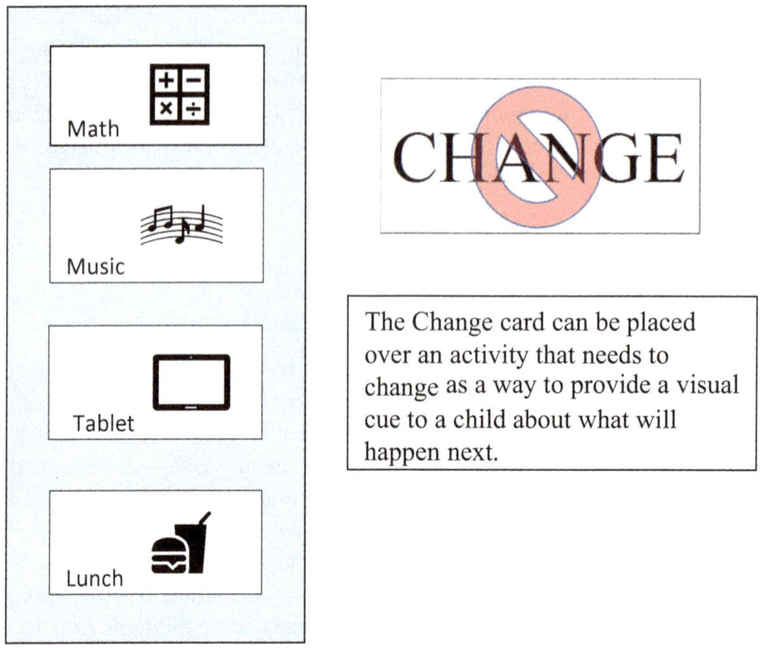

Fig. 4.1 Examples of visual schedules

Engaging in physical exercise can also reduce RRB (Bahrami, Movahedi, Marandi, & Abedi, 2012; Kasner, Reid, & MacDonald, 2012; Schmitz Olin et al., 2017). Some research shows an immediate effect, with RRB reduced immediately after a period of exercise. Other studies show more global reductions in RRB after a period of exercise training.

Finally, treatment of sleep problems can lead to reduced RRBs (Malow et al., 2012, 2014; Reed et al., 2009). Approaches including educating parents about sleep hygiene, behavioral interventions to decrease insomnia, and melatonin have all shown promise as ways to improve sleep that also lead to decreases in repetitive and other challenging behavior.

Changing Consequences to RRB

Many studies have explored how to change the consequences associated with RRBs. Harrop and colleagues (2016) studied family reactions to RRB in the home and found that caregivers respond to about half of the RRB their children displayed. These caregivers were more likely to redirect behaviors that involved objects (e.g., visually inspecting objects and shaking objects) than to motor or verbal behaviors (e.g., flapping hands or repetitive sounds). Parents' physical and verbal strategies to stop the child from engagement in the behaviors were rated as the most effective in stopping RRBs (Harrop, Gulsrud, Shih, Hovsepyan, & Kasari, 2016). Examples of approaches that aim to reduce RRB by changing consequences include blocking or response interruption and redirection, differential reinforcement, as well as exposure and response prevention. These are each described below.

Response interruption and redirection involves interrupting an RRB and redirecting the child to a different action (Ahearn, Clark, MacDonald, & In Chung, 2007; Boyd et al., 2011; Koegel, Firestone, Kramme, & Dunlap, 1974; Liu-gitz & Banda, 2010). For example, a father sees his daughter holding a block close to her eye. He then physically interrupts this behavior by placing his hands over her hand and the object, and redirects her to a different behavior, such as placing the block on another to begin making a tower. This approach can both reduce stereotyped behavior and increase more adaptive behavior.

Differential reinforcement entails reinforcement of certain behaviors (e.g., adaptive skills and varying play skills) while not reinforcing other behaviors (e.g., RRB). It can target a range of goals, such as increasing flexible and novel engagement with routines and toys (Azrin, Besalel, Jamner, & Caputo, 1988; Boyd et al., 2011; Miller & Neuringer, 2000). For example, a teacher responds with specific verbal praise whenever seeing a child using a toy in a new way while ignoring repetitive use of the toy.

Finally, exposure and response prevention (ERP; (Huppert & Franklin, 2005) is a CBT approach to reducing symptoms in people with obsessive compulsive disorder (OCD). This approach has been evaluated in children with ASD because of the partial overlap in symptoms between ASD and OCD (e.g., individuals with both conditions can be observed engaging in repetitive behavior such as opening and closing doors; see Klin et al., 2007; Postorino et al., 2017; Scahill & Challa, 2016 for reviews on the similarities and differences between RRBs and OCD symptoms). ERP involves building up skills to handle challenging or fearful situations, and then gradually exposing the child step-by-step to that situation. Thus, the specific RRB characteristics targeted for children with ASD have been rigidity and need for sameness. Consider a child who gets upset when he wants to complete a jigsaw puzzle in a particular order and becomes upset when he is unable to complete it that way. This intervention would entail step-by-step exposure to completing a puzzle in a different way. Results have shown that these approaches reduce rigidity and accompanying anxiety in children with ASD (Boyd, Woodard, & Bodfish, 2013; Eilers & Hayes, 2015; Reaven & Hepburn, 2003), though they have only been tested with older children to date.

Parent Training

RRBs can be difficult for parents to deal with in daily life (Harrop, McBee, et al., 2016). Thus, it is important to ensure parents and caregivers are equipped with a strong understanding of these symptoms as well as approaches that can be useful to daily life. Teaching parents about behavioral inflexibility in ASD, providing parent to parent support, and teaching parents evidence-supported strategies to prevent and respond to RRBs can be helpful (Boyd et al., 2011; Grahame et al., 2015; Lin & Koegel, 2018).

Incorporating Child RRBs in Learning Activities

A common strategy across a range of intervention approaches entails using one RRB characteristic, circumscribed interests, as a way to engage and reward children with ASD. For example, a 4-year-old child in a preschool class loves to play with blocks and cars but refuses to participate in art activities. One strategy to increase his participation in art might be to include cars in the art activity by dipping wheels in paint and rolling the cars on paper to make a pattern. By using this child's special interest in cars, the teacher increases his engagement in art and provides more opportunities for peer interaction as the child is able to participate in a group activity. Research supports this strategy (Boyd, Conroy, Mancil, Nakao, & Alter, 2007; Gunn & Delafield-Butt, 2016). This approach also reflects the notion that the talents that may develop from these interests (e.g., a strong vocabulary of dinosaur names or states and capitals) are valuable, positive, and a true strength for the individual with ASD.

Pharmacotherapies

Despite considerable research on the efficacy of a range of medications on RRBs, only buspirone currently shows promise to reduce these symptoms in children with ASD. Buspirone is a serotonin agonist generally used to treat anxiety in children and has been associated with improvement in RRBs (Chugani et al., 2016). Other medications have not led to reduction in RRB symptoms, including serotonin receptor inhibitors (Accordino, Kidd, Politte, Henry, & Mcdougle, 2016; Carrasco, Volkmar, & Bloch, 2012).

Conclusion

RRBs are present early in life and can cause significant impairment in development and lead to increase in parent stress and other mental health challenges in children with ASD. Several focused intervention practices including prevention of RRB and changing consequences to RRB are effective for reducing RRB, and supporting parents may have lasting positive effects on the child and family. In addition, some RRBs, such as circumscribed interests provide a way to reach and engage with a child who may be challenging to engage in typical ways. These interests may also develop into strengths to be promoted throughout life.

References

Abel, E. A., Schwichtenberg, A. J., Brodhead, M. T., & Christ, S. L. (2018). Sleep and challenging behaviors in the context of intensive behavioral intervention for children with autism. *Journal of Autism and Developmental Disorders, 48*(11), 3871–3884. https://doi.org/10.1007/s10803-018-3648-0

Accordino, R. E., Kidd, C., Politte, L. C., Henry, C. A., & Mcdougle, C. J. (2016). Expert opinion on pharmacotherapy psychopharmacological interventions in autism spectrum disorder Psychopharmacological interventions in autism spectrum disorder. *Expert Opinion on Pharmacotherapy, 17*(7), 937–952. https://doi.org/10.1517/14656566.2016.1154536

Ahearn, W. H., Clark, K. M., MacDonald, R. P., & In Chung, B. (2007). Assessing and treating vocal stereotypy in children with autism. *Journal of Applied Behavior Analysis, 40*(2), 263–275. https://doi.org/10.1901/jaba.2007.30-06

American Psychiatric Association. (2013). *Diagnostic and statistical manual or mental disorders (5th ed.).* doi: https://doi.org/10.1176/appi.books.9780890425596.744053.

Ausderau, K. K., Furlong, M., Sideris, J., Bulluck, J., Little, L. M., Watson, L. R., ... Baranek, G. T. (2014). Sensory subtypes in children with autism spectrum disorder: Latent profile transition analysis using a national survey of sensory features. *Journal of Child Psychology and Psychiatry, and Allied Disciplines, 55*(8), 935–944. https://doi.org/10.1111/jcpp.12219

Azrin, N. H., Besalel, V. A., Jamner, J. P., & Caputo, J. N. (1988). Comparative study of behavioral methods of treating severe self-injury. *Behavioral Residential Treatment, 3*(2), 119–152.

Bahrami, F., Movahedi, A., Marandi, S. M., & Abedi, A. (2012). Kata techniques training consistently decreases stereotypy in children with autism spectrum disorder. *Research in Developmental Disabilities, 33*(4), 1183–1193. https://doi.org/10.1016/j.ridd.2012.01.018

Bishop, S. L., Hus, V., Duncan, A., Huerta, M., Gotham, K., Pickles, A., ... Lord, C. (2013). Subcategories of restricted and repetitive behaviors in children with autism spectrum disorders. *Journal of Autism and Developmental Disorders, 43*(6), 1287–1297. https://doi.org/10.1007/s10803-012-1671-0

Bishop, S. L., Richler, J., Cain, A. C., & Lord, C. (2007). Predictors of perceived negative impact in mothers of children with autism spectrum disorder. *American Journal of Mental Retardation: AJMR, 112*(6), 450–461. https://doi.org/10.1352/0895-8017(2007)112[450:POPNII]2.0.CO;2

Bishop, S. L., Richler, J., & Lord, C. (2006). Association between restricted and repetitive behaviors and nonverbal IQ in children with autism spectrum disorders. *Child Neuropsychology, 12*(4–5), 247–267. https://doi.org/10.1080/09297040600630288

Bodfish, J. W., Symons, F. J., Parker, D. E., & Lewis, M. H. (2000). Varieties of repetitive behavior in autism: Comparisons to mental retardation. *Journal of Autism and Developmental Disorders, 30*(3), 237–243.

Boyd, B. A., Conroy, M. A., Mancil, G. R., Nakao, T., & Alter, P. J. (2007). Effects of circumscribed interests on the social behaviors of children with autism spectrum disorders. *Journal of Autism and Developmental Disorders, 37*(8), 1550–1561. https://doi.org/10.1007/s10803-006-0286-8

Boyd, B. A., Hume, K., McBee, M. T., Alessandri, M., Gutierrez, A., Johnson, L. A., ... Odom, S. L. (2014). Comparative efficacy of LEAP, TEACCH and non-model-specific special education programs for preschoolers with autism spectrum disorders. *Journal of Autism and Developmental Disorders, 44*(2), 366–380. https://doi.org/10.1007/s10803-013-1877-9

Boyd, B. A., McDonough, S. G., & Bodfish, J. W. (2012). Evidence-based behavioral interventions for repetitive behaviors in autism. *Journal of Autism and Developmental Disorders, 42*(6), 1236–1248. https://doi.org/10.1007/s10803-011-1284-z

Boyd, B. A., McDonough, S. G., Rupp, B., Khan, F., & Bodfish, J. W. (2011). Effects of a family-implemented treatment on the repetitive behaviors of children with autism. *Journal of Autism and Developmental Disorders, 41*(10), 1330–1341. https://doi.org/10.1007/s10803-010-1156-y

Boyd, B. A., Woodard, C. R., & Bodfish, J. W. (2013). Feasibility of exposure response prevention to treat repetitive behaviors of children with autism and an intellectual disability: A brief report. *Autism: The International Journal of Research and Practice, 17*(2), 196–204. https://doi.org/10.1177/1362361311414066

Carrasco, M., Volkmar, F. R., & Bloch, M. H. (2012). Pharmacologic treatment of repetitive behaviors in autism spectrum disorders: Evidence of publication bias. *Pediatrics, 129*(5), e1301–e1310. https://doi.org/10.1542/peds.2011-3285

Chugani, D. C., Chugani, H. T., Wiznitzer, M., Parikh, S., Evans, P. A., Hansen, R. L., … Hirtz, D. (2016). Efficacy of low-dose buspirone for restricted and repetitive behavior in young children with autism spectrum disorder: A randomized trial. *Journal of Pediatrics, 170*, 45–53e4. https://doi.org/10.1016/j.jpeds.2015.11.033

Dawson, G., Rogers, S., Munson, J., Smith, M., Winter, J., Greenson, J., … Varley, J. (2010). Randomized, controlled trial of an intervention for toddlers with autism: The early start denver model. *Pediatrics, 125*(1), e17–e23. https://doi.org/10.1542/peds.2009-0958

Dichter, G. S., Felder, J. N., Green, S. R., Rittenberg, A. M., Sasson, N. J., & Bodfish, J. W. (2012). Reward circuitry function in autism spectrum disorders. *Social Cognitive and Affective Neuroscience, 7*(2), 160–172. https://doi.org/10.1093/scan/nsq095

Eilers, H. J., & Hayes, S. C. (2015). Exposure and response prevention therapy with cognitive defusion exercises to reduce repetitive and restrictive behaviors displayed by children with autism spectrum disorder. *Research in Autism Spectrum Disorders, 19*, 18–31. https://doi.org/10.1016/j.rasd.2014.12.014

Elison, J. T., Wolff, J. J., Reznick, J. S., Botteron, K. N., Estes, A. M., Gu, H., … Piven, J. (2014). Repetitive behavior in 12-month-olds later classified with autism spectrum disorder. *Journal of the American Academy of Child and Adolescent Psychiatry, 53*(11), 1216–1224. https://doi.org/10.1016/j.jaac.2014.08.004

Estes, A., Munson, J., Rogers, S. J., Greenson, J., Winter, J., & Dawson, G. (2015). Long-term outcomes of early intervention in 6-year-old children with autism spectrum disorder. *Journal of the American Academy of Child and Adolescent Psychiatry, 54*(7), 580–587. https://doi.org/10.1016/j.jaac.2015.04.005

Evans, D. W., Leckman, J. F., Carter, A., Reznick, S. J., Henshaw, D., King, R. A., & Pauls, D. (1997). Ritual, habit, and perfectionism: The prevalence and development of compulsive-like behavior in normal young children. *Child Development, 68*(1), 58–68.

Grahame, V., Brett, D., Dixon, L., McConachie, H., Lowry, J., Rodgers, J., … Le Couteur, A. (2015). Managing repetitive behaviours in young children with autism spectrum disorder (ASD): Pilot randomised controlled trial of a new parent group intervention. *Journal of Autism and Developmental Disorders, 45*(10), 3168–3182. https://doi.org/10.1007/s10803-015-2474-x

Gunn, K. C. M., & Delafield-Butt, J. T. (2016). Teaching children with autism spectrum disorder with restricted interests. *Review of Educational Research, 86*(2), 408–430. https://doi.org/10.3102/0034654315604027

Harrop, C., Gulsrud, A., & Kasari, C. (2015). Does gender moderate core deficits in ASD? An investigation into restricted and repetitive behaviors in girls and boys with ASD. *Journal of Autism and Developmental Disorders, 45*(11), 3644–3655. https://doi.org/10.1007/s10803-015-2511-9

Harrop, C., Gulsrud, A., Shih, W., Hovsepyan, L., & Kasari, C. (2016). Characterizing caregiver responses to restricted and repetitive behaviors in toddlers with autism spectrum disorder. *Autism, 20*(3), 330–342. https://doi.org/10.1177/1362361315580443

Harrop, C., McBee, M., & Boyd, B. A. (2016). How are child restricted and repetitive behaviors associated with caregiver stress over time? A parallel process multilevel growth model. *Journal of Autism and Developmental Disorders, 46*(5), 1773–1783. https://doi.org/10.1007/s10803-016-2707-7

Hayes, S. A., & Watson, S. L. (2013). The impact of parenting stress: A meta-analysis of studies comparing the experience of parenting stress in parents of children with and without autism spectrum disorder. *Journal of Autism and Developmental Disorders, 43*(3), 629–642. https://doi.org/10.1007/s10803-012-1604-y

Hollway, J. A., & Aman, M. G. (2011). Sleep correlates of pervasive developmental disorders: A review of the literature. *Research in Developmental Disabilities, 32*(5), 1399–1421. https://doi.org/10.1016/j.ridd.2011.04.001

Horner, R. H., Day, H. M., & Day, J. R. (2006). Using neutralizing routines to reduce problem behaviors. *Journal of Applied Behavior Analysis, 30*(4), 601–614. https://doi.org/10.1901/jaba.1997.30-601

Hundley, R. J., Shui, A., & Malow, B. A. (2016). Relationship between subtypes of restricted and repetitive behaviors and sleep disturbance in autism spectrum disorder. *Journal of Autism and Developmental Disorders, 46*(11), 3448–3457. https://doi.org/10.1007/s10803-016-2884-4

Huppert, J. D., & Franklin, M. E. (2005). Cognitive behavioral therapy for obsessive-compulsive disorder: An update. *Current Psychiatry Reports, 7*(4), 268–273. Retrieved from http://www.ncbi.nlm.nih.gov/pubmed/16098280.

Kanner, L. (1943). Autistic disturbances of affective contact. *The Nervous Child, 2*, 217–250.

Kasner, M., Reid, G., & MacDonald, C. (2012). Evidence-based practice: Quality indicator analysis of antecedent exercise in autism spectrum disorders. *Research in Autism Spectrum Disorders, 6*(4), 1418–1425. https://doi.org/10.1016/j.rasd.2012.02.001

Kennedy, C. H., Meyer, K. A., Knowles, T., & Shukla, S. (2000). Analyzing the multiple functions of stereotypical behavior for students with autism: Implications for assessment and treatment. *Journal of Applied Behavior Analysis, 33*(4), 559–571.

Klin, A., Danovitch, J. H., Merz, A. B., & Volkmar, F. R. (2007). Circumscribed interests in higher functioning individuals with autism spectrum disorders: An exploratory study. *Research and Practice for Persons with Severe Disabilities, 32*(2), 89–100. https://doi.org/10.2511/rpsd.32.2.89

Klin, A., Jones, W., Schultz, R., Volkmar, F., & Cohen, D. (2002). Visual fixation patterns during viewing of naturalistic social situations as predictors of social competence in individuals with autism. *Archives of General Psychiatry, 59*(9), 809. https://doi.org/10.1001/archpsyc.59.9.809

Knutsen, J., Crossman, M., Perrin, J., Shui, A., & Kuhlthau, K. (2019). Sex differences in restricted repetitive behaviors and interests in children with autism spectrum disorder: An Autism Treatment Network study. *Autism, 23*(4), 858–868. https://doi.org/10.1177/1362361318786490

Koegel, R. L., Firestone, P. B., Kramme, K. W., & Dunlap, G. (1974). Increasing spontaneous play by suppressing sel-stimulation in autistic children. *Journal of Applied Behavior Analysis, 7*(4), 521–528.

Lam, K. S. L., Bodfish, J. W., & Piven, J. (2008). Evidence for three subtypes of repetitive behavior in autism that differ in familiality and association with other symptoms. *Journal of Child Psychology and Psychiatry, and Allied Disciplines, 49*(11), 1193–1200. https://doi.org/10.1111/j.1469-7610.2008.01944.x

Lecavalier, L., Leone, S., & Wiltz, J. (2006). The impact of behaviour problems on caregiver stress in young people with autism spectrum disorders. *Journal of Intellectual Disability Research, 50*(3), 172–183. https://doi.org/10.1111/j.1365-2788.2005.00732.x

Lee, S., Odom, S. L., & Loftin, R. (2007). Social engagement with peers and stereotypic behavior of children with autism. *Journal of Positive Behavior Interventions, 9*(2), 67–79.

Lequia, J., Machalicek, W., & Rispoli, M. J. (2012). Effects of activity schedules on challenging behavior exhibited in children with autism spectrum disorders: A systematic review. *Research in Autism Spectrum Disorders, 6*(1), 480–492. https://doi.org/10.1016/j.rasd.2011.07.008

Lin, C. E., & Koegel, R. (2018). Treatment for higher-order restricted repetitive behaviors (H-RRB) in children with autism spectrum disorder. *Journal of Autism and Developmental Disorders, 48*(11), 3831–3845. https://doi.org/10.1007/s10803-018-3637-3

Liu-gitz, L., & Banda, D. R. (2010). A replication of the rird strategy to decrease vocal stereotypy in a student with autism. *Behavioral Interventions, 25*, 77–87. https://doi.org/10.1002/bin

Loftin, R. L., Odom, S. L., & Lantz, J. F. (2008). Social interaction and repetitive motor behaviors. *Journal of Autism and Developmental Disorders, 38*, 1124–1135. https://doi.org/10.1007/s10803-007-0499-5

Lord, C. (1995). Follow-up of two-year-olds referred for possible autism. *Journal of Child Psychology and Psychiatry, 36*(8), 1365–1382. https://doi.org/10.1111/j.1469-7610.1995.tb01669.x

Malow, B., Adkins, K. W., McGrew, S. G., Wang, L., Goldman, S. E., Fawkes, D., & Burnette, C. (2012). Melatonin for sleep in children with autism: A controlled trial examining dose, tolerability, and outcomes. *Journal of Autism and Developmental Disorders, 42*(8), 1729–1737; author reply 1738. https://doi.org/10.1007/s10803-011-1418-3

Malow, B., Adkins, K. W., Reynolds, A., Weiss, S. K., Loh, A., Fawkes, D., … Clemons, T. (2014). Parent-based sleep education for children with autism spectrum disorders. *Journal of Autism and Developmental Disorders, 44*(1), 216–228. https://doi.org/10.1007/s10803-013-1866-z

Mesibov, G. B., Shea, V., & Schopler, E. (2006). *The TEACCH approach to autism spectrum disorders*. New York, NY: Springer.

Miller, N., & Neuringer, A. (2000). Reinforcing variability in adolescents with autism. *Journal of Applied Behavior Analysis, 33*(2), 151–165. https://doi.org/10.1901/jaba.2000.33-151

Morgan, L., Wetherby, A. M., & Barber, A. (2008). Repetitive and stereotyped movements in children with autism spectrum disorders late in the second year of life. *Journal of Child Psychology and Psychiatry, 49*(8), 826–837. https://doi.org/10.1111/j.1469-7610.2008.01904.x

Osborne, L. A., McHugh, L., Saunders, J., & Reed, P. (2008). Parenting stress reduces the effectiveness of early teaching interventions for autistic spectrum disorders. *Journal of Autism and Developmental Disorders, 38*(6), 1092–1103. https://doi.org/10.1007/s10803-007-0497-7

Pierce, K., Glad, K. S., & Schreibman, L. (1997). Social perception in children with autism: An attentional deficit? *Journal of Autism and Developmental Disorders, 27*(3), 265–282. Retrieved from http://www.ncbi.nlm.nih.gov/pubmed/9229258.

Postorino, V., Kerns, C. M., Vivanti, G., Bradshaw, J., Siracusano, M., & Mazzone, L. (2017). Anxiety disorders and obsessive-compulsive disorder in individuals with autism spectrum disorder. *Current Psychiatry Reports, 19*(12), 92. https://doi.org/10.1007/s11920-017-0846-y

Reaven, J., & Hepburn, S. (2003). Cognitive-behavioral treatment of obsessive-compulsive disorder in a child with Asperger syndrome: A case report. *Autism, 7*(2), 145–164.

Reed, H. E., McGrew, S. G., Artibee, K., Surdkya, K., Goldman, S. E., Frank, K., … Malow, B. (2009). Parent-based sleep education workshops in autism. *Journal of Child Neurology, 24*(8), 936–945. https://doi.org/10.1177/0883073808331348

Reichow, B., Hume, K., Barton, E. E., & Boyd, B. A. (2018). Early intensive behavioral intervention (EIBI) for young children with autism spectrum disorders (ASD). *The Cochrane Database of Systematic Reviews, 5*, CD009260. https://doi.org/10.1002/14651858.CD009260.pub3

Richdale, A. L., & Schreck, K. A. (2009). Sleep problems in autism spectrum disorders: Prevalence, nature, & possible biopsychosocial aetiologies. *Sleep Medicine Reviews, 13*(6), 403–411. https://doi.org/10.1016/j.smrv.2009.02.003

Richler, J., Huerta, M., Bishop, S. L., & Lord, C. (2010). Developmental trajectories of restricted and repetitive behaviors and interests in children with autism spectrum disorders. *Development and Psychopathology, 22*(1), 55–69. https://doi.org/10.1017/S0954579409990265

Rispoli, M., Camargo, S., Machalicek, W., Lang, R., & Sigafoos, J. (2014). Functional communication training in the treatment of problem behavior maintained by access to rituals. *Journal of Applied Behavior Analysis, 47*(3), 580–593. https://doi.org/10.1002/jaba.130

Scahill, L., & Challa, S. A. (2016). Repetitive behavior in children with autism spectrum disorder: Similarities and differences with obsessive-compulsive disorder. In L. Mazzone & B. Vitiello (Eds.), *Psychiatric symptoms and comorbidities in autism spectrum disorders*. Berlin: Springer.

Schertz, H. H., Odom, S. L., Baggett, K. M., & Sideris, J. H. (2016). Parent-reported repetitive behavior in toddlers on the autism spectrum. *Journal of Autism and Developmental Disorders, 46*(10), 3308–3316. https://doi.org/10.1007/s10803-016-2870-x

Schmitz Olin, S., McFadden, B. A., Golem, D. L., Pellegrino, J. K., Walker, A. J., Sanders, D. J., & Arent, S. M. (2017). The effects of exercise dose on stereotypical behavior in children with autism. *Medicine and Science in Sports and Exercise, 49*(5), 983–990. https://doi.org/10.1249/MSS.0000000000001197

Shafer, R. L., Newell, K. M., Lewis, M. H., & Bodfish, J. W. (2017). A cohesive framework for motor stereotypy in typical and atypical development: The role of sensorimotor integration. *Frontiers in Integrative Neuroscience, 11*, 1–8. https://doi.org/10.3389/fnint.2017.00019

Stone, W. L., Lee, E. B., Ashford, L., Brissie, J., Hepburn, S. L., Coonrod, E. E., & Weiss, B. H. (1999). Can autism be diagnosed accurately in children under 3 years? *Journal of Child Psychology and Psychiatry, and Allied Disciplines, 40*(2), 219–226. Retrieved from http://www.ncbi.nlm.nih.gov/pubmed/10188704.

Tiger, J. H., Hanley, G. P., & Bruzek, J. (2008). Functional communication training: A review and practical guide. *Behavior Analysis in Practice, 1*(1), 16–23. Retrieved from www.abainternational.

Troyb, E., Knoch, K., Herlihy, L., Stevens, M. C., Chen, C. M., Barton, M., … Fein, D. (2016). Restricted and repetitive behaviors as predictors of outcome in autism spectrum disorders. *Journal of Autism and Developmental Disorders, 46*(4), 1282–1296. https://doi.org/10.1007/s10803-015-2668-2

Turner, M. (1999). Annotation: Repetitive behaviour in autism: A review of psychological research. *Journal of Child Psychology and Psychiatry, 40*(6), 839–849. https://doi.org/10.1111/1469-7610.00502

Turner-Brown, L. M., Baranek, G. T., Reznick, J. S., Watson, L. R., & Crais, E. R. (2013). The first year inventory: A longitudinal follow-up of 12-month-old to 3-year-old children. *Autism, 17*(5), 527–540. https://doi.org/10.1177/1362361312439633

Van Wijngaarden-Cremers, P. J. M., Van Eeten, E., Groen, W. B., Van Deurzen, P. A., Oosterling, I. J., & Van Der Gaag, R. J. (2014). Gender and age differences in the core triad of impairments in autism spectrum disorders: A systematic review and meta-analysis. *Journal of Autism and Developmental Disorders, 44*(3), 627–635. https://doi.org/10.1007/s10803-013-1913-9

Watt, N., Wetherby, A. M., Barber, A., & Morgan, L. (2008). Repetitive and stereotyped behaviors in children with autism spectrum disorders in the second year of life. *Journal of Autism and Developmental Disorders, 38*(8), 1518–1533. https://doi.org/10.1007/s10803-007-0532-8

Wolff, J. J., Botteron, K. N., Dager, S. R., Elison, J. T., Estes, A. M., Gu, H., … Piven, J. (2014). Longitudinal patterns of repetitive behavior in toddlers with autism. *Journal of Child Psychology and Psychiatry, and Allied Disciplines, 55*(8), 945–953. https://doi.org/10.1111/jcpp.12207

Wolff, J. J., Boyd, B. A., & Elison, J. T. (2016). A quantitative measure of restricted and repetitive behaviors for early childhood. *Journal of Neurodevelopmental Disorders, 8*(1), 1–10. https://doi.org/10.1186/s11689-016-9161-x

Chapter 5
Applied Behavior Analytic Approaches to Early Intervention for Children with Autism

Giacomo Vivanti and Melanie Pellecchia

Many early intervention programs for children with ASD are based on the principles of applied behavior analysis (ABA). This chapter will cover the basic principles of ABA, as well as the strategies and procedures used in the ABA-based early intervention program for ASD called "early intensive behavioral intervention (EIBI)," while an in-depth discussion about naturalistic applications of ABA for ASD early intervention will be the focus of the next chapter.

As mentioned in Chap. 1, applied behavior analysis is a scientific discipline (rather than a specific treatment or a curriculum) which investigates the variables that influence an individual's behavior, with a focus on the improvement of behaviors considered to be important for the individual's functioning and well-being (Baer et al., 1968). Within the field of ABA the term "behavior" applies to any observable and measureable act performed by an individual, in contrast to the traditional use of the term to refer to how a person behaves. Talking, running, eating, laughing, screaming, and hitting are all forms of behavior within this frame, because one can observe and measure the occurrence of each of them. The goal of applied behavior analysis is to carefully measure the occurrence of socially significant behavior and modify the behavior using systematic "environmental contingencies," i.e., modifying the circumstances or stimuli that create or encourage the behavior.

The following vignette exemplifies a common situation in which a socially important behavior, a child's verbal response, is influenced by two key variables; what happens before the child's behavior and what happens after. During a play routine, a caregiver says "ready, set …" while looking expectantly at her child with

G. Vivanti (✉)
AJ Drexel Autism Institute, Drexel University, Philadelphia, PA, USA
e-mail: gv89@drexel.edu

M. Pellecchia
Department of Psychiatry, Perelman School of Medicine, University of Pennsylvania, Philadelphia, PA, USA

G. Vivanti et al. (eds.), *Clinical Guide to Early Interventions for Children with Autism*, Best Practices in Child and Adolescent Behavioral Health Care,
https://doi.org/10.1007/978-3-030-41160-2_5

her hands positioned to tickle the child's abdomen. The child responds to the caregiver saying "go!" The caregiver smiles and starts tickling the child. The child laughs, and says again "go!" to get more tickles. In this situation, there are three important elements that maintain the child's behavior, an *antecedent* (the caregiver saying "ready, set"), a *behavior* (the child saying "go"), and a *consequence* (the parent tickles the child). This is often referred to as the A–B–Cs of behavior. Within an ABA framework, the *antecedent* (A) is an event that occurs before a *behavior* (B), and the *consequence* (C) is an event that follows the behavior. The example illustrates a phenomenon known as operant conditioning, a learning process that reliably predicts the behavior of any living organism based on the universal law that behaviors followed by reinforcement will have a higher probability of occurring in the future, and behaviors followed by punishment have a lower probability of occurring in the future (Skinner, 1965). Operant conditioning is used in ASD early intervention as the framework for understanding and, if needed, modifying, the antecedent–behavior–consequence (ABC) contingencies underlying the child's behavior. This allows us to answer the question "why does the child engage in a particular behavior?"—a question that, in the ABA field would be framed as "which variables *reinforce* or *maintain* the behavior?" Answering this question allows one to design interventions to increase or decrease the occurrence of specific behaviors, such as using the word "help" to replace the undesirable behavior of biting one's own hand. The goal, therefore, is to shape a child's behavioral repertoire to equip her or him with functional skills and reduce behaviors that can be harmful to self or others (e.g., aggression and self-harm).

The concepts of reinforcement and punishment are often used differently outside of the field of ABA. In lay terms, reinforcement is often used interchangeably with the term "reward," and is used to describe a *desired* or *preferred* consequence for a behavior. Within ABA, the term reinforcement implies the use of a *consequence* that *increases* the likelihood of a certain behavior occurring again in the future. Similarly, the term punishment is often used to describe an *undesired* consequence for a behavior. Within ABA the term punishment only applies to *consequences* that *decrease* the future likelihood of a behavior. For example, if a child is sent to his room for arguing with his sister, but he continues to argue with his sister in the future, the consequence of being sent to his room is not a punishment because it did not decrease the future rates of arguing, although most would say that the boy was being "punished."

The application of ABA in the field of ASD early interventions has generated sophisticated approaches and technologies to measure and modify the behavior of young children with ASD in order to promote the acquisition of important skills (e.g., requesting) and decrease challenging behaviors (e.g., self-harm). Empirical work supporting these techniques originated in the 1960s, when behavioral principles were first used to successfully teach novel behaviors or discourage unwanted behaviors of individuals with disabilities, challenging the notion that severe challenging behavior could not be modified (Wolf, Risley, & Mees, 1964). Furthermore, research pioneered by Carr and Durand in the 1980s indicated that many challenging behaviors observed in children with ASD served a communicative function, providing the foundation for successfully teaching socially appropriate communication to replace challenging behavior (Carr & Durand, 1985).

The various applications of ABA share seven key principles, outlined in Box 5.1. Importantly, there are many acronyms and terms that are frequently used (and sometimes misused, or used imprecisely) in this complex field. Box 5.2 illustrates the meaning of some of the most frequently used ABA concepts.

Box 5.1:
In 1968, Baer and colleagues articulated seven dimensions that guide practices in applied behavior analytic interventions. These dimensions continue to frame the provision of ABA and include: (1) *Applied*: the applied aspect of ABA emphasizes that interventions should have a practical value and be applied to behaviors that have a socially significant impact for the quality of life of the individual; (2) *Behavioral*: interventions use clear, unambiguous operational definitions of the target behavior (e.g., "refusing to complete assigned work" as opposed to "being disobedient"); (3) *Analytic*: rooted in data-based decision-making, with data systematically collected, reviewed, and analyzed to support decisions on whether interventions should continue, be modified, faded, changed, or stopped; (4) *Technological*: procedures need to be clearly operationalized so that they can be implemented across settings by anyone and results can be replicated; (5) *Conceptually systematic*: interventions are consistent with principles of behavior validated by empirical research; (6) *Effective*: the implementation of procedures needs to be monitored and analyzed to determine if they are having the expected impact on the target behavior; and (7) *Generality*: behavior change should last over time, appear in novel settings, and with many different people.

Box 5.2: Frequently Used Acronyms in the ABA Literature
ABA—Applied behavior analysis; a discipline focused on the factors that influence socially significant behavior, whereby Applied refers to the social importance of targeted behaviors, Behavior refers to the focus on observable phenomena, and Analysis refers to evidence of an interaction between an independent variable (an intervention) and a dependent variable (the behavior of concern).

BACB—Behavior Analyst Certification Board; the certifying body that defines the training and testing necessary to certify professionals working in the field of behavior analysis.

BCBA—A board-certified behavior analyst; this individual holds a master's degree, has completed 1500 h of supervised field work, passed a competency exam, and is required to obtain continuing education.

BCaBA—A board-certified associate behavior analyst; this individual holds a Bachelor's degree, has completed 1000 h of supervised field work under a BCBA, passed a competency exam, and receives ongoing supervision from a BCBA.

RBT—A registered behavior technician; this individual implements behavioral interventions and has completed BACB-approved training, passed a competency exam, and receives ongoing supervision from a BCBA.

DTT—Discrete trial training; a structured teaching arrangement in which isolated opportunities to practice a skill are provided by an instructor; this term is sometimes used erroneously as a synonym for ABA.

EIBI—Early intensive behavioral intervention; a comprehensive intervention for young children with ASD that utilizes principles of ABA and is implemented for an intensive number of hours each week (e.g., 10–35 h/week).

FCT—Functional communication training; a communication intervention designed to teach appropriate communication for individuals with limited communication skills. FCT involves identifying the function (or purpose) of an individual's maladaptive communication behavior (e.g., banging the head against wall to request attention), and teaching alternative appropriate behaviors that serve the same function (e.g., saying the word "help," or touching the adult's shoulder to gain attention).

FBA—Functional Behavior Assessment; a systematic method of assessment to gather information about the purpose (function) of a challenging behavior.

BIP—Behavior intervention plan; an intervention plan based on the results of a functional behavior assessment to decrease undesired behavior and increase appropriate behavior.

Treatment Techniques in Applied Behavior Analytic Approaches to ASD Early Intervention

ABA techniques are often used in the context of focused interventions targeting a circumscribed set of behaviors (e.g., parent training to teach how to request for help) as well as in comprehensive packages designed to address multiple areas of need, such as the approach referred to as early intensive behavioral intervention (EIBI). EIBI is a comprehensive treatment approach for children with ASD, which is based on the principles of applied behavior analysis, initiated at a young age (<5 years) and delivered intensively (10–35 h/week) in an individualized 1:1 child–adult instructional format. EIBI includes specific goals derived from assessment results, the use of manualized instructional procedures and fidelity systems to guide implementation, and the use of data collection systems to facilitate continuous progress monitoring.

There are several approaches to instruction commonly used within EIBI, ranging from highly structured didactic approaches to naturalistic play-based strategies. The structured component within EIBI is known as discrete trial training (DTT; Krug et al., 1979; Lovaas, 1981; Smith, 2001). During a "discrete trial," the child receives individual instruction in a learning environment designed to minimize distraction (e.g., a table where only materials relevant to the task at hand are available), and target skills are broken down in "discrete" components that are taught in isolation. Learning trials include a specific antecedent (e.g., the verbal instruction "show me dog") designed to elicit a specific behavior (the child pointing to the picture of a dog). These are repeated multiple times in a row. Correct responses are systematically reinforced (e.g., the child is given his favorite toy or a candy) and praised, and the trial is repeated until a predefined criterion is met (e.g., 80–100% of correct responses).

DTT procedures were informed by research conducted by Lovaas and colleagues suggesting that children with ASD have attentional, cognitive, and sensory difficulties that hinder processing of multiple cues at the same time. Therefore, the use of instructional cues that are concise and unambiguous and the provision of multiple repetition of the same antecedent–behavior–consequence sequences serve to increase attention to specific instructional cues and promote skill acquisition (Lovaas et al., 1979; Lovaas & Smith, 1989; Mayville & Mulick, 2011). Another rationale informing DTT procedures is the notion that unlike typical children, those with ASD might not find social praise alone (e.g., the adult saying "good job!") to be intrinsically reinforcing—therefore, extrinsic rewards, such as edible treats or access to toys, are often used to motivate children with ASD (Lovaas, 1981). These, however, are delivered in conjunction with social praise, so that the child can learn over time to "pair" (associate) social praise with the positive experience related to the nonsocial reinforcers.

Importantly, DTT is not synonymous with ABA, and most EIBI programs include a combination of DTT and unstructured or naturalistic approaches to instruction (e.g., Howard et al., 2005). Naturalistic behavioral instruction typically consists of sessions that occur in the child's natural environment (instead of a setting carefully crafted to be free of distraction like in DTT). This approach to instruction is usually play-based and uses items that are motivating to the child to guide the teaching interaction. These sessions are initiated and paced by the child, take place in a variety of locations, and employ a variety of teaching materials. The child chooses the instructional object or activity, and the reinforcer is related to the response (e.g., providing access to a car for correctly identifying a car). This type of instruction involves following the child's lead and capturing and contriving teachable moments related to the context. Environmental arrangement is a critical aspect of this approach, such as, for example, placing a preferred toy in sight but out of the child's reach as a method to create an opportunity for the child to request for the toy.

Within EIBI, skills are often taught within the DTT format first, and then generalized to other settings using naturalistic behavioral approaches. These naturalistic approaches were adopted within EIBI in response to critiques that skills taught within a DTT format do not readily generalize to other settings or teaching interactions. An in-depth discussion of naturalistic interventions will be provided in Chap. 6.

In addition to the broad treatment strategies described above, scientific research in the field has generated numerous other techniques that have been incorporated into EIBI. These include:

Prompts and Prompt Fading

A prompt is a cue meant to facilitate the occurrence of a certain response. Prompts can take many forms, such as verbal, physical, gestural, or visual. Examples include showing a child a picture of a toilet as a prompt for him to request to go to the bathroom (visual prompt), or placing a child's hand on the faucet to prompt him to turn on the water (physical). Prompts are systematically faded, or removed, as an individual demonstrates independence with the response, e.g., pointing to the faucet instead of placing the child's hand on the faucet as the child demonstrates success with turning on the water (Walker, 2008).

Chaining

Chaining is a procedure for teaching a complex set of behaviors in which the steps in a behavior chain are taught individually over time until all the steps are completed. For example, when teaching a child to wash his hands—first teaching the child to turn on the water, and then once the child independently turns on the water, adding the step of pumping the soap dispenser, and then adding rubbing hands together, etc., until all the steps in the handwashing routine are taught (Bancroft et al., 2011).

Task Analysis

Task analysis is the process of breaking a complex skill down into smaller units that can be taught individually. For example, in a school setting, teaching a child the arrival routine can be facilitated by identifying the smaller units which make up the routine (go to cubby, take off coat, hang up coat, open backpack, take out homework, put away homework, hang up backpack). Chaining is often used to teach the steps identified through the task analysis (Libby et al., 2008).

Differential Reinforcement

Differential reinforcement is a procedure for providing reinforcement for behaviors that meet a specific criterion, while withholding reinforcement for all other behaviors that do not meet this criterion (for example, providing reinforcement when a child says "ball," but withholding reinforcement when a child say "buh."; Karsten & Carr, 2009).

Shaping

Shaping is a procedure whereby differential reinforcement is used to systematically and gradually reinforce successive approximations to the targeted response, such as, for example, providing reinforcement when a child says "cookie," and then only providing reinforcement when the child says "want cookie," and then only providing reinforcement when the child says "I want cookie." (Ricciardi et al., 2006).

Noncontingent Reinforcement (NCR)

Noncontingent Reinforcement (NCR) is a procedure designed to reduce challenging behaviors. When using NCR, reinforcement is provided on a specified time interval, instead of in the presence of a specific behavior. For example, a child who engages in aggressive behavior in order to obtain attention would receive attention every 5 min, rather than only receiving attention in the presence of a particular behavior. The reasoning underlying the use of NCR is that providing the child with attention on a regular set interval would decrease his motivation to engage in challenging behavior in order to obtain attention (Smith et al., 2019).

Functional Communication Training

Functional Communication Training (FCT) is an intervention in which an appropriate communicative behavior (e.g., verbally requesting, pointing, using a picture) is taught as a replacement for challenging behaviors used by the child to achieve the same purpose. For example, FCT can be used to teach a child to point to a symbol card that represents taking a break when she/he wants to take a break, instead of swiping books off of the table when she/he wants to take a break (Durand & Carr, 1992).

Extinction

Extinction involves the discontinuation of reinforcement for a previously reinforced behavior (i.e., a behavior that once received reinforcement but no longer does). The goal of extinction is to decrease the occurrence of undesired behavior. For example, a child who previously received a treat when he cried no longer receives a treat in the presence of crying. In this example, the crying behavior is under extinction (Jin et al., 2013).

High P Procedure/Behavioral Momentum

In this procedure, a series of easy tasks are presented in quick succession followed by a more difficult/target task. The theory underlying the High P (high probability) procedure is that an individual is likely to respond to a difficult task when it is immediately preceded by tasks that they can complete easily (Mace et al., 1988).

Evidence Supporting Applied Behavior Analytic Approaches to ASD Early Interventions

Applied behavior analysis emphasizes the use of objective and clearly defined descriptions of treatment targets and intervention techniques, which allows for replication of procedures by others. The emphasis on technological precision in this field has generated a wealth of empirical research, including pioneering evidence on the successful use of ABA approaches for ASD early intervention. This evidence includes numerous single-subject design studies supporting the evidence of specific behavioral techniques on improving target behaviors (National Autism Center (2015). Further, several studies based on a group design have tested the efficacy of this approach as a comprehensive package. One prominent example is the Lovaas study (Lovaas, 1987) measuring the outcomes of 19 preschoolers who had received 40 h/week of individualized intervention for 2 years, compared to 19 peers who were delivered the same intervention for 10 h or less/week, and a "community treatment as usual" comparison group. Results indicated that approximately half of the participants in the intensive treatment group had achieved normal intellectual functioning, including mainstream educational placement without assistance, while the two comparison groups showed limited gains. Gains in the intensive treatment group were maintained at a follow-up conducted when participants averaged 13 years of age (McEachin et al., 1993). The study sparked both optimism, as it pointed to the potential for children with ASD to achieve very positive outcomes in response to intervention, and controversies, due to the emphasis on "normalization" of intellectual functioning as the benchmark for positive outcomes, and methodological shortcomings, such as the lack of randomized assignment of participants to intervention conditions.

To address this latter criticism, Smith and colleagues conducted a randomized controlled trial aimed to replicate the Lovaas study, the first study using this design in the field of ASD early intervention (Smith et al., 2000). Results confirmed superior gains for children receiving EIBI compared to peers in the control group, although to a lesser degree compared to the findings reported in the Lovaas study. Additional research, mostly based on single-subject design or nonrandomized group studies, documented substantial improvements in the areas of cognitive functioning, adaptive functioning, language development, problem behavior, and, to a lesser degree, social communication and reciprocity (Green, 1996; Anderson et al., 1987;

Birnbrauer & Leach, 1993; Smith et al., 2000; Weiss, 1999; Howard et al., 2005; Makrygianni et al., 2018; Smith & Iadarola, 2015). All studies have reported marked variability in outcome, with some children demonstrating significant gains across a range of developmental, behavioral, and social outcomes, and other children demonstrating minimal to no progress following treatment—a finding that parallels the evidence for all ASD early interventions (Eldevik et al., 2010; Howlin & Charman, 2011; Smith et al., 2015). As comparative research in the field is virtually nonexistent, it remains to be established whether this approach produces superior benefits compared to other evidence-supported approaches, or is particularly beneficial for children with ASD who have specific characteristics (Vivanti, 2017).

Overall, the use of ABA strategies in early intervention for ASD is recommended by many expert panels and task forces (e.g., National Research Council, 2001), although the strength of evidence for EIBI varies depending on the evaluation parameters that are used (Smith & Iadarola, 2015; see also Vivanti, 2017). For example, a recent review based on the GRADE system, which only considers randomized controlled trials as conclusive evidence, has indicated that the quality of research evidence supporting EIBI is less than optimal (Reichow et al., 2019; see also Green & Garg, 2018). Conversely, reviews that include evidence from different study designs (and in particular single-subject studies, upon which most ABA literature is based) came to the opposite conclusions (e.g., Eldevik et al., 2012; Makrygianni et al., 2018; Smith & Iadarola, 2015). For example, many techniques identified as "evidence-based practices" according to comprehensive reviews of the National Standards Project and the National Professional Development Center on Autism Spectrum Disorder (2014) are based on ABA (Odom et al., 2010; Wong et al., 2015), and EIBI is endorsed by numerous agencies such as the American Academy of Pediatrics, the American Psychological Association, and the Autism Society of America. As mentioned in Chap. 1, there remains controversy about several aspects of EIBI, including the level of inference that can be derived from nonrandomized designs (see Smith et al., 2007; Vivanti et al., 2018), the logistical and financial barriers related to delivering treatment for many hours per week, the evidence supporting the need for such intensity (Pellecchia et al., 2019), and whether aspects of EIBI (DTT in particular) are consistent with processes that appear to facilitate learning in typical development and generalization in nonintervention contexts (e.g., child-driven active experiential learning, and engagement in a continuous flow of back-and-forth social engagement between child and adult during daily routines; Schreibman et al., 2015; see Chap. 9). Procedures designed to address some of these concerns are covered in the next chapter. Additionally, as mentioned in Chap. 1, the neurodiversity movement has frequently challenged ABA approaches based on their focus on "normalization," which is seen as prioritizing "conformity" at the expenses of diversity (Gruson-Wood, 2016). While the influence of the neurodiversity approach on intervention is in its infancy, there is increasing effort in the intervention community to include key stakeholders, such as individuals with ASD and their families, in the decision-making related to what should be defined as desirable goals and outcomes for intervention, and how interventions should be designed and implemented (Pellicano & Stears, 2011; Vivanti & Volkmar, 2019).

Despite these criticisms, the use of basic ABA principles, such as reinforcing children for desired behavior, remains a paramount component of most, if not all, validated approaches to ASD early intervention. Additionally, research has consistently shown the efficacy of these procedures for teaching critical and potentially life-saving skills such as using appropriate means to communicate instead of self-injurious behavior. As an illustration of the far-reaching relevance of this body of literature, the Individuals with Disabilities Education Act (IDEA, 1997/2004) requires that interventions based on functional behavior assessment are developed to target challenging behaviors and improve communication in children with disabilities.

Who Can Deliver Applied Behavior Analytic Interventions?

Applied Behavior Analytic interventions should be delivered by professionals or paraprofessionals who have education and supervised training aligned with the task list created by the Behavior Analyst Certification Board (BACB). In the United States, certain states require that BCBAs are supervised by licensed psychologists, but there is state-to-state variation in supervision requirements. Though many professionals holding a BCBA certificate have experience with young children with ASD, the BCBA certification does not necessarily guarantee that a provider has experience with young children with ASD. Therefore, in the context of ASD early intervention, it is advisable to identify practitioners with expertise in ASD and child development.

Additionally, in the United States, different licensure requirements for practicing behavior analysis are adopted in different states, and in some states private insurance companies and Medicaid have the mandate to cover ABA services for individuals with ASD. Unfortunately, the professional certification process (BACB) and state licensing practices are not always aligned. As an example, some states provide a behavioral interventionist license without requiring the applicant complete the education or training required by the BACB (www.bacb.com/licensure-regulation/), and other states require documentation of training and licensure in a related field.

As the number of individuals who are diagnosed with ASD has increased in the past decade, there is shortage of qualified professionals who can provide ABA services and there are individuals that claim to be using ABA when in fact they are not certified or licensed to do so. Therefore, it is important that consumers make informed decisions and examine the qualifications of those offering ABA treatment, and that legislation continues to support training and dissemination efforts to provide effective treatment for those with ASD.

Conclusions

Early intensive behavioral intervention has gained widespread acceptance as an effective treatment for young children with ASD. As described above, EIBI includes many different intervention techniques and approaches to intervention that are based on the principles of ABA. Most often, EIBI is delivered as part of a comprehensive treatment package including an array of different techniques and a combination of structured and naturalistic approaches to instruction. Given the range of different techniques included within EIBI, there is often confusion for parents and researchers alike regarding the best approach to use for any given child with ASD. Unfortunately, the research regarding the type of behavioral approach best suited for individual children, given their individual clinical profile, is lacking. When recommending EIBI treatment packages clinicians should consider each child's developmental profile, and align the treatment goals and treatment approach with developmentally appropriate practice. Further, consideration of each child's family context, and therapeutic services provided in addition to the child's EIBI (e.g., speech and/or occupational therapy) should be considered to ensure alignment with child and family needs and across therapeutic modalities.

References

Anderson, S.R. , Avery, D.L. , DiPietro, E.K. , Edwards, G.L. , & Christian, W.P. (1987). Intensive home-based early intervention with autistic children. *Education and Treatment of Children, 10*, 352–366.

Baer, D., Wolf, M., & Risley, T. (1968). Some current dimensions of applied behavior analysis. *Journal of Applied Behavior Analysis, 1*, 91–97.

Bancroft, S. L., Weiss, J. S., Libby, M. E., & Ahearn, W. H. (2011). A comparison of procedural variations in teaching behavior chains: Manual guidance, trainer completion, and no completion of untrained steps. *Journal of applied behavior analysis, 44*(3), 559–569.

Birnbrauer, J. S., & Leach, D. J. (1993). The Murdoch early intervention program after 2 years. *Behaviour change, 10*(2), 63–74.

Carr, E. G., & Durand, V. M. (1985). Reducing behavior problems through functional communication training. *Journal of Applied Behavior Analysis, 18*, 111–126.

Durand, V. M., & Carr, E. G. (1992). An analysis of maintenance following functional communication training. *Journal of Applied Behavior Analysis, 25*(4), 777–794.

Eldevik, S., Hastings, R. P., Hughes, J. C., Jahr, E., Eikeseth, S., & Cross, S. (2010). Using participant data to extend the evidence base for intensive behavioral intervention for children with autism. *American Journal on Intellectual and Developmental Disabilities, 115*(5), 381–405.

Eldevik, S., Hastings, R. P., Jahr, E., & Hughes, J. C. (2012). Outcomes of behavioral intervention for children with autism in mainstream pre-school settings. *Journal of autism and developmental disorders, 42*(2), 210–220.

Green, J., & Garg, S. (2018). Annual Research Review: The state of autism intervention science: Progress, target psychological and biological mechanisms and future prospects. *Journal of Child Psychology and Psychiatry, 59*(4), 424–443.

Gruson-Wood, J. F. (2016). Autism, expert discourses, and subjectification: A critical examination of applied behavioural therapies. *Studies in Social Justice, 10*(1), 38–58.

Green, G. (1996). Early behavioral intervention for autism: What does research tell us? In C. Maurice, G. Green, & S. C. Luce (Eds.), Behavioral intervention for young children with autism: A manual for parents and professionals (p. 29–44). PRO-ED.

Howlin, P., & Charman, T. (2011). Autism spectrum disorders, interventions and outcomes. In P. Howlin, T. Charman, & M. Ghaziuddin (Eds.), *The SAGE handbook of developmental disorders*. London: SAGE.

Howard, J. S., Sparkman, C. R., Cohen, H. G., Green, G., & Stanislaw, H. (2005). A comparison of intensive behavior analytic and eclectic treatments for young children with autism. *Research in developmental disabilities, 26*(4), 359–383.

Individuals with Disabilities Education Improvement Act (IDEA) (2004). H.R. Res. 108–446, 108th Cong., 1350 H. R. (enacted).

Individuals with Disability Education Act (1997). H.R. Res. H. R. 5, 105th Cong., 601 House of Representatives 1 (enacted).

Jin, C. S., Hanley, G. P., & Beaulieu, L. (2013). An individualized and comprehensive approach to treating sleep problems in young children. *Journal of Applied Behavior Analysis, 46*(1), 161–180.

Krug, D. A., Arick, J., Almond, P., Rosenblum, J., Scanlon, C., & Border, M. (1979). Evaluation of a program of systematic instructional procedures for pre-verbal autistic children. *Improving Human Performance, 8*, 29–41.

Karsten, A. M., & Carr, J. E. (2009). The effects of differential reinforcement of unprompted responding on the skill acquisition of children with autism. *Journal of Applied Behavior Analysis, 42*(2), 327–334.

Libby, M. E., Weiss, J. S., Bancroft, S., & Ahearn, W. H. (2008). A comparison of most-to-least and least-to-most prompting on the acquisition of solitary plays kills. *Behavior analysis in practice, 1*(1), 37–43.

Lovaas, O. I., Koegel, R. L., & Schreibman, L. (1979). Stimulus overselectivity in autism: A review of research. *Psychological Bulletin, 86*(6), 1236.

Lovaas, O. I., & Smith, T. (1989). A comprehensive behavioral theory of autistic children: Paradigm for research and treatment. *Journal of Behavior Therapy and Experimental Psychiatry, 20*(1), 17–29.

Lovaas, I. (1981). The ME book. Austin, TX: Pro-Ed.

Lovaas, O. I. (1987). Behavioral treatment and normal educational and intellectual functioning in young autistic children. *Journal of consulting and clinical psychology, 55*(1), 3.

Makrygianni, M. K., Gena, A., Katoudi, S., & Galanis, P. (2018). The effectiveness of applied behavior analytic interventions for children with Autism Spectrum Disorder: A meta-analytic study. *Research in Autism Spectrum Disorders, 51*, 18–31.

Mayville, E. A., & Mulick, J. A. (2011). *Behavioral foundations of effective autism treatment*. Cambridge: Sloan Pub.

Mace, F. C., Hock, M. L., Lalli, J. S., West, B. J., Belfiore, P., Pinter, E., & Brown, D. K. (1988). Behavioral momentum in the treatment of noncompliance. *Journal of Applied Behavior Analysis, 21*(2), 123–141.

McEachin, J. J., Smith, T., & Lovaas, O. (1993). Long-term outcome for children with autism who received early intensive behavioral treatment. *American journal of mental retardation, 97*, 359–359.

National Autism Center. (2015). National Standards Report: The national standards project—Addressing the need for evidence-based practice guidelines for autism spectrum disorders, Phase 2. Retrieved from https://www.nationalautismcenter.org/national-standards-project/results-reports/

National Professional Development Center on Autism Spectrum Disorder (2014). What criteria determined whether an intervention was effective? Retrieved from http://autismpdc.fpg.unc.edu/what-criteria-determined-if-intervention-was-effective

National Research Council (2001). Educating children with autism. National Academies Press.

Odom, S. L., Collet-Klingenberg, L., Rogers, S. J., & Hatton, D. D. (2010). Evidence-based practices in interventions for children and youth with autism spectrum disorders. *Preventing School Failure: Alternative Education for Children and Youth, 54*(4), 275–282.

Pellecchia, M., Iadarola, S., & Stahmer, A. C. (2019). How meaningful is more? Considerations regarding intensity in early intensive behavioral intervention. *Autism: The International Journal of Research and Practice, 23*(5), 1075–1078.

Pellicano, E., & Stears, M. (2011). Bridging autism, science and society: Moving toward an ethically informed approach to autism research. *Autism Research, 4*(4), 271–282. https://doi.org/10.1002/aur.201

Ricciardi, J. N., Luiselli, J. K., & Camare, M. (2006). Shaping approach responses as intervention for specific phobia in a child with autism. *Journal of Applied Behavior Analysis, 39*(4), 445–448.

Reichow, B., Barton, E. E., Boyd, B. A., & Hume, K. (2019). Early intensive behavioral intervention (EIBI) for young children with autism spectrum disorders (ASD): A systematic review. *Campbell Systematic Reviews, 10*(1), 1–116.

Skinner, B. F. (1965). Science and human behavior. New York, Macmillian.

Smith, T. (2001). Discrete trial training in the treatment of autism. *Focus on Autism and Other Developmental Disabilities, 16*(2), 86–92.

Smith, T., Groen, A. D., & Wynn, J. W. (2000). Randomized trial of intensive early intervention for children with pervasive developmental disorder. *American Journal on Mental Retardation, 105*, 269–285.

Smith, T., & Iadarola, S. (2015). Evidence base update for autism spectrum disorder. *Journal of Clinical Child & Adolescent Psychology, 44*(6), 897–922.

Smith, T., Klorman, R., & Mruzek, D. W. (2015). Predicting outcome of community-based early intensive behavioral intervention for children with autism. *Journal of Abnormal Child Psychology, 43*(7), 1271–1282.

Smith, H. M., Gadke, D. L., Stratton, K. K., Ripple, H., & Reisener, C. D. (2019). Providing noncontingent access to music in addition to escape extinction as a treatment for liquid refusal in a child with autism. Behavior Analysis: *Research and Practice, 19*(1), 94.

Smith, T., Scahill, L., Dawson, G., Guthrie, D., Lord, C., Odom, S., ... & Wagner, A. (2007). Designing research studies on psychosocial interventions in autism. *Journal of autism and developmental disorders, 37*(2), 354–366.

Schreibman, L., Dawson, G., Stahmer, A. C., Landa, R., Rogers, S. J., McGee, G. G., ... & McNerney, E. (2015). Naturalistic developmental behavioral interventions: Empirically validated treatments for autism spectrum disorder. *Journal of autism and developmental disorders, 45*(8), 2411–2428.

Vivanti, G. (2017). Individualizing and combining treatments in autism spectrum disorder: Four elements for a theory-driven research agenda. *Current Directions in Psychological Science, 26*(2), 114–119.

Vivanti, G., Kasari, C., Green, J., Mandell, D., Maye, M., & Hudry, K. (2018). Implementing and evaluating early intervention for children with autism: Where are the gaps and what should we do?. *Autism Research, 11*(1), 16–23.

Vivanti, G., & Volkmar, F. R. (2019). National Guideline for the Assessment and Diagnosis of Autism Spectrum Disorders in Australia (Whitehouse, Evans et al.2018). Journal of autism and developmental disorders.

Wong, C., Odom, S. L., Hume, K. A., Cox, A. W., Fettig, A., Kucharczyk, S., … Schultz, T. R. (2015). Evidence-based practices for children, youth, and young adults with autism spectrum disorder: A comprehensive review. *Journal of Autism and Developmental Disorders, 45*(7), 1951–1966.

Wolf, M. M., Risley, T., & Mees, H. (1964). Application of operant conditioning procedures to the behavior problems of an autistic child. *Behaviour Research and Therapy, 1*(2–4), 305–312.

Walker, G. (2008). Constant and progressive time delay procedures for teaching children with autism: A literature review. *Journal of Autism and Developmental Disorders, 38*(2), 261–275.

Weiss, M. J. (1999). Differential rates of skill acquisition and outcomes of early intensive behavioral intervention for autism. *Behavioral Interventions: Theory &Practice in Residential & Community-Based Clinical Programs, 14*(1), 3–22.

Chapter 6
Naturalistic Developmental Behavioral Interventions for Children with Autism

Giacomo Vivanti and Hongxuan Nicole Zhong

"Naturalistic developmental behavioral interventions" (NDBIs) is an umbrella term used to describe early intervention approaches that blend behavioral and developmental strategies and use a naturalistic format to address the learning needs of children with autism spectrum disorder (ASD). While the term was coined by Schreibman and colleagues in 2015, NDBI approaches have a long tradition in the ASD field, originating from the attempt to address some of the perceived limitations of behavioral approaches originally designed for older children, and to incorporate knowledge from developmental psychology to maximize developmental outcomes such as language, play, and socialization (Koegel, O'Dell, & Koegel, 1987; McGee, Krantz, Mason, & McClannahan, 1983; Rogers & Lewis, 1989; Schreibman et al., 2015). In the first section of this chapter, we will describe features that are common across NDBI approaches as well as differences and areas of overlap between NDBIs and the standard ABA approaches described in Chap. 5. Subsequently, we will review the principles, strategies, and empirical support for the different ASD early intervention models that fall under the NDBI umbrella.

Key Features of Naturalistic Developmental Interventions

Similar to the comprehensive approaches based on standard applied behavioral analytic techniques, such as EIBI (see Chap. 5), interventions based on the NDBI framework emphasize the importance of (a) starting treatment early in life; (b) delivering treatment in an intensive manner, with many learning opportunities provided throughout the child's day; (c) drawing on evidence-supported practices and

G. Vivanti (✉) · H. N. Zhong
AJ Drexel Autism Institute, Drexel University, Philadelphia, PA, USA
e-mail: gv89@drexel.edu

G. Vivanti et al. (eds.), *Clinical Guide to Early Interventions for Children with Autism*, Best Practices in Child and Adolescent Behavioral Health Care,
https://doi.org/10.1007/978-3-030-41160-2_6

manualized procedures; (d) tailoring treatment objectives on the individual child's profile of strength and needs; (e) monitoring treatment progress through systematic evaluations of child's behavior change; (f) monitoring fidelity of treatment implementation (i.e., the degree to which the intervention is delivered as intended) through the use of fidelity tools that measure adherence to operationally defined intervention procedures; and (g) involving caregivers in decision making. Additionally, like the approaches described in Chap. 5, NDBIs use operant conditioning techniques to promote the acquisition of novel behaviors, including the use of the "antecedent–behavior–consequence" (ABC) contingency structure to systematically cue and reward the child's behavior. However, NDBIs diverge from EIBI in the format of instruction delivery and teaching content, which are informed by the naturalistic and developmental principles listed below.

Naturalistic Principles

The "naturalistic" component of the NDBIs reflects the nonartificial nature of (a) the physical and social context in which instruction takes place, (b) the instructional cues given to the child, and (c) the consequence (reinforcement) delivered by the adult to encourage (reinforce) the child's behavior. With regard to the first aspect, instruction in NDBI is commonly delivered in a physical environment that looks similar to the environment where young children without ASD learn. Rather than engineering the physical space to prioritize attention to an adult-defined task (e.g., by eliminating all distractions, making only objects relevant to the task at hand available, or using "self-explanatory" materials and tasks), NDBI programs use toys, materials, and activities that are similar to the ones a typical child is likely to encounter in their environment. The rationale for this approach is to facilitate learning in response to everyday routines and stimuli rather than a highly structured "therapy room" situation, so that the child has frequent opportunities to generalize acquired skills in everyday contexts, has experience interacting within complex, dynamic environments that mirror nontherapeutic interactions, and has learning experiences during activities and routines that are shared with others (e.g., meals, bath time, playground activities, play routines at home or in daycares).

Importantly, while NDBIs aim to reduce the discrepancy between the setting in which instruction takes place and the context of typical daily experiences, materials and activities are still organized in a way that maximizes child learning and participation to the activity. This is frequently achieved by managing the quantity and nature of "competing stimuli" that are present in the activity, arranging the space to facilitate face-to-face interaction and attention to the adult contingent responses to the child's behavior, and strategically drawing attention to materials to facilitate increasingly complex interactions. This might include giving the child access to only half of the blocks or puzzle pieces in a container to facilitate turn-taking, using objects that require assistance, playfully obstructing access to preferred materials or placing them out of reach to facilitate requesting, expectant waiting (e.g., before placing the last block on a tall block tower) to facilitate emotion sharing (e.g., the suspense before the tower falls), drawing attention to specific actions/materials, and pacing activities to facilitate sustained interest. Therefore, the naturalistic focus coexists with a high degree of adult control on the stimuli provided to the child. Additionally, the degree of structure might be increased or decreased based on child needs and progress (e.g., Vivanti, Duncan, Dawson, & Rogers, 2017).

The "naturalistic" component of NDBI also refers to the strategies adults use to facilitate particular kinds of interactions. While standard procedures in EIBI use concise, stripped-down instruction that clearly defines the target behavior (such the adult telling the child "match" or "push"), NDBI programs emphasize the use of "natural" language, that is, the kind of communication that would be used for young children without ASD—such as saying "ready, set, go!" with a highly emotional tone of voice. The rationale for this "naturalistic language" format is to facilitate generalization of child learning in response to stimuli that the child is more likely to be exposed to in ordinary contexts and daily routines. Further, recent research suggests that use of "telegraphic speech" in caregivers' does not facilitate child language development (Sandbank & Yoder, 2016).

Additionally, the use of a highly animated tone of voice and body language when delivering instructional cues is based on developmental research showing that typically developing children learn best in response to affectively rich interactions (Kuhl, 2007), and that children with ASD show an attenuated, but not absent, response to social affect (Rogers, Vivanti, & Rocha, 2017). Therefore, the use of naturally sounding language associated with an affectively rich display of gestures, emotional facial and vocal expressions, and animated body language serves the purpose of enhancing the child's engagement with the therapist or parent and the activity and facilitating learning in response to stimuli and situations that are similar to those experienced by other children.

Finally, the naturalistic component of NDBIs refers to how the child behavior is reinforced (i.e., rewarded) with delivery of "natural" consequences being preferred to unrelated rewards. For example, in order to reinforce the child's use of the word "up," the adult will lift the child up, rather than rewarding the child with food or an unrelated object for correct use of the word "up". An additional rationale for the provision of intrinsic reinforcement rather than external reward is that the back-and-forth flow of the interaction is not disrupted by introducing materials unrelated to the ongoing interaction (e.g., a tablet during a peek-a-boo routine used to target eye contact).

In summary, the naturalistic component of NDBIs involves targeting skills in the context of "ordinary" and culturally relevant shared experiences and routines, with multiple instructional cues and materials, to facilitate learning and acquisition of responses within the daily contexts where the targeted behaviors are meant to be used (Vivanti, 2019). This approach is analogous to teaching a child how to swim directly in the water rather than first practicing the motions outside of the water.

Developmental Principles

The "developmental" piece of NDBIs is reflected in the selection of intervention targets (what is being taught) as well as the strategies used to target treatment objectives. Intervention targets are informed by research on the developmental sequences and prerequisites for the acquisition of specific skills. For example, research has shown that joint attention, imitation, and functional play are key precursors to language and social cognition in typical and atypical development (Charman, 2003; Poon, Watson, Baranek, & Poe, 2012; Tomasello, 2019; Vivanti & Hamilton, 2014) as acquisition of these skills enables the child to participate in social exchanges that further contribute to his or her learning (e.g., learning the meaning of new words by following the adults' pointing gesture during a visit at the zoo, or learning to play with a drum by imitating a peer during a "music and movement" routine in daycare). As research has shown that learning in children with ASD appears to follow developmental sequences that, at least in some domains, are similar to those observed in typical development (Mundy, 2016; Tager-Flusberg et al., 1990), NDBIs emphasize targeting "pivotal" (i.e., foundational) skills that create the social infrastructure upon which language, social skills, and cognition are developed (Kasari, Gulsrud, Paparella, Hellemann, & Berry, 2015; Koegel, Koegel, Harrower, & Carter, 1999).

This approach requires consideration of the developmental sequences along which complex skills unfold in human development, that is, teaching what "comes first" developmentally in order to create a foundation for more advanced skills. As we will discuss in the section on research supporting different NDBIs, empirical research confirmed that targeting precursors to language and social development facilitates "collateral" acquisition of more advanced behaviors even when those are not directly targeted by therapy (Kasari, Paparella, Freeman, & Jahromi, 2008; Whalen, Schreibman, & Ingersoll, 2006).

Developmental principles also emphasize targeting behaviors that are in the so-called "zone of proximal development" (Vygotsky, 1930–1934/1978), that is, the skill level that is just beyond the child's current repertoire (see also Chap. 9). This requires the consideration of the child's chronological and developmental age in the selection of developmentally appropriate targets (i.e., behaviors that the child is ready to learn based on its current developmental stage). For example, a developmentally appropriate goal for a nonverbal child who is reaching toward an object with an open hand for requesting is to teach a pointing gesture, rather than the three-word sentence "I want ___." This process is facilitated by connecting new behaviors to the child's current developmental level (e.g., facilitating the pointing gesture in the same context in which the child is reaching), which requires the assessment of children's present behavioral repertoire and selection of developmentally informed "next-step" targets. For very young children this is typically accomplished within simple routines such as tickling games, peek-a-boo, clapping games, song routines, or bubbles or balloon games, during which contingencies between antecedent stimuli (e.g., the adult saying "pop!" during a bubbles game), the child's behavior (the child touching the bubble), and a rewarding experience (the bubble pops and the adult smiles at the child) are highly predictable, emotionally engaging, and salient. Behavioral strategies such as shaping (reinforcing approximations to the target behavior), prompting (inserting a verbal, visual, or physical cue between the instruction and the target behavior), and fading (gradually removing the prompts used to support the spontaneous occurrence of the target behavior and avoid "prompt dependency") are also frequently used to facilitate the transition from the current behavioral repertoire to the "next level." This, in turn, provides the foundation for participation in more sophisticated "symbol-infused" routines in which the cause-and-effect focus gradually is replaced by symbolic activities (e.g., drawing, symbolic play), and verbal language (whether spoken or augmented and alternative means) becomes the primary communication modality (Adamson, Bakeman, & Deckner, 2004).

One key notion informing NDBIs is that the construction of behavioral expertise through early intervention has the potential to shape brain development as the organization and specialization of the brain are particularly open to change during preschool years. Therefore, the provision of early intervention during early sensitive stages of brain plasticity might allow for a deeper impact of these social learning experiences on the developing brain (although importantly, learning experiences change brain structure and function throughout the lifespan, and individuals with ASD can learn new skills at any stage of their lives).

Furthermore, learning in typical development is facilitated by affective engagement and emotional connectedness between the learner and the adult delivering instruction. For example, children are more likely to learn novel words or actions from someone who is playfully engaged with them compared to a situation where the exact same words and actions come from a nonengaging adult (Kuhl, 2007; Nielsen, 2006). Therefore, NDBIs consider affective engagement and social–emotional connectedness between child and adult not just as a desirable attribute that precede the act of learning (i.e., building rapport before starting a teaching trial) but rather as an active component of effective learning.

Additionally, NDBIs are informed by research documenting that during early development, typical children are more likely to learn in response to self-initiated goals and self-driven interests (Legare, 2014; Saylor & Ganea, 2018). For example, young children are more likely to learn names for objects that they are interested in compared to those of objects they are not interested in (Begus, Gliga, & Southgate, 2014). Additionally, they are more likely to learn cause–effect associations in response to a self-generated action, for example, activating a cause–effect toy, compared to observing another person activating the toy (Kushnir, Wellman, & Gelman, 2009). Consequently, NDBIs attempt to promote active experiential learning by facilitating and reinforcing child initiative and spontaneity, and building learning opportunities on activities that stem from the child's own goals, sought-out materials, and preferred routines.

Importantly, the indication of "following the child's lead" in NDBIs does not mean that the adult's role is to encourage *any* behavior spontaneously produced by the child. Maladaptive behaviors are systematically analyzed and reduced following the behavioral strategies discussed in the previous chapter, and behaviors that are not conducive to social learning (e.g., engagement in solitary activities with electronic toys) are also discouraged. Rather, learning episodes in NDBIs take place during routines that incorporate both child goals and adult scaffolding of novel behaviors, shared control of materials, turn-taking, and a balance between child and adult contributions to the interaction. For example, if a child spontaneously starts drawing dots on a piece of paper using a red marker, the adult will join and imitate the child's behavior using a different marker to attract his attention, and subsequently will model novel behaviors (e.g., drawing lines instead of circles) to expand the child behavioral repertoire while still considering the child's interest in markers.

The focus on the child's intrinsic motivation is particularly important in the context of teaching social communication and language. NDBIs are informed by developmental research on the social–pragmatic function of language, that is, the notion that language in typical development is a collaborative activity that serves social-affiliative motives such as the desire to share interest about something (Tomasello, 2010). In typical development, the information that is shared during early child–adult interactions is the mutual pleasure for being part of the interaction, which is conveyed through nonverbal means such as mutual gaze and emotional facial expressions. In the second year of life, children start sharing information about external objects/events that attract their interest (e.g., a balloon flying) using gestures, such as pointing, which are frequently followed by the caregiver's contingent labeling of the object, for example, "a balloon!" (Mundy, 2016). These early emerging preverbal conversations characterized by mutual social-affective engagement and a shared frame of reference are considered to be the infrastructure upon which verbal language emerges (Bloom, 2002; Kuhl, 2014). Based on this body of literature, NDBI approaches target language within a "conversational" back-and-forth flow of verbal and nonverbal exchanges that may center around and build on common themes, whereby child and adult communicate, negotiate, and achieve shared goals while manifesting shared enjoyment in the interaction. Therefore, instead of breaking down complex behaviors such as a conversation into smaller units to be targeted one at the time through discrete trials (e.g., saying the word "three"), NDIBIs start from creating a nonverbal conversation structure upon which a verbal repertoire is built (e.g., adult and child push buttons on a pop-up toy as the adult initially says "one … two … three!, and subsequently only "one … two …"). This is based on the notion that language is facilitated (rather than hindered) by engaging the child in a "communicatively rich" situation that involves multiple modalities and interactive goals (including manifestations of affect as well as verbal and nonverbal cues).

In summary, NDBIs are informed by developmental research showing that children learn best when engaged in affectively rich "conversational" routines that build on the child's goals and whereby the child experiences the natural contingencies of their self-initiated behavior (e.g., the caregiver labeling objects they are looking at) in the context of activities and situations that are similar to those experienced in typical daily and play routines. Within this general framework, several different approaches have been developed that take into account developmental research on typical learning processes while adopting specific strategies to address the symptoms of ASD. In the remainder of the chapter, we will focus on the different NDBI approaches to ASD early intervention, focusing on both intervention procedures and scientific support for each model.

Early Start Denver Model (ESDM)

ESDM (Rogers & Dawson, 2010b) is a comprehensive intervention for young children with autism ages 12–48 months that includes a manualized set of treatment procedures and a curriculum that addresses multiple developmental areas with a focus on the core deficits seen in toddlers and preschoolers with ASD (social orientation, affect sharing and attunement, imitation, joint attention, verbal and nonverbal communication, as well as functional and symbolic play). The ESDM originates from the Denver Model, an autism intervention model developed by Rogers and colleagues in the 1980s (Rogers, Lewis, & Reis, 1987) and later expanded into the "Early Start Denver Model" (ESDM; Rogers & Dawson, 2010b), which included additional treatment procedures and a developmentally informed curriculum checklist (ESDM Curriculum Checklist; Rogers & Dawson, 2010a). ESDM is designed for implementation across multiple settings and delivery formats, including therapist-delivered, parent-mediated, and teacher-delivered group-based programs in daycare or preschool settings (Rogers & Dawson, 2010b; Rogers, Dawson, & Vismara, 2012; Vivanti et al., 2017).

Theoretical Basis

The theoretical foundations of the ESDM include the cascade model of ASD proposed by Rogers and Pennington (1991) according to which early symptoms of ASD hinder the development of the processes that facilitate bodily and emotional engagement during early interactions, such as imitation, reciprocal vocalization, and sharing of affect. Reduced social engagement, in turn, disrupts the development of neural specialization and behavioral expertise in the social communication domain. Additional theoretical principles are based on the social motivation framework of ASD proposed by Dawson et al. (2004; Dawson & Bernier, 2007), suggesting that symptoms of ASD might be linked to a deficiency in experiencing social engagement as intrinsically rewarding. Additionally, the ESDM is informed by the naturalistic application of applied behavior analysis developed by Koegel and colleagues in their pioneering work on pivotal response training (PRT; Koegel, O'Dell, & Koegel, 1987), which focuses on addressing child motivation, spontaneity, social initiation, and response generalization.

Practice and Implementation

In the ESDM, measurable learning objectives are developed from a comprehensive assessment of the child's profile of strengths and needs using the ESDM curriculum checklist (Rogers & Dawson, 2010a), which evaluates each child's behavioral repertoire across multiple developmental domains. The child's progress is systematically recorded, mastery of all objectives is assessed every 12 weeks using the same checklist, and new learning objectives are generated based on the assessment results. Teaching episodes in the ESDM are embedded within joint activity routines (see Chap. 3), which include a set-up phase, in which the child chooses the activity; a theme in which the child and the adult participate equally in the activity chosen by the child, creating a predictable and enjoyable routine; variations that expand the theme; and a closing phase, marking the ending of the current activity followed by a transition to the next one. This joint activity structure is designed to address both the social impairments (through the joint engagement component) and the flexibility difficulties (through the systematic introduction of variations on the theme) that define ASD, while also providing opportunities to target multiple objectives capitalizing on the child's spontaneous interest for specific activities/materials. During joint activity routines, a variety of evidence-based instructional techniques are deployed to target learning goals, including the use of "antecedent–behavior–consequence (ABC)" sequences, shaping, fading, prompting, and chaining, active management of affect, arousal, and motivation, and the use of warm, playful shared interactions as a context for learning. Decision trees are used to readjust the program when progress is slower than expected in one or more areas, including increasing structure and reinforcers' strength and introducing augmentative communication tools. A fidelity tool is used to monitor treatment adherence.

Empirical Support

Research supporting the ESDM includes several randomized controlled trials, single-subject design studies, and quasi-experimental studies indicating positive treatment effects in the area of language/communication, with more mixed results in the area of cognitive and adaptive functioning. Intervention outcomes are more favorable in response to intensive, therapist-implemented delivery than short-term parent-mediated formats. The most relevant studies that tested the ESDM are described in Table 6.1.

Table 6.1 Selected research studies on the ESDM

Study	Design	Treatment characteristics	Sample	Main results
Dawson et al. (2010)	Randomized controlled trial	1:1 therapist-implemented; 20 h/week for 2 years	Enrollment: $N = 48$ ESDM group: $n = 24$ ($M_{age} = 23.9$ months, $SD = 4.0$) Community group (treatment as usual): $n = 24$ ($M_{age} = 23.1$ months, $SD = 3.9$) Two-year follow-up: $N = 45$ ESDM group: $n = 24$ ($M_{age} = 52.4$ months, $SD = 3.4$) Community group: $n = 21$ ($M_{age} = 52.1$ months, $SD = 4.3$)	Compared to the community group, children in the ESDM group showed more improvements in cognitive ability and adaptive behavior
Rogers, Estes, et al. (2012)	Randomized controlled trial	Parent-implemented; 1 h/week for 12 weeks	Enrollment: $N = 98$ ESDM treatment group: $n = 49$ ($M_{age} = 21.02$ months, $SD = 3.51$) Community group (treatment as usual): $n = 49$ ($M_{age} = 20.94$ months, $SD = 3.42$) Posttreatment (after 12 weeks): $N = 98$ ESDM treatment group: $n = 49$ ($M_{age} = 24.77$ months, $SD = 3.15$) Community group: $n = 49$ ($M_{age} = 24.49$ months, $SD = 3.43$)	No significant group differences in child outcomes Parents in both groups improved interaction skills. Significantly stronger parent–therapist working alliance were reported in the ESDM group
Vivanti et al. (2014)	Quasi-experimental controlled trial	Group–ESDM implemented with staff–child ratio of 1:3; 15–25 h/week for 12 months	Enrollment: $N = 57$ ESDM treatment group: $n = 27$ ($M_{age} = 40.30$ months, $SD = 9.55$) Community group ("generic" treatment program for autism): $n = 30$ ($M_{age} = 41.97$ months, $SD = 6.71$	Children in both groups improved cognitive ability, adaptive behavior, and social skills (ADOS social affect) Improvements in overall cognitive and receptive language skills were significantly higher in children receiving the ESDM

(continued)

Table 6.1 (continued)

Study	Design	Treatment characteristics	Sample	Main results
Estes et al. (2015)	School-age follow up of the Dawson et al. (2010) RCT	Same as the Dawson et al. (2010) study	Children who participated in the Dawson et al. (2010) study were assessed 2 years after the intervention ended. $N = 39$, on average 6 years of age, $M_{age} = 72.9$ months, $SD = 2.6$	Two years after the Dawson et al. 2010 trial ended, children in the ESDM group maintained skills previously acquired in overall cognitive ability, adaptive behavior, symptom severity, and challenging behavior. Changes in core autism symptoms (ADOS) and adaptive functioning occurring from the end of intervention to the follow-up evaluation were superior in the ESDM group
Vismara et al. (2018)	Randomized controlled trial	Telehealth parent-implemented; parents were randomized to the ESDM group or a treatment as usual group; parents received 1.5 h telehealth training/week for 12 weeks. Follow-up 12 weeks after the intervention ended	Enrollment: $N = 32$ ESDM treatment group: $n = 17$ ($M_{age} = 31.9$ months, $SD = 10.4$) Community group (treatment as usual): $n = 15$ ($M_{age} = 27.2$ months, $SD = 7.9$) Posttreatment: $N = 24$ ESDM treatment group: $n = 14$ Community group: $n = 10$ Follow-up: $N = 24$ ESDM treatment group: $n = 14$ Community group: $n = 10$	Parents in the ESDM group achieved fidelity of implementation and showed higher satisfaction with and confidence to use the program and website resources than community parents after the treatment and at the follow-up. Children in both groups improved their social communication skills across time regardless of parent treatment fidelity
Colombi et al. (2018)	Quasi-experimental controlled trial	1:1 therapist-implemented; 6 h/week over 6 months	Pretreatment: $N = 92$ ESDM treatment group: $n = 22$, between the age of 18 and 48 months ($M_{age} = 31.1$ months, $SD = 8.0$) Community group (treatment as usual): $n = 70$ ($M_{age} = 35.2$ months, $SD = 7.6$)	Both groups improved in cognitive ability, adaptive behavior, and social skills after 3 months and 6 months. Children in the ESDM group made greater gains in cognitive and social skills after 3 and 6 months and larger improvements in adaptive behavior after 3 months of treatment

Zhou et al. (2018)	Quasi-experimental controlled trial	Parent-implemented; Parents received 1.5 h coaching/week for 26 weeks (weekly treatment hours unknown)	Enrollment: $N = 43$ ESDM treatment group: $n = 23$ ($M_{age} = 26.65$ months, $SD = 3.37$) Community group (treatment as usual): $n = 20$ ($M_{age} = 26.43$ months, $SD = 4.52$) Posttreatment: $N = 43$ ESDM treatment group: $n = 23$ ($M_{age} = 34.93$ months, $SD = 3.00$) Community group: $n = 20$ ($M_{age} = 34.15$ months, $SD = 4.67$)	The ESDM group demonstrated greater improvements in social affect, social communication, and symbolic play as compared with the community group
Vivanti et al. (2019)	Randomized controlled trial	Children randomized to receive group–ESDM either in specialized or inclusive settings, with staff–child ratio of 1:3-4; >15 h/week for 10–11 months	Enrollment: $N = 44$ Group–ESDM in inclusive setting: $n = 22$ ($M_{age} = 24.73$ months, $SD = 4.72$) Group–ESDM in specialized setting: $n = 22$ ($M_{age} = 26.36$ months, $SD = 4.64$)	Children showed improvements in spontaneous vocalization, social interaction, and imitation and across distal measures of verbal cognition, adaptive behavior, and autism symptoms regardless of intervention setting Parents of children in both intervention settings reported decreased stress
Rogers et al. (2019)	Multisite randomized controlled trial	1:1 therapist-implemented; 15 h/week for 24 months. Parents received 4 h of parent coaching/month for 24 months.	Enrollment: $N = 118$ ESDM treatment group: $n = 55$ ($M_{age} = 20.58$ months, $SD = 3.37$) Community group (treatment as usual): $n = 63$ ($M_{age} = 20.70$ months, $SD = 3.21$) Posttreatment: $N = 81$ ESDM treatment group: $n = 45$ ($M_{age} = 48.53$ months, $SD = 3.05$) Community group: $n = 36$ ($M_{age} = 48.75$ months, $SD = 3.77$)	Better language outcomes for the ESDM group, no group differences in cognitive or adaptive functioning

Pivotal Response Treatment (PRT)

PRT (Koegel & Koegel, 2006) is a behavioral treatment approach for children with ASD as young as 24 months of age, developed by Robert L. Koegel and Lynn Kern Koegel in the 1980s (Koegel et al. 1987). PRT is focused on the child's motivation to learn and interact with others in their natural environment as well as the "pivotal" skills of self-initiations, responding to multiple cues, self-management, and empathy (Koegel, Ashbaugh, & Koegel, 2016). The concept of "pivotal" skills refers to abilities which, when successfully acquired, can facilitate widespread learning across multiple developmental areas. By targeting those foundational skills, PRT is designed to facilitate collateral improvements in other areas of development (e.g., communication, language, play, and social behaviors) and to decrease episodes of distress or disengagement. PRT techniques can be embedded in daily activities and implemented in a variety of settings, including home (Hardan et al., 2015; Schreibman, Kaneko, & Koegel, 1991; Vernon et al., 2019), and school (Suhrheinrich, 2011; Suhrheinrich, Stahmer, & Schreibman, 2007).

Theoretical Basis

PRT is informed by the notion that ASD symptoms cause social–communicative attempts of children with ASD not to be reinforced during social interactions. As a consequence children with ASD fail to experience response–reinforcer contingencies, resulting in developing "learned helplessness" in the social domain (Koegel et al., 2016). Such learned helplessness decreases the likelihood that the child will initiate and respond to social stimuli, thus interfering with the acquisition of new skills. In order to address these deficits, PRT is designed to increase an individual's motivation to engage with others in social interactions by strengthening the response-reinforcement contingency. Motivational strategies are designed to improve the child's overall responsiveness, engagement, and affect, drawing from ABA principles and techniques (e.g., reinforcement, antecedent control, prompting, fading, shaping, and chaining) embedded within child-led activities and naturally occurring learning opportunities.

Practice and Implementation

PRT targets motivation, self-initiations of social interactions, responding to multiple cues, self-management skills, and empathy within naturalistic interactions. Strategies designed to increase the child's motivation include taking into account the child's preferences, allowing children to choose materials and activities, reinforcing attempts, varying tasks frequently, and interspersing maintenance and acquisition tasks (i.e., tasks that the child already masters and tasks that present new challenges). Improvement in pivotal skills is expected to create a motivational and learning foundation for widespread and generalized gains in developmentally downstream domains, including language, play, and cognitive and adaptive skills. Parent training is an integral component of the program.

Empirical Support

While most of the studies evaluating PRT have used single-subject designs (Koegel, et al., 1987), several group studies, including randomized controlled trials and quasi-experimental studies, have been recently published with results indicating improvements in targeted skills in many treated children. Evidence of collateral improvements in nontargeted areas is more mixed (Verschuur et al., 2014). Relevant group-based studies that tested PRT are described in Table 6.2—see also Verschuur et al., 2014, for a comprehensive literature review.

Table 6.2 Selected early intervention research studies on PRT

Study	Design	Treatment characteristics	Sample	Main results
Schreibman et al. (1991)	Randomized group design	Parent-implemented (19 parents of children with autism were randomly assigned into PRT group or discrete trial training group) Duration and intensity unknown	Enrollment: $N = 19$, ranging from 2.8 to 12 years old ($M_{age} = 7.2$ years)	Parents in the PRT treatment group showed more positive affect compared to those receiving traditional discrete trial training
Hardan et al. (2015)	Randomized controlled trial	Parent-implemented (parents were randomized to PRT or psychoeducation groups); daily for 12 weeks	Enrollment: $N = 48$ PRT treatment group: $n = 25$ ($M_{age} = 4.1$ years, $SD = 1.2$) Parents psychoeducation group: $n = 23$ ($M_{age} = 4.1$ years, $SD = 1.3$)	Children in the PRT group showed significantly greater improvements in frequency of utterances, in comparison with children in the psychoeducation group
Vernon et al. (2019)	Randomized controlled trial	1:1 therapist-implemented; 8 h for 26 months; parents received training 2 h/week	Enrollment: $N = 23$ Enhanced-PRT group (pivotal response intervention for social motivation): $n = 12$ ($M_{age} = 35.75$ months, $SD = 9.31$) Wait-list group (treatment as usual): $n = 11$ ($M_{age} = 34.45$ months, $SD = 10.08$)	In the PRT treatment group, more improvements in symptom severity, cognitive skills, language skills, adaptive skills. In the wait-list group, no significant gains were reported on any measures

JASPER (Joint Attention, Symbolic Play, Engagement, and Regulation)

JASPER is a manualized treatment approach for young children with developmental disabilities, including ASD (Kasari, Freeman, & Paparella, 2006; Kasari et al., 2015; Kasari, Gulsrud, Wong, Kwon, & Locke, 2010). JASPER focuses on increasing joint attention, imitation, and play as these behaviors provide a foundation for the development of other skills that are impaired in ASD, including social communication. This is achieved through a range of naturalistic developmental behavioral strategies (e.g., modeling, imitating, increasing the child's joint engagement with caregivers or interventionists, and planning activities based on the interests of the child) integrated into developmentally appropriate play activities. JASPER can be implemented by parents (Harrop, Gulsrud, Shih, Hovsepyan, & Kasari, 2017; Kasari et al., 2015), teachers (Chang, Shire, Shih, Gelfand, & Kasari, 2016; Lawton & Kasari, 2012; Shire et al., 2017), or clinicians/therapists (Shire et al., 2019).

Theoretical Basis

JASPER targets core skill deficits observed in young children with ASD, including joint attention, symbolic play, engagement, and regulation (Kasari et al., 2006; Kasari et al., 2015; Kasari et al., 2010). Strategies to improve joint attention skills (e.g., sharing attention with others through pointing, showing, and coordinating visual attention between people and objects) are designed to facilitate the development of social engagement and later spoken language (Kasari et al., 2006; Kasari et al., 2010; Wong, 2013). Similarly, JASPER is designed to target symbolic play in order to facilitate collateral improvements in social and communication functioning, given the link between symbolic play and the development of language and social functioning in typical and atypical development (Kasari et al., 2006; Kasari et al., 2005; Kasari et al., 2014). Additionally, as joint engagement is associated with cognitive, social, and communication development (Goods, Ishijima, Chang, & Kasari, 2013; Shire et al., 2019; Wong, 2013), JASPER targets joint engagement to promote social communication and learning opportunities. Supporting emotion and behavior regulation is also emphasized within JASPER as these developmental domains are critical to the advancement of social communication and play (Shire et al., 2019).

Practice and Implementation

In JASPER, joint attention, symbolic play, engagement, and regulation are targeted using naturalistic developmental behavioral strategies such as following the child's lead and interest, modeling and prompting for joint attention, imitating the child's actions on toys to obtain her or his attention, facilitating and expanding play, narrating the child's play behaviors, and giving corrective feedback during developmentally appropriate play activities (Kasari et al., 2006; Kasari et al., 2014; Kasari et al., 2008). In addition, environmental manipulations (e.g., strategically arranging environmental antecedents and consequences) are used to facilitate the child's spontaneous social and communicative bids (Kasari et al., 2006; Kasari et al., 2014; Kasari et al., 2008).

Empirical Support

As detailed in Table 6.3, several studies based on randomized designs support the effectiveness of JASPER in improving joint engagement, joint attention, language, and play skills for young children with ASD.

Early Social Interaction (ESI)

ESI (Wetherby & Woods, 2006) is a comprehensive early intervention model that focuses on a collaborative coaching approach to empower parents to teach important skills to their child in natural environments (Wetherby et al., 2014; Wetherby & Woods, 2006).

Theoretical Basis

ESI has a family-centered capacity-building focus (Wetherby et al., 2018), which emphasizes equipping families with strategies to address their child's developmental needs. Additionally, the model is based on empirical research and clinical investigations of communicative functions in ASD (Wetherby, 1986; Wetherby & Prutting, 1984) and addresses the relationship among communication, social–emotional development, and emotion regulation (Prizant & Wetherby, 1990). Within ESI, parents are actively engaged throughout the assessment and intervention process, facilitating collaborative decision making on treatment planning and active reflection on the use of intervention strategies. Parents are encouraged to incorporate teaching strategies to target developmentally appropriate treatment goals at home or in the community during daily routines important to the family. The purpose of teaching in naturalistic environments is to increase the child's participation in everyday activities and the involvement of the child's family in the community. The naturalistic focus of ESI is also designed to promote the generalization of skills and reduce the amount of professional time needed for service provision (Wetherby et al., 2014; Wetherby & Woods, 2006).

Table 6.3 Selected research studies on the efficacy of the JASPER

Study	Design	Treatment characteristics	Sample	Main results
Lawton and Kasari (2012)	Randomized controlled trial	Teacher-implemented; daily for half-day for 6 weeks	JASPER group: $n = 9$ ($M_{age} = 46.0$ months, $SD = 5.00$) Comparison group (treatment as usual): $n = 7$ ($M_{age} = 43.01$ months, $SD = 6.00$)	Children receiving JASPER demonstrated increased joint attention and joint engagement than the comparison group
Goods et al. (2013)	Randomized controlled trial	1:1 therapist-implemented; 30 min twice/week for 12 weeks	Enrollment: $N = 15$ JASPER group: $n = 7$ ($M_{age} = 48.73$ months, $SD = 11.68$) Comparison group (treatment as usual): $n = 8$ ($M_{age} = 54.68$ months, $SD = 10.25$) Posttreatment: $N = 11$ JASPER group: $n = 5$ ($M_{age} = 58.84$ months, $SD = 10.98$) Comparison group: $n = 6$ ($M_{age} = 60.55$ months, $SD = 9.36$)	Children in the JASPER group demonstrated more diversity of spontaneous play and use of requesting gestures as compared to children in the comparison group
Kasari et al. (2014)	Randomized controlled trial	Parent/caregiver-implemented; 2 h/week for 3 months with 3-month follow-up	Baseline: $N = 112$ JASPER group: Caregiver-mediated module (CMM) $n = 60$ ($M_{age} = 41.9$ months, $SD = 10.0$) Comparison group: Caregiver education module (CEM) $n = 52$ ($M_{age} = 42.8$ months, $SD = 10.21$)	Children in the JASPER group demonstrated greater improvements in joint engagement and initiations of joint attention compared to the comparison group. Children receiving the JASPER maintained joint engagement over time. Children in both groups retained initiations of joint attention over time. Children in the JASPER treatment group also improved symbolic play skills but not functional play skills

Kasari et al. (2015)	Randomized controlled trials	Parent-implemented; 1 h/week for 10 weeks	Enrollment: $N = 86$ JASPER group: $n = 43$ ($M_{age} = 30.7$ months, $SD = 3.5$) Psychoeducation group: $n = 43$ ($M_{age} = 32.3$ months, $SD = 2.7$)	Children in the JASPER group showed a significant increase in joint engagement compared to the psychoeducation group. The improvement maintained at the 6-month follow-up
Chang et al. (2016)	Randomized trial (at the school level)	Teacher-implemented; staff-child ratio = 1:2; daily for 3 months with 1-month follow-up. Six classrooms with one teacher and one assistant in each of them	Enrollment: $N = 66$ JASPER group: $n = 38$ ($M_{age} = 48.87$ months, $SD = 6.30$) Comparison group (treatment as usual): $n = 28$ ($M_{age} = 51.64$ months, $SD = 6.46$) Posttreatment: $N = 63$ JASPER treatment group: $n = 35$ Comparison group: $n = 28$ Follow-up: $N = 62$ JASPER group: $n = 34$ Comparison group: $n = 28$	Children in the JASPER treatment group made significant improvements in initiations of joint engagement, joint attention gestures and language, and play skills, as well as cognitive ability over children in the comparison group
Gulsrud, Hellemann, Shire, and Kasari (2016)	Randomized controlled trial	Same as the Kasari et al. (2015) study	Same as the Kasari et al. (2015) study	Children in the JASPER treatment group demonstrated greater increase in joint engagement than those in the psychoeducation group
Shire, Gulsrud, and Kasari (2016)	Randomized controlled trial	Same as the Kasari et al. (2015) study	Same as the Kasari et al. (2015) study with one child being excluded due to missing data at entry	Children in JASPER treatment group significantly increased responsive behavior compared to the psychoeducation intervention
Harrop et al. (2017)	Randomized controlled trial	Same as the Kasari et al. (2015) study	Same as the Kasari et al. (2015) study	No group differences were found in restricted and repetitive behaviors after treatment
Shire et al. (2017)	Randomized trial (at the classroom level)	Teaching assistant-implemented; about 2 h/day for 10 weeks with 1-month follow-up; a session had 8–10 children with each child paired with a teaching assistant	Enrollment: $N = 115$ JASPER group: $n = 56$ ($M_{age} = 31.71$ months, $SD = 2.94$) Comparison group (treatment as usual): $n = 59$ ($M_{age} = 31.54$ months, $SD = 3.17$)	Children receiving JASPER demonstrated larger improvements in joint engagement, joint attention, and play skills compared to comparison group. The developmental gains were maintained at the one-month follow-up

Practice and Implementation

Parents collaborate with professionals to create an individualized treatment plan for their child and are coached to use intervention strategies in daily activities throughout the day (Wetherby et al., 2014). ESI uses a manualized curriculum-based assessment based on the SCERTS (Social Communication, Emotional Regulation, and Transactional Supports) intervention to identify developmentally appropriate goals and monitor progress (Prizant, Wetherby, Rubin, Laurent, & Rydell, 2006; Wetherby et al., 2018). SCERTS focuses on three dimensions that are foundational to the development of children with ASD, including (1) social communication, with treatment goals including expanding the use of gestures, sounds, and words, initiating spontaneous verbal and nonverbal communication, understanding the meaning of words, initiating and responding to joint attention, increasing functional object use and pretend play, and extending reciprocity in interaction; (2) emotional regulation, with relevant intervention targets including expressing emotion, expanding self-regulatory strategies to calm self when dysregulated, using communication to help regulate emotion when frustrated or help is needed, and using regulatory strategies to stay engaged in activities and handle new and changing situations; and (3) transactional supports, that is, the specific teaching strategies and learning supports for parents (Wetherby et al., 2018).

After treatment goals are identified, the coach and the parent work collaboratively to (a) identify what works for the parent–child dyad using observation, direct teaching, and modeling, (b) practice imbedding intervention with the guide of the therapist and direct feedback, (c) continue practicing with parent-led sessions and reflection on the engagement of the parent and child, and (d) increase parent independence (Wetherby et al., 2014; Wetherby et al., 2018). The coach ensures that the objects, equipment, and materials are appropriate for the routine and observational data are collected periodically for progress monitoring.

Empirical Support

As displayed on Table 6.4, empirical support for ESI includes a quasi-experimental study and a randomized controlled trial that compared different dosages and formats of the same intervention. Results support the effectiveness of this approach in promoting gains in communication, daily living, and social skills for very young children with ASD.

Table 6.4 Research studies on the early social interaction (ESI)

Study	Design	Treatment characteristics	Sample	Main results
Wetherby and Woods (2006)	Quasi experimental study	Parent-implemented (therapist-assisted with two home visits/week); daily for 12 months (weekly treatment hours unknown)	Enrollment: Pre-ESI group: $n = 17$ ($M_{age} = 18.19$ months, $SD = 3.85$) Posttreatment: $N = 35$ Post-ESI group: $n = 17$ ($M_{age} = 30.72$ months, $SD = 3.66$) Comparison group (no treatment) $n = 18$ ($M_{age} = 31.61$ months, $SD = 3.45$)	From baseline to posttreatment, children in the ESI treatment group significantly improved social communication skills. Compared to the control group at posttreatment, children in the ESI treatment demonstrated better performance in social signals, rate of communicating, communicative functions, and understanding
Wetherby et al. (2014)	Randomized controlled trial	Parents randomized to individual-ESI or group-ESI coaching. Both groups are encouraged to incorporate intervention strategies into daily routine activities for at least 25 h/week for 9 months	Enrollment: $N = 82$ Individual–ESI coaching group: $n = 42$ ($M_{age} = 19.64$ months, $SD = 1.93$) Group–ESI coaching group: $n = 40$ ($M_{age} = 19.58$ months, $SD = 1.42$)	Children receiving individual–ESI showed improvement in social communication at a faster rate than those in group-ESI. Parents of children in individual–ESI reported significantly better communication, daily living, and social skills as compared to group–ESI. Children in individual–ESI improved receptive language skills significantly. In comparison, those in group–ESI showed no change

Project ImPACT (Improving Parents as Communication Teachers)

Project ImPACT is a parent training curriculum designed to target social communication skills for young children with autism up to 6 years of age (Ingersoll & Dvortcsak, 2010). The program utilizes a naturalistic approach that includes behavioral and developmental strategies integrated into play activities and daily routines. Parents use these strategies in partnership with an interventionist to promote social engagement, language, social imitation, and play.

Theoretical Basis

Project ImPACT draws from research on the effectiveness of parent training in enhancing child developmental outcomes, promoting generalization and maintenance of targeted skills, and reducing parental stress and depression (Ingersoll & Dvortcsak, 2010). Against this background, Project ImPACT provides parents with a systematic guide to teach their child social communication skills using developmental strategies and ABA-based techniques (e.g., prompting, shaping, and reinforcement).

Practice and Implementation

Project ImPACT teaches parents interactive teaching techniques and direct teaching techniques, which form a three-layer pyramid (Ingersoll & Dvortcsak, 2010). The four interactive teaching techniques at the base of the pyramid (i.e., *follow your child's lead*, *imitate your child*, *animation*, and *modeling and expanding language*) are the foundation for the treatment, serving to improve the child's motivation and engagement as well as adult responsiveness. Once the parent has become proficient at these, the interactive teaching techniques at the middle layer (i.e., *playful obstruction*, *balanced turns*, and *communicative temptations*) are subsequently introduced to facilitate spontaneous communication. Lastly, the top layer of the pyramid includes the direct teaching techniques, which involve the use of prompting and reinforcement for teaching the child more advanced social communication goals.

Empirical Support

As shown in Table 6.5, empirical support for Project ImPACT includes one quasi-experimental study and two randomized studies suggesting improvements in social communication for treated children.

Table 6.5 Research studies on the efficacy of project ImPACT

Study	Design	Treatment characteristics	Sample	Main results
Ingersoll and Berger (2015)	Randomized controlled trial	Parent-implemented; parents randomized to self-directed vs. therapist-assisted	Enrollment: $N = 27$ Self-directed group: $n = 13$ ($M_{age} = 46.08$ months, $SD = 13.18$) Therapist-assisted group $n = 14$ ($M_{age} = 41.57$ months, $SD = 12.24$)	Compared to the self-directed group, parents in the therapist-assisted group were more likely to engage with ImPACT online (a telehealth-based parent-mediated intervention). The program completion rate was significantly higher in the therapist-assisted group than the self-directed group
Stadnick, Stahmer, and Brookman-Frazee (2015)	Nonrandomized group design	Parent-implemented; parents received training 1 h/week for 12 weeks	Enrollment: $N = 30$ Project ImPACT group: $n = 16$ ($M_{age} = 46.75$ months, $SD = 25.88$) Community group (treatment as usual): $n = 14$ ($M_{age} = 64.07$ months, $SD = 22.32$)	Children in the project ImPACT group made significant improvements in communication skills
Ingersoll, Wainer, Berger, Pickard, and Bonter (2016)	Randomized controlled trial	Same as the Ingersoll and Berger (2015) study: Parent-implemented; parents were expected to use online training resources without or with the assistance of a therapist (self-directed vs. therapist-assisted)	Same sample as the Ingersoll and Berger (2015) study: Enrollment: $N = 27$ Self-directed group: $n = 13$ ($M_{age} = 46.08$ months, $SD = 13.18$) Therapist-assisted group $n = 14$ ($M_{age} = 41.57$ months, $SD = 12.24$)	Children in both groups increased scores on language measures; those in the therapist-assisted group made greater gains. Children in the therapist-assisted group showed improvements in social skills. Compared to the self-directed group, parents in the therapist-assisted group demonstrated greater improvements in implementation fidelity and positive perceptions of their child

Incidental Teaching (IT)

Incidental teaching (IT) is an intervention approach which targets the acquisition of spoken language during naturally occurring adult–child interactions. The most distinctive feature of IT is that all interactions during the intervention must be initiated by the child. The concept of IT was originally created by Betty Hart and Todd Risley in the 1970s (Hart & Risley, 1978) and further developed by Gail McGee in the 1990s (McGee, 2005; McGee, Morrier, & Daly, 1999). IT can be implemented by parents, teachers, or therapists.

Theoretical Basis

Incidental teaching emphasizes the importance of family involvement and child social engagement in facilitating language learning and inclusion of children with ASD. Treatment techniques in incidental teaching are based on the notion that children with ASD have difficulty initiating social communication. Therefore, teaching strategies are designed to be embedded in fun play activities that capitalize on the child's interests, motivations, and attentional focus. ABA principles are incorporated within such play activities in natural environments.

Practice and Implementation

IT is used to teach children with ASD communication skills such as responding to social interactions, labeling items, and requesting objects (Neely, Rispoli, Gerow, & Hong, 2016). Building on the child's self-initiations, the interventionist observes the child's preferred objects/activities and captures "teachable moments" (i.e., learning opportunities) to teach the targeted behaviors (McGee et al., 1999). Within the IT framework, materials are typically placed out of reach but within sight in order to create opportunities for the child to request. In a typical teaching episode, once the child shows interest in the materials, the interventionist places his/her hand on the child's hand and looks expectantly to wait for an appropriate response (e.g., verbalization or gesture). In the absence of an appropriate response, the interventionist asks "What do you want?" and provides further prompts as needed (e.g., asking specific questions such as "What color car do you want?" making gestures, and modeling the desired response) to encourage the child's response (McGee et al., 1999). Natural consequences (e.g., access to desired materials, assistance, or adult attention) are systematically provided to reinforce the child's communicative efforts.

Empirical Support

Several single-subject studies (e.g., McGee & Daly, 2007) suggest that children with ASD can improve their language skills through incidental teaching techniques. However, no group-based studies on the effectiveness of this approach are available.

Enhanced Milieu Teaching (EMT)

EMT (Hemmeter & Kaiser, 1994) is an early language intervention approach designed for young children with language impairments, including children with ASD (Kaiser, Hancock, & Nietfeld, 2000). Building on child interests and initiation, the interventionist catches "teachable moments" to model and prompt specific language skills during everyday interactions in a natural and functional context (Kaiser et al., 2000; Olive et al., 2007). EMT can be delivered by parents in the home environment (Hemmeter & Kaiser, 1994; Kaiser et al., 2000), by teachers in the child's classroom (Drasgow, 2007; Olive et al., 2007), or by therapists in home or clinic settings (Hampton, Kaiser, & Roberts, 2017; Hancock & Kaiser, 2002).

Theoretical Basis

The EMT model incorporates three components, which include (a) environmental arrangement, (b) responsive interaction, and (c) milieu teaching (Hancock & Kaiser, 2002; Kaiser et al., 2000). Environmental arrangements are utilized to increase the level of engagement and facilitate learning. Adult responsiveness to the child's communicative attempts is emphasized as parent–child interactions provide natural opportunities for language learning (Hampton et al., 2017; Hemmeter & Kaiser, 1994; Roberts & Kaiser, 2012). EMT also draws strategies from a program called milieu teaching (Hart & Rogers-Warren, 1978), a set of procedures designed to embed language learning opportunities within the child's natural environment by capitalizing on a child's interest in and motivation to gain access to specific materials.

Practice and Implementation

EMT aims to improve social communication skills using responsive interaction strategies and behavioral teaching procedures during naturalistic interactions (Hancock & Kaiser, 2002; Kaiser & Roberts, 2013; Olive et al., 2007). Techniques include following the child's lead, taking turns, imitating the child's play behaviors and vocalizations, and expanding on the child's utterances to increase child communication, modeling language, prompting the child's communication targets, reinforcing communication by providing access to requested objects, and using time delay (see Chap. 5) to elicit language (Hart & Rogers-Warren, 1978; Kaiser et al., 2000). In addition, manipulation of the environment (e.g., putting materials out of reach to promote requesting) is used (Hancock & Kaiser, 2002; Kaiser et al., 2000). These language teaching procedures are embedded throughout play-based therapy sessions.

Empirical Support

As detailed in Table 6.6, there is some initial support for the efficacy of EMT in improving some dimensions of language in young children with communication difficulties as well as in school age children with ASD (Hampton et al., 2017), while evidence of treatment effects on language for young children with ASD is limited.

Reciprocal Imitation Training (RIT)

Reciprocal imitation training (RIT; Ingersoll, 2008) is a treatment approach focused on teaching imitation to young children with ASD. RIT incorporates teaching strategies targeting the flexible and social use of imitation during natural play activities and daily routines. Parents (Ingersoll & Gergans, 2007), therapists (Ingersoll, 2010, 2012), and the child's siblings (Walton & Ingersoll, 2012) can be trained as treatment providers to implement RIT.

Theoretical Basis

RIT is rooted on the notion that imitation in early childhood development is critical to the development of cognitive and social communication (e.g., language, play, and joint attention), serving both a learning function (acquisition of new knowledge) and a social-affiliative function (Vivanti & Hamilton, 2014). As children with ASD exhibit significant deficits in imitation skills that interfere with their learning and social functioning (including imitation of body movements, object use, vocalizations, and facial expressions), RIT focuses on teaching imitation to young children with ASD to support cognitive and social development.

Practice and Implementation

RIT (Ingersoll, 2008) targets the social use of imitation (e.g., object and gesture imitation) in young children with autism during play interactions. ABA based techniques including modeling, prompting, and contingent reinforcement are

Table 6.6 Research studies on enhanced milieu teaching (EMT)

Study	Design	Treatment characteristics	Sample	Main results
Kaiser and Roberts (2013)	Randomized group design	"Therapist-only" EMT group: two therapists, 24 30-min sessions in clinic and one therapist, 12 20-min sessions at home; 6-month and 12-month follow-ups. "Parent and therapist" EMT group: Therapist- and parent-implemented, 24 30-min sessions in clinic and parent-implemented, 12 20-min sessions at home; 6-month and 12-month follow-ups	Children with developmental delay, autism spectrum disorders, or Down syndrome Enrollment: $N = 77$ "Therapist-only" EMT group: $n = 38$ ($M_{age} = 41.32$ months, $SD = 7.30$) "Parent and therapist" EMT group: $n = 39$ ($M_{age} = 40.05$ months, $SD = 8.76$)	No group differences were found in language skills
Roberts and Kaiser (2015)	Randomized controlled trial	Caregiver-implemented; four training workshops, 24 treatment sessions across 3 months (two sessions/week: One 20-min session in the clinic and daily at home for an average of 17 h/week)	Toddlers with *language delays*, excluding children with intellectual disability, hearing loss, a major medical condition, or autism spectrum disorder Enrollment: $N = 97$ EMT group: $n = 45$ ($M_{age} = 30.3$ months, $SD = 5.0$) Comparison group (treatment as usual): $n = 52$ ($M_{age} = 30.6$ months, $SD = 5.1$)	The use of all language facilitation strategies significantly improved in caregivers in the EMT group. Children in the EMT group demonstrated significantly better receptive language skills compared to the comparison group. No group differences in expressive language skills
Curtis, Kaiser, Estabrook, and Roberts (2017)	Randomized controlled trial follow-up	Same as the Roberts and Kaiser (2015) study	Same sample from the Roberts and Kaiser (2015) study	After the intervention ended for 12 months, parents of children in the EMT treatment group reported lower rates of externalizing and internalizing behaviors for the children
Hampton et al. (2017)	Randomized controlled trial follow-up	Same as the Roberts and Kaiser (2015) study	Same sample from the Roberts and Kaiser (2015) study	No group differences in expressive or receptive language skills at either the 6- or 12-month follow-ups

incorporated for teaching imitation within naturalistic social interactions. In order to increase the child's use of eye contact, joint attention, and reciprocity in preparation for imitation, the child's play partner (e.g., caregiver) is expected to contingently imitate the child's actions on toys with a duplicate set of toys, the child's gestures and body movements, and vocalizations (Ingersoll, 2008, 2010, 2012). The play partner is also trained to use developmentally appropriate language to describe the child's play behaviors or to create sound effects in response to the play activities. In teaching imitation, the therapist models an action, paired with a verbal marker to describe the action. Gesture imitation is taught by the play partner demonstrating a meaningful gesture (e.g., affective, object, attributes, and conventional action gestures) as related to the child's play (Ingersoll, 2010). Modeled actions/gestures vary across toys/materials in order to avoid rigid associations between actions and specific toys. Both social reinforcement (e.g., praise) and tangible reinforcement (e.g., access to materials) are used in the intervention.

Empirical Support

As displayed in Table 6.7, there is initial support for the efficacy of RIT in improving elicited and spontaneous imitation (Ingersoll, 2010) as well as joint attention initiations and social–emotional functioning (Ingersoll, 2012).

Table 6.7 Research studies on the efficacy of the reciprocal imitation training (RIT)

Study	Design	Treatment characteristics	Sample	Main results
Ingersoll (2010)	Randomized controlled trial	1–1 therapist-implemented; 3 h/week for 10 weeks	Enrollment: $N = 21$ RIT treatment group: $n = 11$ ($M_{age} = 41.36$ months, $SD = 4.30$) Community group (treatment as usual): $n = 10$ ($M_{age} = 37.20$ months, $SD = 7.36$)	Children in the RIT treatment group made more improvements in elicited and spontaneous imitation
Ingersoll (2012)	Randomized controlled trial	1–1 therapist-implemented; 3 h/week for 10 weeks	Enrollment: $N = 27$ RIT treatment group: $n = 14$ ($M_{age} = 39.3$ months, $SD = 7.3$) Community group (treatment as usual): $n = 13$ ($M_{age} = 36.5$ months, $SD = 8.0$)	Children in the RIT treatment group made more improvements in joint attention initiations at the end of the treatment and at a 2- to 3-month follow-up, compared to the community group. Children in the RIT treatment group also improved social–emotional functioning significantly more than the community group did at the follow-up

Early Achievements (EA)

Early achievements (Landa, Holman, O'Neill, & Stuart, 2011; Landa & Kalb, 2012) is an intervention approach designed to address the learning challenges of young children with ASD or other social and communication disorders. A comprehensive developmental curriculum called Assessment, Evaluation, and Programming System for Infants and Children (AEPS; Bricker, 2002) is utilized for treatment planning, and strategies informed by developmental and behavioral research are delivered in naturalistic settings.

Theoretical Basis

The EA intervention is grounded in research suggesting that child's school readiness can be facilitated through intervention strategies that promote the development of communication, symbolic, linguistic, concept and event representation, reciprocal social engagement with peers, and perspective taking (Landa, 2016).

Practice and Implementation

The EA intervention involves naturalistic developmental behavioral intervention strategies whereby the interventionist creates opportunities for the child's spontaneous communication by following the child's attentional lead and expanding on their play and use of language. Frequent "orchestrated opportunities" are deliberately created for social engagement using various strategies such as modeling, labeling, and imitating the children's actions. The interventionist further encourages the child to imitate peers and adults, to respond to joint attention, and to share their positive affect with others.

Empirical Support

As detailed in Table 6.8, the EA intervention was evaluated in a randomized controlled trial (Landa et al., 2011), which reported treatment effects on socially engaged imitation with gains generalized into different contexts and maintained at the 6-month follow-up. Gains for initiation of joint attention and shared positive affect were similar in the treatment and control groups.

Table 6.8 Research on the efficacy of early achievements (EA)

Study	Design	Treatment characteristics	Sample	Main results
Landa et al. (2011)	Randomized controlled trial	Teacher/therapist-implemented (adult to child ratio = 3:5); 2.5 h/day for 4 days/week for 6 months	Treatment group: $n = 24$ ($M_{age} = 28.6$ months, $SD = 2.6$) Comparison group (regular treatment): $n = 24$ ($M_{age} = 28.9$ months, $SD = 2.8$)	Children in the treatment group showed increased socially engaged imitation after the intervention. Generalization in unfamiliar contexts and maintenance of the skill at the follow-up were also reported. Children in both groups demonstrated similar improvements in initiation of joint attention and shared positive affect

Adapted Response Teaching

Adapted response teaching (ART; Baranek et al., 2015) is a relationship-based intervention aimed at increasing parent responsiveness and, consequently, child developmental outcomes in 1-year-old infants who have an older sibling with ASD, due to their increased likelihood of being later diagnosed with ASD or experiencing developmental delays. It is adapted from the Responsive Teaching Curriculum (Mahoney & MacDonald, 2007), which teaches parents the utilization of highly responsive interactions with their children within daily routines to promote cognition, communication, and social–emotional functioning. ART is primarily designed to be implemented by parents in home environments (Baranek et al., 2015; Watson et al., 2017).

Theoretical Basis

ART is based on two primary theoretical foundations (Watson et al., 2017). First, by targeting pivotal behaviors (e.g., intentional communication, joint attention, and social play), the intervention aims to promote downstream benefits across cognition, language, communication, socialization, and adaptive behavior (Baranek et al., 2015; Watson et al., 2017). In addition, increasing parent responsiveness is critical to the development of communication, language, emotional regulation, sensory regulation, and attention regulation (Watson et al., 2017). Thus, ART was designed to increase the caregivers' responsiveness and sensitivity to their child in order to promote child's development in these areas.

Practice and Implementation

ART is designed to target intervention objectives falling into two broad categories, including the social–communication domain (i.e., social play, joint activity, joint attention, vocalization, intentionality, and conversation) and sensory regulatory domain (i.e., self-regulation, attention and arousal, exploration, engagement, adaptability and coping, and cooperation; Baranek et al., 2015). These "pivotal" domains are known to provide a foundation for later social and cognitive development (Baranek et al., 2015). Parents are trained to use responsive teaching strategies reflecting five dimensions (i.e., reciprocity, contingency, control, affect, and match) during daily routine activities (Baranek et al., 2015; Watson et al., 2017). Responsive strategies used to teach social communication include imitating the child's actions and vocalizations, repeating activity the child enjoys, being animated, communicating at the child's level and without asking questions, and expanding on the child's play (Watson et al., 2017). In order to teach sensory regulatory skills, parents are encouraged to match the child's pace, follow the child's lead, mirror the child's play behavior and use parallel play to join an activity, treating the child's emotions as meaningful and legitimate, and giving frequent opportunities to make choices. A family action plan is created in order to assist parents in implementing and reflecting on the responsive teaching strategies used in daily interactions with their child (Baranek et al., 2015; Watson et al., 2017).

Empirical Support

In the context of ASD early intervention, ART has been tested by randomized trials that included infants presenting early signs of ASD identified through early screening. Evidence for intervention effectiveness, as shown in Table 6.9, is mixed.

Table 6.9 Research studies on the efficacy of adapted responsive teaching (ART)

Study	Design	Treatment characteristics	Sample	Main results
Baranek et al. (2015)	Randomized controlled trial	Parent-implemented; parents received an average of 27.6 training sessions at home with an average of 5.8 additional contacts with a therapist across a 6- to 8-month period; treatment delivered between parent training sessions (weekly treatment hours unknown)	Infants at risk of autism spectrum disorder Enrollment: $N = 16$ ART treatment group: $n = 11$ ($M_{age} = 15.22$ months, $SD = 1.2$) Comparison group (treatment as usual): $n = 5$ ($M_{age} = 15.6$ months, $SD = 1.3$)	Infants in the ART group showed improved social adaptive behavior, including communication and socialization, compared to the treatment-as-usual group. Parents of the infants in the ART group were less directive
Watson et al. (2017)	Randomized controlled trial	Parent-implemented; parents received 24.9 training sessions at home with an average of 2.4 additional contacts with a therapist across a 6- to 8-month period; treatment was delivered between parent training sessions (weekly treatment hours unknown)	Infants at risk of autism spectrum disorder Enrollment: $N = 87$ ART treatment group: $n = 45$ ($M_{age} = 13.8$ months, $SD = 0.71$) Comparison (treatment as usual): $n = 42$ ($M_{age} = 13.7$ months, $SD = 0.79$)	No main effects of ART on child social–communication, sensory-regulatory, adaptive, and autism symptomology. Parents in the ART group demonstrated greater parental responsiveness compared to the treatment-as-usual group

Conclusions

In this chapter, we have examined a variety of early intervention approaches that adhere to the Naturalistic Developmental Behavioral Intervention (NDBI) framework. These interventions are informed by the notion that developmental sequences and processes of early learning supporting typical development are also observed in ASD, although autism symptoms and associated features affect developmental rate and learning patterns in specific domains. Consequently, NDBIs attempt to embed behavioral strategies within the back-and-forth flow of social interaction that characterize early child–adult exchanges (Mundy, 2016; Rogers et al., 2017). Within this framework, the various interventions described here are based on different theoretical orientations and hypothesized mechanisms of change, although they present with remarkable similarities in their practical implementation (to the point that questions have been raised on the need for such numerous "brand names" in the field; Vivanti et al., 2018).

Nevertheless, important differences among the models discussed here include whether they address specific "pivotal" areas such as imitation or social communication (e.g., PRT, JASPER, RIT) or are designed to be comprehensive in scope with treatment targets covering nonsocial domains such as cognitive, motor, and adaptive functioning (e.g., ESDM, ESI). Additionally, the strength of evidence differs across approaches, ranging from support from large randomized trials (e.g., JASPER, ESDM) to preliminary evidence based on nonrandomized designs (e.g., incidental teaching). Additionally, some NDBI interventions have been implemented and evaluated across different age groups (e.g., PRT) while others have been designed to address the needs for very young children (e.g., ESI, ART). While evidence for effectiveness is generally favorable, benefits are more frequently reported in areas that are directly targeted by the intervention, and variability across outcome measures and participants are substantial.

It is also important to acknowledge that our list of NDBI models might not be exhaustive, and intervention programs might exist that do not explicitly use the term NDBI but are broadly consistent with the NDBI principles nonetheless (e.g., Schertz, Odom, Baggett, & Sideris, 2013). Additionally, other ASD early interventions have been implemented and evaluated that involve a developmental focus but do not fit within the NDBI category as they do not include behaviorally based procedures. Notable examples include the Developmental, Individual Difference, Relationship-Based (DIR) Model, which focuses relationship and interactions, emotional development, and individual differences in sensory modulation, processing, and motor planning (Greenspan & Weider, 1998), and the Preschool Autism Communication Trial (PACT), which uses parent coaching to increase parental sensitivity and responsiveness to the child's communication and facilitate adaptation of the parents' communication style to the level of their child's understanding (Green et al., 2010). This latter approach is supported by very well-designed research suggesting treatment-related changes in parental responsivity as well as reduced autism symptom severity for treated children (Pickles et al., 2016).

Finally, while NDBIs are partly designed to address some perceived limitations of standard ABA approaches such as EIBI, both approaches appear to be beneficial to children with ASD. The paucity of direct comparison studies, together with the variability in outcomes across models, and the increasing incorporation of naturalistic strategies in ABA-based approaches make it difficult to provide strong conclusions regarding the superiority of one approach versus the other. Understanding for whom, and for what skills, more naturalistic versus more structured approaches are helpful is a critical clinical and research challenge, which will be discussed in the following chapters.

References

Adamson, L. B., Bakeman, R., & Deckner, D. F. (2004). The development of symbol-infused joint engagement. *Child Development, 75*, 1171–1187. https://doi.org/10.1111/j.1467-8624.2004.00732.x

Baranek, G. T., Watson, L. R., Turner-Brown, L., Field, S. H., Crais, E. R., Wakeford, L., … Reznick, J. S. (2015). Preliminary efficacy of adapted responsive teaching for infants at risk of autism spectrum disorder in a community sample. *Autism Research and Treatment, 386951*, 1–16. https://doi.org/10.1155/2015/386951

Begus, K., Gliga, T., & Southgate, V. (2014). Infants learn what they want to learn: Responding to infant pointing leads to superior learning. *PLoS One, 9*, e108817. https://doi.org/10.1371/journal.pone.0108817

Bloom, P. (2002). Mindreading, communication and the learning of names for things. *Mind & Language, 17*, 37–54. https://doi.org/10.1111/1468-0017.00188

Bricker, D. (2002). *Assessment, evaluation, and programming system for infants and children: Birth to three years* (2nd ed.). Baltimore, MD: Brookes Publishing.

Chang, Y.-C., Shire, S. Y., Shih, W., Gelfand, C., & Kasari, C. (2016). Preschool deployment of evidence-based social communication intervention: JASPER in the classroom. *Journal of Autism and Developmental Disorders, 46*, 2211–2223. https://doi.org/10.1007/s10803-016-2752-2

Charman, T. (2003). Why is joint attention a pivotal skill in autism? *Philosophical Transactions of the Royal Society of London. Series B, Biological Sciences, 358*, 315–324. https://doi.org/10.1098/rstb.2002.1199

Colombi, C., Narzisi, A., Ruta, L., Cigala, V., Gagliano, A., Pioggia, G., … Prima Pietra, T. (2018). Implementation of the Early Start Denver Model in an Italian community. *Autism, 22*, 126–133. https://doi.org/10.1177/1362361316665792

Curtis, P. R., Kaiser, A. P., Estabrook, R., & Roberts, M. Y. (2017). The longitudinal effects of early language intervention on children's problem behaviors. *Child Development, 90*, 576–592. https://doi.org/10.1111/cdev.12942

Dawson, G., & Bernier, R. (2007). Social brain circuitry in autism. In D. Coch, G. Dawson, & K. Fischer (Eds.), *Human behavior and the developing brain*. New York: Guilford Press.

Dawson, G., Rogers, S., Munson, J., Smith, M., Winter, J., Greenson, J., … Varley, J. (2010). Randomized, controlled trial of an intervention for toddlers with autism: The Early Start Denver Model. *Pediatrics, 125*, e17–e23. https://doi.org/10.1542/peds.2009-0958

Dawson, G., Toth, K., Abbott, R., Osterling, J., Munson, J., Estes, A., & Liaw, J. (2004). Early social attention impairments in autism: Social orienting, joint attention, and attention to distress. *Developmental Psychology, 40*(2), 271.

Drasgow, E. (2007). Using enhanced milieu teaching and a voice-output communication aid to increase independent requesting by three children with autism. *Evidence-Based Communication Assessment and Intervention, 1*, 134–135. https://doi.org/10.1080/17489530701701435

Estes, A., Munson, J., Rogers, S. J., Greenson, J., Winter, J., & Dawson, G. (2015). Long-term outcomes of early intervention in 6-year-old children with autism Spectrum disorder. *Journal of the American Academy of Child & Adolescent Psychiatry, 54*, 580–587. https://doi.org/10.1016/j.jaac.2015.04.005

Goods, K. S., Ishijima, E., Chang, Y.-C., & Kasari, C. (2013). Preschool based JASPER intervention in minimally verbal children with autism: Pilot RCT. *Journal of Autism and Developmental Disorders, 43*, 1050–1056. https://doi.org/10.1007/s10803-012-1644-3

Green, J., Charman, T., McConachie, H., Aldred, C., Slonims, V., Howlin, P., … Barrett, B. (2010). Parent-mediated communication-focused treatment in children with autism (PACT): A randomised controlled trial. *The Lancet, 375*(9732), 2152–2160.

Greenspan, S. I., & Weider, S. (1998). *The child with special needs: Encouraging intellectual and emotional growth*. Cambridge, MA: DeCapo Press.

Gulsrud, A. C., Hellemann, G., Shire, S., & Kasari, C. (2016). Isolating active ingredients in a parent-mediated social communication intervention for toddlers with autism Spectrum disorder. *Journal of Child Psychology and Psychiatry, 57*, 606–613. https://doi.org/10.1111/jcpp.12481

Hampton, L. H., Kaiser, A. P., & Roberts, M. Y. (2017). One-year language outcomes in toddlers with language delays: An RCT follow-up. *Pediatrics, 140*, e20163646. https://doi.org/10.1542/peds.2016-3646

Hancock, T. B., & Kaiser, A. P. (2002). The effects of trainer-implemented enhanced milieu teaching on the social communication of children with autism. *Topics in Early Childhood Special Education, 22*, 39–54. https://doi.org/10.1177/027112140202200104

Hardan, A. Y., Gengoux, G. W., Berquist, K. L., Libove, R. A., Ardel, C. M., Phillips, J., … Minjarez, M. B. (2015). A randomized controlled trial of pivotal response treatment group for parents of children with autism. *Journal of Child Psychology and Psychiatry, 56*, 884–892. https://doi.org/10.1111/jcpp.12354

Harrop, C., Gulsrud, A., Shih, W., Hovsepyan, L., & Kasari, C. (2017). The impact of caregiver-mediated JASPER on child restricted and repetitive behaviors and caregiver responses. *Autism Research, 10*, 983–992. https://doi.org/10.1002/aur.1732

Hart, B., & Risley, T. R. (1978). Promoting productive language through incidental teaching. *Education and Urban Society, 10*, 407–429. https://doi.org/10.1177/001312457801000402

Hart, B., & Rogers-Warren, A. (1978). A milieu approach to teaching language. In R. Schiefelbusch (Ed.), *Language intervention strategies* (pp. 193–235). Baltimore, MD: University Park Press.

Hemmeter, M. L., & Kaiser, A. P. (1994). Enhanced milieu teaching: Effects of parent-implemented language intervention. *Journal of Early Intervention, 18*, 269–289. https://doi.org/10.1177/105381519401800303

Ingersoll, B. R. (2008). The social role of imitation in autism: Implications for the treatment of imitation deficits. *Infants & Young Children, 21*, 107–119. https://doi.org/10.1097/01.IYC.0000314482.24087.14

Ingersoll, B. R. (2010). Brief report: Pilot randomized controlled trial of reciprocal imitation training for teaching elicited and spontaneous imitation to children with autism. *Journal of Autism and Developmental Disorders, 40*, 1154–1160. https://doi.org/10.1007/s10803-010-0966-2

Ingersoll, B. R. (2012). Brief report: Effect of a focused imitation intervention on social functioning in children with autism. *Journal of Autism and Developmental Disorders, 42*, 1768–1773. https://doi.org/10.1007/s10803-011-1423-6

Ingersoll, B. R., & Berger, N. I. (2015). Parent engagement with a telehealth-based parent-mediated intervention program for children with autism Spectrum Disorders: Predictors of program use and parent outcomes. *Journal of Medical Internet Research, 17*(e227), 221–215. https://doi.org/10.2196/jmir.4913

Ingersoll, B. R., & Dvortcsak, A. (2010). *Teaching social communication: A practitioner's guide to parent training for children with autism* (Vol. 12, p. 33). New York, NY: Guilford Press.

Ingersoll, B. R., & Gergans, S. (2007). The effect of a parent-implemented imitation intervention on spontaneous imitation skills in young children with autism. *Research in Developmental Disabilities, 28*, 163–175. https://doi.org/10.1016/j.ridd.2006.02.004

Ingersoll, B. R., Wainer, A. L., Berger, N. I., Pickard, K. E., & Bonter, N. (2016). Comparison of a self-directed and therapist-assisted telehealth parent-mediated intervention for children with ASD: A pilot RCT. *Journal of Autism and Developmental Disorders, 46*, 2275–2284. https://doi.org/10.1007/s10803-016-2755-z

Kaiser, A. P., Hancock, T. B., & Nietfeld, J. P. (2000). The effects of parent-implemented enhanced milieu teaching on the social communication of children who have autism. *Early Education & Development, 11*, 423–446. https://doi.org/10.1207/s15566935eed1104_4

Kaiser, A. P., & Roberts, M. Y. (2013). Parent-implemented enhanced milieu teaching with preschool children who have intellectual disabilities. *Journal of Speech, Language, and Hearing Research, 56*, 295–309. https://doi.org/10.1044/1092-4388(2012/11-0231)

Kasari, C., Freeman, S., & Paparella, T. (2006). Joint attention and symbolic play in young children with autism: A randomized controlled intervention study. *Journal of Child Psychology and Psychiatry, 47*, 611–620. https://doi.org/10.1111/j.1469-7610.2005.01567.x

Kasari, C., Freeman, S., Paparella, T., Wong, C., Kwon, S., & Gulsrud, A. (2005). Early intervention on core deficits in autism. *Clinical Neuropsychiatry, 2*, 380–388.

Kasari, C., Gulsrud, A., Paparella, T., Hellemann, G., & Berry, K. (2015). Randomized comparative efficacy study of parent-mediated interventions for toddlers with autism. *Journal of Consulting and Clinical Psychology, 83*, 554–563. https://doi.org/10.1037/a0039080

Kasari, C., Gulsrud, A. C., Wong, C., Kwon, S., & Locke, J. (2010). Randomized controlled caregiver mediated joint engagement intervention for toddlers with autism. *Journal of Autism and Developmental Disorders, 40*, 1045–1056. https://doi.org/10.1007/s10803-010-0955-5

Kasari, C., Lawton, K., Shih, W., Barker, T. V., Landa, R., Lord, C., … Senturk, D. (2014). Caregiver-mediated intervention for low-resourced preschoolers with autism: An RCT. *Pediatrics, 134*, e72–e79. https://doi.org/10.1542/peds.2013-3229

Kasari, C., Paparella, T., Freeman, S., & Jahromi, L. B. (2008). Language outcome in autism: Randomized comparison of joint attention and play interventions. *Journal of Consulting and Clinical Psychology, 76*, 125–137. https://doi.org/10.1037/0022-006X.76.1.125

Koegel, L. K., Ashbaugh, K., & Koegel, R. L. (2016). Pivotal response treatment. In R. Lang, T. B. Hancock, & N. N. Singh (Eds.), *Early intervention for young children with autism Spectrum disorder* (pp. 85–112). Cham: Springer International Publishing.

Koegel, L. K., Koegel, R. L., Harrower, J. K., & Carter, C. M. (1999). Pivotal response intervention I: Overview of approach. *Journal of the Association for Persons with Severe Handicaps, 24*, 174–185. https://doi.org/10.2511/rpsd.24.3.174

Koegel, R. L., & Koegel, L. K. (2006). *Pivotal response treatments for autism: Communication, social & academic development*. Baltimore, MD: Paul H. Brookes.

Koegel, R. L., O'Dell, M. C., & Koegel, L. K. (1987). A natural language teaching paradigm for nonverbal autistic children. *Journal of Autism and Developmental Disorders, 17*, 187–200. https://doi.org/10.1007/BF01495055

Kuhl, P. K. (2007). Is speech learning 'gated' by the social brain? *Developmental Science, 10*, 110–120. https://doi.org/10.1111/j.1467-7687.2007.00572.x

Kuhl, P. K. (2014). Early language learning and the social brain. *Cold Spring Harbor Symposia on Quantitative Biology, 79*, 211–220.

Kushnir, T., Wellman, H. M., & Gelman, S. A. (2009). A self-agency bias in preschoolers' causal inferences. *Developmental Psychology, 45*, 597–603. https://doi.org/10.1037/a0014727

Landa, R. J. (2016). *IES grant: An efficacy trial of the Early Achievements comprehensive intervention for preschoolers with autism.* Retrieved from https://ies.ed.gov/funding/grantsearch/details.asp?ID=1876.

Landa, R. J., Holman, K. C., O'Neill, A. H., & Stuart, E. A. (2011). Intervention targeting development of socially synchronous engagement in toddlers with autism spectrum disorder: A randomized controlled trial. *Journal of Child Psychology and Psychiatry, 52*, 13–21. https://doi.org/10.1111/j.1469-7610.2010.02288.x

Landa, R. J., & Kalb, L. G. (2012). Long-term outcomes of toddlers with autism Spectrum Disorders exposed to short-term intervention. *Pediatrics, 130*, S186–S190. https://doi.org/10.1542/peds.2012-0900Q

Lawton, K., & Kasari, C. (2012). Teacher-implemented joint attention intervention: Pilot randomized controlled study for preschoolers with autism. *Journal of Consulting and Clinical Psychology, 80*, 687–693. https://doi.org/10.1037/a0028506

Legare, C. H. (2014). The contributions of explanation and exploration to children's scientific reasoning. *Child Development Perspectives, 8*, 101–106. https://doi.org/10.1111/cdep.12070

Mahoney, G., & MacDonald, J. D. (2007). *Autism and developmental delays in young children: The responsive teaching curriculum for parents and professionals*. Austin, TX: PRO-ED.

McGee, G. G. (2005). Incidental teaching. In M. Hersen, G. Sugai, & R. H. Horner (Eds.), *Encyclopedia of behavior modification and cognitive behavior therapy: Educational applications* (Vol. 3, pp. 1359–1362). Thousand Oaks, CA: Sage Publications.

McGee, G. G., Krantz, P. J., Mason, D., & McClannahan, L. E. (1983). A modified incidental-teaching procedure for autistic youth: Acquisition and generalization of receptive object labels. *Journal of Applied Behavior Analysis, 16*, 329–338. https://doi.org/10.1901/jaba.1983.16-329

McGee, G. G., Morrier, M. J., & Daly, T. (1999). An incidental teaching approach to early intervention for toddlers with autism. *Journal of the Association for Persons with Severe Handicaps, 24*, 133–146. https://doi.org/10.2511/rpsd.24.3.133

Mundy, P. (2016). *Autism and joint attention: Development, neuroscience, and clinical fundamentals*. New York, NY: Guilford Publications.

McGee, G. G., & Daly, T. (2007). Incidental teaching of age-appropriate social phrases to children with autism. *Research and Practice for Persons with Severe Disabilities, 32*(2), 112–123.

Neely, L., Rispoli, M., Gerow, S., & Hong, E. R. (2016). Preparing interventionists via telepractice in incidental teaching for children with autism. *Journal of Behavioral Education, 25*, 393–416. https://doi.org/10.1007/s10864-016-9250-7

Nielsen, M. (2006). Copying actions and copying outcomes: Social learning through the second year. *Developmental Psychology, 42*, 555–565. https://doi.org/10.1037/0012-1649.42.3.555

Olive, M. L., de la Cruz, B., Davis, T. N., Chan, J. M., Lang, R. B., O'Reilly, M. F., & Dickson, S. M. (2007). The effects of enhanced milieu teaching and a voice output communication aid on the requesting of three children with autism. *Journal of Autism and Developmental Disorders, 37*, 1505–1513. https://doi.org/10.1007/s10803-006-0243-6

Pickles, A., Le Couteur, A., Leadbitter, K., Salomone, E., Cole-Fletcher, R., Tobin, H., … Aldred, C. (2016). Parent-mediated social communication therapy for young children with autism (PACT): Long-term follow-up of a randomised controlled trial. *The Lancet, 388*(10059), 2501–2509.

Poon, K. K., Watson, L. R., Baranek, G. T., & Poe, M. D. (2012). To what extent do joint attention, imitation, and object play behaviors in infancy predict later communication and intellectual functioning in ASD. *Journal of Autism and Developmental Disorders, 42*, 1064–1074. https://doi.org/10.1007/s10803-011-1349-z

Prizant, B., Wetherby, A., Rubin, E., Laurent, A., & Rydell, P. (2006). *The SCERTS model: A comprehensive educational approach for children with autism spectrum disorders*. Baltimore, MD: Brookes.

Prizant, B. M., & Wetherby, A. M. (1990). Toward an integrated view of early language and communication development and socioemotional development. *Topics in Language Disorders, 10*(4), 1–16.

Roberts, M. Y., & Kaiser, A. P. (2012). Assessing the effects of a parent-implemented language intervention for children with language impairments using empirical benchmarks: A pilot study. *Journal of Speech, Language, and Hearing Research, 55*, 1655–1670. https://doi.org/10.1044/1092-4388(2012/11-0236)

Roberts, M. Y., & Kaiser, A. P. (2015). Early intervention for toddlers with language delays: A randomized controlled trial. *Pediatrics, 135*, 686–693. https://doi.org/10.1542/peds.2014-2134

Rogers, S. J., & Dawson, G. (2010a). Chapter 2: An overview of the early start Denver model. In *Early start Denver model for young children with autism: Promoting language, learning, and engagement* (pp. 14–34). New York, NY: The Guilford Press.

Rogers, S. J., & Dawson, G. (2010b). *Early start Denver model for young children with autism: Promoting language, learning, and engagement*. New York, NY: The Guilford Press.

Rogers, S. J., Dawson, G., & Vismara, L. A. (2012). *An early start for your child with autism: Using everyday activities to help kids connect, communicate, and learn*. New York, NY: Guilford Press.

Rogers, S. J., Estes, A., Lord, C., Munson, J., Rocha, M., Winter, J., … Talbott, M. (2019). A multisite randomized controlled two-phase trial of the early start Denver model compared to treatment as usual. *Journal of the American Academy of Child & Adolescent Psychiatry, 58*(9), 853–865. https://doi.org/10.1016/j.jaac.2019.01.004

Rogers, S. J., Estes, A., Lord, C., Vismara, L., Winter, J., Fitzpatrick, A., … Dawson, G. (2012). Effects of a brief early start Denver model (ESDM)–based parent intervention on toddlers at risk for autism Spectrum Disorders: A randomized controlled trial. *Journal of the American Academy of Child & Adolescent Psychiatry, 51*, 1052–1065. https://doi.org/10.1016/j.jaac.2012.08.003

Rogers, S. J., & Lewis, H. (1989). An effective day treatment model for young children with pervasive developmental disorders. *Journal of the American Academy of Child & Adolescent Psychiatry, 28*, 207–214. https://doi.org/10.1097/00004583-198903000-00010

Rogers, S. J., Lewis, H. C., & Reis, K. (1987). An effective procedure for training early special education teams to implement a model program. *Journal of the Division for Early Childhood, 11*, 180–188. https://doi.org/10.1177/105381518701100210

Rogers, S. J., & Pennington, B. F. (1991). A theoretical approach to the deficits in infantile autism. *Development and Psychopathology, 3*, 137–162. https://doi.org/10.1017/S0954579400000043

Rogers, S. J., Vivanti, G., & Rocha, M. (2017). Helping young children with autism Spectrum disorder develop social ability: The early start Denver model approach. In J. Leaf (Ed.), *Handbook of social skills and autism Spectrum disorder*. Cham: Springer International Publishing.

Sandbank, M., & Yoder, P. (2016). The association between parental mean length of utterance and language outcomes in children with disabilities: A correlational meta-analysis. *American Journal of Speech-Language Pathology, 25*(2), 240–251.

Saylor, M. M., & Ganea, P. A. (2018). *Active learning from infancy to childhood: Social motivation, cognition, and linguistic mechanisms*. New York, NY: Springer International.

Schertz, H. H., Odom, S. L., Baggett, K. M., & Sideris, J. H. (2013). Effects of joint attention mediated learning for toddlers with autism spectrum disorders: An initial randomized controlled study. *Early Childhood Research Quarterly, 28*, 249–258. https://doi.org/10.1016/j.ecresq.2012.06.006

Schreibman, L., Dawson, G., Stahmer, A. C., Landa, R., Rogers, S. J., McGee, G. G., … Halladay, A. (2015). Naturalistic developmental behavioral interventions: Empirically validated treatments for autism Spectrum disorder. *Journal of Autism and Developmental Disorders, 45*, 2411–2428. https://doi.org/10.1007/s10803-015-2407-8

Schreibman, L., Kaneko, W. M., & Koegel, R. L. (1991). Positive affect of parents of autistic children: A comparison across two teaching techniques. *Behavior Therapy, 22*, 479–490. https://doi.org/10.1016/S0005-7894(05)80340-5

Shire, S. Y., Chang, Y. C., Shih, W., Bracaglia, S., Kodjoe, M., & Kasari, C. (2017). Hybrid implementation model of community-partnered early intervention for toddlers with autism: A randomized trial. *Journal of Child Psychology and Psychiatry, 58*, 612–622. https://doi.org/10.1111/jcpp.12672

Shire, S. Y., Gulsrud, A., & Kasari, C. (2016). Increasing responsive parent-child interactions and joint engagement: Comparing the influence of parent-mediated intervention and parent psychoeducation. *Journal of Autism and Developmental Disorders, 46*, 1737–1747. https://doi.org/10.1007/s10803-016-2702-z

Shire, S. Y., Shih, W., Chang, Y.-C., Bracaglia, S., Kodjoe, M., & Kasari, C. (2019). Sustained community implementation of JASPER intervention with toddlers with autism. *Journal of Autism and Developmental Disorders, 49*, 1863–1875. https://doi.org/10.1007/s10803-018-03875-0

Stadnick, N. A., Stahmer, A., & Brookman-Frazee, L. (2015). Preliminary effectiveness of project ImPACT: A parent-mediated intervention for children with autism Spectrum disorder delivered in a community program. *Journal of Autism and Developmental Disorders, 45*, 2092–2104. https://doi.org/10.1007/s10803-015-2376-y

Suhrheinrich, J. (2011). Training teachers to use pivotal response training with children with autism: Coaching as a critical component. *Teacher Education and Special Education, 34*, 339–349. https://doi.org/10.1177/0888406411406553

Suhrheinrich, J., Stahmer, A. C., & Schreibman, L. (2007). A preliminary assessment of teachers' implementation of pivotal response training. *The Journal of Speech and Language Pathology–Applied Behavior Analysis, 2*, 1–13. https://doi.org/10.1037/h0100202

Tager-Flusberg, H., Calkins, S., Nolin, T., Baumberger, T., Anderson, M., & Chadwick-Dias, A. (1990). A longitudinal study of language acquisition in autistic and down syndrome children. *Journal of Autism and Developmental Disorders, 20*, 1–21. https://doi.org/10.1007/BF02206853

Tomasello, M. (2010). *Origins of human communication*. Cambridge, MA: MIT Press.

Tomasello, M. (2019). *Becoming human: A theory of ontogeny*. Cambridge, MA: Belknap Press of Harvard University Press.

Vernon, T. W., Holden, A. N., Barrett, A. C., Bradshaw, J., Ko, J. A., McGarry, E. S., … Disorders, D. (2019). A pilot randomized clinical trial of an enhanced pivotal response treatment approach for young children with Autism: The PRISM model. *Journal of Autism and Developmental Disorders, 49*, 2358–2373. https://doi.org/10.1007/s10803-019-03909-1

Vismara, L. A., McCormick, C. E. B., Wagner, A. L., Monlux, K., Nadhan, A., & Young, G. S. (2018). Telehealth parent training in the early start Denver model: Results from a randomized controlled study. *Focus on Autism and Other Developmental Disabilities, 33*, 67–79. https://doi.org/10.1177/1088357616651064

Vivanti, G. (2019). Towards a culturally informed approach to implementing autism early intervention. *Pediatric Medicine, 2*, 20. https://doi.org/10.21037/pm.2019.06.0

Vivanti, G., Dissanayake, C., Duncan, E., Feary, J., Capes, K., Upson, S., … Victorian ASELCC Team. (2019). Outcomes of children receiving Group-Early Start Denver Model in an inclusive versus autism-specific setting: A pilot randomized controlled trial. *Autism, 23*(5), 1165–1175. https://doi.org/10.1177/1362361318801341

Vivanti, G., Duncan, E., Dawson, G., & Rogers, S. J. (2017). *Implementing the group-based early start Denver model for preschoolers with autism*. Cham: Springer International Publishing.

Vivanti, G., & Hamilton, A. (2014). Imitation in autism spectrum disorders. In F. Volkmar, R. Paul, S. Rogers, & K. Pelphrey (Eds.), *The handbook of autism and developmental Disorders, 4th edition, Vol 1—Diagnosis, development and brain mechanisms* (pp. 278–301). New York, NY: Wiley.

Vivanti, G., Kasari, C., Green, J., Mandell, D., Maye, M., & Hudry, K. (2018). Implementing and evaluating early intervention for children with autism: Where are the gaps and what should we do?. *Autism Research, 11*(1), 16–23. https://doi.org/10.1002/aur.1900

Vivanti, G., Paynter, J., Duncan, E., Fothergill, H., Dissanayake, C., Rogers, S. J., & Victorian ASELCC Team. (2014). Effectiveness and feasibility of the early start Denver model implemented in a group-based community childcare setting. *Journal of Autism and Developmental Disorders, 44*, 3140–3153. https://doi.org/10.1007/s10803-014-2168-9

Vygotsky, L. (1930–1934/1978). *Mind in society: The development of higher psychological processes* (A. R. Luria, M. Lopez-Morillas & M. Cole [with J. V. Wertsch], Trans.) Cambridge, Mass.: Harvard University Press.

Verschuur, R., Didden, R., Lang, R., Sigafoos, J., & Huskens, B. (2014). Pivotal response treatment for children with autism spectrum disorders: A systematic review. *Review Journal of Autism and Developmental Disorders, 1*(1), 34–61.

Walton, K. M., & Ingersoll, B. R. (2012). Evaluation of a sibling-mediated imitation intervention for young children with autism. *Journal of Positive Behavior Interventions, 14*, 241–253. https://doi.org/10.1177/1098300712437044

Watson, L. R., Crais, E. R., Baranek, G. T., Turner-Brown, L., Sideris, J., Wakeford, L., … Nowell, S. W. (2017). Parent-mediated intervention for one-year-olds screened as at-risk for autism Spectrum disorder: A randomized controlled trial. *Journal of Autism and Developmental Disorders, 47*, 3520–3540. https://doi.org/10.1007/s10803-017-3268-0

Wetherby, A. M., Guthrie, W., Woods, J., Schatschneider, C., Holland, R. D., Morgan, L., & Lord, C. (2014). Parent-implemented social intervention for toddlers with autism: An RCT. *Pediatrics, 134*, 1084–1093. https://doi.org/10.1542/peds.2014-0757

Wetherby, A. M., & Prutting, C. A. (1984). Profiles of communicative and cognitive-social abilities in autistic children. *Journal of Speech, Language, and Hearing Research, 27*(3), 364–377.

Wetherby, A. M., Woods, J., Guthrie, W., Delehanty, A., Brown, J. A., Morgan, L., … Lord, C. (2018). Changing developmental trajectories of toddlers with autism Spectrum disorder: Strategies for bridging research to community practice. *Journal of Speech, Language, and Hearing Research, 61*, 2615–2628. https://doi.org/10.1044/2018_JSLHR-L-RSAUT-18-0028

Wetherby, A. M., & Woods, J. J. (2006). Early social interaction project for children with autism Spectrum Disorders beginning in the second year of life: A preliminary study. *Topics in Early Childhood Special Education, 26*, 67–82. https://doi.org/10.1177/02711214060260020201

Whalen, C., Schreibman, L., & Ingersoll, B. (2006). The collateral effects of joint attention training on social initiations, positive affect, imitation, and spontaneous speech for young children with autism. *Journal of Autism and Developmental Disorders, 36*, 655–664. https://doi.org/10.1007/s10803-006-0108-z

Wong, C. S. (2013). A play and joint attention intervention for teachers of young children with autism: A randomized controlled pilot study. *Autism, 17*, 340–357. https://doi.org/10.1177/1362361312474723

Zhou, B., Xu, Q., Li, H., Zhang, Y., Wang, Y., Rogers, S. J., & Xu, X. (2018). Effects of parent-implemented early start Denver model intervention on Chinese toddlers with autism Spectrum disorder: A non-randomized controlled trial. *Autism Research, 11*, 654–666. https://doi.org/10.1002/aur.1917

Chapter 7
The TEACCH Approach and Other Visually Based Approaches for Children with Autism

Lauren Turner-Brown and Kara Hume

Introduction

The TEACCH approach as well as other visually based approaches to early intervention for children with ASD considers that the child with ASD has strengths and weaknesses, and that using areas of strength, such as understanding visual information, may help when teaching skills in an area of weakness. For example, Picture Exchange Communication System (PECS; Bondy & Frost, 1998) teaches children to exchange a picture that represents a word with an adult to communicate when that child is not able to verbally express what he or she wants. Below, we review the TEACCH approach for young children as well as other visual approaches used in ASD early intervention.

The TEACCH Approach

The TEACCH Autism Program started studying autism and developing approaches for teaching individuals with ASD in the late 1960s. Structured TEACCHing was the broad approach developed based on research of Dr. Eric Schopler to accomplish two primary goals: (1) to teach a child as many independent skills and routines as possible and (2) to modify the environment to make it more meaningful for a child. Principles that contribute to this approach include understanding the "culture" of

L. Turner-Brown (✉)
UNC TEACCH Autism Program, The University of North Carolina School of Medicine, Chapel Hill, NC, USA
e-mail: ltb@laurenturnerbrownphd.com

K. Hume
School of Education, The University of North Carolina at Chapel Hill, Chapel Hill, NC, USA

G. Vivanti et al. (eds.), *Clinical Guide to Early Interventions for Children with Autism*, Best Practices in Child and Adolescent Behavioral Health Care,
https://doi.org/10.1007/978-3-030-41160-2_7

autism, or the way the individual with ASD sees and interprets his or her world, understanding individual needs of the child, using visual strategies to support learning, and using special interests or talents to promote engagement (Mesibov, Shea, & Schopler, 2005). When this approach was first developed, children with ASD were diagnosed at older ages; thus more recent work has addressed how to apply these principles and Structured TEACCHing strategies to younger children (Ozonoff & Cathcart, 1998; Turner-Brown, Hume, Boyd, & Kainz, 2019; Welterlin, 2009), and, most recently in a manualized parent coaching manual called Family Implemented TEACCH for Toddlers (FITT; Hume, Turner-Brown, & Boyd, 2013). A description of how Structured TEACCHing for young children with ASD and their families follows along with examples of structure that can be used to support the development of receptive and expressive communication, play, and social skills.

Structured TEACCHing Goals for Young Children

To understand Structured TEACCHing with young children, we first review the goals of the approach followed by the specific strategies employed. A primary *goal* of Structured TEACCHing has always been teaching children and older learners with ASD as many independent skills as possible. Independence has proven to be a key skill for optimal outcomes in adulthood. However, for children as young as 12–18 months, independence is not typically a skill area named by caregivers and professionals as a priority. While many young children wish to assert their independence during this period and caregivers can support this desire when possible, toddlerhood is mostly a time to emphasize and build learning and relationships. Thus, the primary goal for Structured TEACCHing when used with young children is to support engagement (Turner-Brown et al., 2019), defined as *being actively and productively involved in activity.*

Structured TEACCHing with young children supports engagement with: (1) people, especially caregivers and family members, to support the development of communication and social interaction skills; (2) toys/objects, to support the development of play skills, which creates opportunities for social interaction and supports many types of learning; and (3) toys/objects and people together, to support the development of "*coordinated or joint attention*," which is the child's ability to share attention between the caregiver and some other object or event in the immediate location.

A second goal of Structured TEACCHing with young children involves modifying the environment to make it understandable and meaningful for the individual with ASD. This goal is identical to goals for older learners. Modifying the environment often entails adding visual cues and supports to help answer six questions that often lead young children with ASD to be confused or frustrated:

1. Where am I supposed to be?
2. What am I supposed to do?

3. How should I do it?
4. How long will I do this or how many should I do?
5. How will I know that I am making progress and when I am finished?
6. What will happen next?

The use of visuals is particularly important with young children, both with and without ASD, because young children are not developmentally ready to process abstract or complicated verbal ideas. Important ideas such as time (e.g., how long activities will last, what it means if we are "leaving in 5 min"), sequencing (such as what activities come "before" and "after"), and sharing (such as offering or giving a toy to others) are abstract. When teaching these concepts to young children with ASD, concrete and visual cues such as an object or picture represent the abstract idea.

Structured TEACCHing Components

Using Structured TEACCHing with young children with ASD and their families requires incorporating common principles of early intervention. First, partnering with caregivers is a key when providing intervention to young children. This is central to the TEACCH philosophy (see Drs. Schopler and Reichler's (1971) then groundbreaking notion of "parents as co-therapists.") Next, it is important to provide services and offer supports in natural environments. These include families' homes, early care and education programs, and other community settings where young children spend the most time. Last, it is essential that skills are taught through participating in everyday activities and routines. Teaching caregivers how to use Structured TEACCHing strategies across daily routines, such as bath time, play time, and meal time, allows the child to have opportunities for intervention every day, throughout the day, without requiring daily visits from an interventionist, specialized equipment, or travel to a medical or clinical setting. The four components or types of structure used with young children and their families are discussed below.

Physical Organization of the Environment

The first component of Structured TEACCHing is physical organization of the environment. An organized environment with carefully arranged intervention spaces may support children who become distracted easily or have difficulty in processing information. Organizing the physical environment also supports active engagement.

There are two primary strategies for physically organizing the home environment to maximize engagement. The first is to use physical and visual boundaries to better define space and expectations for young children. Clarifying spaces in the home helps young children better understand what activities will occur in each different area in the home (e.g., this is where we eat, this is where you play, this is where you get dressed). These boundaries are not meant to contain a child rather to serve as a concrete reminder of where to be and what the expectations are in each space. The FITT manualized approach coaches parents to establish two areas for different types of play with young children—an area for *table-based play* (e.g., puzzles, ring stackers, shape sorters, paints, or markers) and an area for *floor-based play* (such as balls, trucks and cars, bubbles). The table-based play area serves as a location to introduce new play activities or teach new skills. A designated location for teaching new skills helps in creating positive routines around learning, which helps young children accept new activities and materials. Other spaces are created based on what routines or skill areas caregivers would most like to target. For example, if caregivers identify sitting at the table during dinner as a priority skill to target, then creating a physically organized space at the table would be recommended. Similarly, if caregivers would like support during bath time, bedtime, book time, or potty time, those spaces would be organized to help clarify expectations.

The second step is to determine where the spaces should be established and what physical and visual boundaries may be needed to help the child better understand the space. This process involves parent–therapist brainstorming to determine what is necessary. Consider Ryan, a 2-year-old with ASD who always stops when he walks past the entertainment center to stare at his reflection. Parents might consider a physical boundary in his play area that prevents him from walking past this reflective glass during play time. Or, consider Jane, whose older siblings often watch TV in the afternoons in a family room. Jane's parents might choose to set up an area in a different room to play with her because distractions are fewer. See below for examples of physically organized spaces (Fig. 7.1).

Physical and visual boundaries can be used in other areas of the home to clarify spaces and expectations. For example, if a family would like the child to sit at the table during meal time rather than run out of the room, caregivers may choose to

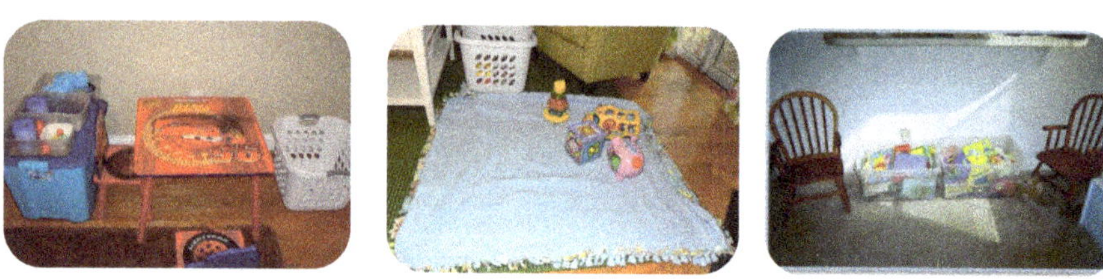

Table based play area.

A parent or therapist sits against the wall. The child sits in his chair and sees the activities he will do to his left. He completes the activities at the table, then places them in a finished basket to the right.

Floor based play area.

A blanket and toys provide visual cues to the child to let her know where she will play with her caregiver.

Book area.

Books are at eye level and accessible with a carpet area for reading

Fig. 7.1 Physical organization of the home

tuck the child's seat closest to the wall rather than out in the middle of the kitchen. The wall may serve as physical boundary reminding the child of the expectation to stay at the table.

A second strategy of physical organization is to minimize distractions. Limiting distractions encourages the child to increase attention to the other person and play materials rather than attending to other sights and sounds in the environment. This could involve limiting the number of toys visible or available to young children when playing together. For example, while a father and his son are building with blocks, covering, or putting away other play materials, such as balls or trucks, may increase the child's attention to the blocks. Minimizing distractions may also include turning off screens (such as computers, tablets, smart phones, televisions) for periods of the day in the home, using visual boundaries such as shelves, or placing covers over items that are not currently in use.

Schedules

The second major component of Structured TEACCHing is the use of a schedule. Providing visual information for children about where to go and when to go there is an important strategy for supporting the child's understanding of communication and expectations. Visual information can attract and hold a child's attention, provide a concrete form of representation of important ideas, and support strengths in visual processing. Schedules also support children with limited receptive language skills.

There are several considerations for using schedules with young children with ASD. First, young children are not likely able to understand a schedule that uses abstract representations such as line drawings, words, or even photographs. The most appropriate schedule form for young children is the use of objects—either functional objects that will be used in the scheduled activity, such as a sippy cup to use at meal time, or representational objects that represent where the child is going, such as a set of toy keys that represents transitioning to the car.

Next, young children are not ready to process long sequences of schedule information; instead, they best understand one piece of information at a time. This information is communicated through a transition object—a concrete way to show the child where he is going next. Each activity or location is represented by a specific object. For example, if a child has difficulty transitioning to the changing table during diaper changes, caregivers may select a diaper as a transition object. When it is time to transition for a diaper change the caregiver will give the diaper to the child and say, "Time for diaper change" and help the child get to the correct location. In time, with the consistent use of transition objects, young children will learn what the transition object means, and transition difficulties will decrease as understanding improves.

Sample Transition Objects

- *Favorite bath toy or washcloth*: Bath
- *Diaper*: Diaper change/Bathroom
- *Puzzle piece*: Table-based play
- *Toothbrush*: Brushing teeth
- *Favorite toy*: Floor-based play
- *Book*: Reading time/book area
- *Placemat*: Mealtime
- *Pillow/stuffed animal*: Bedtime
- *Special toy or CD*: Going for a ride in the car
- *DVD case*: TV time
- *Sand shovel*: Going out to the playground
- *Soap container*: Washing hands

For some young children, a very short sequence of two objects or photos, called a "*first/then schedule*" may be used to help them understand when a favorite activity is going to return. For example, if a child has difficulty transitioning away from a favorite DVD to come play on the floor with a caregiver, two objects may be presented. First, the transition object used for floor-play is presented and next to it is the DVD cover, indicating that first the child will play, and then he can return to the DVD (Fig. 7.2).

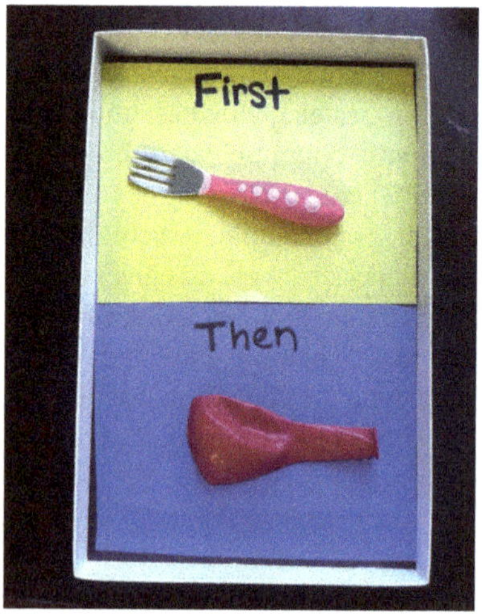

Fig. 7.2 First-then object schedule. This schedule shows the child what is coming first and next. First, he will eat lunch, then he will play balloons with his mom

Activity Systems

The third component of Structured TEACCHing is an activity system. An activity system helps children better understand what to do once they arrive at a designated space or location, such as the table-based play space or the bathroom. The activity system shows the child what activities will be completed, how long the activities will take, how he will know that the activities are finished, and what will happen next. These systems are sometimes termed "*work systems*" (Hume, Plavnick, & Odom, 2012), but "*activity systems*" were coined when the approach was used with young children to reduce the connotation that children were "working" and emphasize the wide range of activities that could benefit from this organizational system.

Activity systems are used during table-based play routine by placing the activities that the caregiver and child will do together on the child's left and a "*finished*" basket on the child's right (a left-to-right activity system, see image 1 above). The finished basket is a designated location where children put their activities when they are finished with them. Caregivers and interventionists teach the system to the child by emphasizing that activities are taken from the child's left, completed together at the table, then put in the finished basket on the right. This allows the child to see how many activities will be completed and what the activities are. Also, they can see that activities are finished when they are in the finished basket. Children also learn that a transition object after the structured activities will direct them to the "what's next" activity, typically playing on the floor or moving to a caregiver-selected routine like snack or outside play.

Activity systems are also used during other routines in the home, to support engagement in daily routines such as dressing, tooth brushing, and taking a bath. For example, a 3-year-old boy, Louis, with ASD cries every day when his mother tries to get him dressed. An activity system would clarify for Louis what he is supposed to do, how long it will last, how he knows he is finished, and what activity is coming next. Specifically, laying the clothes out in a left-to-right fashion allows Louis to see how many steps are required, and as each piece of clothing is put on, he can see that progress is being made. A transition object such as a favorite book at the end of the line of clothes helps Ryan know what preferred activity is coming next (Fig. 7.3).

Visually Structuring Activities and Cues

Finally, the last component of Structured TEACCHing is visually structuring activities and cues. With older children, this component often entails making "tasks" that promote independence. For young children, the focus is on using visual structure to support learning across developmental domains (e.g., early learning, imitation, play, etc.). Activities typically have a clear beginning and end, include a sensory component like preferred sounds or textures, are highly motiving, and build on the child's strengths.

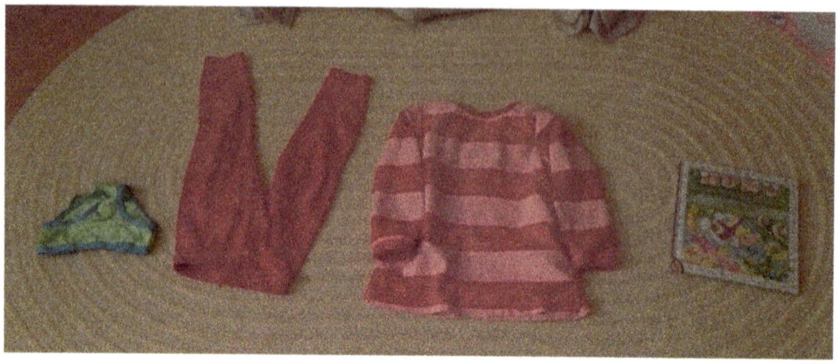

Fig. 7.3 Daily routine activity system. Organizing each item of clothing provides visual cues to a child about how much she needs to do, and what she will do when she finishes getting dressed

These activities incorporate elements of visual instructions, visual organization, and visual clarity. See images below for examples of these elements of visual structure.

Visual instructions such as a series of photos may be used to teach a multistep play activity. For example, when teaching a child with ASD a play routine with a baby doll, interventionists or caregivers may take a series of photos of activities to do with a doll (such as put baby in tub, wash baby, dry baby). Single photos may also be used to provide support for young children as they are learning functional and symbolic play routines (e.g., a farm animal completes an action, such as the pig jumps, the horse sleeps).

Visually organizing the activities can include stabilizing them on a tray, providing containers for extra parts and pieces, and reducing the number of parts and pieces.

Visual clarity of toys and activities means providing cues or highlighting within a play activity to emphasize its most important parts and pieces.

In addition to these principles, activities often *incorporate the child's interests*, a key Structured TEACCHing principle. Adapting play materials to incorporate individual interests can be an important first step to help young children with ASD to engage with new materials or play in new ways. For example, if a child does not typically engage with Duplos®/Legos® but is interested in characters from Sesame Street®, adding pictures of favorite characters to the blocks can increase his interest and motivation to learn to play with them (Fig. 7.4).

Blending Structured TEACCHing with Other Approaches

To summarize, therapists and parents use structure to develop table, floor, and daily living routines that promote active engagement in the child with ASD. Visual approaches support the child's understanding of these routines and his ability to transition between activities. Next, therapists and parents develop goals that target areas of development most affected by ASD. Imitation skills are an example of skills taught in Family Implemented TEACCH for Toddlers (Hume et al., 2013;

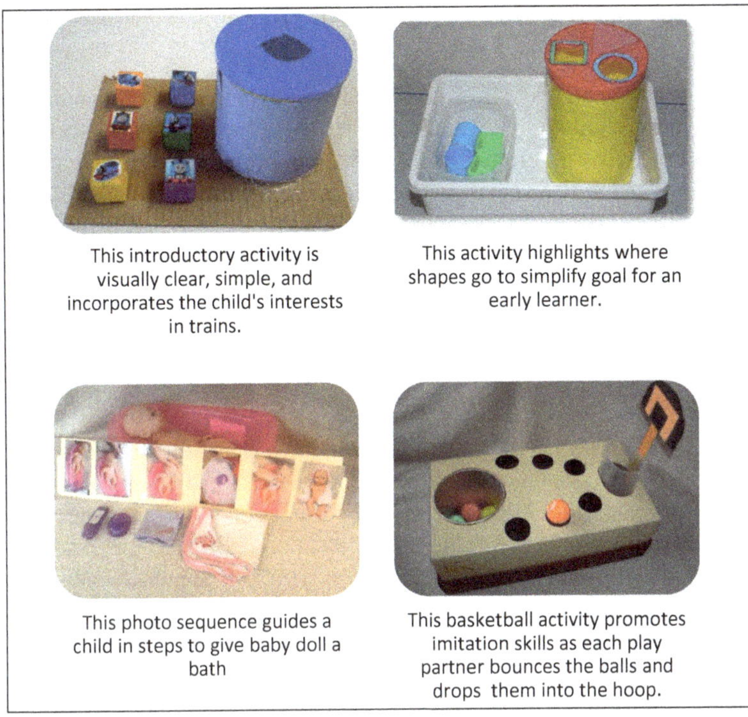

Fig. 7.4 Visually structured activities

Turner-Brown et al., 2019). Therapists and parents begin by conducting informal assessments to determine what interests the child, where she might show emerging skills. Treatment goals can develop from this assessment and may be targeted using highly structured activities if necessary but will also incorporate naturalistic activities and strategies, such as Reciprocal Imitation Training (Ingersoll, 2010) to ensure skills generalize beyond a structured activity.

TEACCH Summary

Providing support for young children with ASD and their families is crucial because children are receiving diagnoses at younger ages, and effective early intervention is proven to improve developmental outcomes. Structured TEACCHing principles and the four elements of structure, adapted to be developmentally appropriate for young children, can serve as important tools for teaching a number of skill areas, including coordinated attention, expressive communication, and play skills. By specifically partnering with parents in natural environments and applying Structured TEACCHing strategies to daily routines, this intervention model ensures that the goal of engagement is supported throughout the child's day.

Other Visual and Augmentative Approaches

Visual and/or augmentative approaches can be quite helpful in teaching communication to young children with ASD. Rather than focus only on speech, these approaches emphasize the importance of directing communication in a variety of forms to others and utilize visual cues or electronically generated sounds to support the child. Three examples of these approaches are PECS, speech-generating devices, and video modeling.

Picture Exchange Communication System

PECS (Bondy & Frost, 1998) is one approach that has proven effective in teaching children a range of communication skills (see Wong et al., 2015, for a review). This approach is designed for children with limited functional communication skills to initiation as well as back and forth communication. PECS is one example of an alternative and augmentative communication system. The approach entails teaching a child to give a partner a picture of an item in exchange for the actual item. For example, if a child wants to play with a toy train, he would give the communicative partner a picture of a train, and the partner would then give the child the actual train. PECS uses behavioral strategies to build the exchange skill and expand upon the vocabulary and length of communication. Research has shown improvements in communication and social skills in young children who learn this approach (Carr & Felce, 2007; Dogoe, Banda, & Lock, 2010; Jurgens, Anderson, & Moore, 2009) as well as to older learners (see Wong et al., 2015, for a review).

Speech-Generating Devices

Speech-generating devices include a range of devices that speak electronically when a child pressed a button. At a simple form, there may be one button to push to request "more," and the device speaks "more." In a more complex form, the child could press three picture buttons or icons that represent more, bubbles, and please, and the device would speak that phrase. Studies have shown that the use of speech generated devices promotes spontaneous language in minimally verbal children with ASD when paired with a naturalistic developmental behavioral approach (Almirall et al., 2016; Kasari et al., 2014). Use of these devices can also promote peer interactions in preschool aged children (Thiemann-Bourque, Feldmiller, Hoffman, & Johner, 2018).

Video Modeling

Another visual approach that can lead to gains in communication, social, play, and daily living skills is video modeling. In this approach, individuals are presented with videos that demonstrate skills or behaviors being taught. For example, a child might watch a video of children taking turns appropriately to learn how to take turns with his peers. Or, a parent might watch a video of how he plays with his son and get feedback or tips about ways to engage his child in more complex ways (e.g., video self-modeling). In an early intervention context, video modeling can improve play skills (e.g., Dueñas, Plavnick, & Bak, 2019; Hine & Wolery, 2006). In these studies, young children watch videos of children playing and then show increases in varied play with peers in their school setting. With older children and even adults, video modeling can lead to changes in a range of skills and behavior, including conversations, self-help, and parenting (see Wong et al., 2015, and Hong et al., 2016, for a review).

Summary

In summary, the TEACCH approach as well as other augmentative communication approaches can support young children with ASD by supporting areas of relative weakness, such as understanding language or using speech. It is promising that these approaches can be used with other approaches to support children and families.

References

Almirall, D., DiStefano, C., Chang, Y.-C., Shire, S., Kaiser, A., Lu, X., … Kasari, C. (2016). Longitudinal effects of adaptive interventions with a speech-generating device in minimally verbal children with ASD. *Journal of Clinical Child & Adolescent Psychology, 45*(4), 442–456. https://doi.org/10.1080/15374416.2016.1138407

Bondy, A., & Frost, L. (1998). The picture exchange communication system. *Seminars in Speech and Language, 19*(04), 373–389. https://doi.org/10.1055/s-2008-1064055

Carr, D., & Felce, J. (2007). The effects of PECS teaching to Hase III on the communicative interactions between children with autism and their teachers. *Journal of Autism and Developmental Disorders, 37*(4), 724–737.

Dogoe, M. S., Banda, D. R., & Lock, R. H. (2010). Acquisition and generalization of the picture exchange communication system behaviors across settings, persons, and stimulus classes with three students with autism. *Education and Training in Autism and Developmental Disabilities, 45*(2), 216–229.

Dueñas, A. D., Plavnick, J. B., & Bak, M. Y. S. (2019). Effects of joint video modeling on unscripted play behavior of children with autism spectrum disorder. *Journal of Autism and Developmental Disorders, 49*(1), 236–247. https://doi.org/10.1007/s10803-018-3719-2

Hine, J. F., & Wolery, M. (2006). Using point-of-view video modeling to teach play to preschoolers with autism. *Topics in Early Childhood Special Education, 26*(2), 83–93. https://doi.org/10.1177/02711214060260020301

Hong, E. R., Ganz, J. B., Mason, R., Morin, K., Davis, J. L., Ninci, J., … Gilliland, W. D. (2016). The effects of video modeling in teaching functional living skills to persons with ASD: A meta-analysis of single-case studies. *Research in Developmental Disabilities, 57*, 158–169. https://doi.org/10.1016/j.ridd.2016.07.001

Hume, K., Plavnick, J., & Odom, S. L. (2012). Promoting task accuracy and independence in students with autism across educational setting through the use of individual work systems. *Journal of Autism and Developmental Disorders, 42*(10), 2084–2099. https://doi.org/10.1007/s10803-012-1457-4

Hume, K., Turner-Brown, L., & Boyd, B. A. (2013). *Family implemented TEACCH for toddlers.*

Ingersoll, B. (2010). Brief report: Pilot randomized controlled trial of reciprocal imitation training for teaching elicited and spontaneous imitation to children with autism. *Journal of Autism and Developmental Disorders, 40*(9), 1154–1160. https://doi.org/10.1007/s10803-010-0966-2

Jurgens, A., Anderson, A., & Moore, D. W. (2009). The effect of teaching PECTS to a child with autism on verbal behaviour, play, and social fuctioning. *Behavior Change, 26*(1), 66.

Kasari, C., Kaiser, A., Goods, K., Nietfeld, J., Mathy, P., Landa, R., … Almirall, D. (2014). Communication interventions for minimally verbal children with autism: a sequential multiple assignment randomized trial. *Journal of the American Academy of Child & Adolescent Psychiatry, 53*(6), 635–646. https://doi.org/10.1016/j.jaac.2014.01.019

Mesibov, G. B., Shea, V., & Schopler, E. (2005). *The TEACCH approach to autism spectrum disorders.* Retrieved from https://www.worldcat.org/title/teacch-approach-to-autism-spectrum-disorders/oclc/55634429.

Ozonoff, S., & Cathcart, K. (1998). Effectiveness of a home program intervention for young children with autism. *Journal of Autism and Developmental Disorders, 28*(1), 25–32. Retrieved from http://www.ncbi.nlm.nih.gov/pubmed/9546299

Schopler, E., & Reichler, R. J. (1971). Parents as cotherapists in the treatment of psychotic children. *Journal of Autism and Childhood Schizophrenia, 1*(1), 87–102. https://doi.org/10.1007/BF01537746

Thiemann-Bourque, K., Feldmiller, S., Hoffman, L., & Johner, S. (2018). Incorporating a peer-mediated approach into speech-generating device intervention: effects on communication of preschoolers with autism spectrum disorder. *Journal of Speech, Language, and Hearing Research, 61*(8), 2045–2061. https://doi.org/10.1044/2018_JSLHR-L-17-0424

Turner-Brown, L., Hume, K., Boyd, B. A., & Kainz, K. (2019). Preliminary efficacy of family implemented TEACCH for toddlers: Effects on parents and their toddlers with autism spectrum disorder. *Journal of Autism and Developmental Disorders, 49*(7), 2685–2698. https://doi.org/10.1007/s10803-016-2812-7

Welterlin, A. (2009). *The Home TEACCHing Program: A study of the efficacy of a parent training early intervention model.* Retrieved from https://rucore.libraries.rutgers.edu/rutgers-lib/26147/.

Wong, C., Odom, S. L., Hume, K. A., Cox, A. W., Fettig, A., Kucharczyk, S., … Schultz, T. R. (2015). Evidence-based practices for children, youth, and young adults with autism spectrum disorder: A comprehensive review. *Journal of Autism and Developmental Disorders, 45*(7), 1951–1966. https://doi.org/10.1007/s10803-014-2351-z

Chapter 8
Choosing the "Right" Program for Each Child in Autism Early Intervention

Giacomo Vivanti and Pamela Paragas

In the previous chapters, we have described a plethora of early intervention approaches and techniques that have at least some evidence suggesting benefits for children with ASD. Being able to choose among different interventions is, in principle, desirable, given the heterogeneity of learning strengths and needs in children with ASD. Nevertheless, families and professionals are faced with many challenges when navigating treatment options, including (a) selecting the "right" intervention for the particular child, as different children with ASD have different needs, and might respond differently to different interventions and (b) selecting the right intervention provider in the community, given that the same intervention can be implemented differently by different providers.

Selecting the Right Intervention

Even when guidance is given to discern between evidence-supported and unsupported interventions, the issue of which intervention should be chosen for an individual child remains a dilemma for families and professionals alike. Will this particular child benefit more from receiving EIBI, JASPER, or ESDM? These interventions, like the other evidence-supported approaches described in the previous chapters, have been shown to "work" at the group level (i.e., when comparing the average progress of a group of children receiving the intervention versus a comparison group), but outcomes vary from child to child. For example, research has suggested that improvements following EIBI are very rapid for approximately 20–30% of children, very slow for 10–20% of children, and in between the two extremes for

G. Vivanti (✉) · P. Paragas
AJ Drexel Autism Institute, Drexel University, Philadelphia, PA, USA
e-mail: gv89@drexel.edu

G. Vivanti et al. (eds.), *Clinical Guide to Early Interventions for Children with Autism*, Best Practices in Child and Adolescent Behavioral Health Care,
https://doi.org/10.1007/978-3-030-41160-2_8

most children (Eldevik et al., 2010; Smith et al., 2015). Similar variability is documented following NDBI approaches (Tiede & Walton, 2019) and delivery of "non-branded" early intervention services in the community (Noyes-Grosser et al., 2018).

This does not mean necessarily that some children are just "fast learners" and others "slow learners"—rather, intervention outcomes are shaped by the interplay between child and intervention characteristics. Although all evidence-supported interventions include procedures to individualize the treatment program to the learning profile of each child, they differ across a number of key treatment strategies (e.g., emphasis on verbal versus visually conveyed instructions, child-lead vs. adult-directed models) and objectives (e.g., focus on cognitive vs. social skills). As children with ASD vary in their learning strengths, needs, and preferences, and different intervention approaches vary in their teaching procedures, outcomes will be optimal when the right fit is identified between the child's learning profile and treatment teaching techniques. For example, it is plausible that a child who seems to learn best in response to visually presented information (e.g., pictures) and has difficulties with changes in routine might benefit an intervention that uses picture-based schedules showing the sequence of activities that will occur during her or his day.

Family priorities, beliefs, and needs are also an important consideration when selecting interventions. Different approaches use instructional techniques (e.g., play-based vs. structured adult-directed teaching) that may fit differently with a family's educational style and cultural values about educating children. Similarly, different parent coaching formats might be more or less compatible with the caregivers' learning style and availability (e.g., small groups sessions vs. 1:1 supervision in which the parent is asked to implement educational strategies and receives live feedback).

Nevertheless, establishing the best fit between child/family features and the teaching procedures involved in different approaches is not easy, given the complexity of child and family learning styles, preferences and needs, the limited knowledge on "what works for whom" in ASD early intervention, and the variability in intervention options across contexts. Currently, research suggests that the specific intervention approach that children with ASD receive in the community depends mostly on the geographical proximity to a specific provider and the theoretical orientation of that provider rather than consideration of child or family characteristics (Green, 2007; Hebert, 2014).

However, research efforts in this area are increasing, providing insight on the factors that can be considered when selecting among different intervention options (Stahmer, Schreibman, & Cunningham, 2011; Vivanti et al., 2014). For example, there is initial evidence that pivotal response training (PRT) might be particularly beneficial for children who engage more with toys, approach people more often, and show positive affect more frequently (Fossum et al., 2018; Koegel et al., 1999; Sherer & Schreibman, 2005; Schreibman, Stahmer, Barlett, & Dufek, 2009). This profile was found to predict response to PRT but not DTT (Schreibman, Stahmer, Barlett, & Dufek, 2009). Vivanti et al. (2013) also found that engagement with toys, together with imitation and response to joint attention (but not social attention), predicted positive response to the Early Start Denver Model. Conversely, Yoder and

Stone (2006) reported that children who engaged more with objects responded better to an intervention based on PECS (see Chap. 7) compared to a naturalistic intervention, while children who were less interested in objects had better outcomes in response to a naturalistic intervention compared to the PECS intervention. Additional research found that children showing low interest in objects benefitted most from the "Hanen More Than Words" intervention, a parent-mediated naturalistic approach focused on language (Carter et al., 2011). Finally, larger gains in response to DTT and EIBI have been documented in children who are more socially engaged and responsive to social reinforcers such as praise (Klintwall & Eikeseth, 2012; Klintwall et al., 2015; Smith et al., 2015).

These findings provide an initial indication of interventions that can be particularly beneficial for children with specific profiles as well as skills that should be targeted in order for children to benefit optimally from specific approaches. However, the evidence base is too preliminary to make conclusive recommendations on the intervention a particular child should receive in order to achieve optimal outcomes. Methodological complexities include variability in the outcome measures used to characterize children's learning profiles and define intervention response and, for most studies, lack of comparison groups that allow for a determination of whether children who are not optimally responsive to one intervention will benefit more from an alternative intervention. For example, low scores in IQ, language, and adaptive and social functioning predict poorer response across different early interventions. However, as poor performance on standardized tests can reflect a variety of factors, including difficulties in test-taking skills (e.g., understanding verbal instructions, compliance, attention to relevant features of the task), it is important to identify the specific barriers and strengths that make children more or less amenable to benefit from different interventions. For example, rather than concluding that a child will be a "poor responder" to an early intervention model because she or he has a low IQ score, it is helpful to identify and target the constraint responsible for the low performance in the IQ test (e.g., difficulties engaging in tasks mediated by verbal instructions) to ensure the child is "equipped" for learning in response to early intervention models that require this prerequisite. Importantly, however, targeting "readiness" skills should not result in children missing the opportunity to participate in high-quality interventions that provide rich learning opportunities. Rather, therapists should calibrate instruction to the child's current level of ability/understanding while at the same time working toward moving to the next level. For example, for a child who has low performance in IQ testing due to difficulties with understanding verbal instructions, it might be helpful to use augmentative alternative communication strategies (see Chap. 7) to facilitate learning across multiple goals and domains while also targeting toward language understanding.

In the absence of a conclusive evidence-base on "what works for whom," several scholars have suggested clinical guidelines on matching children to interventions based on the theoretical fit between child and family factors and what different interventions are designed to achieve. For example, Siegel (1999) suggested that approaches based on DTT are best suited for children who are not motivated by novelty, social reward, or peer affiliation and have difficulties learning "incidentally" from nonstructured interactions. Additionally, according to the same author, TEACCH would best serve children who need a high degree of predictability, and whose primary difficulty is in comprehending and expressing verbal and nonverbal communication, but learn best in response to visually mediated information. Finally, Siegel suggests that developmental approaches are best suited for children who engage more frequently in self-initiated actions and are more motivated by novelty and social interaction. In other words, approaches that emphasize "following the child's lead" might be best for children who offer many leads to follow, particularly in the social domain, while those relying on a high degree of repetition and structure might be ideal for children with a preference for predictability and struggle with novelty and unstructured situations. Similarly, preference for verbal versus visual instruction and social versus nonsocial reinforcers can inform assignment to more versus less naturalistic approaches.

While most children with ASD will show a constellation of deficits and preferences across these different dimensions rather than a "clean" profile of preference for visual versus verbal instruction, response to social versus nonsocial reinforcers and motivation for predictability versus novelty, consideration of these features can help practitioners decide which approach may be most suited for them. As mentioned earlier, it is important for all children with ASD to receive interventions that are both tailored to their existing strengths and provide opportunities to grow in areas of relative weakness, so that catering to specific learning preferences (e.g., using images to communicate) does not deprive children from the opportunity to gain expertise in multiple modalities and domains.

Additionally, regardless of any a priori reasoning on what approach works best for the child, treatment progress in response to the selected intervention should be consistently monitored and intervention strategies should be changed if data indicate that the teaching program is not facilitating child learning. Slow learning rate in a child receiving evidence-based intervention does not mean that the child cannot learn or that the intervention is ineffective for all children—rather, it means that the selected teaching strategies, despite the theoretical fit for the child, do not meet the child's learning needs and preferences. In this case, it is imperative to take action and introduce new evidence-based approaches that differ from what has been tried already rather than persist indefinitely on the basis of the clinician's philosophical adherence to a specific model.

Selecting the Right Provider

Once a decision is made on which intervention seems to be the best fit for the child's learning needs and strengths, another complex challenge is choosing the right provider for that intervention. While information on the effectiveness of interventions is based on the results of carefully conducted clinical trials, families typically access interventions through services available in their community. The range of services available to young children varies considerably across contexts (see Chap. 10 for more information on this topic), and many of the intervention approaches described in the previous chapters are not widespread across communities.

Additionally, community implementation of interventions is highly variable and can substantially deviate from the manualized procedures and fidelity criteria used in clinical trials (Stahmer et al., 2005). This, in turn, comes with the risk of diminished effectiveness (Nahmias et al., 2019). Further, community providers often pick and choose intervention strategies from a variety of approaches, including both evidence-based and unsupported interventions, rather than adhering to one specific intervention package (Drahota, Aarons, & Stahmer, 2012). Although flexibility and drawing from various sources of knowledge might appear preferable than adhesion to a single approach, unsystematic deviations from a protocol and mixing strategies (including unsupported ones) come with the risk of "diluting" intervention effectiveness (Vivanti, 2017).

Therefore, when choosing among different interventions in the community, one should consider not only the scientific evidence for the "brand name" intervention offered by the provider (e.g., EIBI, ESDM, or JASPER) but also the degree to which such intervention is delivered as intended. As implementing intervention models with high fidelity requires understanding of the evidence base, extensive training, and appropriate resources, important criteria to guide choice of the intervention provider are whether (a) all the intervention practices offered by the provider are supported by scientific evidence (see Chap. 2 for details on criteria used to established whether intervention are evidence-supported); (b) staff delivering the intervention has received formal training/certification in the intervention they offer; (c) intervention fidelity (i.e., the degree to which intervention is delivered as intended, or at least maintains the aspects of the intervention thought to be most important) is systematically monitored; (d) resources are available to accomplish the intervention goals (e.g., availability of typically developing children for an ABA program targeting social skills or whether a parent coaching intervention is offered after work hours, thus allowing working caregivers to participate in the program).

Additionally, when providers offer an eclectic model that combines different practices, it is important that a clearly defined plan exists on the specific goals targeted by the different practices (Kasari & Smith, 2013). For example, an evidence-based parent coaching program focused on management of disruptive behavior might be combined with therapist-delivered implementation of an alternative augmentative communication system to target functional communication. In this case, the combination of these different interventions, if implemented at fidelity by trained clinicians, might result in a complementary effect (as the two approaches address different areas of need) or even a synergistic one (improvements in child communication increase the success of the behavioral management intervention). However, the combination of strategies can be problematic when inconsistent procedures are used to target the same goal—for example, if disruptive behaviors are at times addressed through planned ignoring and other times through removing a token from the child's token board (see Chaps. 5, 6, and 8 for details on these strategies). In these cases, strategies might work against one another, and exposure to inconsistent responses and teaching methods can be detrimental to child learning.

Conclusions

In summary, identifying intervention programs that are optimally tailored to the specific child and family needs does not rely on an exact science but requires the appreciation of the child's learning needs (including barriers originating from co-occurring difficulties that are not part of the core deficits of ASD, such as deficits in motor skill, difficulties with eating or sleeping behaviors) and resources that might help children respond to the teaching style and goals offered by the intervention. This, in turn, requires a fine-grained knowledge of what the child needs to learn (which will inform treatment objectives), how the child learns best (which will inform treatment strategies), what the family's goals and resources are, and fine-grained understanding of what interventions are designed to achieve and how and what they require on the child and family's part. Additionally, regardless of the theoretical reasoning for recommending a specific approach, professionals need to maintain an open-minded and data-driven attitude and change intervention strategies when data show limited intervention progress. Finally, it is important to appreciate that the same intervention approach can be implemented differently by different providers. Therefore, factors such as the intervention provider's level of training, fidelity of implementation, and consistency of intervention procedures should be considered when choosing among treatment options. Finally, there are several intervention strategies and goals that cut across models and are critically important for the success of the intervention being delivered regardless of the specific approach. These are discussed in detail in the following chapter.

References

Carter, A. S., Messinger, D. S., Stone, W. L., Celimli, S., Nahmias, A. S., & Yoder, P. (2011). A randomized controlled trial of Hanen's 'More Than Words' in toddlers with early autism symptoms. *Journal of Child Psychology and Psychiatry, 52*(7), 741–752.

Drahota, A., Aarons, G. A., & Stahmer, A. C. (2012). Developing the autism model of implementation for autism spectrum disorder community providers: Study protocol. *Implementation Science, 7*(1), 85.

Eldevik, S., Hastings, R. P., Hughes, J. C., Jahr, E., Eikeseth, S., & Cross, S. (2010). Using participant data to extend the evidence base for intensive behavioral intervention for children with autism. *American Journal on Intellectual and Developmental Disabilities, 115*(5), 381–405.

Fossum, K. L., Williams, L., Garon, N., Bryson, S. E., & Smith, I. M. (2018). Pivotal response treatment for preschoolers with autism spectrum disorder: Defining a predictor profile. *Autism Research, 11*(1), 153–165.

Green, V. A. (2007). Parental experience with treatments for autism. *Journal of Developmental and Physical Disabilities, 19*(2), 91–101.

Hebert, E. B. (2014). Factors affecting parental decision-making regarding interventions for their child with autism. *Focus on Autism and Other Developmental Disabilities, 29*(2), 111–124.

Kasari, C., & Smith, T. (2013). Interventions in schools for children with autism spectrum disorder: Methods and recommendations. *Autism, 17*(3), 254–267.

Klintwall, L., & Eikeseth, S. (2012). Number and controllability of reinforcers as predictors of individual outcome for children with autism receiving early and intensive behavioral intervention: A preliminary study. *Research in Autism Spectrum Disorders, 6*(1), 493–499.

Klintwall, L., Macari, S., Eikeseth, S., & Chawarska, K. (2015). Interest level in 2-year-olds with autism spectrum disorder predicts rate of verbal, nonverbal, and adaptive skill acquisition. *Autism, 19*(8), 925–933.

Koegel, L. K., Koegel, R. L., Shoshan, Y., & McNerney, E. (1999). Pivotal response intervention II: Preliminary long-term outcome data. *Journal of the Association for Persons with Severe Handicaps, 24*(3), 186–198.

Nahmias, A. S., Pellecchia, M., Stahmer, A. C., & Mandell, D. S. (2019). Effectiveness of community-based early intervention for children with autism spectrum disorder: a meta-analysis. *Journal of Child Psychology and Psychiatry, 60*(11), 1200–1209.

Noyes-Grosser, D. M., Elbaum, B., Wu, Y., Siegenthaler, K. M., Cavalari, R. S., Gillis, J. M., & Romanczyk, R. G. (2018). Early intervention outcomes for toddlers with autism spectrum disorder and their families. *Infants & Young Children, 31*(3), 177–199.

Schreibman, L., Stahmer, A. C., Barlett, V. C., & Dufek, S. (2009). Brief report: Toward refinement of a predictive behavioral profile for treatment outcome in children with autism. *Research in Autism Spectrum Disorders, 3*(1), 163–172.

Sherer, M. R., & Schreibman, L. (2005). Individual behavioral profiles and predictors of treatment effectiveness for children with autism. *Journal of Consulting and Clinical Psychology, 73*(3), 525.

Siegel, B. (1999). Autistic learning disabilities and individualizing treatment for autistic spectrum disorders. *Infants & Young Children, 12*(2), 27–36.

Smith, T., Klorman, R., & Mruzek, D. W. (2015). Predicting outcome of community-based early intensive behavioral intervention for children with autism. *Journal of Abnormal Child Psychology, 43*(7), 1271–1282.

Stahmer, A. C., Schreibman, L., & Cunningham, A. B. (2011). Toward a technology of treatment individualization for young children with autism spectrum disorders. *Brain Research, 1380*, 229–239.

Stahmer, A. C., Collings, N. M., & Palinkas, L. A. (2005). Early intervention practices for children with autism: Descriptions from community providers. *Focus on Autism and Other Developmental Disabilities, 20*(2), 66–79.

Tiede, G., & Walton, K. M. (2019). Meta-analysis of naturalistic developmental behavioral interventions for young children with autism spectrum disorder. *Autism, 23*(8), 2080–2095.

Vivanti, G., Prior, M., Williams, K., & Dissanayake, C. (2014). Predictors of outcomes in autism early intervention: Why don't we know more? *Frontiers in Pediatrics, 2*, 58.

Vivanti, G. (2017). Individualizing and combining treatments in autism spectrum disorder: four elements for a theory-driven research agenda. *Current Directions in Psychological Science, 26*(2), 114–119.

Vivanti, G., Dissanayake, C., Zierhut, C., Rogers, S. J., & Victorian ASELCC Team. (2013). Brief report: Predictors of outcomes in the Early Start Denver Model delivered in a group setting. *Journal of Autism and Developmental Disorders, 43*(7), 1717–1724.

Yoder, P., & Stone, W. L. (2006). A randomized comparison of the effect of two prelinguistic communication interventions on the acquisition of spoken communication in preschoolers with ASD. *Journal of Speech, Language, and Hearing Research, 49*(4), 698–711.

Chapter 9
Beyond Monolithic Packages: Important Strategies Across Early Interventions for Children with Autism

Kristen Bottema-Beutel and Shannon Crowley

Promoting Active Child Engagement

As described in Chaps. 3 and 6, children's development can be supported by engagement with caregivers and other social partners. In these interactions, caregivers scaffold increasingly complex forms of social interaction often in the context of play activities (Bakeman & Adamson, 1984; Bruner, 1982). Developmental theory has long suggested that the mechanism by which caregiver–child play and other forms of social engagement has beneficial impacts on development involves children's active role in shaping and sometimes leading the interactions and activities in which they are engaged (Piaget & Inhelder, 1971). This principle also applies to development in children with ASD. As such, active child engagement is the premise of many early interventions, especially those targeting social communication development (e.g., Kasari et al., 2015).

To ensure that children with ASD are actively engaged within intervention contexts, interactions with interventionists or caregivers should be characterized by shared control, mutual regulation, and creativity. This can mean that adults do things such as follow the child's lead during toy play activities (imitate the child's actions on toys, or take on a play persona parallel to the child's selected persona), verbally expand on the child's spontaneous interactional overtures (following a child point by saying, "yes, I see the duck!"), and engage in creative word play using onomatopoeic sounds to draw the child into the interaction (playfully animating the duck and saying "quack quack quack!" in a back and forth exchange). Intervention research has also shown that "responsive" practices such as mirrored pacing (imitating the children's actions shortly after the child has produced them) and communicative

K. Bottema-Beutel (✉) · S. Crowley
Lynch School of Education and Human Development, Boston College, Chestnut Hill, MA, USA
e-mail: botteabe@bc.edu

G. Vivanti et al. (eds.), *Clinical Guide to Early Interventions for Children with Autism*, Best Practices in Child and Adolescent Behavioral Health Care,
https://doi.org/10.1007/978-3-030-41160-2_9

synchrony (communicating about what the child is doing) are linked to children's gains in language (Green & Garg, 2018). Further, the intervention context itself should incorporate preferred materials and child interests into activities (Gulsrud et al., 2016; Schreibman et al., 2015). Capitalizing on the child's interests will maximize children's motivation to communicate with caregivers about materials in the environment, enact complex play schemes during play, and actively participate during daily activities.

Importantly, although interventionists and caregivers may have explicit goals in mind when scaffolding engagement with children with ASD, the specific details of how the interaction is to proceed should not be entirely defined in advance or expected to strictly conform to a "correct" standard. Interactions that are overly constraining in terms of children's expected modes of participation can lead to passive participation, suppress active engagement, or can even be met with resistance which will ultimately undermine children's display of interactional competence (Sterponi & Fasulo, 2010).

Caregiver Coaching

Many early interventions that were originally developed in clinics with trained professionals acting as interventionists have now been adapted so that they can be implemented by caregivers in the child's home; these are referred to as parent-mediated interventions. Nevill, Lecavalier, and Stratis (2016) recently conducted a meta-analysis of these interventions and showed positive albeit modest effects on overall symptoms associated with ASD, socialization, communication, and cognition. A benefit of caregivers acting as interventionists is that, at least theoretically, intervention strategies can be used much more frequently and fused into family routines (more on this in the next section). In order for caregivers to effectively carry out intervention procedures, they must be adequately coached by professionals who have expertise in intervention techniques. This type of training is usually referred to as caregiver coaching and is now an emerging area within early intervention research. Much of the caregiver coaching research has focused on NDBI or developmental interventions (see Chap. 6) that focus on caregiver–child interactive routines as the primary intervention context (e.g., Green et al., 2010; Kasari et al., 2015). As such, one of the primary areas of focus for caregiver coaching is maximizing caregiver responsivity to children's interactional overtures.

Caregiver coaching can be delivered in a variety of modalities, such as in-person or via video conferencing or other online technologies (see Sutherland, Trembath, & Roberts, 2018), and in a variety of instructional formats, including 1:1 or small group sessions. Most coaching models involve some amount of instruction on intervention strategies, multiple opportunities for the caregiver to practice using the strategies with the child, and feedback on the quality of caregiver's implementation of each strategy. The "dose" of caregiver training can also vary considerably with sessions lasting 30 min to 3 h and occurring weekly to monthly over several months.

Many parent-mediated intervention programs emphasize that similar to young children who are the ultimate receivers of the intervention caregivers must have an active role in the coaching process to effectively learn to implement intervention strategies (Wetherby et al., 2018). This means that caregivers are involved in setting appropriate child goals, specifying how general intervention procedures will be adapted to the individual child, characterizing their own responsivity to children's overtures, and identifying children's responses to the intervention procedures (Nevill et al., 2016). In a randomized controlled trial, Shire, Gulsrud, and Kasari (2016) demonstrated that an intervention actively engaging parents in ways to be more responsive interaction partners produced superior outcomes to a didactic teaching approach that focused on similar content (see also Rogers et al., 2019).

Incorporate Interaction Strategies into Everyday Routines

As caregivers learn interaction strategies that accommodate their child's cognitive, communicative, and sensory profiles, these strategies can be incorporated into everyday routines and activities that already, or could potentially, involve the child (Landa & Sharpless, 2018; Rogers et al., 2019). For example, caregivers might expand on children's initiations during meal and snack times, imitate children's actions on toys during play routines at home, or incorporate visual supports into bathing, dressing, or clean-up routines.

There are several advantages to leveraging the child's everyday environment to support children's development as compared to exclusively relying on intervention sessions in clinical or other decontextualized settings. First, when caregivers are able to adapt everyday routines to be more accommodating to their children with ASD, it improves the child's ability to access and participate in routines that have cultural and familial significance. Second, as mentioned in Chap. 6, clinical environments can be overly stripped down (i.e., exclude any stimuli thought to be superfluous to learning) and can utilize stimuli that do not change in quality from session to session. This can make it difficult for children to generalize what they have learned in clinical settings to settings that are more relevant to the child's life, such as the home (Schreibman et al., 2015). Third, everyday routines by definition occur with high frequency and are repeated across days and weeks, giving children many more learning opportunities than can be provided in clinic visits. At least theoretically, more learning opportunities will translate to greater developmental gains.

While initial research into interventions that include a strong home component has shown some promise (e.g., Green et al., 2010; Kasari et al., 2015), there is a caveat to recruiting caregivers as interventionists. Doing so can lead to situations where caregivers are made to feel that *all* interactions with the child should serve a therapeutic role, requiring caregivers to exclusively function as therapists (with children always positioned in the role of pupil). To avoid this outcome, special effort should be made by intervention providers so that the strategies caregivers are encouraged to use are culturally relevant, acceptable to the family, and easily integrated into the caregivers' natural interaction styles and daily routines (Vivanti, 2019).

Thoughtful Environmental Arrangements

Interventionists and caregivers can arrange the physical intervention and home environment in a thoughtful way that accommodates the cognitive and sensory profiles of the child. The TEACCH approach, described in detail in Chap. 7, is based on a set of instructional strategies and systematic arrangements of the environment that account for the individualized needs and preferences of children with ASD (Mesibov & Shea, 2010). Although this approach is typically used in classroom settings, the visual support strategies and environmental arrangements can be adapted for early intervention contexts. In particular, these supports can foster meaningful interactions between the child and adult, help children more independently engage in important tasks, and have better access to their environment (Welterlin, Turner-Brown, Harris, Mesibov, & Delmolino, 2012).

Arrangements to Support Sensory Differences

Some individuals with ASD are reported to have differences in their perception of and response to sensory information. Interventionists and caregivers should be mindful about the child's' sensory processing patterns and adapt the physical organization of the setting to accommodate their individual sensory profiles (Ganz, 2007). Children who display a hyporesponsiveness to sensory stimuli are less likely to process sensory information from the environment and could benefit from more intensive stimulation in intervention settings and within the home. Using brightly colored materials, playing music, or promoting physical activity can help children become actively engage with others (Dunn, 2007).

On the other hand, children who are hyperresponsive to sensory stimuli can be more easily distractible and sensitive to sensory information from the environment. Interventionists can cover windows or have the children sit with their backs to doors and windows to accommodate visual sensitivity (Mesibov & Shea, 2010). In addition, caregivers could plan for more quiet time throughout the day if children can become overstimulated by noise and physical activity.

Supporting Transitions

The restricted and repetitive behaviors or interests that are characteristic of ASD can include an insistence on sameness or inflexible adherence to routines (American Psychiatric Association, 2013; Chap. 4). These features can make it difficult for children to transition between activities OR cope with unexpected changes in their schedule. However, the implementation of multimodal supports such as text, visual cues, and oral language can be used to convey expectations and serve as reminders regarding the child's schedule of activities (Sterling-Turner & Jordan, 2007). For example, a timer can be used for the child to visualize how much time is left in a particular play activity, and visual schedules comprised of picture cards arranged in a sequence can be implemented to help children anticipate future activities (D'Elia et al., 2014).

Balancing Between Structure and Novelty

Young children with ASD often show a preference for sameness in their environment, activity schedules, and interactional routines with others (APA, 2013). Intervention programs may seek to accommodate this preference by maintaining a uniform physical arrangement of the intervention space, providing similar materials such as the same set of toys from session to session, engaging in consistently ordered intervention activities, and encouraging interventionists to use similar interaction styles tailored to individual children's preferences. Providing such structure can be critical for ensuring that children are comfortable with intervention routines (especially for children who may become dysregulated with unexpected schedule changes or sensory stimulation). However, maintaining too much structure can result in overdependence on sameness that can prevent the child from learning new skills, generalizing the skills they have learned to contexts outside the intervention, or developing an ability to be flexible.

To mitigate this concern, intervention programs should promote a balance between providing structural adaptations that maintain the child's emotional regulation while also introducing novelty that will encourage growth and development. This can be both at a "macro" level, such as changing the sequence of intervention activities or providing new sets of toys in addition to more familiar toys or the "micro" level such as expanding on the child's existing play and language routines to introduce new elements (Chang et al., 2016).

Developmental Sequencing of Intervention Goals

Interventions that are able to influence children's growth beyond what is directly taught in the intervention tend to focus on goals that are developmentally sequenced (Yoder et al., 2013). Appropriate goals are initially selected to reflect the child's cognitive, social, and communication profile (see Chaps. 3 and 6), which should be established using assessment procedures that have been validated for developmental domain. Vygotsky's concept of the "Zone of Proximal Development" (ZPD; Vygotsky, 1930–1934/1978) is helpful for determining appropriate starting points for intervention (see Chaps. 1 and 6). The ZPD is defined as competencies just beyond what the child can do independently but can achieve with support (often provided by the interventionist, or some other more competent social partner). Once these goals are achieved, new goals are then set that reflect progression through a cascading developmental trajectory where subsequent milestones build on previously achieved milestones. Descriptions of developmental trajectories are usually based on research conducted on typical child populations but can also include deviations from typical paths that commonly occur in ASD populations (Rogers, 2006).

While this approach is promising for facilitating children's long-term growth, there are two potential barriers to implementing developmental strategies within interventions for children with ASD. First, developmental pathways are better described in some domains as compared to others. For example, much is known about the development of social communication in both child development, more generally, and in children with ASD, in particular (see Chap. 3 for a description of this trajectory). On the other hand, there is less consensus on the developmental origins or pathways of processes with the RRB domain (see Chap. 4) in children with ASD (Poljac, Hoofs, Princen, & Poljac, 2017; Rogers & Ozonoff, 2005). This means that for some domains of development, there is an insufficient understanding of how developmental milestones build on one another to appropriately sequence intervention goals using this framework.

Second, there is some evidence that children with ASD do not always follow (or need to follow) a typically developing sequence for some domains, and there is significant variation within the ASD population in terms of developmental trajectories (Lord, Bishop, & Anderson, 2015). While there is evidence that interventions can be implemented that support children with ASD in achieving social communicative milestones that follow a typical child trajectory (Wetherby et al., 2018), there is also some evidence that "environmental demands" can guide intervention targets in many cases with less emphasis on developmental pathways (Bottema-Beutel et al., 2014). That is, interventionists can consider the types of new skills or competencies that will aid the child in better accessing their environment, regardless of a known developmental progression of these skills. This is especially the case when developmental sequences are not well defined.

Data Collection to Guide Goal Selection and Inform Decision Making

All early intervention programs for children with ASD should involve some means of collecting and analyzing data on child progress to ensure that the intervention is working as intended. Specific data collection procedures will vary depending on the nature of the intervention and the targeted developmental domain or child behavior. Some intervention traditions, such as EIBI (see Chap. 5), have highly developed methods for operationalizing and measuring target behavior and for making intervention decisions based on collected data. These interventions typically use observational procedures to assess children's current behavioral profiles as well as the environmental variables that influence the child's behavior. Once the intervention has been implemented, these methods are also used to determine if there are decreases or increases in the level, trend, or variability of the occurrence of a specific behavior or set of behaviors to determine whether or not an intervention was successful.

Other traditions, especially those that do not target discrete behaviors, may take a more eclectic approach to data collection. Informal and formal observations, interviews, standardized assessments, and document reviews may be used to determine children's developmental levels across a variety of domains, and developmentally appropriate goals are then selected. Similar procedures may be used to monitor intervention progress although it is important that a specific protocol is established to consistently measure the phenomena of interest before, during, and after intervention implementation to monitor children's development. Similar to behavioral approaches, developmental interventions should attend to the absolute value indicated by measurement procedures (e.g., a child's standardized score on an assessment of social functioning to determine whether the child is at the expected level given their age) as well as growth rates to determine if progress is being made at a sufficient pace.

During and after the implementation of an intervention, formative and summative assessments are also used to determine if intervention procedures should be modified or discarded and replaced by entirely new interventions to better meet children's needs. Decision making should use data collected from a variety of stakeholders in addition to direct observation of the child with attention paid to the feasibility of implementing the intervention as well as its effects on the child. Finally, it is important to measure intervention *fidelity*, that is, the extent to which the intervention was implemented as planned (see Chap. 8). This is usually done by observing the intervention in progress by someone other than the interventionist. If the intervention did not follow prespecified procedures or was not administered in the correct "dosage" or level of intensity, this should be addressed before a determination is made about the adequacy of the planned intervention.

Providing Meaningful, Natural Reinforcement

A critical component of behavioral interventions is the provision of reinforcement. As described in Chap. 5, reinforcement is any stimulus following a child behavior that increases the probability that the child will produce the behavior again in the future (Skinner, 1963). Originally, extrinsic reinforcers that were unrelated to the behavior the child produced, such as treats or stickers, were the primary means of reinforcement (Lovaas, 1987). However, interrupting social routines by providing external rewards unrelated to the activity may result in overdependence on the reinforcement, disruption of the activity flow, and an inability to generalize newly learned skills to contexts that do not involve reinforcement.

Instead, caregivers or interventionists should aim to naturalistically embed reinforcement that the child perceives as internally motivating into social activities (Schreibman et al., 2015). For example, if a caregiver and child are engaged in a play routine and the child spontaneously requests a doll, the adult should help the child retrieve the doll as a means to reinforce the child's request for help. In addition to responding to the child's request, the caregiver should be socially attentive to the child, which will reinforce joint engagement more generally (Rogers, 2013). In contrast to external reinforcement, naturally embedded reinforcement is contextually meaningful. When activities provide opportunities to engage in interactions that are inherently reinforcing, this provides a context for the child to understand the social-interactive functions of their behavior and develop agency in shaping joint engagement routines. However, external reinforcement should be considered when children show limited learning in response to intrinsic reinforcement, and failure to learn a new behavior/refrain from a current behavior pose an immediate danger to the child (e.g., if a child is being encouraged to wear protective clothing or sunscreen during outdoor time on a sunny day). Some interventions (e.g., Rogers & Dawson, 2010) include a decision tree to guide selection of reinforcers based on intervention progress, following a hierarchy from more intrinsic to more external reinforcers.

Task Analysis to Teach Functional Skills

Many EIBI strategies for young children with ASD involve the adult explicitly providing the child with instructions on how to accurately produce a new behavior. To teach more complex skills, it may be necessary to use task analysis, a procedure in which skills are broken down into simpler components or steps. Learning complex skills in smaller components that systematically build on one another, as opposed to learning skills in a single step, can be less overwhelming for the child and can ultimately improve skills acquisition.

When task analysis procedures are developed, a few key ideas should be kept in mind. First, steps can be represented using photographs or other pictorial systems for children who are not yet reading text or able to identify sight words (see Chap. 7). This will provide the child with visual reminders of how to complete each step (Eldevik, Hastings, Jahr, & Hughes, 2012). Second, task analyses are often paired with prompt hierarchies to cue the child to complete each step and reinforcement systems to shape the child's correct execution of task components. Prompt hierarchies often proceed with a "least to most" progression, beginning with gestures (e.g., pointing at the tooth brush holder to remind the child to retrieve the tooth brush) and ending with hand-over-hand assistance (e.g., guiding the child's hand to grasp the tooth brush). This ensures that the child receives just enough but not too much support in completing the task (Gulsrud et al., 2016). Finally, task analyses are most effective for teaching functional skills that can be sensibly broken down into discrete steps, such as bathing, dressing, brushing teeth. For some domains, particularly those involving social engagement, breaking processes down into discrete components changes the meaning of the social experience. For example, teaching the child to rotely memorize a social script can result in interactions that appear ritualized and stilted and bear little resemblance to naturally occurring interactions that are dynamic and fluid (Bottema-Beutel, Park, & Kim, 2018).

Fading Intervention Supports Over Time

Prior to the implementation of an intervention, plans should be made to systematically fade interventionist or caregiver provision of supports where possible. This can include decreasing the amount, intensity, or adult control over several different types of supports, including environmental supports (e.g., allowing the child to organize and initiate the use of visual schedules and sensory accommodations), reinforcement (providing longer intervals between reinforcements, especially extrinsic reinforcement not related to a given activity), and scaffolding provided by caregivers during engagement routines (e.g., allowing the child to retrieve and arrange activity materials, waiting for the child to initiate turn-taking routines).

Gradually fading supports over the course of early intervention is important for several reasons. First, failure to do so can result in overreliance on adult-provided support, which can unnecessarily limit children's independence (Hume, Loftin, & Lantz, 2009). This also means that children may have difficulty transitioning between early intervention and K–12 education, a context where children are expected to be more independent. Finally, fading caregiver scaffolding during joint engagement routines can allow the child greater agency and control of the interaction with less reliance on the caregiver to initiate and maintain interactions. This will prepare the child for eventually engaging with same-age peers, who may be less apt to provide scaffolding during joint engagement.

Conclusion

To date, there are a variety of early intervention strategies that appear to be associated with positive adaptive and/or developmental outcomes for children with ASD. High-quality interventions may use some or all of the strategies described in this chapter, which are then individualized to meet the unique needs of children and families. Intervention strategies should also be selected and adapted according to the social and cultural context as well as the specific environment in which the intervention is to be implemented.

References

American Psychiatric Association. (2013). Diagnostic and statistical manual or mental disorders. In *Diagnostic and Statistical Manual of Mental Disorders, 5th Edition*.

Bakeman, R., & Adamson, L. B. (1984). Coordinating attention to people and objects in mother-infant and peer-infant interaction. *Child Development, 55*(4), 1278–1289.

Bottema-Beutel, K., Park, H., & Kim, S. Y. (2018). Commentary on social skills training curricula for individuals with ASD: Social interaction, authenticity, and stigma. *Journal of Autism and Developmental Disorders, 48*(3), 953–964.

Bottema-Beutel, K., Yoder, P., Woynoroski, T., & Sandbank, M. (2014). Targeted intervention for social-communication symptoms in preschoolers. In F. R. Volkmar, R. Paul, S. J. Rogers, & K. A. Pelphrey (Eds.), *Handbook of autism and pervasive developmental disorders*. Hoboken, NJ: Wiley & Sons.

Bruner, J. (1982). The organization of action and the nature of the adult-infant transaction. In E. Tronick (Ed.), *Social interchange in infancy: Affect, cognition, and communication*. Baltimore: University Park Press.

Chang, Y. C., Shire, S. Y., Shih, W., Gelfand, C., & Kasari, C. (2016). Preschool deployment of evidence-based social communication intervention: JASPER in the classroom. *Journal of Autism and Developmental Disorders, 46*(6), 2211–2223.

D'Elia, L., Valeri, G., Sonnino, F., Fontana, I., Mammone, A., & Vicari, S. (2014). A longitudinal study of the TEACCH program in different settings: The potential benefits of low intensity intervention in preschool children with autism spectrum disorder. *Journal of Autism and Developmental Disorders, 44*(3), 615–626.

Dunn, W. (2007). Supporting children to participate successfully in everyday life by using sensory processing knowledge. *Infants and Young Children, 20*(2), 84–101.

Eldevik, S., Hastings, R. P., Jahr, E., & Hughes, J. C. (2012). Outcomes of behavioral intervention for children with autism in mainstream pre-school settings. *Journal of Autism and Developmental Disorders, 42*(2), 210–220.

Ganz, J. B. (2007). Classroom structuring methods and strategies for children. *Exceptionality, 15*(4), 249–260.

Green, J., Charman, T., McConachie, H., Aldred, C., Slonims, V., Howlin, P., … Barrett, B. (2010). Parent-mediated communication-focused treatment in children with autism (PACT): A randomised controlled trial. *The Lancet, 375*(9732), 2152–2160.

Green, J., & Garg, S. (2018). Annual research review: The state of autism intervention science: Progress, target psychological and biological mechanisms and future prospects. *Journal of Child Psychology and Psychiatry, 59*(4), 424–443.

Gulsrud, A. C., Hellemann, G., Shire, S., & Kasari, C. (2016). Isolating active ingredients in a parent-mediated social communication intervention for toddlers with autism spectrum disorder. *Journal of Child Psychology and Psychiatry, 57*(5), 606–613.

Hume, K., Loftin, R., & Lantz, J. (2009). Increasing independence in autism spectrum disorders: A review of three focused interventions. *Journal of Autism and Developmental Disorders, 39*(9), 1329–1338.

Kasari, C., Gulsrud, A., Paparella, T., Hellemann, G., & Berry, K. (2015). Randomized comparative efficacy study of parent-mediated interventions for toddlers with autism. *Journal of Consulting and Clinical Psychology, 83*(3), 554–563.

Landa, R. J., & Sharpless, J. P. (2018). Caregiver-mediated intervention and the achievements for little learners model. In *Handbook of parent-implemented interventions for very young children with autism* (pp. 339–356). Cham: Springer.

Lord, C., Bishop, S., & Anderson, D. (2015). Developmental trajectories as autism phenotypes. *American Journal of Medical Genetics Part C: Seminars in Medical Genetics, 169*(2), 198–208.

Lovaas, O. I. (1987). Behavioral treatment and normal educational and intellectual functioning in young autistic children. *Journal of Consulting and Clinical Psychology, 55*(1), 3–9.

Mesibov, G. B., & Shea, V. (2010). The TEACCH program in the era of evidence-based practice. *Journal of Autism and Developmental Disorders, 40*, 570–579.

Nevill, R. E., Lecavalier, L., & Stratis, E. A. (2016). Meta-analysis of parent-mediated interventions for children with autism spectrum disorder. *Autism, 22*(2), 84–98.

Piaget, J., & Inhelder, B. (1971). *Psychology of the child*. New York: Basic Books.

Poljac, E., Hoofs, V., Princen, M. M., & Poljac, E. (2017). Understanding behavioural rigidity in autism spectrum conditions: The role of intentional control. *Journal of Autism and Developmental Disorders, 47*(3), 714–727.

Rogers, S. J. (2006). Evidence-based interventions for language development in young children with autism. In T. Charman & W. Stone (Eds.), *Social and communication development in autism spectrum disorders* (pp. 143–179). New York, NY: The Guilford Press.

Rogers, S. J. (2013). Early start Denver model. In F. R. Volkmar (Ed.), *Encyclopedia of autism spectrum disorders*. New York, NY: Springer.

Rogers, S. J., Estes, A., Vismara, L., Munson, J., Zierhut, C., Greenson, J., ... Whelan, F. (2019). Enhancing low-intensity coaching in parent implemented Early Start Denver Model intervention for early autism: A randomized comparison treatment trial. *Journal of Autism and Developmental Disorders, 49*(2), 632–646.

Rogers, S. J., & Ozonoff, S. (2005). Annotation: What do we know about sensory dysfunction in autism? A critical review of the empirical evidence. *Journal of Child Psychology and Psychiatry, 46*(12), 1255–1268.

Rogers, S. J., & Dawson, G. (2010). *Early Start Denver Model for young children with autism: Promoting language, learning, and engagement.* Guilford Press.

Schreibman, L., Dawson, G., Stahmer, A. C., Landa, R., Rogers, S. J., McGee, G. G., ... McNerney, E. (2015). Naturalistic developmental behavioral interventions: Empirically validated treatments for autism spectrum disorder. *Journal of Autism and Developmental Disorders, 45*(8), 2411–2428.

Shire, S. Y., Gulsrud, A., & Kasari, C. (2016). Increasing responsive parent-child interactions and joint engagement: Comparing the influence of parent-mediated intervention and parent psychoeducation. *Journal of Autism and Developmental Disorders, 46*(5), 1737–1747.

Skinner, B. F. (1963). Operant behavior. *American Psychologist, 18*(8), 503–515.

Sterling-Turner, H. E., & Jordan, S. S. (2007). Interventions addressing transition difficulties for individuals with autism. *Psychology in the Schools, 44*(7), 681–690.

Sterponi, L., & Fasulo, A. (2010). "How to go on": Intersubjectivity and progressivity in the communication of a child with autism. *Ethos, 38*(1), 116–142.

Sutherland, R., Trembath, D., & Roberts, J. (2018). Telehealth and autism: A systematic search and review of the literature. *International Journal of Speech-Language Pathology, 20*(3), 324–336.

Vivanti, G. (2019). Towards a culturally informed approach to implementing autism early intervention. *Pediatric Medicine, 2*, 20. https://doi.org/10.21037/pm.2019.06.0

Vygotsky, L. (1930–1934/1978). Vygotsky, L. S. (1978). *Mind in society: The development of higher psychological processes* (A. R. Luria, M. Lopez-Morillas & M. Cole [with J. V. Wertsch], Trans.) Cambridge, Mass.: Harvard University Press.

Welterlin, A., Turner-Brown, L. M., Harris, S., Mesibov, G., & Delmolino, L. (2012). The home TEACCHing program for toddlers with autism. *Journal of Autism and Developmental Disorders, 42*, 1827–1835.

Wetherby, A. M., Woods, J., Guthrie, W., Delehanty, A., Brown, J. A., Morgan, L., ... Lord, C. (2018). Changing developmental trajectories of toddlers with autism spectrum disorder: Strategies for bridging research to community practice. *Journal of Speech, Language, and Hearing Research, 61*(11), 2615–2628.

Yoder, P. J., Bottema-Beutel, K., Woynaroski, T., Chandrasekhar, R., & Sandbank, M. (2013). Social communication intervention effects vary by dependent variable type in preschoolers with autism spectrum disorders. *Evidence-based Communication Assessment and Intervention, 7*(4), 150–174.

Chapter 10
Understanding Legislation, Health Insurance, and Disparities in Service Provision in Autism Early Intervention

Kristen Bottema-Beutel, Josephine Cuda, and So Yoon Kim

Individuals with Disabilities Education Act

In the United States, the provision of educational services to children with disabilities from birth to 21 years of age is mandated by the Individuals with Disabilities Education Act (IDEA, 2004). Under this law, children with disabilities are eligible to receive a free (i.e., publicly funded) and appropriate public education (FAPE), which would result in meaningful benefit to the child. IDEA also specifies a preference that children receive these services in a least restrictive environment (LRE), which for school age children means placement in classrooms alongside their typically developing peers as opposed to segregated settings. Finally, IDEA provides procedural safeguards that outline referral, assessment, education planning, service provision, and progress monitoring processes. Below, we provide an overview of this federal law in relation to both early intervention services prior to school entry (Part C and Extended Part C), and school-based services (Part B).

Early Intervention Services Under IDEA Part C

Under Part C of IDEA, eligible children under the age of 3 may receive early intervention services, which are preferentially delivered in the home setting with the participation of caregivers. The services provided vary by state, and may include combinations of parent- and practitioner-provided interventions, with different states favoring different modes of delivery and types of services (Stahmer &

K. Bottema-Beutel (✉) · J. Cuda · S. Y. Kim
Lynch School of Education and Human Development, Boston College,
Chestnut Hill, MA, USA
e-mail: botteabe@bc.edu

G. Vivanti et al. (eds.), *Clinical Guide to Early Interventions for Children with Autism*, Best Practices in Child and Adolescent Behavioral Health Care,
https://doi.org/10.1007/978-3-030-41160-2_10

Mandell, 2007). There are two categories of eligibility under which children may qualify for early intervention services. The first category applied to children who exhibit developmental delays, and the second applied to children with established conditions putting them at substantial risk of developmental delay. Given that a reliable ASD diagnosis is not usually made until after age 2, many children with ASD become eligible under the developmental delay category prior to an ASD diagnosis. Eligibility under this category involves a determination as to whether or not the child is experiencing delays (with thresholds set by individual states) in at least one of five categories: cognitive, social–emotional, speech and language, adaptive, and physical development (Early Childhood Technical Assistance Center, n.d.). Although most states use federal guidelines at least in part to establish eligibility criteria, there is some variation from state to state that seems to translate to variation in the proportion of young children with ASD who receive early intervention (Barton et al., 2016).

Once children are found eligible for early intervention services, service providers work with families to develop an individualized family service plan (IFSP) that can include services provided to both the child and the caregivers. These often include, but are not limited to, applied behavior analysis, speech therapy, occupational therapy, or other psychosocial treatments. IDEA Part C stipulates that these plans should be tailored to meet the needs of individual children, and should consider parents' input in regards to service selection. However, early intervention providers are not required to implement services desired by the family if they are able to provide other services that would convey the same benefit. There is also a lack of clarity in federal law regarding service intensity (i.e., the number of treatment hours) that must be provided through early intervention, which reflects a lack of research evidence in this regard (Dicker, 2013). The American Academy of Pediatrics recommends at least 25 h/week of intervention services with low child to teacher ratios, which should be delivered year round (Myers & Johnson, 2007). Even given these recommendations, there is no explicit provision that IFSPs must provide this level of intensity for every child.

Transition to School Under IDEA Part B

Some states offer transitional services from age 3 to kindergarten enrollment, known as "Extended Part C." These services are meant to support the transition between early intervention services and entry into the school system. If children are not receiving Extended Part C services or have aged out of these services, they then transition to IDEA Part B services. IDEA Part B is the section of federal law that mandates special education services for children and youth ages 3–21. This law lists 13 specific disability categories under which children may be eligible to receive educational interventions, one of which is autism. Children either transition from an IFSP into an individualized education program (IEP) developed by a team of school professionals, administrators, and the child's caregivers, or are referred for an evaluation once they reach school age to determine eligibility. Because services are generally more comprehensive and family centered under Part C as compared to Part B, there is sometimes conflict during the transition periods as families work with schools to determine which services will continue through the child's school-based program, and which will be revised or discontinued (Dicker, 2013). Similar to Part C services, school-based services can include various types of programming, which can be delivered by classroom teachers or other licensed (and in some cases unlicensed) professionals. Because of the LRE provision of IDEA, many more children with ASD are educated alongside their typically developing peers than have been in the past (Morningstar, Kurth, & Johnson, 2017).

Just as is the case with IDEA Part C services, court cases have determined that Part B educational services need only provide meaningful benefit and are not required to be the best services possible (Dicker, 2013). Because federal dollars only account for a small portion of special education funding and the remaining costs are left to states, there is wide state-by-state variation in educational supports provided to children and youth with ASD. We discuss this issue in more detail in the final sections of this chapter.

Insurance Coverage for Diagnostic and Early Intervention Services

Given the support needs of children with ASD, which can include services directly related to the diagnosis as well as any and accompanying health conditions, healthcare costs are substantially higher for these children as compared to children who are typically developing (Buescher, Cidav, Knapp, & Mandell, 2014). Services provided to children with ASD in the United States can be covered by a combination of school agencies, insurance providers, and Medicaid, a federal and state program that helps with medical costs for some people with limited income and resources (Dicker, 2013). As of 2017, 46 U.S. states and the District of Columbia have passed legislation mandating insurance funding for ASD diagnostic services and interventions (National Conference of State Legislatures, 2018). Prior to these mandates, insurers often denied coverage for ASD-related services, citing a lack of clear evidence of effectiveness for most interventions (Mandell et al., 2016). These new mandates appear to have increased service utilization and the proportion of spending by insurers, and this is especially true for families who spend more on services (Candon et al., 2019).

However, even given that legislative mandates are widespread across states, there still remains ample variability in the nature of services covered, and the extent to which services are covered by private insurers. Due to federal restrictions, insurance coverage is limited to families with fully insured plans, which means those who are self-insured may not be covered (Candon et al., 2019). There is also variability across states in expenditure caps, which can range as low as $12,000 and as high as

$50,000 (Mandell et al., 2016). Because of limitations in study designs, it is not clear if insurance mandates have improved service access across all SES strata, but this might not the case given that low SES families are least likely to be insured. Due to a variety of factors, including barriers posed by insurers, the number of children with ASD who receive insurer-covered services is well below what would be expected given the prevalence of ASD (Mandell et al., 2016). Still, improvements in access to care under state insurance mandates are expected to continue into the future (Mandell et al., 2016).

At present, there is a lack of clarity and continued debate in regards to whether specific services should be covered by insurance providers, by local school systems, or be paid out of pocket by families (Bilaver, Cushing, & Cutler, 2016; Holland, 2010). Many states explicitly specify insurance coverage of applied behavioral analysis but leave requirements for other intervention and service types more vague (NCSL, 2018). This can lead families toward services that are more likely to be covered, regardless of their appropriateness or effectiveness.

Regional Variation in Service Access and Utilization

Another factor contributing to variability in service provision for children with ASD in the United States is geographic location. Programming enacted through Part C of IDEA is supported by way of federal formula grants, which are proportionally determined based upon the number of children under 3 years of age reported to reside in a given state (Noyes-Grosser et al., 2018). Federal funding contingent on population data is one reason for geographic differences in access to services, which is often stratified on rural and urban/suburban lines. For example, attaining an early diagnosis is often more difficult in rural as compared to urban or suburban areas (Antezana, Scarpa, Valdespino, Albright, & Richey, 2017; Kalkbrenner, Daniels, Emch, Morrissey, Poole, & Chen, 2011; Singh, Moody, Rigles, & Smith, 2018). Additionally, parents living in rural communities report reduced service availability than did those residing in urban environments (Centers for Disease Control, 2011). Delays in receiving diagnoses and support services often occur in rural areas due to limited overall awareness, inadequate screening procedures, and increased demands on families to travel greater distances to locations more equipped with available supports (Antezana et al., 2017).

Due to limitations in the health care systems within rural communities, families often rely more heavily on other sources, like the school community, for service support. One corollary of this is that, according to the SPSD, rural parents demonstrate lower rates of communicating concerns with healthcare providers as compared to nonrural parents. Within rural communities, healthcare providers are also more likely to encourage parents to consult school personnel than do healthcare providers within urban communities (Antezana et al., 2017; Centers for Disease Control, 2011).

There may also be differences between rural and urban/suburban communities in terms of the supports they most value. For example, within more metropolitan regions, behavior supports are held in higher regard than in rural communities while rural communities place a higher value on speech and language therapies than do families in nonrural areas (Murphy & Ruble, 2012). This difference can be explained by how readily available families perceive such services within their communities. Speech and language therapies are available on-site in most schools while behavior support services are generally provided in off-site clinics or through privately contracted professionals in the home. As noted previously, it is generally preferable for children to receive early intervention services in the home; however, within rural communities this can be particularly challenging. Qualified professionals often reside considerable distances from rural families, requiring significant travel time for service provision (Meadan, Meyer, Snodgrass, & Halle, 2013; Mello et al., 2016). There is also variability in the types of service providers more easily accessible within communities. Speech language pathologists (SLPs) are more prevalent across both rural and metropolitan regions while board-certified behavior analysts (BCBAs) are more representative in nonrural areas (Mello et al., 2016). It is possible that this discrepancy is explained by BCBA being a relatively new profession in comparison to SLP, and thereby BCBAs have a less widespread presence than SLPs (Mello et al., 2016).

To counter these challenges, video-, teleconferencing, and other internet-based technologies are increasingly used to train educators and caretakers within rural communities on how to implement best practices at home and in the classroom (Boisvert, Lang, & Andrianopoulos, 2010; Gibson, Pennington, Stenhoff, & Hopper, 2010; Meadan, Meyer, Snodgrass, & Halle, 2013). Such "telehealth" methods are also useful for service providers to observe, assess, or screen a child remotely, and develop plans and interventions regarding his or her behavior, communication, and/or academic success (Gibson et al., 2010). While these pathways to service and consultation certainly have limitations, they offer the potential for meaningful access to rural communities that otherwise might have very little.

Ethnic and Racial Disparities in Access to Diagnosis and Support Services

Although there is no evidence that suggests racial or ethnic differences in either incidence or prevalence of ASD either in the United States or globally (Bertrand et al., 2001; Mandell, Listerud, Levy, Pinto-Martin, 2002), researchers have consistently found racial and ethnic variation in the rates of ASD diagnosis and documentation of ASD (Liptak et al., 2008; Magaña, Lopez, Aguinaga & Morton, 2013; Mandell et al., 2009; Zuckerman et al., 2014). For instance, Mandell et al. (2009) reported that non-White children (i.e., African American, Hispanic, Asian and other ethnicities) were less likely than White children to have documentation of an ASD diagnosis.

Furthermore, while the prevalence of having documentation of an ASD diagnosis was consistently lower for African American children than for White children across children of all IQ levels, in Hispanic and Asian populations, the disparity in documentation was even greater among children with IQs lower than 70 (Mandell et al., 2009).

Mandell et al. (2002) discussed the reasons why early diagnosis and having accurate documentation of ASD are essential. First, early interventions in response to timely diagnosis have demonstrated positive changes in children's development outcomes as many interventions are considered more effective with younger children (Vivanti et al., 2016). Second, due to the heightened risk of having a subsequent child with ASD, parents stand to derive substantial benefit from early diagnosis of their first child. Third, the Individuals with Disabilities Act (PL 94–142) mandates the public education system to provide children with special education and related services. Early identification is important to give time for schools to properly plan to provide FAPE to eligible students.

Early diagnosis is also important because the current healthcare system requires documentation of diagnosis in order to access mental health–related and psychiatric services. For example, children with ASD who lived in regions with low percentages of White residents were less likely to use psychotropic medications than children with ASD who lived in regions with high percentages of White residents (Mandell et al., 2009). Magaña et al. (2013) reported that Latino families received significantly fewer special services such as children's recreational programs, psychological services, family support services (respite), or intensive autism therapy than White families and voiced the need for improvements in such unmet services. Furthermore, Latino families with limited English proficiency more frequently reported experiencing barriers related to ASD knowledge, lower trust in service providers, and fewer therapy hours than non-Latino White families (Zuckerman et al., 2017).

Latino children with ASD are diagnosed later (2.5 years later) and less frequently than non-Latino White children with similar clinical autistic symptoms (Mandell et al., 2002; Zuckerman et al., 2014). However, when diagnosed, Latino children with ASD have been shown to have more severe autistic symptoms than non-Latino White children (Mandell et al., 2002). Relatedly, Mandell et al. (2002) also reported that African American children with ASD receive a diagnosis at older ages and are more likely to be misdiagnosed as having a conduct disorder or adjustment disorder than White children, while Latino children are more likely to be misdiagnosed as having specific language impairment.

Taken together, these reports indicate that lower rates of ASD diagnosis and delayed diagnosis among ethnic and racial minorities can be explained by contextual or environmental factors rather than clinical presentation. Differences in access to support or advocacy systems, cultural differences such as conceptualization of ASD among non-White parents (Zuckerman et al., 2014), language barriers, families' and school authorities' interpretations of symptoms, lack of awareness of available services, and absence of services or institutions that provide culturally sensitive support (Alegría et al., 2007) have all been cited as limitations in providing proper diagnostic services to ethnic and racial minorities.

Meanwhile, Smedley et al. (2003) attribute ethnic and racial disparities to federal laws and policies controlling healthcare provision. For instance, immigration status has been highlighted as a potential factor in the racial and ethnic disparities in diagnosis and service provision. Latino families with children with ASD voiced that they were unwilling to visit healthcare facilities due to fear of exposing their immigration status (Alegría et al., 2007). Furthermore, Fountain and Bearman (2011) reported that when policies protecting client privacy in regards to immigration status were in place in California, the rates of ASD diagnosis of Latino children and White children were similar, but when they were not in place, the rates of ASD diagnosis of Latino children were significantly lower than those of White children. Therefore, the underrepresentation of ASD among minority populations is also susceptible to the effects of state and federal immigrant policies (Fountain and Bearman 2011; Mandell et al., 2002).

Implications

In the Standards for Culturally and Linguistically Appropriate Services, the U.S. Department of Health and Human Services (DHHS) Office of Minority Health (OMH) instructed healthcare institutions to consider healthcare as "a cultural construct, arising from beliefs about the nature of disease and the human body" and cultural issues as "central in the delivery of health services treatment and preventive interventions" (U.S. DHHS, 2010, p. 80863 as cited in Smedley et al., 2003). Therefore, because culture and language influence how health is conceptualized, and how healthcare supports are provided and received, Smedley et al. (2003) have argued that increased responsiveness to culture and language will improve the quality of care not only for minority patients but all patients.

While more state and federal guidelines are requiring healthcare systems to be sensitive to the growing diversity of U.S. healthcare consumers, Smedley et al. (2003) offer additional recommendations for alleviating ethnic and racial disparities. For instance, they urge healthcare institutions, legislators, and regulators to develop policies that (a) bolster stable healthcare provider-patient relationships (e.g., accessibility of primary care providers, reasonable patient loads for primary physicians), (b) increase the proportion of healthcare professionals who are ethnic and racial minorities, (c) provide more funding and resources to the U.S. DHHS Office of Civil Rights to address and enforce civil rights laws, and (d) equalize access to insurance plans by encouraging public healthcare insurance programs like Medicare to provide higher quality plans to ethnic and racial minorities.

Conclusion

In the United States, federal law provides for diagnostic and support services for eligible children with ASD and their families. However, these services are not distributed equally across a variety of demographic variables including race, ethnicity, immigration status, and geographic location. Health insurance and educational systems should cover the costs of services deemed necessary, but there are wide variations by state. Healthcare workers and other support providers should be aware these disparities and develop and implement policies that will mitigate these effects.

References

Alegría, M., Mulvaney-Day, N., Woo, M., Torres, M., Gao, S., & Oddo, V. (2007). Correlates of past-year mental health service use among Latinos: Results from the national Latino and Asian American study. *American Journal of Public Health, 97*(1), 76–83.

Antezana, L., Scarpa, A., Valdespino, A., Albright, J., & Richey, J. A. (2017). Rural trends in diagnosis and services for autism spectrum disorder. *Frontiers in Psychology, 8*, 590.

Barton, E. E., Harris, B., Leech, N., Stiff, L., Choi, G., & Joel, T. (2016). An analysis of state autism educational assessment practices and requirements. *Journal of Autism and Developmental Disorders, 46*(3), 737–748.

Bertrand, J., Mars, A., Boyle, C., Bove, F., Yeargin-Allsopp, M., & Decoufle, P. (2001). Prevalence of autism in a United States population: The Brick Township, New Jersey, investigation. *Pediatrics, 108*, 1155–1161.

Bilaver, L. A., Cushing, L. S., & Cutler, A. T. (2016). Prevalence and correlates of educational intervention utilization among children with autism spectrum disorder. *Journal of Autism and Developmental Disorders, 46*(2), 561–571.

Boisvert, M., Lang, R., Andrianopoulos, M., & Boscardin, M. L. (2010). Telepractice in the assessment and treatment of individuals with autism spectrum disorders: A systematic review. *Developmental Neurorehabilitation, 13*(6), 423–432.

Buescher, A. V., Cidav, Z., Knapp, M., & Mandell, D. S. (2014). Costs of autism spectrum disorders in the United Kingdom and the United States. *JAMA Pediatrics, 168*(8), 721–728.

Candon, M. K., Barry, C. L., Marcus, S. C., Epstein, A. J., Kennedy-Hendricks, A., Xie, M., & Mandell, D. S. (2019). Insurance mandates and out-of-pocket spending for children with autism spectrum disorder. *Pediatrics, 143*(1), e20180654.

Centers for Disease Control and Prevention, National Center for Health Statistics, State and Local Area Integrated Telephone Survey. (2011). *Survey of pathways to diagnosis and services frequently asked questions*. Retrieved Mar 2019, from http://www.cdc.gov/nchs/slaits/spds.htm.

Dicker, S. (2013). Entering the spectrum: The challenge of early intervention law for children with autism spectrum disorders. *Infants and Young Children, 26*(3), 192–203.

Early Childhood Technical Assistance Center. (n.d.). *Part C eligibility*. Retreived Mar 2019, from https://ectacenter.org/topics/earlyid/partcelig.asp.

Fountain, C., & Bearman, P. (2011). Risk as social context: Immigration policy and autism in California. *Sociological Forum, 26*(2), 215–240.

Gibson, J. L., Pennington, R. C., Stenhoff, D. M., & Hopper, J. S. (2010). Using desktop videoconferencing to deliver interventions to a preschool student with autism. *Topics in Early Childhood Special Education, 29*(4), 214–225.

Holland, C. D. (2010). Autism, insurance, and the IDEA: Providing a comprehensive legal framework. *Cornell Law Review, 95*(6), 1253–1282.

Individuals with Disabilities Education Act, 20 U.S.C. § 1400. (2004).

Kalkbrenner, A. E., Daniels, J. L., Emch, M., Morrissey, J., Poole, C., & Chen, J. C. (2011). Geographic access to health services and diagnosis with an autism spectrum disorder. *Annals of Epidemiology, 21*(4), 304–310.

Liptak, G. S., Benzoni, L. B., Mruzek, D. W., Nolan, K. W., Thingvoll, M. A., Wade, C. M., & Fryer, G. E. (2008). Disparities in diagnosis and access to health services for children with autism: Data from the National Survey of Children's Health. *Journal of Developmental and Behavioral Pediatrics, 29*(3), 152–160.

Magaña, S., Lopez, K., Aguinaga, A., & Morton, H. (2013). Access to diagnosis and treatment services among Latino children with autism spectrum disorders. *Journal of Intellectual and Developmental Disability, 51*(3), 141–153.

Mandell, D. S., Barry, C. L., Marcus, S. C., Xie, M., Shea, K., Mullan, K., & Epstein, A. J. (2016). Effects of autism spectrum disorder insurance mandates on the treated prevalence of autism spectrum disorder. *JAMA Pediatrics, 170*(9), 887–893.

Mandell, D. S., Listerud, J., Levy, S. E., & Pinto-Martin, J. A. (2002). Race differences in the age at diagnosis among Medicaid-eligible children with autism. *Journal of the American Academy of Child and Adolescent Psychiatry, 41*(12), 1447–1453.

Mandell, D. S., Wiggins, L. D., Carpenter, L. A., Daniels, J., DiGuiseppi, C., Durkin, M. S., ... Kirby, R. S. (2009). Racial/ethnic disparities in the identification of children with autism spectrum disorders. *American Journal of Public Health, 99*(3), 493–498.

Meadan, H., Meyer, L. E., Snodgrass, M. R., & Halle, J. W. (2013). Coaching parents of young children with autism in rural areas using internet-based technologies: A pilot program. *Rural Special Education Quarterly, 32*(3), 3–10.

Mello, M. P., Goldman, S. E., Urbano, R. C., & Hodapp, R. M. (2016). Services for children with autism spectrum disorder: Comparing rural and non-rural communities. *Education and Training in Autism and Developmental Disabilities, 51*, 355–365.

Morningstar, M. E., Kurth, J. A., & Johnson, P. E. (2017). Examining national trends in educational placements for students with significant disabilities. *Remedial and Special Education, 38*(1), 3–12.

Murphy, M. A., & Ruble, L. A. (2012). A comparative study of rurality and urbanicity on access to and satisfaction with services for children with autism spectrum disorders. *Rural Special Education Quarterly, 31*(3), 3–11.

Myers, S. M., & Johnson, C. P. (2007). Management of children with autism spectrum disorders. *Pediatrics, 120*(5), 1162–1182.

National Conference of State Legislatures. (2018, August). *Autism and insurance coverage: State laws*. Retrieved Mar 2019, from http://www.ncsl.org/research/health/autism-and-insurance-coverage-state-laws.aspx.

Noyes-Grosser, D. M., Benham, R., & Osbahr, T. (2018). Implementing services for children with ASD and their families within state early intervention programs: A view from two states–opportunities, challenges, and future directions. In *Handbook of parent-implemented interventions for very young children with Autism* (pp. 459–481). Cham: Springer.

Singh, R. L., Moody, E. J., Rigles, B., & Smith, E. B. (2018). What it takes to raise children with autism in a rural state. *Advances in Neurodevelopmental Disorders*, 1–12.

Smedley, B. D., Stith, A. Y., Nelson, A. R., & Institute of Medicine (U.S.). (2003). *Unequal treatment: Confronting racial and ethnic disparities in health care*. Washington, DC: National Academy Press.

Stahmer, A. C., & Mandell, D. S. (2007). State infant/toddler program policies for eligibility and services provision for young children with autism. *Administration and Policy in Mental Health and Mental Health Services Research, 34*(1), 29–37.

U.S. DHHS. Healthy People. (2010). *Understanding and Improving Health* (p. 2000). Washington, DC: U.S. DHHS.

Vivanti, G., Dissanayake, C., & Victorian ASELCC Team. (2016). Outcome for children receiving the Early Start Denver Model before and after 48 months. *Journal of Autism and Developmental Disorders, 46*(7), 2441–2449.

Zuckerman, K., Sinche, B., Mejia, A., Cobian, M., Becker, T., & Nicolaidis, C. (2014). Latino parents' perspectives of barriers to autism diagnosis. *Academic Pediatrics, 14*(3), 301–308.

Zuckerman, K. E., Lindly, O. J., Reyes, N. M., Chavez, A. E., Macias, K., Smith, K. N., & Reynolds, A. (2017). Disparities in diagnosis and treatment of autism in Latino and Non-Latino White families. *Pediatrics, 139*(5), e20163010.

Correction to: Clinical Guide to Early Interventions for Children with Autism

Giacomo Vivanti, Kristen Bottema-Beutel, and Lauren Turner-Brown

Correction to: Chapter 3 and 4 in: G. Vivanti et al. (eds.), *Clinical Guide to Early Interventions for Children with Autism*, Best Practices in Child and Adolescent Behavioral Health Care, https://doi.org/10.1007/978-3-030-41160-2

Mary Kate Frisch provided her valuable contribution to chapter 4 "Understanding and Addressing Restricted and Repetitive Behaviors in Children with Autism" of this book. However, the author's name was inadvertently added to chapter 3 instead of chapter 4. This error has been corrected in this version of the book.

The updated online version of this chapter can be found at
https://doi.org/10.1007/978-3-030-41160-2_3
https://doi.org/10.1007/978-3-030-41160-2_4

G. Vivanti et al. (eds.), *Clinical Guide to Early Interventions for Children with Autism*, Best Practices in Child and Adolescent Behavioral Health Care,
https://doi.org/10.1007/978-3-030-41160-2_11

Index

G. Vivanti et al. (eds.), *Clinical Guide to Early Interventions for Children with Autism*, Best Practices in Child and Adolescent Behavioral Health Care,
https://doi.org/10.1007/978-3-030-41160-2

F

www.ingramcontent.com/pod-product-compliance
Lightning Source LLC
Chambersburg PA
CBHW060942280126
38801CB00003B/29
* 9 7 8 3 0 3 0 4 1 1 5 9 6 *